Surface changes		
	Scale White flaki... superficial horny layer (indicates epidermal pathology)		
	Excoriation Scratch mark (a sign of itching = pruritus)		**Lichenification** Thickening of the epidermis with exaggerated skin markings (bark-like), usually due to repeated rubbing

	Vascular changes		
	Telangiectasia Easily visible superficial blood vessels (blanches)		**Spider naevus** A single telangiectatic arteriole in the skin
	Purpura (non-blanching): extravasation of blood into skin (usually around 2mm in diameter)		**Petechiae** Pinhead-sized areas of purpura
	Ecchymosis A 'bruise'. Purpura >2mm in diameter		**Erythema** Blanching reddening of the skin due to local vasodilatation

Further terminology

- Eruption: rash.
- Cyst: an epithelial-lined cavity filled with fluid or semi-solid material.
- Milium (milia): the tiny, firm, white papule is an intradermal cyst.
- Open comedone: dark, plugged, dilated pilosebaceous orifice (blackhead).
- Closed comedone: pale, pinhead-sized papule in pilosebaceous orifice (whitehead).
- Hyperkeratotic: thickened horny layer, difficult to detach scale.
- Scar: dermal fibrous tissue replaces normal architecture.
- Haematoma: localized deep swelling from bleeding.
- Hyperpigmented (dark): usually increased melanin or iron in skin.
- Depigmented: lost all pigment, e.g. vitiligo.
- Hypopigmented (pale): less melanin or colour obscured, e.g. by oedema.
- Morbilliform rash: erythematous macules and papules of 2–10mm in diameter, with tendency to confluence (as in measles).
- Cribriform: spaces, perforations, or holes like a sieve. Often applied to the pattern of scarring seen in pyoderma gangrenosum.

OXFORD MEDICAL PUBLICATIONS

Oxford Handbook of
Medical
Dermatology

Published and forthcoming Oxford Handbooks

Oxford Handbook of
Medical Dermatology

Second Edition

Susan Burge
Honorary Consultant Dermatologist
Oxford University Hospitals NHS Foundation Trust
and Honorary Senior Clinical Lecturer, University of
Oxford, UK

Rubeta Matin
Consultant Dermatologist
Oxford University Hospitals NHS Foundation Trust
and Honorary Senior Clinical Lecturer, University of
Oxford, UK

Dinny Wallis
Consultant Rheumatologist
University Hospital Southampton NHS Foundation
Trust, UK

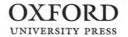

OXFORD
UNIVERSITY PRESS

OXFORD
UNIVERSITY PRESS

Great Clarendon Street, Oxford, OX2 6DP,
United Kingdom

Oxford University Press is a department of the University of Oxford.
It furthers the University's objective of excellence in research, scholarship,
and education by publishing worldwide. Oxford is a registered trade mark of
Oxford University Press in the UK and in certain other countries

First Edition published 2011
Second Edition published 2016

Impression: 5

Published in the United States of America by Oxford University Press
198 Madison Avenue, New York, NY 10016, United States of America

British Library Cataloguing in Publication Data

Data available

Library of Congress Control Number: 2016936807

ISBN 978–0–19–874792–5

Printed and bound in Italy by L.E.G.O. S.p.A. Lavis (TN)

Foreword to the second edition

If you are faced with a challenging skin problem, then pull this brilliant and magical book from your bag, or search it with your electronic device: the answer will be there. It is packed with top tips, information gems and clinical pearls. Whether you are a student needing a logical and clear way to understand dermatology, if you are in primary care faced with a diagnosis that requires a quick refresh of your memory, or a hospital doctor or dermatology trainee dealing with emergencies and complex cases, this book will become your friend and companion.

This new edition introduces fresh new writing on eczema and tumours, a new chapter on genetic skin diseases and expansion of the tropical diseases section. Dinny Wallis has updated the rheumatology disorders and vasculitis. Rubeta Matin has joined the team from Oxford bringing expertise in immunosuppression. The whole book is right up to date so experienced consultant dermatologists will find it a useful quick reference for managing complex diseases. The text flows and draws in the reader who will quickly be absorbed, oblivious to passing time.

The question and answer format, the text boxes and the clarity of the writing make the second edition of Sue Burge's *Oxford Handbook of Medical Dermatology* the go-to small dermatology textbook. The British Society of Medical Dermatology gives this as a prize to the best UK trainees at their meeting each year. This is the book to get if you truly wish to understand dermatology.

Nick Levell
President: British Association of Dermatologists (2016–18);
Director of Dermatology, Consultant Dermatologist,
Norfolk and Norwich University Hospital;
Specialty National Lead (Dermatology), National Institute
of Health Research, UK

Foreword to the first edition

Dr Susan Burge and I first (really) met as senior registrars to the Department of Dermatology in Oxford in 1981. It soon became apparent to me that Susan's most commonly asked question was 'why?', always spoken in a most expressive Northern Irish accent. Usually there was no easy answer which of course indicated why she had asked the question in the first place. If an answer was preferred it had to make sense, be logical and simple. Any flannel would meet with short shrift! This story reflects the (senior) author's enquiring mind and need for knowledge to be imparted in a sound, simple and logical way. It therefore comes as no surprise that the format of the new textbook is prompted by questions: What should I look for? What should I do?

Dermatology is arguably the most clinical of all medical specialties because it relies less on investigation and more on good old fashioned observation and interpretation of symptoms and signs for diagnosis. Dermatology practice is sometimes criticized for being simply a 'spot diagnosis' and for using outdated Latin terminology. The diagnosis and management of skin disease, however, demands a logical ordering and structuring of clinical information in such a way that makes it a most stimulating intellectual exercise which has few equals among other medical specialties.

In this new book Susan and Dinny, who is currently in specialist training in rheumatology, bring a refreshingly new approach to learning dermatology. The combination of old and young authors (forgive me Susan!) brings a nice balance of wisdom and practicality—exactly what the junior doctor requires.

Professor Peter Mortimer
Professor of Dermatological Medicine to the University of London,
Consultant Skin Physician to St George's Hospital, London,
and the Royal Marsden Hospital,
London

Preface

The second edition of this Handbook still provides a practical introduction to dermatology, with an emphasis on the medical aspects of the specialty. Skin problems are hugely variable (>2500 diagnoses), but we hope this little book will help you to make sense of what you find and will provide you with a framework for analysing clinical signs, so that you develop your diagnostic expertise. Dermatology trainees should find the book particularly useful, as may hospital doctors in other medical specialties faced with assessing skin problems, but it also includes much that will be of value to those working in the community and to medical students.

The content has been updated, and we have tried to make it even more comprehensive. We include a new chapter on dermatogenetics and have added to other sections, particularly those on skin in infancy and childhood, cutaneous reactions to drugs, skin tumours, and skin and rheumatology.

We discuss common and important skin problems, such as skin failure and emergency dermatology, eczema, psoriasis, blisters, vasculitis, and pustular rashes, but also include some fascinating rarities that we hope may inspire you to read more. Each topic includes answers to the clinical questions 'What should I ask?', 'What should I look for?', and 'What should I do?'. Management guidelines have been incorporated, where possible.

The expanded tumour chapter will help you to recognize and manage skin tumours, including those in immunosuppressed individuals, as well as to advise on photoprotection, but the Handbook does not include information on surgical techniques in dermatology.

Chapters on skin problems in the medical specialties should be of particular interest to physicians working in those disciplines. We introduce skin conditions that you may encounter when working in specialties such as rheumatology, haematology, nephrology, endocrinology, and gastroenterology. The section on medical management introduces topical treatments, occlusion, and wet dressings, as well as discussing the systemic drugs commonly used in dermatology.

Illustrations complement the text, but the emphasis is on enabling you to make sense of the findings using your clinical skills, rather than matching findings to pictures.

We hope that you will find this book useful when you are asked to see someone with a puzzling skin problem and that there will be a place for it in your pocket, in the outpatient clinic, or on the ward.

Please send back your comments or criticisms, so that we can improve the book in future editions. You can send your comments to us via the OUP website ♒ http://www.oup.co.uk.

Acknowledgements

Once more, we would like to thank the Oxford dermatology trainees (now consultants) who inspired the book. It is still used in our regular Tuesday morning teaching.

We are very grateful to these colleagues who provided invaluable advice on individual chapters and answered our questions so patiently:
Andrew Brent and Chris Conlon (infections)
Fiona Browne (genetics)
James Burge (neurology)
Caroline Champagne (hair)
Susan Cooper (eczema and mucosal disorders)
Sarah Felton and Sheru George (photodermatology)
Rachael Morris-Jones (infestations and parasites)
Celia Moss (neurofibromatosis)
Graham Ogg (immunology)
Vanessa Venning (blisters)
Sarah Walsh (severe drug reactions).

Contents

Symbols and abbreviations

➔	cross reference
◠	website
❶	warning
⚠	warning
►►	don't dawdle
☀	controversial topic
⚠☀	rare but fascinating
1°	primary
2°	secondary
~	approximately
=	equal to
>	greater than
<	less than
≥	equal to or greater than
+/-	plus/minus
%	percent
α	alpha
β	beta
δ	delta
γ	gamma
κ	kappa
♀	female
♂	male
°C	degree Celsius
®	registered trademark
™	trademark
AAT	α-1-antitrypsin
ABPI	ankle–brachial pressure index
ACE	angiotensin-converting enzyme
ACR	American College of Rheumatology
ACTH	adrenocorticotrophic hormone
AD	autosomal dominant

ADHD	attention-deficit/hyperactivity disorder
AGEP	acute generalized exanthematous pustulosis
AIDS	acquired immune deficiency syndrome
AJCC	American Joint Committee on Cancer
AMP	antimicrobial peptide
ANA	antinuclear antibody
ANCA	anti-neutrophil cytoplasmic antibody
APECED	autoimmune polyendocrinopathy–candidiasis–ectodermal dystrophy
AR	autosomal recessive
AST	aspartate aminotransferase
ATLL	adult T-cell leukaemia/lymphoma
AV	arteriovenous
BAD	British Association of Dermatologists
BCC	basal cell carcinoma
BCG	bacille Calmette–Guérin
bd	*bis die* (twice daily)
BMI	body mass index
BMZ	basement membrane zone
BP	bullous pemphigoid
BSA	body surface area
CAPS	cryopyrin-associated periodic syndromes
CCLE	chronic cutaneous lupus erythematosus
CCP	cyclic citrullinated peptide
CFTR	cystic fibrosis transmembrane conductance regulator
CH	congenital haemangioma
CINCA	chronic infantile neurological cutaneous and articular syndrome
CLASI	Cutaneous Lupus Disease Activity and Severity Index
CM	capillary malformation
CMV	cytomegalovirus
CNS	central nervous system
CRP	C-reactive protein
CT	computed tomography

CTCL	cutaneous T-cell lymphoma
CTLA-4	cytotoxic T-lymphocyte-associated protein 4
CXR	chest X-ray
DH	dermatitis herpetiformis
DIC	disseminated intravascular coagulation
DIP	distal interphalangeal
DLE	discoid lupus erythematosus
DLI	donor lymphocyte infusion
DLQI	Dermatology Life Quality Index
DMARD	disease-modifying antirheumatic drug
DMSO	dimethyl sulfoxide
DNA	deoxyribonucleic acid
DRESS	Drug rash, eosinophilia, and systemic symptoms
ds	double-stranded
DSSI	Dermatomyositis Skin Severity Index
DVT	deep venous thrombosis
EASI	Eczema Area and Severity Index
EB	epidermolysis bullosa
EBA	epidermolysis bullosa acquisita
EBV	Epstein–Barr virus
ECG	electrocardiogram
ECM	extracellular matrix
ECP	extracorporeal photopheresis
ED	ectodermal dysplasia
EDS	Ehlers–Danlos syndrome
eGFR	estimated glomerular filtration rate
EGFR	epidermal growth factor receptor
EGPA	eosinophilic granulomatosis with polyangiitis
EKV	erythrokeratoderma variabilis
EKVP	erythrokeratodermia variabilis et progressiva
EM	erythema multiforme
EMPD	extramammary Paget disease
EN	erythema nodosum
ENA	extractable nuclear antigen
ENT	ear, nose, and throat

EPP	erythropoietic protoporphyria
ESR	erythrocyte sedimentation rate
ET	epidermolytic toxins
FAE	fumaric acid ester
FBC	full blood count
FCAS	familial cold auto-inflammatory syndrome
FGFR2	fibroblast growth factor receptor 2
FMF	familial Mediterranean fever
FSH	follicle-stimulating hormone
FTU	fingertip unit
g	gram
G-CSF	granulocyte colony-stimulating factor
GFR	glomerular filtration rate
GI	gastrointestinal
GIT	gastrointestinal tract
GLUT1	glucose transporter 1
GP	general practitioner
GPA	granulomatosis with polyangiitis
G6PD	glucose-6-phosphate dehydrogenase
GPP	generalized pustular psoriasis
GTN	glyceryl trinitrate
GVHD	graft-versus-host disease
HAART	highly active antiretroviral therapy
HBV	hepatitis B virus
HCV	hepatitis C virus
HDL	high-density lipoprotein
HED	hypohidrotic ectodermal dysplasia
HHV	human herpesvirus
HIAA	hydroxyindoleacetic acid
HIDS	hyperimmunoglobulin D syndrome
HIV	human immunodeficiency virus
HLA	human leucocyte antigen
HPV	human papillomavirus
HSCT	haemopoietic stem cell transplant
HSV	herpes simplex virus
HTLV	human T-lymphotropic virus

Hz	hertz
IBD	inflammatory bowel disease
ICU	intensive care unit
IFN	interferon
Ig	immunoglobulin
IL	interleukin
ILVEN	inflammatory linear verrucous epidermal naevus
IM	intramuscular
IMF	immunofluorescence
IP	incontinentia pigmenti
IQ	intelligence quotient
IRIS	immune reconstitution inflammatory syndrome
IU	international unit
IV	intravenous
JAK	janus kinase
kcal	kilocalorie
kDa	kilodalton
KOH	potassium hydroxide
KS	Kaposi sarcoma
L	litre
LDH	lactate dehydrogenase
LDL	low-density lipoprotein
LE	lupus erythematosus
LEKTI	lymphoepithelial Kazal-type 5 serine protease inhibitor
LFT	liver function test
LH	luteinizing hormone
LP	lichen planus
LPC	liquor picis carbonis
LPP	lichen planopilaris
m	metre
M	molar
MALT	mucosa-associated lymphoid tissue
MAPK	mitogen-activated protein kinase
MC1R	melanocortin 1 receptor

MCP	metacarpophalangeal
MCTD	mixed connective tissue disease
MEK	mitogen-activated protein kinase
MEN	multiple endocrine neoplasia
MF	mycosis fungoides
mg	milligram
MHC	major histocompatibility complex
MHRA	Medicines and Healthcare Products Regulatory Agency
mL	millilitre
mm	millimetre
mmol	millimole
6-MP	6-mercaptopurine
MRA	magnetic resonance angiography
MRI	magnetic resonance imaging
MRP6	multidrug resistance-associated protein 6
MRSA	meticillin-resistant *Staphylococcus aureus*
MSSA	meticillin-sensitive *Staphylococcus aureus*
mTOR	mammalian target of rapamycin
NAPSI	Nail Psoriasis Severity Index
NF1	neurofibromatosis type 1
NF2	neurofibromatosis type 2
NF-κB	nuclear factor kappa B
ng	nanogram
NHS	National Health Service
n	nanometre
NTT	non-treponemal test
NOMID	neonatal-onset multisystem inflammatory disease
NSAID	non-steroidal anti-inflammatory drug
NSF	nephrogenic systemic fibrosis
PAN	polyarteritis nodosa
PAPA	pyogenic arthritis, pyoderma gangrenosum, and acne syndrome
PAS	periodic acid–Schiff
PASH	pyoderma gangrenosum, acne, and hidradenitis suppurativa

PASI	Psoriasis Area and Severity Index
PCOS	polycystic ovary syndrome
PCR	polymerase chain reaction
PCT	porphyria cutanea tarda
PDE	phosphodiesterase
PEST	Psoriasis Epidemiology Screening Tool
PET	positron emission tomography
PG	pyoderma gangrenosum
PHACE	Posterior fossa malformations, Haemangioma, Arterial abnormalities, Coarctation of the aorta, and Eye abnormalities
PIIINP	type III procollagen peptide
PIP	proximal interphalangeal
PLE	polymorphic light eruption
POEM	patient-orientated eczema measure
PPK	palmoplantar keratoderma
PRN	*pro re nata* (as required)
PSEK	progressive symmetric erythrokeratoderma
PTH	parathyroid hormone
PUVA	psoralen with ultraviolet A
PVL	Panton–Valentine leukocidin
PWS	port wine stain
PXE	pseudoxanthoma elasticum
qds	*quater die sumendum* (four times daily)
RA	rheumatoid arthritis
RBC	red blood cell
RCLASI	revised Cutaneous Lupus Disease Activity and Severity Index
RDD	Rosai–Dorfman disease
RF	rheumatoid factor
RTR	renal transplant recipient
SCC	squamous cell carcinoma
SCLE	subacute cutaneous lupus erythematosus
SCORAD	SCORing Atopic Dermatitis
SDRIFE	symmetrical drug-related intertriginous and flexural exanthema

SF-MPQ	short-form McGill Pain Questionnaire
SJS	Stevens–Johnson syndrome
SLE	systemic lupus erythematosus
SLICC	Systemic Lupus International Collaborating Clinics
SSM	superficial spreading melanoma
SSRI	selective serotonin reuptake inhibitor
SSSS	staphylococcal scalded skin syndrome
STD	sexually transmitted disease
TB	tuberculosis
tds	*ter die sumendum* (three times daily)
TEN	toxic epidermal necrolysis
TGF	transforming growth factor
TGM1	transglutaminase-1
Th	T-helper
TNF	tumour necrosis factor
TORCH	toxoplasmosis, other, rubella, cytomegalovirus, herpes simplex
TPMT	thiopurine methyltransferase
TRAPS	tumour necrosis factor receptor superfamily 1A-associated periodic fever syndrome
Treg	T-regulatory
TSS	toxic shock syndrome
TT	treponemal test
UAS	urticaria activity score
UK	United Kingdom
USA	United States of America
UV	ultraviolet light
UVA	ultraviolet A
UVA1	ultraviolet A1
UVB	ultraviolet B
UVR	ultraviolet radiation
VAS	visual analogue scale
VLDL	very low-density lipoprotein
VZV	varicella-zoster virus
WCC	white cell count

WHO	World Health Organization
WSP	white soft paraffin
XP	xeroderma pigmentosum

Definitions

Isomorphic response (Koebner phenomenon): appearance of new lesions of a pre-existing disorder at a site of injury.

Isotopic response: occurrence of a new skin disorder exactly at the site of another unrelated and already healed skin disorder.

Pathergy test: hyper-reactivity of the skin to needle-prick.

Nikolsky sign: applying firm sliding pressure to the skin causes the epidermis to separate from the dermis, producing an erosion.

Structure and function of the skin

Contents

Relevant pages in other chapters

For a discussion of adhesion within the epidermis
and at the basement membrane zone, see ➲ Chapter 13,
Adhesion in the epidermis, p. 262.
For pigmentation, melanocytes, and sun protection,
see ➲ Chapter 16, pp. 320–1 and pp. 338–9.

Introduction

The skin is the largest organ in the body and the heaviest—an adult's skin weighs 4–5kg. Skin is not an inert barrier but plays an active part in defending against insults (microbial, physical, and chemical) from the external environment.

In this chapter, we aim to give you an insight into what your skin is doing for you, in the hope that this will encourage you to care for the skin of your patients (and your own skin) with the respect it deserves. An understanding of cutaneous physiology will also help you to analyse what has gone wrong or what might happen in patients with skin problems, including skin failure.

We discuss the structure of the skin and consider how this finely tuned organ functions as a barrier ('keeping the inside in and the outside out') and reduces water loss, is part of the immune system, is a metabolic organ synthesizing vitamin D and cytokines, regulates body temperature, and senses noxious stimuli (skin on the tips of your fingers is particularly sensitive; see Box 1.1).

Most of us will, at some stage, worry about the appearance of our skin, hair, and/or nails. 'Looking good' gives us confidence, and we may try to enhance the appearance (or smell) of our skin if we want to display ourselves to make a positive impression or attract a sexual partner. It is no surprise that fortunes are spent on lotions, potions, and procedures designed to conceal blemishes (actual or imagined) and to restore the appearance of youth. The psychological aspects of skin problems are discussed in more detail in ➔ Chapter 28, pp. 570–1.

Box 1.1 Dermatoglyphics (fingerprints)

- Fingertips, palms, soles, and toes are covered with a pattern of epidermal ridges called dermatoglyphics.
- The three basic patterns (loops, arches, and whorls) are unique to each individual.
- Characteristic dermatoglyphic patterns accompany many chromosomal abnormalities.
- The ridges amplify vibrations when your finger brushes across a rough surface.
- The ridges enhance grip.
- Autosomal dominant adermatoglyphia (*SMARCAD1* mutation)—absence of epidermal ridges, also known as 'immigration delay disease'. Also absent in some rare genodermatoses and in cases of palmoplantar dysaesthesias secondary to chemotherapy drugs.

Summary of functions of the skin

Prevention of water loss
- Stratum corneum—overlapping cells and intercellular lipid.

Immune defence
- Structural integrity of stratum corneum.
- Keratinocytes produce antimicrobial peptides (AMPs) including defensins, cathelicidins, and members of the granin family, e.g. catestatin.
- Langerhans cells trap antigens and migrate to lymph nodes where antigens are presented to T-cells (see ➔ p. 14).
- Cytokines secreted by lymphocytes, macrophages, and keratinocytes regulate inflammatory and immune responses.
- Acid pH of sweat and stratum corneum.
- Fungistatic activity of sebaceous secretions.
- Dermcidin (AMP) produced by eccrine sweat glands activates keratinocytes to produce cytokines/chemokines important in skin immunity.

Protection against ultraviolet damage
- Melanin synthesized by melanocytes protects keratinocyte nuclei from harmful effects of ultraviolet (UV) radiation by absorbing and scattering rays and by scavenging free radicals (see ➔ Chapter 16, pp. 320–1).
- Enzymes repair UV-damaged deoxyribonucleic acid (DNA) (see ➔ Chapter 16, pp. 320–1).

Temperature regulation
- Vasoconstriction and vasodilation control blood flow and transfer of heat to the body surface.
- Evaporation of sweat cools the body.

Synthesis of vitamin D
- Skin is the 1° source of vitamin D. 7-dehydrocholesterol is photoactivated to cholecalciferol (vitamin D_3), which is metabolized in the liver to 25-(OH)D_3 and in the kidney to the active form of vitamin D calcitriol (1,25-(OH)$_2D_3$). Only small amounts of vitamin D are obtained from the diet. Vitamin D is required for calcium absorption and has essential roles in bone metabolism, neuromuscular function, and immune function. Deficiency can lead to rickets (in children), osteomalacia, and osteoporosis (see ➔ Chapter 16, pp. 319–39).

Sensation
- Free nerve endings detect potentially harmful stimuli (heat, pain).
- Specialized end-organs detect pressure, vibration, and touch (see Box 1.1).
- Autonomic nerves supply blood vessels, sweat glands, and arrector pili muscles.

Aesthetic
- The skin has an important role in social interaction.

Epidermis

The epidermis originates from embryonic neuroectodermal cells. The epidermis is a stratified squamous epithelium composed of layers of keratinocytes that differentiate as they move towards the skin surface (see Box 1.2). The epidermis is attached to an underlying collagenous dermis, which contains the blood vessels that nourish the epidermis. Downward projections of epidermal rete pegs interlock with upward projecting dermal papillae, stabilizing the structure and making it difficult to shear the epidermis from the dermis (see Fig. 1.1).

Structure of the epidermis

(See Fig. 1.2.)

* A single layer of columnar keratinocytes in the deepest layer of the epidermis (basal layer) is attached to a basement membrane that is an interface between the epidermis and the underlying dermis. The basal cells are anchored to the basement membrane by adhesion junctions called hemidesmosomes (see ➲ p. 262).
* Regeneration of the epidermis (and hair follicles; see ➲ p. 10) depends on populations of epidermal stem cells.
* The middle layers of the epidermis (spinous or prickle cell layers) have a spiky appearance under a light microscope, because of the intercellular junctions (desmosomes) that are the main adhesive force between adjacent keratinocytes (see ➲ p. 262).
* The outermost horny layer or stratum corneum is composed of layers of flattened keratinocytes (corneocytes) locked together by modified desmosomes (corneodesmosomes) in a lipid matrix.
* All keratinocytes contain keratin intermediate filaments, but the structure of the keratins changes as the cells differentiate (see Box 1.2).
* Melanocytes are dendritic cells that are interspersed amongst the basal keratinocytes (approximate ratio 1:6) (see ➲ pp. 12–3).
* Epidermal Langerhans cells (dendritic antigen-presenting cells) are found throughout the epidermis (see ➲ p. 14).
* Migratory leucocytes are present in small numbers in the epidermis.

Proliferation and shedding

* The thickness of normal epidermis (0.05–0.1mm) is regulated by the balance between proliferation of basal keratinocytes and shedding of cells at the surface (desquamation).
* It takes ~40 days for a keratinocyte to move upwards from the basal layer to the horny layer where, after proteolytic breakdown of adhesion junctions, cells flake off (desquamate) (see Box 1.2).
* The activity of epidermal proteases and their inhibitors regulate cornification and desquamation.

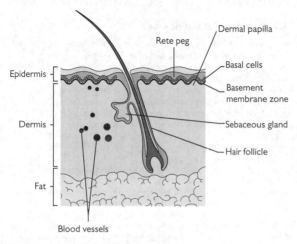

Fig. 1.1 Diagram of skin: epidermis, dermis, and fat.

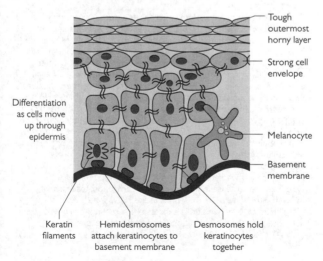

Fig. 1.2 Structure of epidermis.

Differentiation and the skin barrier

Box 1.2 Keeping the outside out

- Each keratinocyte has a cytoskeleton of microfilaments containing actin, microtubules containing tubulin, and intermediate keratin filaments composed of type I and type II keratins (from the Greek 'keras' meaning horn).
- Keratinocytes are held together by desmosomes (see Fig. 1.2). A glycoprotein intercellular substance aids cell cohesion. In acute eczema, hyaluronan secreted by keratinocytes into the intercellular space takes up water and may dilute noxious chemicals (see ➜ pp. 214–16).
- Keratinocytes change (differentiate), as they move from the basal layer towards the skin surface:
  - The types of keratins in the cells and the composition of the desmosomes change.
  - A protein called filaggrin aggregates and cross-links the keratin filaments, giving the keratinocytes internal strength. Loss-of-function mutations in filaggrin are associated with ichthyosis vulgaris, atopic eczema, and food allergies in older children.
  - The cell envelope is strengthened by Ca^{2+}-dependent cross-linking of proteins, such as involucrin and loricrin, and is catalysed by transglutaminase-1 (TGM1). Mutations in *TGM1* cause ichthyosis (abnormalities in the cell envelope and desquamation).
  - Lipid is synthesized by keratinocytes and accumulates in the intercellular space.
  - By the time the keratinocytes reach the outermost horny layer, they have lost their nuclei and subcellular organelles and are densely packed with keratin filaments.
- The outermost horny layer is composed of ~20 layers of flattened horny cells (corneocytes) with tough insoluble cell membranes (cornified envelopes) locked together by corneodesmosomes and a thick intercellular layer of lipids (like mortar). This impermeable layer enables the skin to withstand chemical and mechanical injury and restricts loss of water and electrolytes. Darkly pigmented skin seems to provide a better epidermal barrier than lightly pigmented skin—the stratum corneum is less permeable and more cohesive.
- Permeability of the skin depends primarily on the balance between intercellular cohesion and desquamation in the stratum corneum. Serine proteases, such as kallikreins, degrade corneodesmosomes, so cells can desquamate. Inhibitors, such as lymphoepithelial Kazal-type 5 serine protease inhibitor (LEKTI), control protease activity. In Netherton syndrome, mutations in the *SPINK5* gene encoding LEKTI lead to defective LEKTI expression, unregulated proteolytic activity, increased desquamation, and highly permeable skin (see ➜ Box 31.11, p. 603).

Further reading

Cork MJ et al. J Invest Dermatol 2009;129:1892–908.

Dermis and glands

The dermis is a layer of connective tissue beneath the epidermis. A layer of subcutaneous fat separates the dermis from the underlying fascia and muscle. The dermis has a rich supply of blood vessels, lymphatics, nerves, and sensory receptors. The thickness of the dermis varies with body site and may measure as much as 5mm on the back.

Structural components

- Collagen, mainly type I but some type III, gives the dermis tensile strength. Ageing skin is characterized by reduced collagen synthesis and increased collagen breakdown by matrix metalloproteinases.
- Elastic fibres, containing a core of elastin, supply elasticity and resilience, but elastin functions poorly in aged skin.
- Ground substance of proteoglycans and glycoproteins that binds water and hydrates the dermis.
- Skin appendages: hair follicles, sebaceous glands, eccrine sweat glands, and apocrine sweat glands (see ➜ p. 9, and p. 10).
- Blood vessels: superficial and deep vascular plexuses. Vasodilatation and vasoconstriction help to regulate heat loss.
- Lymphatics: afferent capillaries in dermal papillae pass via a superficial plexus to deeper horizontal plexuses and collecting lymphatics (see ➜ Skin immune system, p. 14).
- Nerve fibres: most sensory nerves end in the dermis, but a few penetrate the epidermis. Free nerve endings detect heat and pain; Pacinian corpuscles detect pressure and vibration, and Meissner corpuscles detect pressure and touch. Autonomic innervation is cholinergic to the eccrine sweat glands, and adrenergic to eccrine and apocrine glands, arterioles, and arrector pili muscle.

Cellular components

- Fibroblasts synthesize proteins, such as collagen and elastin, as well as glycosaminoglycans in the dermal ground substance.
- Dendritic cells (dermal dendritic cells) are involved in antigen presentation (see ➜ p. 14).
- Macrophages scavenge cell debris and foreign material.
- Mast cells: a few near blood vessels. Granules contain inflammatory mediators, such as histamine, prostaglandins, leukotrienes, and other chemokines, that may be involved in inflammatory responses.

Langer lines

Langer lines (cleavage lines) correspond to the alignment of collagen fibres within the dermis. They define the direction along which the skin has least flexibility. Surgical incisions carried out parallel to favourable skin tension lines heal with less scarring.

Eccrine glands

- Eccrine glands cover most of the body surface but are most numerous on the palms and soles.
- A secretory coil deep in the dermis is attached to a duct that conveys sweat to the surface of the skin.
- Glands are innervated by the sympathetic nervous system.
- Eccrine glands secrete water, electrolytes, lactate, urea, and ammonia.
- Sweating helps to regulate body temperature.
- Sweat may have antimicrobial properties; eccrine glands produce dermcidin peptides (antimicrobial peptides)—DCD-1 and DCD-1L.

Apocrine glands

- Apocrine glands are found mainly in the axillae, anogenital region, female breast, eyelids, and external auditory canal.
- A secretory coil in the deep dermis leads to a duct that opens into the upper portion of a hair follicle.
- They produce an oily secretion of protein, carbohydrate, ammonia, and lipid.
- Apocrine glands become active at puberty.
- Sympathetic nerve fibres control secretion.
- The action of bacteria on secretions produces body odour.

Sebaceous glands

- Sebaceous glands are associated with the upper portion of each hair follicle. The hair follicle and associated glands are known as a pilosebaccous unit (see Fig. 1.3).
- The size of glands varies at different body sites. The largest glands are on the face and upper trunk (sites prone to acne).
- Sebocytes secrete lipid-rich sebum with emollient properties.
- Sebocytes produce cathelicidin, which has antimicrobial properties, in response to vitamin D and infectious agents.
- Sebum in the sebaceous duct enters the upper portion of the hair follicle and protects the surface of the skin.

Further reading

Peng Y et al. Ageing Res Rev 2015;19:8–21.

Hair and nails

Hair

- Hair is found all over the body, except for the palms and soles, but the density and size of hair follicles vary at different sites.
- The hair follicle opens onto the surface of the epidermis and is a potential portal of entry for pathogenic microbes.
- The size of the follicle determines the size of the hair shaft (the product of the follicle). Short, fine, soft, non-pigmented vellus hair covers most of the body (you can just feel vellus hair on your forehead), and coarse, pigmented terminal hair grows at sites such as the scalp, eyebrows, eyelashes, limbs, genitalia, and axillae. Androgens influence the hair type—some vellus hair changes to terminal hair in hirsutism (see ➲ p. 474).
- The cylindrical follicular root sheath moulds the shape of the hair shaft.
- A bulge region in the mid portion of the root sheath contains epithelial hair follicle stem cells from which the follicle arises (see Fig. 1.3). These stem cells regulate the hair cycle (see Box 1.3). Damage to stem cells may contribute to irreversible hair loss (scarring alopecia) in inflammatory conditions such as cutaneous lupus erythematosus.
- The hair shaft arises from dividing cells in the bulb at the bottom of the follicle. The shaft gradually keratinizes, producing a highly cohesive structure, as it moves up through the follicle root sheath. Blood vessels and sensory nerves in the associated dermal papilla supply the cells of the hair bulb (see Fig. 1.3).
- Melanocyte stem cells are found in the bulge region from where they migrate to the bulb.
- The arrector pili muscles attach to the mid portion of follicles. These smooth muscles, supplied by adrenergic nerves, make hair 'stand on end' in the cold or during emotional stress (goose pimples).
- The sebaceous and apocrine ducts penetrate the follicular root sheath at the start of the upper third of the follicle.

Nails

- A nail is a plate of keratinized cells (onychocytes) with a free edge.
- The nail plate is formed by specialized keratinocytes in the nail matrix, which lies under the proximal nail fold and extends distally to the lunula but proximally to the insertion of the extensor tendon.
- The nail plate grows forward over a nail bed that is tightly connected to the nail plate.
- Lateral and proximal nail folds cover the sides and base of the nail plate. The cuticle forms a seal between the nail plate and the proximal nail fold.
- Fingernails grow by ~1mm per week (toenails more slowly). If growth in the matrix is slowed by serious illness or drugs, horizontal lines or dents appear at the same place in all nail plates (Beau lines). The lines will only become apparent 8–12 weeks after the insult when the nail plate emerges from under the cuticle. For a diagram of a normal nail, see ➲ Fig. 3.3, p. 47.

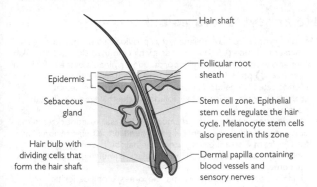

Fig. 1.3 Structure of a hair follicle. The arrector pili muscle (not shown) attaches to the mid portion of the follicle.

Box 1.3 The hair follicle cycle

- Hair grows by 0.3–0.4mm/day. About 85–90% of the 100 000 scalp hairs are growing. Each hair follicle cycles through phases of:
    - Growth (anagen): active phase of hair production (2–6 years on the scalp). The length of hair is determined by the duration of anagen. The duration of anagen is determined genetically.
    - Involution (catagen): conversion from active growth to resting phase (2–4 weeks).
    - Rest (telogen): 15% of scalp hairs are in telogen (2–4 months).
- At the end of telogen, hair is shed, and a new cycle starts. It is normal to lose 100–150 scalp hairs a day.
- Each hair follicle cycle is independent of neighbouring follicles, so humans do not moult, unlike many other mammals.

Further reading

Harries MJ et al. Autoimmun Rev 2009;8:478–83.

Melanocytes and colour

Melanin, synthesized by melanocytes, provides some defence against ultraviolet radiation (UVR) as well as giving colour to skin and hair. Skin colour and ease of tanning are important determinants of the risk of skin cancer (see ➲ pp. 320–1 and p. 346, and Chapters 16 and 17).

* Melanocytes are dendritic cells that migrate from the neural crest to the epidermis and hair follicles in the third month of fetal development.
* Melanocytes are interspersed amongst the basal keratinocytes in the epidermis. Melanocyte stem cells are found in the bulge region of hair follicles from where they migrate to the hair bulb (see Fig. 1.3).
* Melanocytes synthesize both brown/black eumelanin and red/yellow phaeomelanin from tyrosine.
* Melanin is passed in packages (melanosomes) along dendritic processes into keratinocytes (see Fig. 1.2) where melanosomes sit in a cap or 'parasol' over the upper sun-exposed side of the keratinocyte nucleus. Each melanocyte links to a number of keratinocytes, forming an epidermal melanin unit. Melanin provides UV protection by absorbing visible light and UVR (see ➲ pp. 320–1).
* UVR induces tanning by stimulating oxidation of pre-existing melanin, by triggering the synthesis of new melanin, and by changing the distribution of melanosomes (see ➲ pp. 320–1).
* Melanin is the main determinant of the colour of skin and hair (see Box 1.4). The colour depends on the number, size, and distribution of melanosomes within keratinocytes and the type of melanin, rather than the number of melanocytes. Darkly pigmented skin has similar numbers of melanocytes to lightly pigmented skin, but more and slightly differently packaged melanin (melanosomes) within keratinocytes.
* Skin colour is not uniform (see Box 1.5).
* Darkly pigmented skin has better epidermal barrier function than lightly pigmented skin (see Box 1.2).
* Genetic variation in the amino acid sequence of the melanocortin 1 receptor (MC1R) is a major determinant of skin and hair colour. Some variants, e.g. redheads, do not tan in response to sun. Polymorphisms in MC1R variants confer susceptibility to skin cancers (see ➲ p. 347).
* The first step in the synthesis of melanin is hydroxylation of tyrosine to dopaquinone. Oculocutaneous albinism is caused by abnormalities in the function of tyrosinase or other enzymes in the synthetic pathway of melanin.
* Defective migration of melanocytes from the neural crest or abnormalities in the maturation or trafficking of melanosomes may present as a pigmentary disorder.
* Depletion of melanocyte stem cells in hair follicles may contribute to age-related greying of hair.

Box 1.4 Skin colour

- The colour of normal skin comes from a mixture of pigments, but melanin is the main contributor to skin colour.
- Oxyhaemoglobin in blood gives untanned Caucasian skin a pink colour.
- Carotene in subcutaneous fat and the horny layer of the epidermis adds a yellow hue to normal skin.
- Abnormalities in skin colour may result from an imbalance of pigments (e.g. in cyanosis, chloasma, and carotenaemia) or the presence of abnormal pigments (e.g. haemosiderin).
- Genetic abnormalities in the synthetic pathway of melanin present with abnormal skin colour.
- Post-inflammatory hypo- or hyperpigmentation is common, particularly in darker skin.
- Damage to the basal layer of the epidermis (interface or lichenoid reaction) is associated with the release of melanin into the dermis and hyperpigmentation.

Box 1.5 Pigmentary demarcation lines (Voigt–Futcher lines)

Dorsal skin surfaces are more pigmented than ventral surfaces. Lines of demarcation between darker dorsal and paler ventral surfaces are apparent in about 20% of people with dark skin. The lines, which are symmetrical and bilateral, are present from infancy and have no clinical significance.

- Type A: vertical line on the lateral aspect of the upper arm that may extend into the pectoral region (commonest).
- Type B: curved line on back of the thigh (posteromedial) that extends from the perineum to the popliteal fossa and occasionally the ankle.
- Type C: vertical or curved hypopigmented band on the mid chest (contains two parallel lines).
- Type D: vertical line on the posteromedial area of the spine.
- Type E: bilateral hypopigmented streaks, bands, or patches on the upper chest in the zone between the mid third of the clavicle and the periareolar skin.

Facial patterns, which appear around puberty, have been described in the Indian subpopulation:

- Type F: 'V'-shaped hyperpigmented lines between the malar prominence and the temple.
- Type G: 'W'-shaped hyperpigmented lines between the malar prominence and the temple.
- Type H: linear bands of hyperpigmentation from the angle of the mouth to the lateral aspects of the chin.

Further reading

Lin JY and Fisher DE. *Nature* 2007;**445**:843–50.
Somani VK et al. *Indian J Dermatol Venereol Leprol* 2004;**70**:336–41.

Skin immune system

The skin immune system (both innate and adaptive) provides vital defence against external cutaneous pathogens or physical injury.

Keratinocytes

Keratinocytes respond to cutaneous injury or infection by releasing antimicrobial peptides (AMPs), such as β-defensins and cathelicidins, that have broad-spectrum antimicrobial activity against bacteria, fungi, and viruses. AMPs may also reduce the likelihood of microbes entering the skin through follicular openings. AMPs are part of the innate immune system (see Box 1.6). Keratinocytes can also produce a wide range of cytokines: pro- or anti-inflammatory, immunomodulatory, and immunosuppressive. Alarmin cytokines, such as interleukin (IL)-33, can be released in response to cell damage. Cathelicidins induce the production of pro-inflammatory cytokines that enhance cell migration and promote wound healing. Vitamin D$_3$ seems to be involved in the regulation of cathelicidin expression in the epidermis. Keratinocytes are also able to present antigens to T-cells.

Dendritic cells

Dendritic antigen-presenting cells, such as epidermal Langerhans cells and dermal dendritic cells, express major histocompatibility complex (MHC) class II antigens and CD1 on their surface and 'police' the skin. They are part of the 1st line of defence if the skin is breached. The cells trap, ingest, process, and present antigens, in association with MHC (peptide antigens) or CD1 (lipid antigens), to the receptors of T-cells.

Lymphatics

Langerhans cells and dermal dendritic cells that have trapped antigens migrate via afferent lymphatics to draining lymph nodes where the processed antigen is presented to naïve T-cells that have the receptor that will bind that antigen. This triggers the generation of activated and memory T-cells imprinted with specific combinations of adhesion molecules and chemokine receptors that target their migration to the skin.

T-cells

Memory T-cells can be resident in the skin or can patrol the body for foreign antigens, recirculating through lymph nodes, lymphatics, blood vessels, and skin. Endothelial adhesion molecules aid trafficking by tethering flowing T-cells, so they can migrate through endothelial junctions. Chemokine gradients direct migration in the skin.

The receptor of each memory T-lymphocyte will bind to a specific peptide antigen presented on the surface of target cells in association with MHC class I (for CD8$^+$ T-cells) or class II (for CD4$^+$ T-cells). Some T-cells can recognize lipid antigens presented by the CD1 family of molecules. The antigen–MHC complex interacts with the T-cell receptor, which, along with co-stimulatory molecules, triggers the release of cytokines that attract more lymphocytes into the skin to augment the inflammatory response.

Box 1.6 What is the innate immune system?

The innate immune system is the first line of defence against environmental insults. The response is rapid and efficient but is less specific than adaptive immunity and does not improve with repeated exposure.

Receptors (transmembrane and intracellular), such as Toll-like receptors, recognize highly conserved molecular patterns that are common to many classes of pathogen, e.g. components of the wall of microbes.

Activated receptors stimulate the production of cytokines, chemokines, and AMPs. Immune cells, such as innate lymphoid cells (e.g. natural killer cells), and neutrophils are activated and recruited to the site of injury or infection. This innate response kills pathogens, promotes angiogenesis, and initiates repair after injury.

The major components of the skin innate immune system are:
- Intact physical barrier: stratum corneum and intercellular junctions.
- Antigen-presenting cells, keratinocytes, mast cells, innate lymphoid cells and neutrophils.
- AMPs, cytokines, and chemokines.

Further reading

Salimi M and Ogg G. *BMC Dermatol* 2014;**14**:18.
Sigmundsdottir H and Butcher EC. *Nature Immunology* 2008;**9**:981–7.

The history
in dermatology

Contents

Relevant pages in other chapters

The dermatological history: 1

Setting the scene

Introduce yourself; make the patient comfortable; ensure privacy (difficult on a ward), and allow sufficient time to establish rapport and for the patient to explain what has happened. Remember that skin problems can be embarrassing. Your history will be guided by the nature of the problem—a rash, a leg ulcer, or a skin tumour—but 'Please tell me about your skin problem' is a good opening question.

Finding out what the patient means

Clarify what the patient means by words such as blemish, wheal, hive, scar, or blister. Patients, as well as many doctors, find it difficult to describe rashes. You may think that you know what is meant, but make sure you use these words to describe the same thing as the patient. For example, some people call any raised lesion a 'blister' but do not mean a bump filled with clear fluid, and people may use the word 'scar' to describe post-inflammatory pigmentation without any dermal damage. Even 'sunburn' means different things to different people. Some people use this term to describe getting a suntan.

Sometimes the rash will have changed or even disappeared, and you will have nothing but the patient's description to help you make a diagnosis, so the description should be as accurate as possible (see Box 2.1). The patient may bring photographs to clinic.

Getting on the same wavelength

Clarify the patient's preconceptions about the cause of the problem, as well as their expectations of the consultation and your role. It is helpful to know more about the patient's perception of the current severity of the condition, particularly in those with fluctuating inflammatory rashes. This may differ markedly from your own assessment (see Box 2.2). You need to understand what matters to the patient, so ask 'What is most important to you?'. This will help you and the patient to set goals when planning investigation and treatment (see ❷ p. 32).

Symptoms, causation, and impact

'How does your rash/skin condition bother you?' is another good open question to start off the discussion (see Box 2.3).

Document the relationship of the condition to work, hobbies, and drugs, including herbal medicines and health foods. Might the rash be related to the menstrual cycle (a catamenial dermatosis)?

Skin conditions can be both disfiguring and embarrassing, and treatments can be messy, unpleasant, and time-consuming, so find out how the skin condition is affecting the life of the patient, as well as that of the family and/or carers.

More information about questions to ask in specific circumstances is given later in this chapter (also see ❷ DLQI under Quality of life, p. 32).

Box 2.1 Questions to ask about a rash

- Where the rash started, appearance at onset, and how it evolved.
- Is the surface smooth or scaly, or is the rash flat or raised?
- The colour of the rash: if red, did the patient notice what happened if he/she applied light pressure, i.e. did it blanch, suggesting an erythema as opposed to purpura?
- Is the rash persistent, or do lesions come and go? Is it cyclical?
- If transient—how long do individual lesions last, and, when they fade, what does the skin look like? Are there any changes in skin colour or any marking (scarring)?
- Are hair, nails, or mucosal surfaces affected?

Box 2.2 Grading the skin condition: the patient's perception

It helps to have some insight into the patient's perception of the severity of his/her skin condition as it is now. Ask the patient to grade the condition:
'You have explained that your rash/skin condition can vary a bit. I would like to get a feel for how bad it is for you today by asking you to grade your skin condition. Let us say that a grade of 10 means it is the worst it has ever been for you and zero means that you have no skin problem. What grade would you give your skin today?'

Box 2.3 Questions to ask when exploring symptoms and impact of a skin condition

- What does the rash feel like? Is the skin tender, itchy, or painful?
- What brings on the itch/pain? What does the patient do about it?
- Itch—try to quantify the impact. Does it affect sleep or concentration?
- Is anyone else itchy? Ask about family and all close contacts, e.g. sexual partner (could it be scabies?).
- Pain: what is the character of the pain? Sharp, dull, throbbing, paraesthesiae, continuous, or intermittent?
- Does the skin ooze clear fluid, pus, or blood?
- Is the skin fragile? Does it bruise easily, or does the skin blister?
- Has the patient noticed a smell from the skin (ulcer)? Patients may welcome a chance to discuss this awkward and embarrassing symptom if you introduce the subject in a sensitive manner.
- What makes the rash better or worse? Is there any relationship to recent travel, work, or hobbies? Does the problem improve or worsen at the weekends or in holidays? Does sunlight make a difference? Any relationship to cosmetics being used or to drugs/health foods?
- How does the skin condition affect activities of everyday living— school, work, or social?
- How long does applying treatment take, and what is the treatment costing?
- Is the skin condition affecting mood?
- Are carers coping, e.g. the parents of a child with eczema?

The dermatological history: 2

Drug history

- What has been prescribed, purchased, begged, or borrowed? Patients may be using a variety of topical preparations, some of which they will not regard as medicaments at all—and they will probably not remember all the names.
- Is the product an ointment (greasy, petroleum jelly-like, sits on the surface of the skin), a cream (white, 'disappears into the skin'), a gel, a foam, or a lotion (liquid)?
- What does the patient do with the treatment? How much is used—how long does the tube or tub last? Where, and how often, is it applied? If the patient has more than one topical preparation, how and where are they used—at the same time or at different times?
- Is any moisturizer being used, and how often is it applied?
- What soaps, cosmetics, or other toiletries are used?
- Is anything added to the bath, e.g. bath salts?
- Is the patient taking other drugs, including recreational drugs, and how does the use of these relate to the onset of the rash?

Past medical history

- Enquire about previous skin problems, in particular has the patient had a similar skin condition before, and, if so, how long did it last, and what was done?
- Is there a history of atopy such as infantile eczema or 'dry skin', asthma, or hay fever?
- Document other medical conditions.

Allergies

- Ensure you know what the patient means if he/she uses the term 'allergy'.
- Has the patient noticed 'reactions' when anything is in contact with the skin, e.g. topical medicaments, jewellery (usually nickel allergy), cosmetics, or perfumes? What sort of reaction and how long did it last? Has allergy been investigated by patch or prick testing?
- Have there been 'reactions' to oral medications? What happened, and what was done?

Social and personal history

- Explore lifestyle, exposure to nicotine and alcohol, sexual history, travel, hobbies, and occupation.

Family history

- Does anyone at home have a similar skin problem? Scabies and skin infections are contagious. Other skin conditions, such as atopic eczema or psoriasis, may have a strong genetic predisposition.
- Draw a family tree if you think that you are dealing with an inherited condition (see ➜ p. 622).

Functional enquiry

Complete the history with a review of all systems (functional enquiry). Itching, ulcers, or purpuric rashes can be manifestations of a systemic disease. A careful history may provide clues to a diagnosis, such as underlying malignancy or connective tissue disease, and guide the examination as well as investigation.

Patients do not always volunteer such additional information without prompting, because they do not relate the skin problem to their other symptoms.

History in patients with allergy

Type I hypersensitivity

Urticaria (hives, wheals, welts) is an immediate type I hypersensitivity reaction that may occur on its own or in association with angio-oedema and/or anaphylaxis. Urticaria is commoner in atopics.

Acute urticaria may be triggered by drugs, e.g. penicillin, or foods, e.g. peanuts, fish. The patient can often identify the allergen. In contrast, it is difficult to pinpoint the trigger in most patients with chronic urticaria. Physical urticarias can be triggered by firm pressure (dermographism), heat, cold, sun, or exercise.

The wheals of urticaria are 2° to dermal oedema. They are raised, smooth, erythematous, and usually itchy. Angio-oedema implies oedema of the deep dermis and subcutaneous tissues, as well as mucosal and submucosal oedema. Patients describe the sudden onset of large tender swellings involving the skin, mucosae, and submucosal tissues (see ➔ Chapter 5, pp. 104–5, and Chapter 11, p. 228 and pp. 230–1).

The history should be directed at finding out exactly what happened to confirm the diagnosis of urticaria and/or angio-oedema, as the rash may not be present when you see the patient (see Boxes 2.4 and 2.5). Does the patient have one or both problems? ⚠ Rarely, angio-oedema can be caused by a deficiency of C1 esterase inhibitor (inherited or acquired), but these patients do *not* have urticaria (see ➔ p. 104).

Prick testing may be helpful to investigate the cause in some cases of acute urticaria, particularly if there is a history suggesting food allergy, but such testing is unlikely to be helpful in chronic urticaria.

Irritant contact dermatitis or type IV hypersensitivity

Dermatitis (eczema) caused by an external agent is known as contact dermatitis. Contact dermatitis may be irritant or, less often, allergic.

Irritant contact dermatitis is caused by chronic exposure to irritants (wet work, detergents, chemicals) and is commonest in individuals with atopic eczema who already have an inadequate skin barrier.

Allergic contact dermatitis is a type IV hypersensitivity. The patient has to be sensitized by prior exposure to the allergen, sometimes for months or years, before the onset of allergy. The eczematous response is maximal 5–7 days after exposure to the allergen. Allergic contact dermatitis is less common in children than in adults. Irritant contact dermatitis is commoner than allergy.

If you suspect an allergic contact dermatitis, direct your history towards elucidating the cause (see Box 2.6) by exploring the relationship of the rash to activities (work, hobbies). Patch testing is the investigation of choice (see ➔ Chapter 10, pp. 214–16).

A 2° allergic contact dermatitis may complicate the picture in an individual with long-standing dermatitis of another type, particularly when many different medicaments or over-the-counter preparations have been used over a prolonged period. Consider this possibility in individuals with chronic problems such as leg ulcers, pruritus ani, hand dermatitis, facial dermatitis, or otitis externa.

Box 2.4 The history in suspected urticaria

- Triggers?
- Confirm the diagnosis by asking about the appearance and behaviour of the rash:
  - Urticarial wheals are raised pink papules or plaques.
  - The wheals may be itchy.
  - The surface of the skin is smooth.
  - The wheals are erythematous, i.e. blanch with light pressure.
  - Individual wheals generally last no more than 24 h (48 h at the very most).
  - Wheals come and go in different places.
  - Wheals fade to leave normal skin.
- What happens if the skin is rubbed—does it wheal? = dermographism

Box 2.5 The history in suspected angio-oedema

- Triggers? Dental procedures or vaginal pressure during sexual intercourse may precipitate attacks of angio-oedema in people with C1 esterase inhibitor deficiency. These patients do not develop urticaria, only angio-oedema.
- The patient may describe one or more of these problems:
  - Sudden onset of deep tender swellings of hands, feet, and genitals.
  - Swelling of lips, tongue, and/or larynx.
  - Puffiness around eyes and lips.
  - Difficulty swallowing or difficulty breathing.
  - Stridor or wheeze.
- Gastrointestinal symptoms, such as vomiting or abdominal pain, occur in patients with C1 esterase inhibitor deficiency.

Box 2.6 The history in suspected contact dermatitis

- Remember that the allergen may be a product that the patient has used for some time.
- Document symptoms (itch?) and appearance (red, scaly, blisters?).
- Explore patients' occupations and hobbies in detail. Find out exactly what they do and with what they are in contact. Do they protect the skin, e.g. with gloves?
- Does the rash improve at weekends or during holidays?
- Is the skin exposed to any prescribed topical medicaments or over-the-counter remedies, and how long have they been used?
- How does the patient care for his/her skin—what is used to wash the skin or to moisturize? What cosmetics are being applied?
- Is the patient atopic? Irritant contact dermatitis is commoner in atopics (dry skin with poor barrier function is easily irritated).

History in patients with hair loss

Hair loss is a cause of great distress and may be difficult or impossible to reverse. Androgenetic alopecia is patterned in men (male-pattern baldness), with loss being most marked on the vertex of the scalp and/or the temples. Women with androgenetic alopecia describe diffuse thinning.

The commonest cause of sudden diffuse shedding is telogen effluvium (see Box 2.7)—a great diagnosis to make, because you can reassure your patient that he/she will not lose all their hair and that the hair will grow back. Drugs may also cause reversible hair loss (see Box 2.8).

What should I ask the patient?

- When did the problem start? Has this happened before?
- Establish if hair was shed suddenly or gradually.
- Is the loss diffuse or in patches?
- Is the loss complete, leaving bald patches, or partial?
- Is hair being lost at other sites, e.g. eyebrows, eyelashes, axillae? Alopecia areata can be widespread—alopecia totalis (all scalp hair) or universalis (all body hair).
- Are teeth or nails abnormal (indication of an ectodermal problem)?
- Is the patient still shedding excess hair? Remember it is normal to shed 100–150 hairs a day, and this may appear to be a lot to an anxious patient, particularly if the hair is long.
- Is the loss associated with other symptoms such as itching or scaling? Eczema and psoriasis are not usually associated with hair loss, but fungal infections certainly are. Some fungal infections cause no inflammation and minimal scale.
- How does the patient care for the hair—hot combs, perms, hair straighteners, colouring?
- Is the hair ever tied back tightly and for how long each day?
- Does the patient pull or pluck the hair?
- Did the patient start any new medications prior to the hair loss? (See Box 2.8.)
- Any exposure to radiation?
- Is there a family history of hair loss?
- Do close contacts have similar problems?
- Was there an event 8–12 weeks prior to the onset of loss, e.g. serious illness that might have triggered telogen effluvium? (See Box 2.7.)
- Has the patient just had a baby? The growing phase (anagen) is prolonged in pregnancy, but hair is shed post-partum.
- Has the patient any other medical problems? Iron deficiency and thyroid disease (hypo- and hyperthyroidism) may be associated with diffuse hair loss.

Box 2.7 The hair cycle and telogen effluvium

Hair grows by 0.3–0.4mm a day, but growth is asynchronous. About 90% of the 100 000 scalp hairs are growing. Each hair follicle cycles through phases of growth (anagen), involution (catagen), and rest (telogen) (see ➲ p. 10). At the end of the telogen phase, hair is shed, and a new cycle is initiated. It is normal to shed 100–150 hairs per day.

Telogen effluvium, 2–3 months after an insult such as severe illness or major surgery, is a common cause of acute diffuse hair loss. The hair follicle switches from a growing phase into a resting phase, and then the hair is shed when the new hair starts to form.

Box 2.8 Drugs causing reversible hair loss

- Anticoagulants.
- Antineoplastic agents.
- Antiretroviral drugs.
- Oral contraceptives.
- Progestin-releasing implants.
- Gonadotropin-releasing hormone agonist.
- Anti-oestrogens and aromatase inhibitors.
- Esterified oestrogens–methyltestosterone replacement therapy.
- Extracorporeal membrane oxygenation.
- Immunosuppressive drugs.
- Interferons.
- Minoxidil.
- Psychotropic drugs:
  - Antidepressants.
  - Anxiolytics.
  - Dopaminergic therapy.
  - Mood stabilizers.
- Retinol (vitamin A)/retinoids.

History in patients with skin tumours

Skin cancers are the commonest type of cancer. The non-melanocytic skin cancers, basal cell carcinoma (BCC; the commonest skin cancer) and squamous cell carcinoma (SCC), are commoner than the melanocytic cancer malignant melanoma, but all are rising in incidence.

Most elderly Caucasian patients have sun-damaged skin and are at risk of skin cancer. In any patient with a cutaneous tumour or an isolated scaly lesion, the history should include specific questions that will help you to decide if this patient is likely to have a skin cancer.

Sun damage and skin cancers are discussed in more detail in ➔ Chapter 16, pp. 320–1 and pp. 336–7, and Chapter 17, pp. 341–63.

The history

Find out:

- How long the patient has had the lesion(s).
- If it is changing (many skin cancers grow slowly, and the patient may not have noticed any recent change).
- If the patient is aware of any reason for the 'bump' to have changed, e.g. a history of trauma.
- If it is symptomatic—some non-melanocytic skin cancers may itch or 'tickle'; some SCCs can be tender or painful.
- If there was a pre-existing mark, such as a brown 'spot' or 'mole', but most malignant melanomas arise *de novo*, not in a pre-existing melanocytic lesion.

Risk factors

Document:

- Skin phototype—what happens to the patient's skin in the sun? (See Table 2.1.)
- History of sunburn, particularly in childhood.
- Chronic sun exposure—explore occupation, hobbies, holiday destinations, time spent in hot climates, e.g. military service or living abroad in childhood. How was the skin protected?
- Previous skin cancers.
- Chronic immunosuppression or chronic photosensitivity, e.g. drug-induced. Both increase the risk of skin cancer.
- Exposure to carcinogens, such as industrial tars or oils, pipe smoking, especially the clay pipes still smoked in India (SCC of the lower lip), X-irradiation, or arsenic (a constituent of some old-fashioned 'tonics' such as Fowler's solution; a contaminant in drinking water drawn from wells in Bangladesh and parts of India and elsewhere, e.g. Taiwan).
- Family history of skin cancers.

Skin phototype

Skin phototype affects the likelihood of burning in the sun, as well as the risk of skin cancer.

Table 2.1 Fitzpatrick classification

Skin type	Response of skin to sun	Appearance
I	Always burns, never tans	White or pale skin, many freckles, blond or red hair, blue or green eyes
II	Burns easily, tans poorly	Pale skin, possibly some freckles, blond hair, blue or green eyes
III	Sometimes burns, tans lightly	Darker white skin, dark hair, brown eyes
IV	Burns minimally, tans easily	Olive skin, brown or black hair, brown eyes. Mediterranean
V	Rarely burns, always tans	Naturally black-brown skin. Often has dark brown eyes and hair. Asian, Latin American, Middle Eastern
VI	Never burns, tans darkly	Naturally black-brown skin. Usually has black-brown eyes and hair. Black African

History in photosensitivity

Photosensitivity is defined as an abnormal cutaneous response involving the interaction between photosensitizing substances and sunlight or filtered or artificial light. People who are photosensitive are easily sunburnt. The skin is uncomfortable or develops a rash when exposed to sunlight or filtered or artificial light. You may suspect photosensitivity from the history or if you find a rash predominantly on sun-exposed surfaces (see ➲ Box 4.6, p. 73). Photosensitivity is most often an acquired problem (see Boxes 2.9 and 2.10).

Sometimes conditions, such as atopic eczema or psoriasis, are made worse by sunlight (photoaggravated).

What should I ask?

Specific questions will help you to pinpoint the type and cause of the photosensitivity.

- At what age did the problem start?
- Were any drugs or topical agents started prior to the onset of the problem? Most cases will present within 6 weeks of starting the drug, but drugs started in late autumn may not cause a rash until the following spring or summer.
- What are the symptoms—itch, pain, burning?
- Is there a rash? What is the distribution, and what does it look like—redness, swelling, blisters, pigmentation?
- How quickly does the problem occur after exposure to sunlight?
- How long does the problem persist—minutes, hours, or days?
- Does the rash leave any pigmentation when it fades?
- What time of year does the problem present—is there any seasonal variation? Symptoms usually commence in the spring.
- What sort of exposure is required to trigger the problem?
  - How much exposure is required to cause the rash?
  - Does sunlight in the United Kingdom (UK) produce the eruption, or does it only happen when the patient is abroad?
  - Does it happen if the light comes through glass, e.g. when sitting next to a window or when driving? Ultraviolet B (UVB), unlike ultraviolet A (UVA) or visible light, cannot penetrate glass (see ➲ p. 320).
  - Does lying on a sunbed (UVA) trigger the problem?
- Is there any evidence of 'hardening', i.e. does the skin become tolerant after repeated exposures to sunlight or a sunbed? Paradoxically, some problems improve, as summer progresses, and the rash may spare chronically exposed skin on the face.
- Are antihistamines, sunscreen creams, or clothing protective?
- What impact does the problem have on the quality of life?
- Is there a history of skin cancer, and did skin cancers occur at an earlier age than one would expect, given the skin type and history of sun exposure? Some photosensitive patients are more prone to skin cancers (see ➲ pp. 336–7).
- What hobbies or occupation does the patient have?
- Is there a family history of photosensitivity?

Box 2.9 Types of photosensitivity

1° photosensitivity (uncommon or rare)
- Idiopathic photodermatoses.
- Cutaneous porphyrias.
- Genophotodermatoses: very rare.

Acquired photosensitivity (phototoxicity or photoallergy)
- Drug-induced (commonest cause of photosensitivity).
- Contact photosensitivity:
  - Soaps, tars, perfumes.
  - Phytophotodermatitis (plants containing psoralen).

Box 2.10 Drugs that cause photosensitivity

Phototoxicity
(common, erythematous like an exaggerated sunburn)
- Phenothiazines, amiodarone, thiazides, non-steroidal anti-inflammatory drugs (NSAIDs), quinine, tetracyclines, sulfonamides, retinoids, psoralens, vemurafenib, voriconazole.

Photoallergy
(eczematous scaly rash, may not occur on 1st exposure)
- Sulfonamides, phenothiazines, thiazides.

Lupus erythematosus
- Hydralazine, procainamide, thiazides.

Pseudoporphyria
- Furosemide, nalidixic acid, amiodarone, ciprofloxacin, bumetanide, NSAIDs.

Lichen planus
(may be photoaggravated)
- Thiazides, quinine.

Pellagra
- Isoniazid.

For more information, see ➔ Box 4.6, p. 73, and Chapter 16, pp. 319–39.

Why the skin condition has not responded to treatment

Patients often say that the treatment 'has not worked'. It is important to explore exactly what is meant by this statement. It is not pleasant using messy ointments, and some people, particularly older people and those living alone, may find it difficult to apply the treatment. It is hardly surprising if patients do not adhere to treatment plans.

What should I ask the patient?

- What does the patient mean by the phrase 'has not worked'—are the patient's expectations realistic? Most skin conditions can be controlled, but cure is the exception, rather than the rule.
- Have you established what matters to the patient by asking 'What is most important to you?'. The answer will help you and the patient to agree treatment goals (see Box 2.11).
- Has the patient given the treatment enough time to 'work'? It may take 3 or 4 months before some treatments have a maximal effect.
- If the patient has stopped the treatment, what was the reason? Were there any problems applying the treatment or reactions to the treatment? Was the patient under the impression that it was a 'course' of treatment that would be stopped, rather than an ongoing treatment?
- Did the patient collect the prescribed medicaments or more medicaments from the general practitioner (GP) after the initial prescription?
- What was prescribed? It is not sufficient to know the name. You need more information before agreeing with the patient that 'it does not work' (see Box 2.12). It will help if the patient can show you the preparations being used—they may not be what you think were prescribed!
- When, where, and how is the preparation applied? Ask open questions to find out exactly what the patient is doing: 'Tell me more about how you use your treatment'.
- How much is being applied, and how often? Underuse is common.
  - Steroid phobia is a common cause of treatment failure. How long does the 30g or 100g tube of steroid ointment last? Some parents may be very reluctant to apply topical steroids to their child's eczematous skin (see ➲ pp. 608–9).
  - Emollients should be used liberally and frequently. Was the patient given a 500g tub?
- It can be particularly confusing for the patient if several topical preparations were prescribed. Are they to be used at the same time or sequentially; all over the skin or just on localized areas?
- Has anyone shown the patient how to use the treatment? There is a knack to applying topical medicaments. Ideally, all patients with chronic skin problems would see a dermatology nurse. The nurse can answer questions, explain (again) what the treatment is likely to do, and show the patient (or carer) how to use the treatments. If you do not have access to a dermatology nurse, you should be prepared to demonstrate the treatments yourself.

Box 2.11 Shared decision-making

Decisions about care should be patient-centred and collaborative. Your role, as a clinician, is to help the patient to understand the options and to reach a decision after considering his values, beliefs, and goals. Patient-centred care, utilizing shared decision-making, is associated with improved patient satisfaction, improved adherence to medication, and better outcomes.

Shared decision-making involves three steps:

1. Explaining/discussing the need to consider alternatives (team talk).
2. Describing the alternatives in more detail (option talk). At this stage, it may be helpful to introduce an option grid: a one-page evidence-based summary of options and frequently asked questions (see Option Grids website, available at ℜ www.optiongrid.org).
3. Helping the patient to explore their personal preferences and to reach a decision (decision talk). But give the patient time to consider all the information—it may be entirely reasonable to defer reaching a decision until another day.

Box 2.12 Questions to ask when exploring what was prescribed

- Is the product a cream, an ointment, or a lotion?
- Ointments have fewer preservatives and are less likely to irritate the skin than creams. They are also more effective than creams in dry, scaly conditions. But some people stop treatment, because they dislike the feel of the greasy film left on the surface of the skin or the mess left on clothes. They may also have the erroneous perception that the ointment does not 'get into the skin'. The answer may be to use an ointment in the evenings and a cream in the daytime.
- Some people find the skin is itchier under an occlusive ointment than under a cream.
- Preservatives in creams can sting inflamed skin or cause transient erythema. People who misinterpret these problems as a sign of 'allergy' will stop the treatment.
- Was the patient prescribed enough of the preparation? Hopefully, a 500g tub of moisturizer (emollient), rather than a small tube? Most medicaments come in 30g or 100g tubes.

Further reading

Elwyn G et al. J Gen Intern Med 2012;27:1361–7 (shared decision-making).
Elwyn G et al. Patient Educ Couns 2013;90:207–12 (Option Grids).
Elwyn G et al. Ann Fam Med 2014;12:270–5 (shared decision-making).

Assessing the impact of skin conditions

Impact of skin diseases

Our appearance affects the way we feel about ourselves and how well we function. The skin is always on show, particularly on the face and hands. If we think that we 'look good', we are more likely to 'feel good' and have confidence.

The psychosocial and physical impact of highly visible inflammatory skin diseases, such as psoriasis, acne, or atopic eczema, may be profound. Skin diseases disrupt school, work, and social life. Low self-esteem, common in teenagers with acne, may affect personal relationships, as well as prospects of employment. Inherited skin diseases, such as epidermolysis bullosa (EB), may be even more devastating. Patients, their families, and friends may find it difficult to cope.

Patients with chronic scaly skin conditions may also have a deep-seated, and probably quite irrational, fear of being contagious. 'I feel like a leper'. This may be reinforced by the reaction of family and/or friends who have an equally deep-seated fear of 'catching something'. The patient withdraws from physical and social contact.

Skin conditions in patients with other medical problems may be the 'last straw', e.g. the intractable itching in chronic liver or renal failure which can be more difficult to control than pain; photosensitivity in diseases, such as systemic lupus erythematosus (SLE), which may have a major impact on normal daily activities; hair loss or pigmentary changes which may be disabling; and highly visible adverse effects of drugs (see ➔ pp. 372–91) or the result of conditions such as chronic graft-versus-host disease (GVHD) (see ➔ pp. 534–6).

Quality of life

Consider measuring quality of life objectively, using a validated questionnaire such as the Dermatology Life Quality Index (DLQI) (⌗ www.cardiff.ac.uk/dermatology/quality-of-life/dermatology-quality-of-life-index-dlqi/) (see Boxes 2.13 and 2.14). This tool will give you insight into patients' perceptions of the impact of their skin conditions on their lives and also help you to assess the effectiveness of interventions such as education, counselling, and, of course, treatment. The reaction of patients is not predictable and sometimes may seem out of proportion to the severity of the skin disease. The DLQI provides insight into that reaction.

The DLQI is self-explanatory and is designed for patients over the age of 16 years. It can be handed to the patient before the consultation and takes 1 or 2min to complete. A similar questionnaire has been validated for use in children. Skindex is another dermatology-specific health-related quality of life instrument that can be self-administered. Tools have been developed for specific conditions, e.g. hand eczema.

Itch severity scale

Itch is the commonest symptom in dermatology, and severe itch may be extremely debilitating. A questionnaire (completed by the patient) quantifies how much of the day itch is a problem, the quality of itch, the intensity of itch, and the impact of itch (including impact on sleep) (see ➔ Further reading).

Box 2.13 Dermatology Life Quality Index® (DLQI)

DERMATOLOGY LIFE QUALITY INDEX

		DLQI
Hospital No:	Date:	
Name:		Score:
Address:	Diagnosis:	

The aim of this questionnaire is to measure how much your skin problem has affected your life OVER THE LAST WEEK. Please tick one for each question.

1.	Over the last week, how **itchy, sore, painful, or stinging** has your skin been?	Very much ☐ A lot ☐ A little ☐ Not at all ☐	
2.	Over the last week, how **embarrassed** or **self-conscious** have you been because of your skin?	Very much ☐ A lot ☐ A little ☐ Not at all ☐	
3.	Over the last week, how much has your skin interfered with your going **shopping** or **looking after your home or garden**?	Very much ☐ A lot ☐ A little ☐ Not at all ☐	Not relevant ☐
4.	Over the last week, how much has your skin influenced the **clothes** you wear?	Very much ☐ A lot ☐ A little ☐ Not at all ☐	Not relevant ☐
5.	Over the last week, how much has your skin affected any **social** or **leisure** activities?	Very much ☐ A lot ☐ A little ☐ Not at all ☐	Not relevant ☐
6.	Over the last week, how much has your skin made it difficult for you to do any **sport**?	Very much ☐ A lot ☐ A little ☐ Not at all ☐	Not relevant ☐
7.	Over the last week, has your skin prevented you from **working or studying**?	Yes ☐ No ☐	Not relevant ☐
8.	Over the last week, how much has your skin created problems with your **partner** or any of your **close friends or relatives**?	A lot ☐ A little ☐ Not at all ☐	
9.	Over the last week, how much has your skin caused any **sexual difficulties**?	Very much ☐ A lot ☐ A little ☐ Not at all ☐	Not relevant ☐
10.	Over the last week, how much of a problem has the **treatment** for your skin been, for example by making your home messy or by taking up time?	Very much ☐ A lot ☐ A little ☐ Not at all ☐	Not relevant ☐

Please check you have answered EVERY question. Thank you.

Box 2.14 Calculating and interpreting the DLQI score
- Very much, scored 3.
- A lot, scored 2.
- A little, scored 1.
- Not at all, scored 0.
- Not relevant, scored 0.

Sum the score of the answers:
- 0–1 = no effect on the patient's life.
- 2–5 = small effect on the patient's life.
- 6–10 = moderate effect on the patient's life.
- 11–20 = very large effect on the patient's life.
- 21–30 = extremely large effect on the patient's life.

Further reading

Chren MM et al. *J Invest Dermatol* 1996;**107**:707–13.
Finlay AY and Khan GT. *Clin Exp Dermatol* 1994;**19**:210–16.
Hongbo Y et al. *J Invest Dermatol* 2005;**125**:659–64.
Majeski CJ et al. *Br J Dermatol* 2007;**156**:667–73 (itch severity scale).

Skin and the psyche

Impact of skin disease on mood

People with skin disease may feel shame or embarrassment and have poor self-image or low self-esteem. Ten percent of people with psoriasis have had suicidal thoughts. Some patients become increasingly introspective, isolated, and depressed. Treatments prescribed for the skin condition, such as systemic corticosteroids, can also affect mood.

But anxiety or depression may be quite unrelated to skin disease, and the potential link between the mood change and the skin problem should be explored in the history.

Dysmorphophobia and dermatological non-disease

Each of us has a clear idea of how we look, but some individuals have a distorted body image.

Dysmorphophobia (body dysmorphic disorder) is a psychiatric condition in which patients have an unshakeable belief that they have a major flaw in their appearance. If present, the lesion is trivial, but some patients have no visible pathology (dermatological non-disease). Most patients lack insight into their behaviour but want a dermatological answer to the intractable problem.

Before diagnosing dysmorphophobia or dermatological non-disease, it is important to be clear what the patient is describing and what they are doing to their skin, e.g. picking may scar the skin, hair plucking induces folliculitis. Many inflammatory skin conditions do fluctuate in severity, and some, such as urticaria, may disappear completely.

Ask the patient to grade the skin problem as it is today, with 10 being the worst possible and zero being normal skin. If the patient says it is dreadful and gives the problem a grade of 10, yet you can see no gross pathology, it is likely that your patient is delusional (see ➔ p. 570).

Delusions of parasitosis

The patient believes that he/she is infested and quite often will have convinced other members of the family that this is the case. He/she may describe a crawling or biting sensation, lumps on the skin, and digging out the 'parasites' to provide relief. You may be given a bag or box containing specimens of these 'parasites' (fragments of skin scale, crust, or hair). For more information, see ➔ Delusions, pp. 570–1.

Also see ➔ Neuropathic itch, pp. 548–9.

Examination of the skin

Contents

Relevant pages in other chapters
Signs of photosensitivity ➔ Box 4.6, p. 73
Blisters ➔ p. 266
Examination of leg ulcer ➔ p. 296

Preparation

Get the basics right, and examination of the skin will be much easier. You should inspect all the skin and aim to describe the signs just as accurately as you would signs in the respiratory or cardiovascular systems. You should be able to interpret what you see, and, although you may not reach a diagnosis, try to pull together a reasonable differential.

Explain what you would like to do, and obtain the patient's consent to examine all the skin, not just the areas that seem to be affected. Ensure the patient is warm and comfortable. You will need to expose the skin, but you can do this in stages, so have a sheet or blanket to hand so that you can cover the patient. Ask if the skin is tender before you begin.

Remember to examine the nails, scalp, hair, and mucous membranes, as well as the skin. Look under dressings, and invite patients to remove make-up, dentures, or wigs. You may need a chaperone, particularly if you are going to examine sensitive areas such as the genitalia. You may also need a nurse to help you with dressings.

Can you see?

Lighting in most clinical areas is inadequate for examining the skin. Ideally, you should be working in bright ambient lighting that is equivalent to daylight, and you should have access to mobile supplementary illumination for some tasks, e.g. inspecting inside the mouth or illuminating awkward skinfolds.

Magnification

Some dermatologists use a hand lens or magnifying loupes for close inspection of skin lesions. Magnification can also help to assess the small blood vessels in the nail folds—you can use an ophthalmoscope with a drop of immersion oil, but a dermatoscope is even better. A dermatoscope can also confirm the diagnosis of scabies by revealing mites in burrows. A dermatoscope is used for assessing pigmented lesions, but it takes expertise to interpret the signs (see ➲ p. 640).

Wood light (black light)

A Wood light emitting UVR in the long-wave UVA region may be used in the assessment of hypo- or hyperpigmentation or some cutaneous infections (see ➲ p. 640).

Recording the signs

Draw pictures, or use a body map, to show the distribution of any rash or tumours (see Fig. 3.1). It is good practice to record the maximum dimensions of any tumour. It may be helpful to record the appearance of a rash or tumour photographically, but do obtain consent before you take clinical photographs.

Use simple diagrams to show your findings

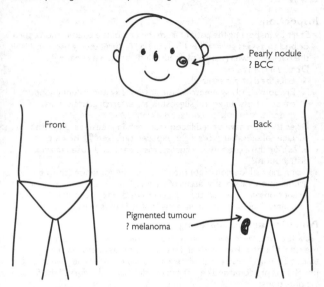

Front

Back

Pearly nodule
? BCC

Pigmented tumour
? melanoma

Fig. 3.1 Recording signs. Include the maximum dimensions of any tumour.

Rashes

Inspection

- Start by inspecting the patient from the end of the examination couch or bed to assess general health. Is this a life-threatening problem? Is the patient unwell (septic, malnourished) or looking healthy?
- Decide if the rash is:
  - Localized or generalized.
  - Predominantly symmetrical, suggesting a systemic (endogenous) cause, or asymmetrical suggesting an external cause such as infection, trauma, or contact dermatitis.
- Does the rash have a predilection for certain areas, e.g. extensor surfaces, flexural surfaces, light-exposed skin (see ➔ Box 4.6, p. 73), or the extremities—fingers, toes, ears, and nose (an acral distribution)?
- Does the rash demonstrate the Koebner phenomenon (show a predilection for scars or areas of trauma)?
- Are lesions grouped, scattered, generalized, linear, annular (in a ring), reticulate (net-like), or serpiginous (snake-like) (see Fig. 3.2)?

Palpation and interpreting the signs

Now look more closely at the individual lesions, and be prepared to feel the skin, but do ask the patient if the rash is tender before you begin. Try to describe a 1° lesion as precisely as possible, and decide whether the problem is predominantly epidermal or dermal. Ask yourself the following questions:

- How does the rash start, and what shape are the 1° lesions?
- Is the border well demarcated or indistinct?
- Is the surface scaly, indicating an epidermal pathology, or smooth suggesting a predominantly dermal pathology? Do not be afraid to gently scratch the surface of the skin.
- Are the lesions raised or flat? Palpate to answer this question.
- What colour is the rash? Does redness blanch with gentle pressure, indicating erythema (increased blood in small vessels), or persist indicating purpura (leakage of blood from the vessels into the dermis)?
- Is the involved skin hotter or cooler than normal?
- If there are blisters, what size are they? Do they rupture easily, suggesting an intra-epidermal blister, or are they tense with a thick roof suggesting a subepidermal blister, with the whole of the epidermis forming the roof? (see ➔ Fig. 13.1, p. 261.) Any milia? These tiny (<3mm), white intradermal keratinous cysts are sometimes found in subepidermal blistering diseases.
- Are there excoriations or erosions 2° to scratching?
- Is the skin thickened (lichenified), suggesting chronic rubbing?
- What happens as lesions evolve? Ask the patient to show you lesions at different stages. Do the lesions leave any colour change or scars?
- Is the problem malodorous, suggesting an anaerobic infection?

For terminology, see ➔ inside front cover.

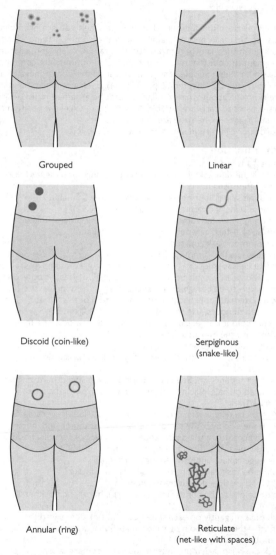

Fig. 3.2 Diagram of signs in the skin and patterns.

Skin tumours

Take an interest in the tumours that you see when you are examining patients, so that you become familiar with the common tumours and can distinguish the many benign 'bumps' that can be safely ignored from the malignant tumour that needs treatment. Skin tumours are common, particularly in older people, and skin cancer is the commonest of all malignancies (see ➌ Chapter 17, pp. 341–64). Seek a second opinion, if you are not sure about what you find. Do not be ashamed to ask—skin cancers diagnosed early are curable. You are in an excellent position to make that diagnosis when you are clerking patients.

Record your clinical findings as accurately as possible.

The examination
(Also see ➌ Box 4.8, p. 83.)

- Check all the skin, taking a particular interest in your patient's back—he/she cannot see it.
- Record the skin colouring (skin phototype) (see ➌ Table 2.1, p. 27).
- Are there signs of chronic sun damage (see Box 3.1)?
- Does one pigmented tumour stand out from the others? Take a careful look—this 'ugly duckling' may be malignant.
- For any tumour, ask yourself:
  - Where has this tumour arisen—epidermis, dermis, or deeper?
  - What cells/tissues are probably involved, e.g. keratinocytes, melanocytes, vascular, fibroblasts, neural, lipocytes, or other?
  - Is it likely to be benign or malignant (might it be a metastasis)?
- Take a systematic approach to the examination of the tumour—for pigmented tumours, use the ABCDE criteria on ➌ p. 354.
  - What colour is it, e.g. brown, purple, erythematous, or a mix?
  - What are the maximal dimensions?
  - Is the outline regular or irregular?
  - Is the surface smooth, shiny (pearly), crusted, keratotic, or ulcerated?
  - Is there a punctum? Seen in epidermoid cysts and other tumours centred on hair follicles such as sebaceous hyperplasia (see Box 3.1).
  - Are there telangiectasia running over the surface (suggests BCC)?
- Stretch the skin over the tumour between your thumb and index finger to accentuate the pearly appearance and borders of a nodular BCC, as well as the thready margin of a superficial BCC.
- Is the edge rolled, undermined, or indurated?
- Could it be vascular—can you compress the tumour?
- Might it be cystic—does it transilluminate?
- Palpate to check the consistency (soft, firm, hard) and thickness (depth).
- Pinch the skin gently on each side—does it 'sink down' into the dermis?—the buttonhole sign in dermatofibromas (see ➌ p. 342).
- Is it mobile or deeply fixed?
- Check the regional lymph nodes if you suspect malignancy.

Chronic sun damage (photoageing)

(See Box 3.1.)

Patients with fair skin, blue eyes, and blond or red hair are most at risk of sun damage and skin cancer. UVR is responsible for many of the signs we associate with old age, including coarse wrinkles and blotchy abnormal pigmentation.

Sun-damaged skin looks old—perhaps the most effective message to give to those addicted to 'cooking' themselves on beaches!

Chronic photosensitivity, e.g. caused by some drugs, is also linked to photoageing and skin cancer.

Box 3.1 **Signs of chronic sun damage**

- Solar lentigines: persistent flat, brown spots (liver spots) on exposed skin, e.g. backs of hands, forearms, face.
- Easy bruising (senile purpura) which resolves, leaving white stellate pseudoscars—most obvious on forearms and backs of hands. Elastic tissue damaged by chronic sun exposure provides the small cutaneous blood vessels with inadequate support.
- Waxy coarse, yellowish skin (solar elastosis) on the forehead, temples, cheeks, and back of the neck, associated with deep furrows.
- Sebaceous hyperplasia: scattered small, yellowish papules on the face. Often misdiagnosed as BCC but lacks marked telangiectasia (check with magnification). Look for a central punctum.
- Favre–Racouchot syndrome: thick, yellowish plaques (solar elastosis) studded with comedones (dilated follicles, blackheads) on the back of the neck and face, particularly the skin around the eyes.
- Telangiectasia on the sides of the neck and cheeks with reddish brown pigmentation. Known as poikiloderma of Civatte and seen most often in women with fair skin.
- Hypopigmented macules, alternating with areas of increased pigment—most obvious on the forearms and bald scalp.
- Dry skin.
- Solar keratoses: erythematous or pigmented rough, hyperkeratotic areas on chronically sun-exposed skin such as bald scalp, face, dorsum of hands.
- Bowen disease (SCC *in situ*) on lower legs: scaly, red patches. Usually asymptomatic. Differentiate from eczema or tinea.
- Skin cancers (BCC, SCC, malignant melanoma).

Scalp and hair

Examining the scalp is part of the general dermatological examination but assumes particular importance in any patient who is complaining of hair thinning, excessive shedding, or balding (complete loss).

Hair loss (alopecia) may be caused by a variety of insults, including fungal infections, drugs, or systemic disease. The loss may be diffuse or localized. Loss manifest by increased shedding may be apparent to the patient but not the physician. Normal hair density may be reduced by as much as 50%, before thinning becomes obvious. The loss may affect hair elsewhere, e.g. eyelashes, eyebrows, beard hair, or body hair (see ➋ p. 94).

Your findings should help you to decide if the pathology is likely to be a non-scarring alopecia (you will still be able to see the hair follicles in the affected area) or scarring alopecia (the hair follicles cannot be seen easily).

What to look for: the scalp

- Is the hair loss complete, and/or is the hair density reduced? Is the loss diffuse or patchy? Is there any sign of regrowth?
- Does the hair loss affect particular parts of the scalp, i.e. is it patterned? Androgenetic alopecia in men predominantly affects the vertex of the scalp and/or the temporal areas. Check the frontal hairline (see ➋ p. 480).
- Does the loss affect white hairs as well as pigmented hairs? White hairs are spared in alopecia areata (see ➋ p. 488).
- Does the scalp appear normal, or is it erythematous or scaly? Are there follicular pustules, perifollicular erythema, or follicular plugging?
- Are there broken hairs? Is the hair shaft smooth or rough?
- Can you see exclamation-mark hairs (short and tapering to a point) at the edge of patches of complete loss—pathognomonic of alopecia areata, but not found very often.
- Do you think there is scarring? (See Box 3.2.)

Hair pull and hair pluck

Telogen effluvium is a common cause of acute diffuse hair loss (➋ Box 2.7, p. 25). The hair becomes less dense, but patients do not lose all their hair, and the scalp looks entirely normal. In contrast, radiotherapy or drugs, such as chemotherapeutic agents, cause growing anagen hairs to fall out. Consider performing a hair pull or hair pluck (see Boxes 3.3 and 3.4).

What to look for: the hair shaft

You have examined the scalp, but you may also need to look at the morphology of individual hairs.

The hairs in some inherited ectodermal conditions are abnormal. Cut off a sample of a few hairs, and examine the hair shafts under a light microscope (or send them to an expert). If the hair shafts are abnormal, does the patient have problems with other ectodermal tissues, e.g. nails, teeth, or sweat glands? (see ➋ p. 634–5.)

Box 3.2 Diagnosis of scarring alopecia

The diagnostic sign is loss of follicular ostia. Use a hand lens or derma-toscope to examine the involved areas of the scalp.

Other signs will depend on the cause but might include:
- Epidermal atrophy—shiny, thin skin that wrinkles excessively if pinched gently.
- Perifollicular hyperkeratosis and perifollicular erythema.
- Boggy swelling and inflammation.
- Follicular plugging or prominent follicular openings without hair.
- Follicular pustules.
- Keloidal scarring.

To confirm the diagnosis, take two deep 4mm punch biopsies, orien-tated parallel to the hair shafts, from hair-bearing skin where the dis-ease is active clinically. Ask your pathologist to section one specimen vertically and the other horizontally.

Box 3.3 Hair pull

This test involves gently pulling a group of 25–50 hairs, while running your fingers from the base to the terminal ends. Normally, only one or two hair shafts are dislodged.

In active telogen effluvium, a gentle hair pull will yield at least ten hairs with each pull. Light microscopy will demonstrate that these are in the telogen phase (see Box 3.4).

A gentle hair pull at the edge of a patch of alopecia areata will also remove hairs if the disease is active.

Box 3.4 Hair pluck or trichogram

A hair pluck involves removing a tuft of 10–20 hairs forcefully (use artery forceps).

The hairs are placed on a glass slide, covered with a glass cover-slip, and the coverslip held in place by adhesive tape. Long hairs may be folded in a figure of eight to fit them under the coverslip. The hair shafts can be examined under the light microscope. Telogen hairs have club-shaped root 'bulbs' without much pigment. Growing anagen hairs have much smaller root bulbs. These bulbs tend to be soft and easily distorted, and they may have tissue adhering to them (root sheaths).

The normal anagen/telogen ratio is 4:1. In telogen effluvium, the ratio is decreased or reversed. More than 25% of the hairs may be in telogen.

Nails

Inspection of fingernails and toenails is an important part of the physical examination. Inspect the nail fold, nail plate, and nail bed (see Fig. 3.3).

Acquired changes may be a manifestation of drugs or systemic disease. Congenital problems may indicate a more widespread ectodermal problem that might also affect hair, teeth, and sweating. Nails may be partially absent, misshapen, or totally lost (see ⊃ p. 634).

Equipment

Side-lighting makes it easier to pick up changes in the surface of the nail plate. Consider magnification with an ophthalmoscope or a dermatoscope to look at the blood vessels in the nail fold.

What to look for

Inspect:

- Nail folds, both lateral and proximal. Is there erythema or swelling?
- Blood vessels in the proximal nail fold. You will need magnification to assess blood vessels, e.g. dermoscopy (see ⊃ p. 38).
- Cuticle: is this present, intact, and firmly attached to the nail plate?
- Shape of the nail plates.
- Colour of the nail plates: punctate white areas are common in normal individuals; linear splinter haemorrhages near the distal free edge of the nail plate in one or two nails may be a sign of trauma. Is any colour change uniform, or does it involve part of the nail?
- Surface of the nail plates: longitudinal grooves are common in the elderly, when they are of no significance.
- Thickness of the nail plates.
- Attachment of the nail plate to the underlying nail bed. Separation (onycholysis) may be caused by problems such as psoriasis.
- Nail beds (look beneath the nail plate). Is there hyperkeratosis or a tumour such as a subungual wart?

Interpretation

Which nails are involved?

The distribution of the nail problem, just as in the skin, will provide some guide to the likely cause. If the abnormality is widespread and symmetrical, it is more likely to have an endogenous than an exogenous explanation.

If just a few nails appear abnormal, particularly if these are toenails, consider whether the changes might be due to trauma or a fungal infection. What does the patient do to his/her nails—biting, manicuring, trauma at work? If infection is a possibility, you may wish to take nail clippings for mycological examination and culture (see ⊃ p. 646).

For more information about the causes of a nail dystrophy, see ⊃ p. 96.

For drug-induced nail problems, see ⊃ pp. 380–1.

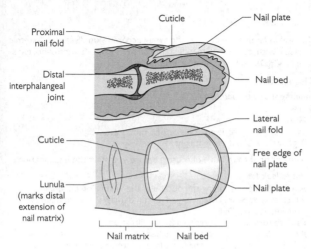

Fig. 3.3 Normal nail. Adapted with permission from De Berker D, Hair and nails. In Warrell, Firth, and Cox, *Oxford Textbook of Medicine* 5th edn, 2010. Oxford: Oxford University Press.

Mucosal surfaces

Mucosal inflammation or ulceration may occur in skin diseases, systemic diseases with cutaneous manifestations, such as graft-versus-host disease (GVHD), and in some drug eruptions.

The mouth

Equipment and preparation

You will need:
- Gloves.
- Two wooden tongue spatulas or oral mirrors.
- A gauze swab and a bright light.

Ask the patient to remove dentures, before you start the examination.

What to look for
- Assess the lips, including the outline of the vermillion border, which may appear rather 'ragged' in sun damage or discoid lupus erythematosus (DLE).
- Palpate tumours or ulcers to assess infiltration.
- Are the lips swollen, scaly, or cracked?
- Lichen planus (LP) gives the lips a lacy, white appearance.
- Look at the hard and soft palate.
- Check the attached gingiva for bright erythema (desquamative gingivitis), bleeding, or ulceration—seen in LP or pemphigus.
- To examine the buccal mucosa, ask the patient to move his/her tongue across to one side of the mouth, so that you can see the opposite side, and repeat this for the other side. Use spatulas to help you to visualize the buccal mucosa. Are asymmetrical areas of erythema or ulcers adjacent to broken teeth? Are pigmented areas near teeth that are filled with amalgam?
- Grasp the tongue gently with a gauze swab, and examine the dorsal and ventral surfaces. Move the tongue to the right and left to examine the retromolar region ('the coffin trap' and a common site of oral cancer).
- Check the dentures, if the signs suggest trauma.

Genitalia

In patients with oral mucosal lesions, you should examine the genitalia where you may find similar mucosal signs. Sometimes these are not symptomatic or the patient may be too embarrassed to complain.

What to look for
- Erythema, swelling, rashes, erosions, ulcers, or pigment change.
  - Assess the labia, the folds between them, and the clitoris.
  - Inspect the scrotum and shaft of the penis.
- Distortion of the normal anatomy or scarring.
  - Does the foreskin retract normally? In uncircumcised patients, pull back the foreskin gently to check for tightening and to inspect the glans.
  - Are the labia majora and minora visible or obliterated by scar tissue?

- Palpate to assess for tenderness and infiltration.
- Is there any discharge from the vagina or penis?
- Inspect the perianal skin and rectal mucosa.

The eye

The eye may be involved in a number of systemic diseases with cutaneous manifestations, including GVHD and connective tissue diseases, but pay particular attention to the eyes in any patient with a history of a red gritty eye, blisters, or mucosal ulcers.

What to look for

- Assess the lids, e.g. the violaceous discoloration of dermatomyositis.
- Are the eyelashes normal? These may be lost in alopecia areata.
- Is there blepharitis, or are there chalazions, e.g. in rosacea?
- Is there ectropion—seen in chronic erythroderma?
- If a patient with ectropion closes the eye, is the cornea covered? If not, refer to an ophthalmologist.
- Is the eye red? For causes of a red eye, see ➜ p. 86.
- Is the eye sticky?
- Is the patient photophobic?
- Is there subconjunctival blistering or scarring? Gently pull down the lower lid to see if the sulcus between bulbar and lid conjunctival surfaces is retained (loss of the sulcus suggests scarring) or surfaces are adhering together because of scars (synechiae). Synechiae may be more obvious if you ask the patient to look laterally and then medially.

Assessing the severity of a rash

Clinicians should consider using an objective tool to assess and monitor the extent and severity of skin involvement in inflammatory conditions such as psoriasis, atopic eczema, lupus erythematosus (LE), or dermatomyositis, particularly when new therapies are being introduced. Objective scoring is equally important in patients with life-threatening problems such as toxic epidermal necrolysis (TEN).

The percentage of body surface area (BSA) affected can be calculated (see Box 3.5), but this provides no other insight into the severity. A number of instruments have been shown to be reliable in specific skin conditions. These clinical scoring systems supplement information provided by a tool like the DLQI that assesses the patient's perception of the impact of the condition on quality of life (see ➔ p. 32). A few systems are mentioned here.

Psoriasis Area and Severity Index (PASI)

One of the best known disease-specific tools for assessing an inflammatory skin disease (see ➔ Chapter 9, pp. 200–1).

Atopic eczema score (SCORAD or EASI)

See ➔ Chapter 31, pp. 606–7.

Cutaneous Lupus Disease Activity and Severity Index (CLASI) and Dermatomyositis Skin Severity Index (DSSI)

Indices validated by both dermatologists and rheumatologists. Changes in scores correlate well with changes in global assessments, as well as with symptoms such as pain or itch (see ➔ p. 404 and p. 410).

Scorten

Severity-of-illness score developed to predict mortality in toxic epidermolysis/Stevens–Johnson syndrome (SJS).

See ➔ p. 119.

Box 3.5 Calculating the body surface area involved

The rule of nines was devised for determining the percentage of the body surface area (BSA) involved in adults with thermal burns (see Fig. 3.4).
It is calculated as follows:

- Head and neck = 9%.
- Anterior chest = 9%.
- Posterior chest = 9%.
- Anterior abdomen = 9%.
- Posterior back and buttocks = 9%.
- Upper limbs = 9% each.
- Lower limbs = 18% each.
- Perineum = 1%.

Alternatively, you can use the patient's palm to measure the BSA. Each palm without fingers = 0.5% of total BSA. (Palm plus fingers and thumb = 1% of total BSA, but this is less reliable than using the palm alone).

Scarisbrick JJ and Morris S. *Br J Dermatol* 2013;**169**:260–5.

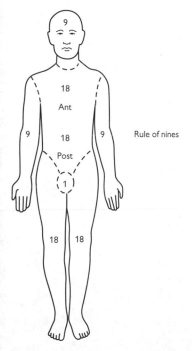

Rule of nines

Fig. 3.4 Wallace rule of nines. Reproduced with permission from Giele H and Cassell O. *Plastic and Reconstructive Surgery*, 2008. Oxford: Oxford University Press.

What is the diagnosis?

Contents

Relevant pages in other chapters
Leg ulcers ➔ Boxes 15.1 and 15.2, p. 295
Skin tumours ➔ Chapter 17, pp. 341–64

Epidemiology of skin disease

The prevalence of the skin problems that you see will be influenced by the setting in which you are working—hospital or community, rural or urban, tropical or temperate, specialty or general—but always remember that common diseases are commonest! Atypical presentations of common skin diseases are much more frequent than typical presentations of rare skin diseases.

In the community, you are more likely to come across skin infections, viral exanthems, skin tumours, and inflammatory dermatoses, such as acne, eczema, psoriasis, or urticaria, than manifestations of systemic disease. Chronic leg ulcers are common in 1° and 2° care, as are drug eruptions. In 2° care, you may see manifestations of systemic disease and acute problems, including conditions that cause skin failure.

But even in the hospital setting, please bear in mind what is common. Do not forget scabies as a cause of itching when you are caring for patients with chronic renal failure, many of whom are going to be itchy; remember fungal infections when you are looking at asymmetrical scaly rashes; exclude infection or trauma when you see blisters; and think of other causes of photosensitivity, e.g. a photosensitizing drug, before diagnosing LE.

What is common?

- Skin infections:
  - Bacterial cellulitis, impetigo.
  - Viral: herpes simplex, varicella-zoster, warts, molluscum.
  - Fungal: dermatophyte, yeast.
- Skin infestations:
  - Scabies, fleas, lice.
- Inflammatory diseases:
  - Acne.
  - Eczema (dermatitis) of any type.
  - Psoriasis.
  - Urticaria.
- Skin tumours:
  - Benign.
  - Premalignant (solar keratoses, Bowen disease).
  - Malignant (BCC, SCC, malignant melanoma).
- Hair loss (alopecia) or gain (hirsutes, hypertrichosis).
- Chronic leg ulcers.
- Pigment change (gain or loss).

Prevalence of skin disease

In 1975, the Lambeth Study of 2180 adults in the UK found that 55.5% of them had a skin condition. The prevalence of individual skin conditions in this community is shown on a bar chart in Fig. 4.1.

In developing countries, skin diseases are a major burden, particularly in children. These are predominantly bacterial infections, fungal infections, and infestations.

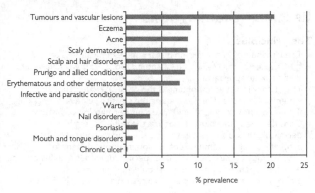

Fig. 4.1 Community prevalence of skin conditions. Data from Lambeth Study (Rea JN et al. Br J Prev Soc Med 1976;**30**:107–14).

Further reading

Schofield JK et al. Br J Dermatol 2011;**165**:1044–50.
Williams HC. Epidemiology of skin disease. In: Burns T et al. (eds) Rook's Textbook of Dermatology, 8th edn, 2010. Oxford: Blackwell Scientific Publications.

Reaching the diagnosis

The principles

- The introductory chapters on history and examination (see
  ⊃ Chapter 2, pp. 17–36, and Chapter 3, pp. 37–51) will help you to
  take a logical approach.
- The history is just as important as the physical examination, but
  experts often take short cuts, using the signs to guide history taking.
  If you are a novice, you should take a full dermatological history.
- Consider the whole patient, not just the skin—after all,
  dermatologists are physicians of the skin and its contents. Systemic
  problems, such as immunosuppression, malnourishment, or
  rheumatological disease, may have specific cutaneous manifestations.
- A rash in a patient who is unwell should alert you to a
  different differential diagnosis than a rash in a patient who is well
  (see ⊃ p. 58).
- Check the mucous membranes, hair, and nails, as well as the skin.
- Remove dressings, so you can see what is beneath them.
- Integrate the information you gather, and formulate a differential
  diagnosis, using analytical rules as well as pattern recognition
  (see Box 4.1).

Box 4.1 Analytical processing and pattern recognition

- Reaching a diagnosis depends partly on ordering and structuring
  information (analytical processing) and partly on pattern
  recognition.
- Experts use their knowledge and previous experience to integrate
  and make sense of clinical information.
- Pattern recognition ('spot diagnosis') is said to be an almost
  unconscious process that involves recognizing similarities between
  cases, based on the overall form of the cases. Expertise is equated
  with rapid, efficient, and accurate pattern recognition.
- Your skills in pattern recognition will improve when you have been
  exposed to many clinical examples of a condition and thought about
  their similarities. Concentrate on the variations in the presentation
  of common skin problems in the first instance. Why is this likely to
  be seborrhoeic dermatitis, and not asteatotic eczema? What makes
  this venous stasis, rather than a fungal infection? Read around the
  conditions that you see, and reflect on the variations you observe
  with your peers.
- To develop your analytical skills, adopt an organized approach to
  each case, so that you gather relevant information (experts know
  what questions to ask), detect important clinical signs (experts
  know what to look for), integrate the information, and formulate
  a differential diagnosis. The introductory chapters on history and
  examination will help you.
- Pattern recognition may have a powerful influence on the eventual
  diagnosis, but even experts use analytical rules as a safeguard
  against error.

A framework for analysing cutaneous signs

- Distribution: symmetrical (suggests an endogenous process) or asymmetrical (consider an external cause).
- Is there a predilection for certain sites, e.g. sun-exposed, acral (cold), flexures, extensors?
- What is the pattern, e.g. unilateral, generalized, grouped, linear (see ➡ pp. 62–3), annular (ring-like), reticulate (may be vascular), serpiginous? (see ➡ Fig. 3.2, p. 41.)
- Surface: scaly (epidermal problem—can scratch off scale), smooth (predominantly dermal), hyperkeratotic (thick horny layer, does not scratch off easily), or crusted (dried exudate—look underneath).
- Colour: red—erythema (blanches) or purpura (non-blanching).
- Hypo- or hyperpigmentation: this may be post-inflammatory.
- Identify a 1° lesion, e.g.:
  - Erythematous macules and papules: 2–10mm in diameter, with a tendency to confluence—morbilliform rash.
  - Erythematous scaly papules (papulosquamous rash) or scaly plaques.
  - Smooth papules or nodules (dermal involvement, e.g. granulomas).
  - Lichenoid papules: these have a purplish colour and a relatively smooth surface.
  - Urticarial wheal: smooth, raised erythematous papules or plaques that last no more than 48h and fade to leave normal skin.
  - Urticated erythema: smooth, raised erythematous papules or plaques that persist for more than 48h.
  - Purpuric macules or papules.
  - Blister: is it thick-walled (subepidermal) or thin-walled and easy to rupture (intra-epidermal)?
  - Pustule.
  - Thick plaque that feels as if the process extends below the dermis into the subcutaneous tissue.
- What does the involved skin feel like—soft, firm, hard (like bone)?
- Identify 2° lesions:
  - Excoriations: sign of scratching.
  - Lichenification: sign of chronic rubbing.
  - Prurigo: nodular reaction to chronic rubbing, typically spares the middle of the back which cannot be reached easily.
  - Erosion, ulcer, or scar.

Generalized rash in a sick patient

Has the patient been travelling? Is the patient immunosuppressed or taking any medication? Has the patient a fever?

Generalized erythematous rash in a sick patient

- Drug rash, eosinophilia, and systemic symptoms (DRESS) (see ➔ pp. 122–3).
- Infection (see Boxes 4.2 and 4.3).
- Erythroderma (red and scaly) 2° to drugs, eczema, psoriasis, or T-cell lymphoma but may be idiopathic (see ➔ p. 108).
- Acute GVHD (see ➔ pp. 532–3)—facial involvement suggests GVHD, rather than a drug reaction.
- Early TEN (see ➔ p. 116).
- Toxic shock syndrome (TSS): may be rapidly fatal (see ➔ p. 101).

Anaphylactic reaction with urticaria

- Reaction to drugs, venoms, or foods (see ➔ pp. 104–5).

Purpura in a sick patient

- Extensive irregularly outlined ecchymoses, bullae, and gangrene: disseminated intravascular coagulation (DIC) (purpura fulminans)—does the patient have meningococcal septicaemia? (see ➔ pp. 102–3.)
- Other infection (see Box 4.4).
- Small-vessel cutaneous vasculitis 2° to infection, drugs, or a systemic vasculitis (see ➔ p. 440).
- Drug reaction, e.g. DRESS (see ➔ pp. 122–3).

Widespread blisters and/or erosions in a sick patient

- Examine the mucosal surfaces (ocular, oral, genital) for blisters or erosions.
- Blisters that rupture easily, leaving erosions: consider staphylococcal scalded skin syndrome (SSSS), SJS, TEN, DRESS, acute GVHD, and pemphigus (may be 2° to drugs, including angiotensin-converting enzyme (ACE) inhibitors) (see ➔ p. 112 and p. 114).
- Generalized herpes simplex infection (eczema herpeticum) or herpes zoster. Vesicles evolve into pustules and become crusted (see ➔ Box 5.11, p. 113).
- Tense blisters: bullous pemphigoid (BP), but patients are usually systemically well, unless there is 2° infection (see ➔ pp. 270–1).

Generalized pustules in a sick patient

- Herpes simplex infection in atopic patient (eczema herpeticum): vesicles evolve into vesicopustules (see ➔ p. 112).
- Varicella-zoster infection (chickenpox): vesicles evolve into vesicopustules (see ➔ pp. 156–7).
- Bacterial infection.
- Sterile pustules: pustular psoriasis, acute generalized exanthematous pustulosis (AGEP) usually 2° to drugs (see ➔ pp. 124–5).

For dermatological emergencies, see ➔ Chapter 5, pp. 99–127.

Box 4.2 Some infections that may present with a morbilliform (measles-like) rash and fever

(see ➲ Chapter 6, pp. 129–48, and Chapter 7, pp. 149–69.)

- Measles (rubeola): also cough, coryza, and Koplik spots on the buccal mucosa.
- Rubella (German measles).
- Erythema infectiosum (parvovirus B19): 'slapped cheek' appearance on the face of children.
- Roseola infantum (human herpesvirus 6, HHV-6) = exanthem subitum: affects children.
- Enterovirus: may have pharyngitis.
- Infectious mononucleosis (Epstein–Barr virus, EBV): malaise, pharyngitis. A rash develops in 90% of patients with EBV who are treated with antibiotics such as amoxicillin.
- Leptospirosis.
- Acute retroviral syndrome (HIV).
- 2° syphilis: weeks to months after initial chancre.
- Typhoid fever: vomiting, diarrhoea, pink papules on trunk = rose spots (culture of rose spots may yield *Salmonella typhi*).
- Streptococcal scarlet fever, staphylococcal toxic shock syndrome.

Box 4.3 Infections that may cause a morbilliform (measles-like) rash and fever in travellers

- Chikungunya fever: Asia, Africa, Indian Ocean.
- Dengue fever: South East Asia, Central America, South America, Caribbean, South East United States of America (USA).
- West Nile virus: Asia, Africa Europe, south-eastern USA.
- O'nyong-nyong fever: sub-Saharan Africa.
- Mayaro virus: South America.
- Sindbis virus: Europe, Africa, Asia, Australia.
- Ross River disease: Australia, Papua New Guinea, Fiji, Samoa.

Box 4.4 Infections that may cause a purpuric rash and fever

- Meningococcal septicaemia.
- Rocky Mountain spotted fever: North America, Central America, and South America.
- Dengue fever: South East Asia, Central America, South America, Caribbean, south-eastern USA.
- Viral haemorrhagic fever: arbovirus/arenavirus infection.
- Yellow fever: sub-Saharan Africa, Amazon basin of South America.
- Epidemic louse-borne typhus.
- Leptospirosis.
- Atypical measles.

Itch

Generalized itch

The history is crucial. You need to decide, for example, if the itch (pruritus, not pruritis!) is a manifestation of a skin problem or an infestation, reflects an underlying systemic disease, or might be neuropathic or psychogenic in origin (see ➜ Box 10.5, p. 223, and Box 28.1, p. 567). What is the character of the itch? Ask about symptoms, such as burning, tingling, hypoaesthesia, or hyperalgesia that might suggest an underlying sensory neuropathy. How much impact is the itch having on the patient? Is it disturbing sleep? Is anyone else itchy? Ask about drugs, including substance abuse.

When you are examining the patient, decide what signs are 2° to scratching or rubbing (excoriations, lichenification, nodules, ulcers, scars) or if you can find evidence of a 1° dermatosis. Patients cannot easily reach the middle of the upper back, and usually this is spared if signs are just 2° to scratching. Look carefully for evidence of scabies (and look a 2nd time if the patient returns still itching).

1° skin condition—the differential includes
- Scabies (are any close contacts itchy?) (see ➜ p. 172).
- Eczema (see ➜ pp. 211–24).
- Psoriasis (see ➜ pp. 189–207).
- Urticaria (the rash may have gone by the time you see the patient). Ask about the rash and how it behaved. Stroke the skin to test for dermographism (a physical urticaria) (see ➜ p. 228, and Fig. 11.2, p. 231).
- Insect bites.
- LP.
- Prurigo nodularis (see ➜ Fig. 10.6, p. 223).
- The prodrome of BP: look for urticated erythema and blisters (see ➜ pp. 270–1).

Itch may be 2° to a systemic disease or drugs
Sensory neuropathy may cause itch or contribute to itch in some of these conditions (see ➜ pp. 548–9). The differential includes:
- Pregnancy-related (see ➜ pp. 584–5).
- Iron deficiency anaemia.
- Hypo- or hyperthyroidism.
- Chronic renal failure.
- Biliary obstruction, including primary biliary cirrhosis.
- Polycythaemia.
- Internal malignancy, including Hodgkin disease.
- Neuropathic: centrally driven neuropathic itch in association with brain tumours, strokes, spinal tumours, and multiple sclerosis. Human immunodeficiency virus (HIV) and diabetes may be associated with neuropathic itch (see ➜ p. 548).

- Drugs may cause pruritus (see ➡ p. 375), including:
  - Statins.
  - ACE inhibitors.
  - Opiates, barbiturates, and recreational drugs.
  - Antidepressants.
  - Oral retinoids.
  - Hydroxyethyl starch products (colloid volume expanders). Attacks of itch may last for years. Withdrawn in the UK in 2013, because of risk of renal damage.

Localized itch

Skin that is persistently rubbed becomes thickened with increased markings (lichenified) or may become hyperpigmented, nodular, or even ulcerated.

Consider:

- Contact dermatitis (see ➡ pp. 214–16).
- Lichen simplex (see ➡ p. 222).
- Picker's nodule (localized prurigo nodularis) (see ➡ p. 222).
- Neuropathic itch such as notalgia paraesthetica affecting the lower border of the scapula or brachioradial pruritus affecting the dorsolateral aspect of the arms (see ➡ pp. 548–9, and Boxes 27.1 and 27.2, p. 548 and p. 549).
- Rarely, localized itch is the presenting sign of an intracranial tumour, e.g. pruritus of the nostrils caused by brain tumours extending to the base of the fourth ventricle, intramedullary tumours causing unilateral itch of the upper limb, brainstem or spinal cord tumours causing itch of the head/neck/upper extremity.
- Trigeminal trophic syndrome (see ➡ Box 27.3, p. 549).

Linear patterns and sharp demarcations

If a rash is linear or displays a sharp cut-off, consider an external cause such as an excoriation, pressure of a waistband, or brushing against a plant (see ➜ Box 16.4, p. 327). External agents usually produce strikingly asymmetrical rashes. Some inflammatory dermatoses, such as LP, psoriasis, or vitiligo, demonstrate the Koebner phenomenon, and the rash develops at sites of trauma, e.g. where the skin has been scratched, and some cutaneous infections may be auto-inoculated into a scratch, e.g. viral warts or molluscum contagiosum. Ask about trauma such as scratching.

Once you have excluded an outside cause, seek an internal explanation, remembering the comment of that distinguished skin pathologist Ian Whimster: '*Some invisible intersegmental boundaries, whose existence we have been taught to expect by comparative anatomy and embryology, are only revealed by disease*'.

Venous or lymphatic drainage

Does the problem follow a vein or lymphatic? Stand the patient up to look for varicose veins. Conditions, such as stasis dermatitis or vitiligo, may follow varicose veins. Thrombophlebitis presents with tender nodules along a vein. The extending red line of lymphangitis is a typical finding in cellulitis, but other infections, including sporotrichosis, may spread along lymphatics, as may a malignant infiltrate.

Dermatome

A dermatome is the cutaneous area supplied by one spinal dorsal nerve root. Almost all areas of the skin are innervated by two or more spinal roots, so that adjacent dermatomes overlap to a large and variable extent, excluding those separated by the ventral axial line (see next section). Herpes zoster involves the skin in a dermatomal pattern (see ➜ p. 156–7 and Fig. 4.2, pp. 64–5).

Embryonic ventral axial line

The embryonic ventral axial line marks the border between the C5/C6 and C8/T1/T2 dermatomes. There is no crossover of sensory nerves or sensory function along this line that separates the cranial and caudal dermatomes. Contiguous dermatomes on either side of the ventral axial line are supplied from discontinuous spinal cord segments: C5 and C6 dorsal; and C8, T1, and T2 ventral (see Fig. 4.2, pp. 64–5).

Some morbilliform drug eruptions show a sharp 'drug line' that corresponds to this axial line, with well-demarcated involvement of the T1, T2, T3 spinal nerve dermatomes, but sparing of the adjacent C5 nerve dermatome.

Pigmentary demarcation lines (Voigt–Futcher lines)

(see ➜ Box 1.5, p. 13.)

The demarcation between darker dorsal and paler ventral surfaces is apparent in about 20% of people with dark skin. Pigmentary demarcation lines in the upper limb that correspond to the ventral axial line (see previous section) were first described by Voigt and Futcher. The lines are normal variants in skin colour that may appear pathological.

Blaschko lines

These lines seem to correspond to the pathways followed by keratino-cytes migrating from the neural crest during embryogenesis. Dermatoses following Blaschko lines suggest keratinocyte mosaicism (see ➜ pp. 620–1, Fig. 32.1, p. 621, and inside back cover). The lines follow a V shape over the spine, an S shape on the front and sides of the trunk that is unlike dermatomes, and a linear pattern on the limbs.

A number of inflammatory conditions can follow Blaschko lines, including lichen striatus (self-limiting inflammatory rash of childhood), linear LP, inflammatory linear verrucous epidermal naevus (ILVEN), and blashki-tis (Blaschko dermatitis)—a rare, self-limiting linear or whorled itching erythematous papulovesicular eruption on the trunk and limbs that may be the adult equivalent of lichen striatus. Rare inherited conditions with cutaneous features following Blaschko lines include incontinentia pig-menti and Goltz syndrome (see ➜ pp. 636–7).

Embryonic cleft

Congenital anomalies in the midline may be associated with the lines of fusion between embryonic tissues.

Wallace line

This demarcation line marks the anatomical boundary on the lateral aspect of the palms and soles where the glabrous (i.e. skin devoid of hair) plantar or palmar skin meets hair-bearing dorsal skin. Some inflammatory problems involving the palms or soles, such as LP, pompholyx (vesicular eczema), or the erythematous rash of Kawasaki disease display a sharp cut-off at the Wallace line.

Langer lines of cleavage

see ➜ p. 8.

Further reading

Lee MW et al. Clin Anat 2008;21:363–73.
Shelley ED et al. J Am Acad Dermatol 1999;40:736–40.
Whimster IW. Transact St Johns Hosp Dermatol Soc 1968;54:11–41.

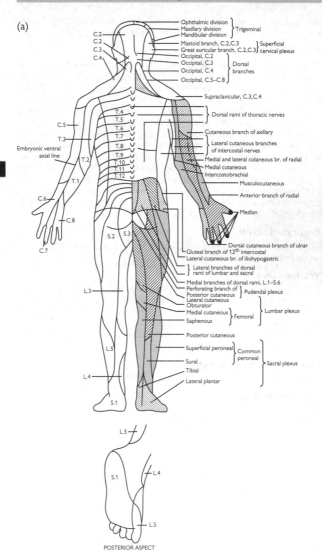

Fig. 4.2 Dermatomes. Reproduced with permission from Longmore, Wilkinson, and Rajagopalan *Oxford Handbook of Clinical Medicine*, 6th edn, 2004, Oxford: Oxford University Press.

(b)

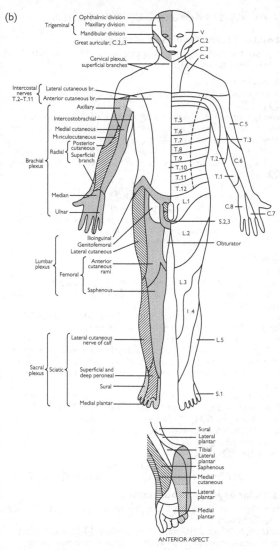

ANTERIOR ASPECT

Fig. 4.2 (Contd.)

Scaly or hyperkeratotic red rashes

Erythematous scaly papules or plaques

Scale suggests the pathology involves the epidermis. Scratch the skin with your fingernail to reveal scaling. Consider:

Relatively localized

- Lichen simplex: localized itchy patch. The skin is thickened (see ➡ p. 222).
- Varicose (gravitational, venous stasis) eczema: usually not terribly itchy. A single patch may develop over a varicosity—stand the patient up to see the dilated vein (see ➡ p. 220).
- Fungal infection: usually asymmetrical and often annular. Scale may be lost if topical corticosteroids have been applied. Not terribly itchy (see ➡ p. 164).
- Herald patch of pityriasis rosea (see ➡ p. 151).
- Irritant or allergic contact dermatitis (see ➡ pp. 214–16).
- Bowen disease: not itchy (see ➡ p. 348–9).
- Red, oozing nipple: atopic eczema or Paget disease (see ➡ p. 360).
- Asymmetric periflexural exanthem of childhood: papular scaly rash, more obvious on one side of the body.

Relatively widespread

(see ➡ Box 4.5.)

- Scabies: itchy papules, nodules, and excoriations (see ➡ p. 172).
- Eczema: endogenous (symmetrical) (see ➡ Chapter 10, pp. 211–24):
  - Atopic: very itchy.
  - Seborrhoeic: scaly, greasy-looking erythema with relatively little itch. Signs may overlap with those of psoriasis. Look for diffuse scale 'dandruff' in the scalp, flaky eyebrows, central facial erythema (nasolabial folds), flexural erythema, and scaly papules in the centre of the chest and back. May have an annular pattern.
  - Discoid (nummular): generally very itchy, and often crusted and weeping.
  - Asteatotic (dry skin): itch is variable. Often limited to the shins.
- Psoriasis: the amount of itch varies (see ➡ pp. 189–208).
- Pityriasis rosea (see ➡ p. 151) or pityriasis versicolor (often pigmented or hypopigmented) (see ➡ pp. 168–9).
- Drug reaction (see ➡ p. 374).
- 2° syphilis (see ➡ p. 146).
- Photodermatitis: uncommon (see ➡ p. 324).
- Cutaneous T-cell lymphoma (CTCL): uncommon (see ➡ pp. 358–9).

Scaly annular erythematous lesions

Look for scale, either following the erythema or at the expanding edge of the ring. Consider:

- Dermatophyte infection (tinea, ringworm) (see ➡ p. 164). Usually localized. (Scale may be lost if topical corticosteroids have been applied.)
- Pityriasis rosea (see ➡ p. 151).

- Seborrhoeic dermatitis (central trunk, flexures, face, scalp)
  (see ➲ p. 219).
- Psoriasis (see ➲ pp. 189–208) or rarely CTCL (see ➲ pp. 358–9).
- Subacute cutaneous LE: remember drugs as a cause. The patient is
  photosensitive, but paradoxically the face is often spared (see
  ➲ p. 402).
- Annular erythema: uncommon—a few lesions (see ➲ pp. 238–9).

Hyperkeratotic papules and plaques

Rough hyperkeratosis, a sign of a thick horny layer, is not removed as
easily as scale by scratching. Is the rash follicular? Consider:

Relatively localized

- Tumours: viral wart, corns (pressure sites), seborrhoeic wart
  (may be numerous), actinic (solar) keratosis (sun-exposed skin),
  keratoacanthoma, SCC (sun-exposed skin) (see ➲ Chapter 17,
  pp. 341–63).
- Keratosis pilaris: perifollicular rash most often on the upper lateral
  arms and thighs, giving the skin a dry rough texture (see ➲ Box 31.11,
  p. 603).
- Lichen simplex: itchy nodules or plaques. On the legs may resemble
  LP—see next bullet point (see ➲ p. 222).
- Hypertrophic LP: itchy purplish nodules or plaques that may become
  very thickened (hypertrophic) on the leg. Resembles lichen simplex.
  Look for LP at other sites, including buccal mucosa (see ➲ p. 224).
- DLE: look for scars, follicular plugging, loss of hair (see ➲ p. 404).
  May only be one or two plaques.

More widespread

- Chronic psoriasis: occasionally very hyperkeratotic, particularly on
  the palms and soles (see ➲ pp. 189–208). Reiter syndrome, which is
  pustular and hyperkeratotic, is probably a variant of psoriasis
  (see ➲ p. 208). Usually very symmetrical.
- Follicular eczema.
- Follicular hyperkeratosis: uncommon. May be caused by some
  inflammatory diseases that target the hair follicle, including LP,
  hereditary conditions, and nutritional deficiency (phrynoderma)
  (see ➲ p. 512).

Box 4.5 Erythroderma

⚠ If the patient is red and scaly all over, and this has developed sud-
denly, the patient may be very unwell. Skin failure is a dermatological
emergency (see ➲ p. 108).
  Consider:
- Eczema, particularly atopic or seborrhoeic.
- Psoriasis.
- Drug eruption.
- Cutaneous T-cell lymphoma.

Smooth erythematous rashes

Smooth erythematous patches, papules, or plaques

Lack of scale suggests the pathology is predominantly dermal, but the signs may have been modified by treatment. Consider:

Relatively localized

(Also see ➔ Red faces, p. 72.)

- Insect bites or papular urticaria (an urticarial reaction to bites).
- Cellulitis: asymmetrical distribution. Hot, tender, erythematous, and swollen. May blister (see ➔ pp. 138–9 and pp. 234–5).
- Acute contact dermatitis: may be smooth and oedematous (sometimes blisters), rather than scaly. Skin may be tender and itchy (see ➔ pp. 214–16).
- Lipodermatosclerosis: tender, indurated erythema on the leg (see ➔ p. 308; for eosinophilic fasciitis, see ➔ p. 421).
- Necrotizing fasciitis: rapidly spreading, poorly demarcated purplish erythema in an ill patient with high temperature, tachycardia, and low blood pressure (see ➔ pp. 126–7).
- Treated or flexural psoriasis: well-demarcated shiny erythema.
- Treated eczema also loses scale.
- Erythema migrans (not always annular) (see ➔ p. 148).
- Carcinoma erysipeloides (spreading erythema on the breast) (see ➔ pp. 360–1).
- Very rarely, an erythematous patch or plaque may overlie a tumour of the bone (plasmacytoma, sarcoma).

More generalized

- Urticaria: crops of itchy erythematous papules or plaques (wheals) that may evolve into rings with normal central skin. Wheals last no more than 48h. The skin is normal when wheals fade. May be associated with angio-oedema (deep swelling). No blisters. Stroke the skin with a spatula to test for dermographism (a physical urticaria) (see ➔ pp. 230–1 and p. 372).
- Morbilliform or anaphylactoid drug eruption: symmetrical (see ➔ p. 372).
- Viral exanthem: symmetrical.
- DRESS (see ➔ p. 122–3): papules coalesce into plaques. May have angio-oedema. Toxic shock syndrome: may be mild or rapidly fatal (see ➔ Box 5.2, p. 101).
- Erythema multiforme (EM): papules that last at least 7 days. May spread into rings with a dusky or blistered centre (target lesions). May have mucosal ulcers (see ➔ p. 111).
- Prodrome of BP: itchy, erythematous, urticated papules. Look for blisters (see ➔ pp. 270–1).
- Scleredema (rare): indurated erythematous skin (see ➔ Box 22.2, p. 467). Eosinophilic cellulitis (Wells syndrome): rare. Painful itchy, erythematous oedematous plaques and nodules. Resembles cellulitis. Tissue and usually circulating eosinophilia.

Smooth annular erythematous lesions

Without scale. Consider:

- Urticaria: transient and fades to leave normal skin. Common.
- BCC (central ulceration): common (see ➡ p. 350).
- Granuloma annulare: fairly common (see ➡ Box 22.3, p. 469).
- LP (little scale): often penis or axillary (see ➡ p. 224).
- Sarcoid (may have some scale). Diascopy reveals yellow-brown 'apple jelly' nodules (see ➡ pp. 524–5). Uncommon.
- Erythema migrans (see ➡ Lyme disease, p. 148): uncommon.

Livedo reticularis: a net-like erythema often on the legs

- Physiological reticulated erythema is continuous and disappears when the skin is warmed. Differentiate from the fixed brownish net-like discoloration that develops after prolonged exposure to external heat—erythema ab igne (see ➡ Fig. 20.5, p. 454).
- Discontinuous reticulate erythema that does not disappear on warming. May be purpuric (retiform purpura). Consider:
  - Occlusive vasculopathy caused by cholesterol emboli or thrombi, e.g. in antiphospholipid syndrome(see ➡ Box 20.10, p. 453, p. 312, p. 314). Look for scars with a telangiectatic margin.
  - Vasculitis affecting medium and/or large vessels (see ➡ pp. 450–1). Look for purpuric nodules or ulcers with a purpuric rim.

Purpura and telangiectasia

Purpura

Exclude trauma, the commonest cause. Is the patient taking aspirin, another platelet inhibitor, or an anticoagulant that might potentiate bleeding into the skin? For discussion of purpura in sick patients, see ➋ pp. 102–3.

Flat (macular) purpura

Leakage of red blood cells (RBCs) without inflammation of vessel walls. Consider:

- Legs: non-specific, associated with inflammatory rashes, e.g. stasis eczema, psoriasis.
- Forearms: minor trauma to sun-damaged atrophic skin with poorly supported vessels, particularly in elderly patients. Also common in patients with atrophic skin 2° to prolonged treatment with oral or very potent topical corticosteroids.
- Scurvy: perifollicular purpura, corkscrew hairs, poor wound healing (see ➋ p. 513).
- Thrombocytopenia or hyperglobulinaemic purpura (see ➋ p. 539).
- Palmoplantar petechiae or purpuric macules in dermatitis herpetiformis (DH) (see ➋ p. 274).

Palpable purpura

- Purpuric papules: small-vessel cutaneous vasculitis, with or without systemic disease (see ➋ p. 440).
- Urticarial vasculitis: erythematous wheals become purpuric and fade to leave bruising (see ➋ p. 443).

Purpura, livedo reticularis, and nodules

- Cholesterol emboli: asymmetrical acral petechiae, subcutaneous nodules, and livedo reticularis (see ➋ p. 452).
- Antiphospholipid syndrome (see ➋ Box 20.10, p. 453).
- Necrotizing vasculitis affecting deeper cutaneous vessels (see ➋ pp. 450–1).
- Extensive irregularly outlined ecchymoses, bullae, and gangrene: DIC with purpura fulminans (see ➋ pp. 102–3).
- Erythematous purpuric plaques with livedo and ulceration at the site of application of ice packs (used to relieve chronic pain). Uncommon.

Telangiectasia (small dilated cutaneous vessels)

- Sun damage (face), rosacea (face) (see Fig. 4.3).
- Oestrogen-related: liver disease, pregnancy, exogenous oestrogens.
- Prolonged use of potent topical corticosteroids.
- Unilateral naevoid telangiectasia: congenital or acquired. Usually in trigeminal or upper cervical dermatomes.
- General essential telangiectasia: usually legs of women.
- Cutaneous collagenous vasculopathy: symmetrical, starts on legs.
- Hereditary haemorrhagic telangiectasia (see ➋ Other rare gastrointestinal conditions, p. 522).

- Mucocutaneous and gastrointestinal (GI) telangiectasia: visible on mucous membranes in adolescence.
- Diffuse or limited cutaneous systemic sclerosis: matt telangiectasia on the face, hands, and/or lips (see ➔ p. 414).
- Poikiloderma, e.g. in chronic dermatomyositis, chronic GVHD, mycosis fungoides (MF).
- Telangiectasia macularis eruptiva perstans (mastocytosis) (see ➔ Box 31.5, p. 593).
- Carcinoid syndrome: rare (see ➔ pp. 520–1).
- Genodermatoses (rare), e.g. Klippel–Trenaunay syndrome, ataxia telangiectasia, xeroderma pigmentosum (XP), Goltz syndrome.

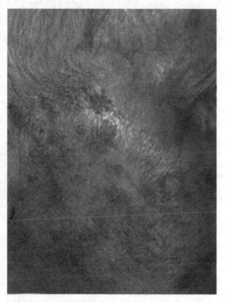

Fig. 4.3 Telangiectasia and solar keratoses in sun-damaged skin.

Red faces

A red face may indicate photosensitivity, but consider other causes:

- *Seborrhoeic dermatitis*: scaly, greasy-looking erythema with little itch. Tends to involve the nasolabial folds, centre of the forehead, and skin behind the ears, as well as other sites (see ➲ p. 219).
- *Cellulitis or erysipelas*: is there fever or malaise? Look for swelling and tenderness, as well as erythema. The rash is often asymmetrical.
- *Contact dermatitis*: is the skin itchy or scaly? Is the face swollen? Any vesicles? Might this be an acute contact dermatitis (irritant or allergic) to a cosmetic? Remember that the product may have been used for some time before the patient is sensitized (see ➲ pp. 214–16).
- *Acne*: pustules, papules, comedones, nodules, scars (see ➲ pp. 242–7).
- *Rosacea*: pustules, as well as telangiectasia, erythema, and swelling, but some patients have much more of one component than another. Comedones are not a feature of rosacea (see ➲ pp. 254–5, and Box 12.3, p. 247). Morbihan disease (late-stage rosacea)—look for persistent erythema and solid oedema of upper 2/3 of the face.
- *Herpes simplex or herpes zoster*: any prodrome of tingling or discomfort? Look for vesicles progressing to small pustules. Herpes zoster presents in a dermatomal distribution.
- *Corticosteroid-induced acneiform rash*: prolonged application of potent topical corticosteroids to the face can produce a telangiectatic rosacea-like eruption with pustules, but no comedones.
- *Angio-oedema*: usually transient. Swelling more marked than erythema. Mucous membranes may be affected (see ➲ p. 104). Subcutaneous emphysema (rare complication of dental treatment) may cause periorbital swelling, mimicking angio-oedema. Check for crepitation.
- *Photosensitivity*: what is the distribution of the redness? Check the eyelids, under the hair, behind the ears, and under the chin. Compare exposed and covered sites (see Box 4.6 and ➲ p. 28 and p. 324).
- *Flushing*: if repeated, may become fixed. Investigation is only required if flushing is of sudden onset and associated with systemic symptoms (see ➲ Box 24.7, p. 521). Ask about triggers. Consider:
  - Blushing: flushing triggered by emotions.
  - Physiological flushing after exercise, heat, hot drinks, alcohol.
  - Menopausal hot flushes (flashes).
  - Rosacea: labile flushing progresses to fixed oedematous erythema, telangiectasia, and pustules (see ➲ pp. 254–5).
  - Carcinoid syndrome (very rare): look for rosacea-like vascular changes, oedema and induration of the face, wheezing, severe diarrhoea, hypotension and tachycardia, features of pellagra (scaly sun-exposed skin, glossitis, angular stomatitis) (see ➲ pp. 520–1).
- *Superior vena cava obstruction*: the face is swollen and red. Look for dilated veins on the neck, chest, and arms. Symptoms include dyspnoea, cough, and headache. Associated with malignancy (bronchial carcinoma, lymphoma) or, less often, thrombosis, e.g. after pacemaker insertion.
- *Other*: cutaneous LE, dermatomyositis.

Box 4.6 Is the patient photosensitive?

What should I look for?

The signs will depend on the cause of photosensitivity but may include erythema, urticaria, papules, blisters, and/or pigmentation. Look for a rash that is maximal on exposed sites and spares covered skin. The skin may be normal between episodes. Chronic sun exposure may induce tolerance, so-called 'hardening', and so, paradoxically, the face may be spared. Drugs are a common cause of photosensitivity (see ➜ Box 16.3, p. 327).

Photosensitive rashes may involve one or more of the following sites:
* The prominences of the forehead, nose, cheeks, particularly over the cheekbones (malar), and chin.
* The back of the neck, if not covered by hair.
* The helix of the ear, if not covered by hair.
* The V on the upper chest where the shirt sits open.
* The extensor surfaces of forearms, the back of the hands.
* The nails: tender onycholysis with a rim of pigmentation (photo-onycholysis) (associated with some drug-induced photosensitivity).
* The dorsum of the feet (if exposed).

Are there signs of chronic sun damage such as freckling on exposed skin (photoageing) or skin cancer (see ➜ p. 43)? Are these signs appropriate for the age and lifestyle of the patient or greater than you would expect?

Is there sparing of covered skin, with a sharp cut-off between involved and uninvolved skin? Check:
* Around the orbit (ask the patient to close his/her eyes to see the eyelids).
* Under the frame of spectacles.
* The upper lip.
* Under the nose.
* Deep wrinkles on the face.
* Below the chin.
* Behind the ears.
* Under the hair—on the forehead or at the back of the neck. Is a spared area exposed, because the hair has been cut recently?
* Under watch straps.
* The distal phalanges, because the hands often sit with fingers curled.
* Between the fingers.
* Under the shoe.

Red legs and leg ulcers

Red leg(s)

Erythematous

- Cellulitis (unlikely to be bilateral): hot, oedematous, and tender.
- Lipodermatosclerosis: often bilateral. Painful, indurated erythema that may simulate cellulitis in acute stages.
- Gravitational eczema: associated with venous stasis and oedema. Stand the patient up to look for varicose veins. Often bilateral.
- Pseudo-Kaposi sarcoma (acroangiodermatitis): purplish patches, papules, and plaques in association with chronic venous stasis (also seen in arteriovenous (AV) malformations or AV fistulae).
- Acute allergic or irritant contact dermatitis (may be bilateral): oedematous, erythematous, and may blister (see ➔ Fig. 10.1, p. 216). Itchy, but also uncomfortable if swollen.
- Deep venous thrombosis (DVT): unilateral swelling with erythema and calf tenderness.
- Lymphoedema: initially erythematous and pitting oedema. Later indurated with thick hyperkeratotic skin. Predisposes to cellulitis (see ➔ pp. 316–17).
- Erythema nodosum (EN): tender erythematous nodules on the shins (see ➔ pp. 458–9).
- Necrobiosis lipoidica: well-defined reddish yellow plaques with telangiectasia, an atrophic centre (that may ulcerate), and a raised erythematous rim (see ➔ p. 468). Associated with insulin-dependent diabetes.
- Livedo reticularis: net-like mottled purplish pattern (see ➔ p. 452, and Fig. 3.2, p. 41). Patients may have leg ulcers and nodular vasculitis or an obstructive vasculopathy (see ➔ p. 452, p. 312, and p. 314). May be purpuric in places (retiform purpura) (see ➔ p. 452). Differentiate from erythema ab igne—fixed brownish reticulate marking where the skin has been repeatedly exposed to heat (see ➔ p. 452).
- Erythermalgia (erythromelalgia erythralgia): painful burning erythema. May be idiopathic, associated with thrombocythaemia, or familial. Involves acral sites (see ➔ p. 551).

Purpuric

- Some flat purpura is not uncommon in inflammatory rashes on legs, e.g. psoriasis, eczema, simply because of leakage of RBCs.
- Capillaritis (pigmented purpura) produces flat purpuric spots (likened to cayenne pepper) and brownish yellow (haemosiderin) pigmentation but does not signify systemic disease. Capillaritis is commonest on the legs. The cause is unknown (rarely, drugs cause capillaritis). Lymphocytic inflammation around capillaries is associated with extravasation of RBCs into the skin.
- Palpable purpura. If purpura is palpable, consider small-vessel cutaneous vasculitis (usually bilateral), and exclude systemic disease (see ➔ p. 440).

- Retiform purpura (purpura in a livedo pattern): seen with occlusive vasculopathies, including cholesterol emboli, antiphospholipid syndrome, deficiency of protein C or protein S, cryoglobulinaemia (see ➲ p. 452).

Chronic leg ulcers

The history and examination should help you to pinpoint the cause of the chronic ulcer. More details are given on ➲ pp. 294–5. Consider:

Common
- Venous ulcers: risk factors include DVT, trauma, operations to hips or knees, obesity, and immobility.
- Arterial disease: look for intermittent claudication, rest pain, night pain, pain worse when the leg is elevated. Occurs in tobacco smokers.
- Mixed AV: symptoms of both venous and arterial disease.
- Neuropathic: develop at sites of pressure—painless ulcers. Commonest on the feet of diabetics.
- Malignancy: do not accept the label 'leg ulcer' without looking under the dressing. BCCs are often misdiagnosed as leg ulcers.

Less common
- Pyoderma gangrenosum (PG): rapidly growing, painful ulcer with an undermined bluish margin. May be associated with rheumatoid arthritis (RA), inflammatory bowel disease (IBD), or myeloproliferative disorders, but 50% of patients have no underlying disease (see ➲ p. 310). Nicorandil-induced ulcers may simulate PG.
- Vasculitis: is the rim purpuric? Associated with connective tissue diseases, particularly RA (see ➲ Box 19.1, p. 395).
- Occlusive vasculopathy (see ➲ pp. 314–15 and p. 452): suggested by the presence of livedo reticularis. Causes include inherited disorders of coagulation—mutations in protein C, protein S, antithrombin III, fibrinogen, or factor V genes.
- Necrobiosis lipoidica: associated with insulin-dependent diabetes (see ➲ p. 468).
- Infection, e.g. deep fungal, treponemal (syphilitic gumma).

Hands, feet, and other extremities

The skin is cool at acral sites such as the hands, feet, ears, and tip of the nose. These sites are also exposed to sun and trauma. Conditions that tend to favour acral sites include:

- Scabies: crusting between fingers and burrows on palms. Blisters on the palms and soles in children (see ➔ p. 172).
- Some infections (see Box 4.7).
- Contact dermatitis (irritant or allergic) is common on hands.
- Chilblains (perniosis): warm erythematous nodules that may become purplish. Itch or cause burning pain. Occur in cold weather in damp temperate climates. Seen most often in the young, especially children, and elderly, but less frequent now homes are centrally heated. Self-limiting. May be associated with acrocyanosis—see later in list.
- Sarcoidosis: may involve the tip of the nose—dusky purplish discoloration and swelling (lupus pernio) (see ➔ p. 524).
- Chronic cutaneous LE: hyperkeratotic papules on fingers (chilblain lupus) or photoaggravated disease on the nose (see ➔ p. 404).
- Raynaud phenomenon (sudden pallor, followed by cyanosis, and finally erythema with swelling and tingling): may affect fingers, toes, nose, and/or earlobes (see ➔ Box 19.18, p. 414, p. 444).
- Acrocyanosis: persistent dusky, mottled discoloration of hands and feet. May be bright red when very cold. Associated with chilblains (see ➔ pp. 444–5).
- Erythromelalgia (erythermalgia, erythralgia): attacks of painful burning erythema affecting feet, legs, and, less often, hands (see ➔ p. 551). May be idiopathic, associated with thrombocythaemia, or familial. Sometimes also associated with acrocyanosis.
- Chemotherapy-induced hand–foot skin reaction (see ➔ p. 382).
- EM is associated with erythematous papules and target lesions on palms and soles. Check mucosae (see ➔ p. 111).
- Acute GVHD: macular blotchy erythema of palms, soles, and face; a common early sign (see ➔ p. 532).
- In systemic sclerosis, fingers are tight and puffy (sclerodactyly)—look for calcinosis and vascular changes in nail folds (see ➔ p. 414).
- Cutaneous vasculitis and occlusive vasculopathy favour cool sites where blood flow is slow—check toes (see ➔ p. 440, p. 452).
- Neutrophilic dermatosis of dorsal hands (see ➔ pp. 518–9).
- Cryoglobulinaemia or cryofibrinogenaemia: mottling, retiform purpura, ulceration, or blotchy cyanosis at acral sites exposed to cold—helices of the ears, as well as fingers and toes. May be associated with Raynaud phenomenon and livedo reticularis (see ➔ pp. 444–5).
- Cholesterol embolus: blue toe or peripheral gangrene associated with livedo reticularis. May have retiform purpura. Seen when arterial catheterization disrupts an atheromatous plaque or after prolonged anticoagulation when a clot becomes friable (see ➔ p. 452).
- Palmoplantar pustulosis: sterile pustules on palms and/or soles (see ➔ p. 198); also see ➔ Zinc deficiency, p. 513).
- In porphyria cutanea tarda (PCT), blisters and erosions on the dorsum of hands (trauma and the skin is fragile) (see ➔ p. 332).

Box 4.7 Infections that may produce acral signs

- Herpes simplex causing a whitlow on a finger (see ➲ p. 152).
- Orf or milker's nodule on a finger (see ➲ pp. 158–9).
- Hand–foot–mouth disease associated with infections by Coxsackie viruses A10 and A16 and with enterovirus 71. Vesicopustules on hands and feet, as well as mucosal ulcers.
- Gianotti–Crosti syndrome (papular acrodermatitis of childhood) (see ➲ p. 150): flat-topped, brownish pink papules or papulovesicles on hands and feet. Most often associated with hepatitis B and Epstein–Barr viral infections in children.
- Purpuric rash in a gloves-and-socks distribution caused by human parvovirus B19 (see ➲ p. 150).
- 2° syphilis: copper-coloured macules on palms (see ➲ p. 146).
- Atypical mycobacterial infection with nodule on finger (see ➲ p. 144).
- Mycobacterial infections favour the nose and ears: leprosy, cutaneous tuberculosis (TB) (lupus vulgaris) (see ➲ p. 144).

Flexural rashes

Intertrigo is another name for a flexural rash but is not a diagnosis. Consider these causes of intertrigo.

Common
- *Candidiasis*: look for a bright red erythema and satellite pustules with a collarette of scale. The rash is often asymmetrical, and the skin is sore, rather than itchy. Candidiasis is commoner in obese patients, those with diabetes, and the immunocompromised. Take swabs to exclude a streptococcal infection. May complicate an irritant dermatitis (see ➲ p. 166).
- *Dermatophyte infection*: the rash gradually spreads out from the flexure. Look for scale at the edge of the erythematous patch. Tinea cruris (groin) is common. Infection is often asymmetrical. Take a scraping from the scaly margin to confirm the diagnosis (see ➲ p. 164).
- *Seborrhoeic dermatitis*: look for 'dandruff' in the scalp (ill-defined diffuse scaling) and behind the ears, or erythematous, greasy, scaly plaques in the centre of the face, centre of the chest, or centre of the back. The features overlap with those of flexural psoriasis (sebopsoriasis). Look for signs of psoriasis in the nails, e.g. pitting, onycholysis, or subungual hyperkeratosis (see ➲ p. 219).
- *Flexural psoriasis*: presents as a well-demarcated, shiny erythema. Skin is moist, rather than scaly. Is there plaque psoriasis on extensors? Check for pitting of the nails or onycholysis, and look in the scalp for scaling plaques. Any family history of psoriasis? (see ➲ p. 194.).
- *Irritant contact dermatitis*: in obese, sweaty, or incontinent patients (see ➲ p. 214).
- *Erythrasma*: look for symmetrical orange-brown, slightly scaly plaques in the flexures. The skin fluoresces coral pink under Wood light (UVA). Caused by infection with *Corynebacterium minutissimum*. Commoner in warm humid climates, diabetes, obesity, and old age (see ➲ p. 132).
- *Streptococcal infection*: bright red, painful perianal rash.

Less common
- *Allergic contact dermatitis*, e.g. to deodorants, clothing dyes: eczema involves the edge of axillae and spares the axillary vault (see ➲ p. 214).
- *Pseudomonas infection*: brownish, scaly rash with painful fissuring. Potentiated by washes with antibacterial lotions (see ➲ p. 132).
- *Hidradenitis suppurativa*: patients present with a history of recurrent 'boils'. Look for comedones, inflamed nodules, pustules, sinuses, and scars (see ➲ p. 250).
- *Acanthosis nigricans*: velvety, hyperpigmented thickening of flexural skin, associated with skin tags. Seen most often in obese Asian patients with insulin resistance ('pseudoacanthosis nigricans') (see ➲ p. 466–7). Presents rarely as a manifestation of an underlying malignancy, usually adenocarcinoma of the stomach (see ➲ p. 546).

Pustules

Pustules are small dome-shaped bumps filled with milky fluid containing neutrophils or sometimes eosinophils. Pustules are often caused by bacterial infection of a hair follicle (folliculitis) but may be sterile. Decide if pustules are arising in association with hair follicles (perifollicular pustules). Vesicles (small blisters that contain clear fluid) may evolve into pustules (vesicopustules) or may simulate pustules, when on palms and soles and covered by a thick horny layer. Puncturing the vesicle to let out some fluid may help, if you are not sure if it is clear or milky.

Common
- Bacterial folliculitis (usually staphylococcal): may be a 2° bacterial folliculitis in conditions such as atopic eczema (see ➔ pp. 134–5).
- Bullous impetigo: superficial vesicles and pustules rapidly rupture, leaving golden crusting (see ➔ p. 136).
- *Candida*: satellite pustules at the margin of the erythematous flexural rash (see ➔ p. 166).
- Irritant or occlusive folliculitis, e.g. with thick applications of greasy emollients (see ➔ Box 6.3, p. 135).
- Acne: follicular lesions with comedones, inflammatory papules, pustules, nodules, cysts, and scars. Involves the face and may involve the trunk (see ➔ p. 242–3).
- Herpes simplex virus, including eczema herpeticum; herpes zoster virus infection (dermatomal): vesicles (the 1° lesion) evolve into pustules or vesicopustules (see ➔ pp. 152–7).
- Periorificial 'dermatitis': pustulovesicular facial rash, most often caused by potent topical corticosteroids (see ➔ pp. 256–7).
- Rosacea: look for erythema, telangiectasia, papules, and oedema (see ➔ p. 254). No comedones. Involves the face but spares the trunk.
- Steroid-induced acne: look for sterile pustules without comedones.

Less common
- Hidradenitis suppurativa: pustules in flexures with grouped comedones, nodules, scars, and sinuses (see ➔ p. 250).
- Chronic palmoplantar pustulosis (sterile non-follicular pustules) (see ➔ p. 198).
- PG may be preceded by a tender pustule (see ➔ p. 310).
- Demodicosis in immunocompromised (see ➔ p. 178).

Rare
- Bowel-associated dermatosis–arthritis syndrome or Sweet syndrome (see ➔ p. 519).
- AGEP: sterile non-follicular pustules (see ➔ p. 124).
- DRESS: morbilliform rash with 'juicy' papules that may coalesce into plaques. Sometimes sterile pustules or vesicles (see ➔ pp. 122–3).
- Pustular psoriasis: waves of non-follicular pustules appear at the edge of erythematous tender plaques or patches. Sick patient with fever and neutrophilia (see ➔ pp. 124–5 and p. 198).
- Subcorneal pustular dermatosis (see ➔ Box 13.4, p. 269).
- Behçet disease (see ➔ pp. 284–5).

Blisters

A blister is a bump, which may be large (bulla) or small (vesicle), filled with clear fluid (serum). Blisters may form just below the stratum corneum, within the epidermis, or within or below the dermo-epidermal junction (see → Fig. 13.1, p. 261). Causes of blisters include:

Fairly localized blisters

Common

- Physical causes:
  - Friction, pressure, ischaemia, scalds or cold injury, sunlight, radiation.
- Cutaneous infections:
  - Viral: herpes simplex or varicella-zoster (shingles); Coxsackie virus A16 (hand–foot–mouth disease).
  - Bacterial: bullous impetigo caused by *Staphylococcus aureus*; blisters in association with oedema 2° to streptococcal infection (cellulitis, erysipelas, and necrotizing fasciitis).
  - Fungal: dermatophyte.
- Insect bites and stings.
- Scabies (vesicles or vesicopustules on the palms or soles in infants).
- Contact dermatitis: irritant or allergic, e.g. nickel sensitivity (see → Fig.10.1, p. 216).
- Pompholyx (itchy vesicles on hands and feet) (see → p. 221).
- Photosensitivity: drug-induced and phytophotodermatitis (see → p. 326, and Box 16.4, p. 327).
- Oedema blisters: sudden peripheral oedema in elderly patients with atrophic skin may cause blisters on the legs.

Uncommon

- Diabetic blister: on legs (see → pp. 466–7).
- Damage to basal cells (lichenoid reaction):
  - EM (see → Chapter 5, p. 111).
  - Fixed drug eruption (see → Chapter 18, p. 378).
- PCT or pseudoporphyria on back of hands (see → pp. 332–4).
- Mastocytoma: a localized increase in mast cells in the skin—seen in infants (see → Box 31.5, p. 593).
- Coma blisters: originally described with barbiturates (see → p. 379).

Rare

- Genetic:
  - EB simplex (see → p. 624–5).
  - Incontinentia pigmenti (see → pp. 636–7).
  - Acrodermatitis enteropathica (see → p. 513).

More widespread blisters

Common

- Eczema:
  - Contact eczema may generalize after starting in a localized pattern.
  - Atopic eczema (exclude infection if you see blistering in atopic eczema).
- Cutaneous infections:
  - Viral: herpes simplex (may generalize in conditions such as atopic eczema) or varicella-zoster (chickenpox); poxvirus (vaccinia).
  - Bacterial: widespread infection in atopic eczema.
- Miliaria (caused by blockage of eccrine ducts and sweating in a hot, humid environment; the itchy vesicles may be superficial or deep).

Uncommon

- Cutaneous infections:
  - Bacterial: SSSS caused by a circulating exotoxin produced by *S. aureus* (see ➔ Fig. 6.2, p. 131 and pp. 136–7).
- Damage to basal cells (lichenoid reaction):
  - SJS (see ➔ p. 116).
  - TEN with full-thickness necrosis of the epidermis (see ➔ p. 116).
  - LP (see ➔ p. 224).
  - Vesiculobullous cutaneous LE (see ➔ Box 19.9, p. 405).
- Autoimmune blistering diseases:
  - BP (commonest of the autoimmune blistering diseases in Western Europe) (see ➔ pp. 270–1).
  - Pemphigus foliaceus and vulgaris (see ➔ pp. 268–9).
  - DH (see ➔ pp. 274–5).
- Bullous cutaneous vasculitis (bullae will be haemorrhagic) (see ➔ p. 440).
- Urticaria pigmentosa (increased mast cells in the skin) (see ➔ Box 31.5, p. 593).
- PCT (sporadic commoner than inherited):
  - Associated with iron overload (haemochromatosis), alcohol, oestrogens, and hepatitis C (see ➔ p. 332–3).

Rare

- Autoimmune blistering diseases, including:
  - Paraneoplastic pemphigus (see ➔ Box 13.4, p. 269).
  - Mucous membrane (cicatricial) pemphigoid (see ➔ p. 272).
  - Pemphigoid gestationis (see ➔ p. 584).
  - Epidermolysis bullosa acquisita (EBA) (see ➔ p. 272).
  - Linear IgA dermatosis (see ➔ p. 272).
- Genetic:
  - Hailey–Hailey disease (see ➔ Box 32.4, p. 629).
  - EB group of diseases (see ➔ p. 624–5).
  - Epidermolytic ichthyosis (see ➔ Box 32.2, p. 627)
  - Cutaneous porphyrias associated with subepidermal blistering:
    —Variegate porphyria.
    —Hereditary coproporphyria.
    —Congenital erythropoietic porphyria.

Nodules and solitary cutaneous ulcers

Nodules suggest involvement of the dermis and sometimes subcutaneous tissues. They may be tender or painless and sometimes ulcerate.

Nodules

- Cysts: epidermoid ('sebaceous' with a punctum—face, trunk, scalp), pilar (no punctum—scalp), dermoid (congenital and usually in midline on the face), acne (inflammatory on the face).
- Thrombophlebitis: tender nodules along a vein.
- Prurigo nodularis: excoriated dome-shaped nodules (see ➔ p. 222).
- Granulomatous, e.g. foreign body with granulomatous reaction, sarcoidosis, rheumatoid nodules (see ➔ pp. 394–5).
- Gouty tophi: hands, elbows, ears (see ➔ Box 19.2, p. 395).
- Calcinosis cutis: hard, white nodule that extrudes chalk-like material. Usually hands or pressure sites. May occur in systemic sclerosis (see ➔ pp. 416–17 and Fig. 19.11, p. 419).
- Tumour (see ➔ pp. 42–3, Chapter 17, pp. 341–63, and Box 4.8), including:
  - BCC, SCC, melanoma.
  - Lipoma, muscle tumour, neural tumour.
  - Vascular tumour.
  - Appendageal tumours.
  - Lymphoma (T-cell or B-cell).
  - Metastatic carcinoma (breast, renal, colon, lung, ovary, gastric).
  - Kaposi sarcoma (KS).
- Infection, including:
  - Furuncle ('boil'): hot, tender, erythematous.
  - Sporotrichosis or atypical mycobacterial infection: nodules spread proximally along a lymphatic.
  - Leprosy, deep fungal infection.
- Xanthoma: elbows, knees, ankles, hands. Yellowish tinge (see ➔ p. 470).
- Panniculitis, e.g. erythema nodosum, traumatic panniculitis, nodular vasculitis (see ➔ Chapter 21, pp. 455–63).
- Perforating disease: rare (see ➔ p. 494 and Box 19.28, p. 431). Nodules with a central keratin plug.
- Multicentric reticulohistiocytosis (rare): symmetrical nodules on fingers, papules around nail folds, destructive arthritis (see ➔ p. 426).

Solitary cutaneous ulcer

For leg ulcers, see ➔ p. 75 and pp. 291–318.

- Trauma: including insect/arthropod bites, intravenous drug abuse, pressure—is the ulcer neuropathic?
- Infection: ecthyma—full-thickness infection of the skin, usually by *S. aureus* or *Streptococcus pyogenes*, with ulceration and crusting (see ➔ p. 137); herpes simplex virus (HSV) infection (see ➔ p. 152).
- Malignant tumour.
- Temporal arteritis: ulcer on the forehead or scalp (see ➔ pp. 450–1).
- Pyoderma gangrenosum. Drug related—nicorandil, hydroxyurea.
- Dermatitis artefacta: deliberate self-harm (see ➔ pp. 566–7).

Box 4.8 Skin checks and skin cancer

Skin cancers are the commonest malignancy. You should carry out a full skin examination when assessing patients. But cutaneous tumours are common, and you need to 'get your eye in', so you know when to refer. For more information, see ➡ Chapter 17, pp. 341–63. These pointers may be helpful:

- Patients with fair skin who burn in the sun are at greatest risk of skin cancers. Chronic immunosuppression with drugs, such as azathioprine, or chronic photosensitivity greatly increase the chances of developing skin cancer (see ➡ p. 346).
- Most skin cancers grow slowly, an important exception being nodular malignant melanoma.
- BCCs and malignant melanomas are usually painless, but some SCCs may be tender, particularly on the ear.
- Most malignant melanomas arise *de novo*, and not from a pre-existing melanocytic naevus.
- Carry out a skin check in all patients. Examine sun-exposed skin on the face, bald scalp, ears, forearms, and back of the hands. Look at the skin on the back and legs, and check behind the ears.
- Look for signs of chronic sun damage, e.g. mottled pigmentation, telangiectasia, yellowing, wrinkling, and keratoses (see ➡ Box 3.1, p. 43). The more sun damage, the greater the likelihood of developing a skin cancer—eventually.
- Remember deeply tanned skin is generally unhappy skin!
- Solar keratoses are common and do not need treatment, unless the keratosis is thickened (indurated) when you should suspect an SCC. But solar keratoses do indicate too much sun exposure, and you should advise your patient accordingly.
- Put the skin on the stretch to see the pearly border of a BCC (the commonest skin cancer).
- Think again before you diagnose melanocytic naevus in an elderly patient. Benign melanocytic naevi, common in youth, gradually regress with age. A pigmented tumour in an elderly patient is much more likely to be a seborrhoeic wart (raised, well-defined margin, 'stuck-on' appearance, rough with a pitted, crinkled surface) or a solar lentigo (flat, smooth, even pigmentation), but it just might be a malignant melanoma.
- Use the ABCDE criteria (see ➡ p. 354) to assess the likelihood of any pigmented lesion being a malignant melanoma, and remember to look twice at moles that stand out from their neighbours—the 'ugly ducklings'.
- Record your findings, including the presence of sun damage and the fact that you carried out a skin check.
- Advise patients how to protect their skin from sun damage to minimize the risk of skin cancer. But temper your advice with a little common sense—we all need some sun to lift our spirits and maintain our vitamin D levels! (See ➡ pp. 346–7.)

Induration

Induration (woody hardness) and thickening suggest deep involvement with fibrosis.

- Scar or changes after radiotherapy (see ➔ pp. 530–1).
- Lipodermatosclerosis (leg in association with venous stasis) (see ➔ p. 308).
- Morphoea, systemic sclerosis, or drug-induced scleroderma (see ➔ p. 414–5 and p. 420).
- Chronic GVHD: sclerodermoid form (see ➔ pp. 534–6).
- Scleredema: associated with infection, diabetes, monoclonal gammopathy. Firm non-pitting oedema of the face, neck, upper back (see ➔ Box 22.2, p. 467).
- Scleromyxoedema: associated with paraproteinaemia, myeloma, lymphoma, and leukaemia (see ➔ Box 26.10, p. 541). Waxy, flesh-coloured papules on the face, trunk, and extremities.
- Nephrogenic systemic fibrosis (see ➔ p. 498). Seen in patients with renal failure exposed to contrast medium containing gadolinium. Features similar to scleromyxoedema (see ➔ Box 26.10, p. 541). Now rare.
- PCT: waxy thickening of sun-exposed skin (see ➔ p. 332).

Eyes, mouth, and genitalia

Causes of a red eye

- Conjunctivitis: redness involves the entire surface of the eye. Examine the conjunctiva, both bulbar and palpebral (lid).
  - If the eye is also sticky, this is likely to be a bacterial or viral conjunctival infection.
- Dry eye. Is the conjunctiva irritated, because the eye is dry? Dry eyes burn and feel gritty. Vision may be blurred. Confirm the diagnosis by performing a Schirmer strip test.
- Allergic conjunctivitis: common in atopic eczema.
- Iritis (anterior uveitis): the eye is painful and photophobic. The eye is not sticky. Redness is most marked around the cornea. Small pupil.
  - Iritis occurs in systemic diseases that may also have cutaneous manifestations including sarcoidosis, IBD, Behçet disease, herpes virus infection, and Lyme disease.

Causes of oral ulcers

⚠ Biopsy any long-standing unexplained ulcer to exclude malignancy.

Common
- Trauma: check teeth and/or dentures.
- Inflammatory:
  - Aphthous ulcers: minor, major, or herpetiform (see ➜ pp. 282–3).
  - Erosive LP (see ➜ p. 286).
- Infections:
  - Herpes simplex, varicella-zoster virus (VZV), hand–foot–mouth disease, *Candida*, syphilis, HIV.
- Drugs:
  - Cytotoxic agents, co-trimoxazole, antithyroid drugs, nicorandil, beta-blockers, clopidogrel, alendronate, protease inhibitors, non-steroidal anti-inflammatory drugs (NSAIDs), anticholinergic bronchodilators, and antihypertensives (captopril, enalapril).
  - Cocaine (ask about recreational drugs).
  - Ulcers heal when the drug is withdrawn.
- Radiation to the head and neck.
- Oral SCC (solitary ulcer, may be asymptomatic).

Uncommon
- Inflammatory:
  - EM, SJS, and TEN (see ➜ p. 111 and pp. 116–21).
  - GVHD (see ➜ pp. 534–6).
  - Eosinophilic ulcer: uncommon benign self-limiting ulcer, probably 2° to trauma. Usually a large ulcer on the tongue.
  - LE (see ➜ pp. 396–400).
  - Behçet disease: rare (see ➜ pp. 284–5).
- Infection in immunosuppressed patients:
  - TB (prevalence increasing as a complication of HIV infection), fungus (*Cryptococcus*, histoplasmosis, *Aspergillus*), leishmaniasis.

Rare
- Inflammatory:
  - Angina bullosa haemorrhagica (blood-filled blisters that rupture).
  - Immunobullous diseases, such as pemphigus vulgaris, which may affect the oral mucosa before the skin (see ➲ p. 268).
  - EB (see ➲ pp. 624–5).

Causes of genital ulcers

⚠ Biopsy any long-standing unexplained ulcer to exclude malignancy.
- Trauma: including sexual abuse.
- Infections:
  - HSV: may be extensive and chronic in immunosuppressed patients (see ➲ pp. 280–1).
  - EBV (see ➲ Box 14.2, p. 281).
  - Ecthyma gangrenosum caused by *Pseudomonas aeruginosa* in immunosuppressed patients (see ➲ p. 137).
  - Syphilis: *Treponema pallidum*.
  - Chancroid: *Haemophilus ducreyi*.
  - Lymphogranuloma venereum: *Chlamydia trachomatis*.
  - Granuloma inguinale (donovanosis): *Klebsiella granulomatis*.
- Inflammatory:
  - Aphthous ulcers: possibly triggered by local injury or infection, including HIV. Most patients also have oral aphthous ulcers (see ➲ p. 282–3). Genital aphthous ulcers usually measure 1–3cm in diameter and may be quite deep and either round or irregular in outline. Patients usually only have a few genital aphthous ulcers (often just one). Large ulcers may heal with scarring.
  - Erosive LP: check the mouth (see ➲ pp. 286–7).
  - EM, SJS, and TEN (see ➲ p. 111 and pp. 116–7).
  - Hidradenitis suppurativa: sinus tracts develop into chronic ulcers (see ➲ p. 250).
  - Crohn disease (see ➲ pp. 508–9).
  - PG (see ➲ p. 310).
  - Drugs: including nicorandil.
  - Behçet disease: rare (see ➲ pp. 284–5).
  - Immunobullous disease such as pemphigoid or pemphigus. The skin is fragile, and genital vesicles rupture rapidly to form painful superficial erosions or ulcers (rare) (see ➲ p. 268–9 and pp. 270–1).
- Malignancy:
  - Carcinoma: BCC or SCC.
  - Leukaemia or lymphoma.
  - Extramammary Paget disease.

Change in skin colour

The commonest cause of change in colour is previous inflammation. Ask when the change appeared (was it present at birth?) and if anything preceded it. A Wood light may determine if the pigment is epidermal or dermal and will accentuate the epidermal change (see ➔ p. 640).

Acquired hyperpigmentation

Strictly speaking, hyperpigmentation means brown skin, but this list encompasses colours ranging from brown to blue or grey.

Common
- Normal racial variation or suntan.
- Stasis dermatitis: the pigment is a mix of melanin and haemosiderin.
- Melasma (usually facial): brown colour caused by melanin (see ➔ Box 30.1, p. 583).
- Post-inflammatory hyperpigmentation, particularly in dark skin. Common after acne or lichenoid eruptions such as LP or cutaneous LE. After lichenoid eruptions, the skin has a greyish tinge, as the pigment is deep in the dermis (see ➔ p. 224).
- Ten percent of normal people have one or two café au lait spots (see ➔ Box 27.6, p. 553).
- Erythema ab igne: repeated local heating of the skin from a hot water bottle or fire causes localized fixed reticulate pigmentation.
- Phytophotodermatitis: linear streaks of brown pigmentation are preceded by erythema and sometimes blisters (see ➔ Fig. 31.11, p. 615).
- Dermatitis neglecta: occasionally, patients avoid touching a patch of skin. The unwashed skin builds up brown scale.
- Drugs, including minocycline, antimalarials, amiodarone, and heavy metals, may give the skin a bluish grey tinge (see ➔ pp. 376–7).

Less common
- Neuropathic itch or chronic rubbing (see ➔ Box 27.2, p. 549).
- Malabsorption, pellagra.
- Cutaneous systemic sclerosis and sclerodermoid chronic GVHD. The skin is thickened, often with perifollicular hypopigmentation (see ➔ p. 414 and Box 26.4, p. 535).
- Pseudo-ochronosis 2° to hydroquinone in skin-lightening creams (may also cause confetti-like loss of pigment).
- Primary biliary cirrhosis, haemochromatosis.

Rare
- Café au lait spots: neurofibromatosis, McCune–Albright syndrome, multiple mucosal neuromas syndrome (see ➔ Box 27.6, p. 553).
- Widespread freckling in children may be associated with XP, multiple lentigines syndrome, Carney complex, and Peutz–Jeghers syndrome (see ➔ p. 613).
- Generalized pigmentation: adrenal insufficiency, Nelson syndrome, ectopic adrenocorticotrophic hormone (ACTH)-producing tumours, POEMS syndrome in plasma cell disorders (see ➔ Box 26.8, p. 540).
- Alkaptonuria: blue black pigment of helices of the ear and sclerae.

Hypopigmentation and depigmentation

Hypopigmented skin: loss of pigment is partial. The tone of the skin is creamy, rather than absolutely white. Depigmented skin is white and fluoresces bright white under Wood light, e.g. vitiligo.

Common

- Pityriasis alba: hypopigmented cheeks in children. Subtle scale.
- Pityriasis versicolor: scaly in the active phase, but macular post-inflammatory hypopigmentation may persist for months, until melanocytes are stimulated by sun exposure.
- Idiopathic guttate hypomelanosis: pale macules on sun-damaged forearms of adults.
- Progressive macular hypomelanosis: common in young Afro-Caribbean adults. Progressive symmetrical hypopigmentation in midline of the trunk.
- Post-inflammatory hypopigmentation: most often in dark skin. Causes, e.g. psoriasis, sarcoidosis, leprosy, pinta, and kwashiorkor.
- Vitiligo: smooth depigmented macules or patches (see ➔ pp. 486–7).
- Halo naevus: children or young adults. A ring of white skin appears around a melanocytic naevus. The brown 'mole' gradually turns pink and eventually disappears, leaving a depigmented macule.
- Scars (may also be hyperpigmented).
- Atrophie blanche: pale scar with a rim of telangiectasia. Leg in venous disease.

Less common

- Contact leukoderma after exposure to chemicals, e.g. aromatic or aliphatic derivatives of phenols or catechols, hydroquinone in skin-lightening creams, betel leaves, fentanyl patches.
- 2° syphilis: hypopigmented macules superimposed on hyperpigmented, reticulate patches (syphilitic leucomelanoderma). Neck, chest, and back. Six months after 1° disease.
- Tuberous sclerosis: oval or confetti-like hypopigmentation (see ➔ pp. 556–7).
- Cutaneous LE: hypo- and hyperpigmentation (see ➔ pp. 396–407).
- Morphoea or cutaneous systemic sclerosis: perifollicular hypopigmentation in thickened skin. May also be hyperpigmentation (see ➔ p. 414 and pp. 420–1).
- Chronic GVHD (see ➔ Box 26.4, p. 535) (also hyperpigmentation).
- Antiphospholipid syndrome: porcelain white scars with telangiectatic rim (like atrophie blanche) (see ➔ Box 20.10, p. 453). Associated with livedo reticularis. Differentiate from Degos disease (see ➔ p. 90).
- Chronic arsenic ingestion: 'raindrop' hypopigmentation.
- Extragenital lichen sclerosus (see ➔ p. 288): crinkly, shiny white papules with follicular plugging. Look for genital disease.
- Naevus depigmentosus: localized hypopigmented skin with discrete, regular, or serrated margins. Stable appearance (also see ➔ p. 641).
- Naevus anaemicus: jagged outline, caused by vasoconstriction (see ➔ p. 562 and p. 641).
- Cutaneous T-cell lymphoma (see ➔ pp. 358–9).

Rare
- Malignant atrophic papulosis (Degos disease). Erythematous papules evolve into porcelain white scars with a rim of telangiectasia. Linked to fatal vascular occlusion in the gastrointestinal tract (GIT) or central nervous system (CNS). Differentiate from antiphospholipid syndrome.
- Pigmentary mosaicism: swirling hypopigmented patches (see ➲ Box 32.7, p. 637).
- Focal dermal hypoplasia of Goltz (see ➲ Box 32.8, p. 637).
- Albinism: total body depigmentation, light blue iris, nystagmus.
- Waardenburg syndrome (a form of piebaldism). Autosomal dominant (AD) inheritance. Symmetrical patches of hypopigmentation on the face, scalp, back, and proximal extremities, with a stripe of normal-coloured skin down the centre of the back. Also white forelock, neurosensory deafness, widening of the bridge of the nose, and heterochromia of the iris.

Further reading

Vachiramon V et al. *Clin Exp Dermatol* 2011;**37**:97–103.

Skin of colour

Signs in dark skin may be difficult to assess, and some conditions are much commoner in certain ethnic groups, while others may present differently (see Box 4.9). Pigmentary disorders may be particularly distressing and disfiguring.

- Traditional medicines, cultural practices, or cosmetics may affect the skin, so ask what the patient is using on the skin.
- Pigmentary demarcation lines may simulate pathology (see ➜ Box 1.5, p. 13).
- Benign melanocytic naevi are common in the nail bed of black patients and produce hyperpigmented linear bands of varying width in the nail plate. These may be single or multiple, and their number tends to increase with age. Pigment does not extend onto the skin of the surrounding nail fold, although some pigment may be visible beneath the translucent cuticle. If pigment is detected in the nail fold (Hutchinson sign), arrange a biopsy to exclude malignant melanoma.
- Some black patients have harmless diffuse nail pigmentation.
- Palms and soles are paler than the rest of the skin in dark-skinned patients.
- Palmar creases tend to be hyperpigmented and, in black patients, may contain punctate conical pits (keratosis punctata).
- Asymptomatic hyperpigmented macules varying in shape and size are common on plantar surfaces in black patients, particularly the ball of the foot and the heel.
- Brown pigmentation of the oral mucosa, including the tongue, buccal mucosa, and palate, is a normal finding in many black patients.
- Gingival tattooing (blue-grey) is common in parts of Africa.
- Periorbital hyperpigmentation is common in the Indo-Asian population. Colour change (may be familial) starts below the eyes around puberty.
- Dermatosis papulosa nigra (1–3mm pigmented, warty papules like small seborrhoeic warts) is common on the cheeks of Africans, African Americans, and dark-skinned South East Asians.
- Redness (erythema) in dark skin may be difficult to assess, and the skin may merely appear slightly darker than normal. Ask the patient to show you what is normal or abnormal. Even erythroderma (generalized erythema) may not be obvious. Look for signs of skin failure such as shivering, thirst, and widespread scaling (see ➜ p. 106).
- Long-lasting post-inflammatory hypopigmentation and/or hyperpigmentation are common after conditions, such as acne, psoriasis, or eczema, as well as after lichenoid inflammatory conditions such as LP or LE. Ask if anything preceded the colour change.
- Prolonged hypopigmentation may be caused by intralesional corticosteroids or very potent topical corticosteroids, but it is much commoner for the colour change to be 2° to the inflammatory skin condition for which the corticosteroids were prescribed.
- Even individuals with dark-coloured skin may be photosensitive, so do not assume anything!

Box 4.9 Presentations commoner in skin of colour

Hair follicles and follicular rashes

- Alopecia related to hair straightening (with chemicals or hot combs) or to tight braiding (traction alopecia) in black patients.
- Pomade acne on the forehead caused by greasy hair oils.
- Acne keloidalis nuchae: firm papules on the nape of the neck or scalp, common in black patients with curly hair.
- Pseudofolliculitis barbae: hyperpigmented papules/pustules on the neck/cheek where skin shaved. Triggered by ingrowing hairs.
- Atopic eczema in a follicular pattern is common in black children, as is follicular accentuation in other inflammatory conditions, including lichen planus and pityriasis versicolor.
- Disseminated and recurrent infundibulofolliculitis: itchy follicular papules on the chest, back, and buttocks of black patients.

Darker colour (often post-inflammatory) (Also see ➲ p. 88.)

- Scaly plaques of psoriasis look blue-black, rather than red.
- LP presents with deeply coloured purple papules in dark skin. LP pigmentosa is commoner in Asian patients and presents with ashy grey macules.
- Pseudo-acanthosis nigricans: hyperpigmentation, velvety thickening, and skin tags in the flexures of obese Asian patients. Associated with diabetes and insulin resistance (see ➲ pp. 466–7).
- Macular amyloidosis: itchy rash with rippled grey-brown pigmentation, often on the upper back. Commoner in Asian patients (see ➲ Box 23.3, p. 497).
- Acquired ochronosis: hyperpigmentation caused by skin-lightening creams containing hydroquinone.
- Suction cups used in the traditional practice of cupping leave circular hyperpigmented macules that may simulate bruising.

Paler colour (often post-inflammatory) (Also see ➲ pp. 89–90.)

- Pityriasis alba: pale oval patches and fine scale. Most often on the face but may involve the trunk. Seen in prepubertal children (see ➲ p. 89).
- Trichrome vitiligo: zones of hypopigmentation, as well as depigmentation and normal pigmentation.
- Leprosy produces anaesthetic macules (see ➲ Box 6.8, p. 145).
- Dyspigmentation with scarring in discoid LE (see ➲ p. 404).
- Confetti-like hypopigmentation on the face caused by skin-lightening creams containing hydroquinone.

Wounds and scars

- Sickle-cell leg ulcers (see ➲ Box 15.2, p. 295).
- Keloids (smooth nodular scars that extend beyond original wound) common on the upper chest, shoulders, and upper back. Avoid taking skin biopsies from these sites in patients with black skin.

Neonates (see ➲ p. 590)

- Mongolian spots (dermal melanocytes). Light blue to slate grey macules, most often lumbosacral. May be multiple. Fade slowly (see ➲ Fig. 31.10, p. 615). Naevus of Ota affects periorbital skin and sclera.
- Transient neonatal pustular melanosis (see ➲ Box 31.4, p. 593).
- Infantile acropustulosis (see ➲ Box 31.4, p. 593). Differentiate from scabies.

Hair: too much or too little

The history and examination in hair problems are described on ➜ p. 24 and p. 44. Excess hair may grow anywhere there are hair follicles. Hair loss may be diffuse, localized, complete (bald patches), or partial (thinning). Scalp may be normal or scaly. Decide if alopecia is non-scarring and potentially reversible, or scarring when loss is irreversible (see ➜ Box 3.2, p. 45).

Hypertrichosis

Definition: excessive hair on any part of the body.
- *Acquired*: generalized, most often drugs (see ➜ p. 380). Rarely indicates systemic disease, including malnutrition (anorexia nervosa; see ➜ pp. 512–13 and p. 572), advanced HIV infection, PCT (see ➜ p. 332), POEMS syndrome (see ➜ Box 26.8, p. 540), and disorders of the CNS. Localized hypertrichosis occurs after chronic cutaneous irritation or inflammation and may develop in association with some tumours (melanocytic naevi, Becker naevi, plexiform neurofibromas, smooth muscle hamartomas).
- *Congenital*: localized hypertrichosis in the midline over the scalp or spine may indicate an underlying neural tube defect, e.g. a hair collar in the scalp or a lumbosacral faun tail (see ➜ p. 594). Hypertrichosis is associated with some rare hereditary diseases, including porphyrias, mucopolysaccharidoses, fetal alcohol syndrome, and Cornelia de Lange syndrome.

Hirsutes

- Increased growth of terminal hairs in ♀ in an androgen-dependent pattern (normal ♂ sexual pattern)—face, lips, chest, arms, thighs. Caused by androgen overproduction, androgenic drugs, or increased sensitivity of the hair follicle to androgens (see ➜ p. 474).

Localized non-scarring alopecia

- Alopecia areata: well-defined areas of loss. The scalp is smooth, not scaly. You may find exclamation-mark hairs. At first, regrowing hair is not pigmented (see ➜ p. 488 and p. 44).
- Tinea capitis (dermatophyte infection, ringworm): scalp is itchy and scaly, and may be inflamed.
- Hair pulling (trichotillomania): short, stubby hairs (<2cm). Longer hairs can be pulled out. Common in children.
- Trauma: hair may be pulled out when thick scale is removed in psoriasis or seborrhoeic dermatitis.
- Traction alopecia: affects the margins of the scalp where hair has been pulled back tightly. No scale or exclamation-mark hairs.

Diffuse non-scarring alopecia

- Telogen effluvium (illness in previous 2–3 months?), post-partum.
- Androgenetic alopecia (see ➲ p. 480).
- Thyroid disease or iron deficiency anaemia.
- Drugs (see ➲ p. 380).
- Rare congenital causes of hypotrichosis include ectodermal dysplasias and disorders in which the hair shaft is abnormal and brittle (see ➲ pp. 634–5).

Scarring alopecia

Follicles may be replaced by a tumour. In inflammatory diseases, such as DLE, damage to follicular stem cells (see ➲ p. 10) probably contributes to permanent hair loss.

Commoner

- Trauma: including radiotherapy.
- Tumours:
  - Benign: naevus sebaceous—present at birth (see ➲ Fig. 31.2, p. 595).
  - Malignant: BCC, SCC, metastatic deposits.
- DLE (see ➲ p. 404).
- Acne keloidalis: most often in black men. Firm follicular papules (keloids) at the nape of the neck and/or occipital scalp. May also have pustules.

Uncommon

- Aplasia cutis: present at birth (see ➲ Box 31.6, p. 595).
- Linear morphoea.
- Lichen planopilaris (variant of LP that affects hair follicles).
- Folliculitis decalvans: erythematous perifollicular pustules and scarring. Cause unclear but may involve *S. aureus*.
- Dissecting cellulitis of scalp: occurs most often in young black-skinned men. Firm, deep nodules become fluctuant, discharge malodorous pus, and develop interconnecting sinuses. May be associated with hidradenitis suppurativa and acne conglobata (see ➲ p. 250).

Funny nails

As with the skin, the distribution of changes points towards the cause. If many nails are affected (symmetry), the problem is likely to be endogenous; if only one nail is affected (asymmetry), the problem is likely to be exogenous. Inflammation of periungual skin in conditions, such as eczema, leads to 2° changes in the nail plate.

Common or important signs

- *Changes in nail colour* (see Box 4.10).
- *Transverse depressions*: temporary loss of mitotic activity in the proximal nail matrix. Think of trauma if only one nail is affected. Some patients damage the nail plate by repeatedly pushing down the cuticle. Beau lines affect all the nails and indicate slowing of nail growth in the previous 1–2 months, e.g. during a serious illness or chemotherapy (see ➲ pp. 380–1). Arrest of all nail matrix activity causes nail shedding (onychomadesis).
- *Nail pitting*: foci of abnormal keratinization of nail matrix. Psoriasis is the commonest cause of coarse pits. Many fine pits occur in alopecia areata. May see pits in eczema.
- *Thinning, longitudinal ridging, and fissuring* (onychorrhexis): diffuse damage to nail matrix. Mild disease is common in older people. Also seen with impaired vascular supply, LP, chronic GVHD, and amyloidosis. May cause permanent loss of the nail plate with dorsal pterygium (adhesion between nail fold and nail bed).
- *Onycholysis*: the nail plate separates from an abnormal nail bed. If distal and only a few nails, consider fungus, trauma, or subungual tumour. How does the patient manicure the nails? Is something being pushed underneath the nail plate to remove accumulated debris? This will damage the nail bed and worsen onycholysis. Psoriasis may cause proximal oil spots or salmon patches, as well as distal onycholysis. Also seen with hyperthyroidism. Drugs, particularly tetracyclines and taxanes, cause painful photo-onycholysis (see ➲ Box 16.3, p. 327).
- *Subungual hyperkeratosis and discoloured thickened nail plate*: fungus, psoriasis. Likely to be a fungal infection if only a few nails. Crumbling starts at the free edge of the nail and moves proximally. Exclude psoriasis by looking for pitting and/or onycholysis in finger nails (see ➲ p. 196).
- *Splinter haemorrhages*: indicate damage to nail bed capillaries. Trauma is likely if only one nail is affected and the haemorrhages are distal, rather than proximal. Splinter haemorrhages may develop when the nail plate is abnormal, e.g. in psoriasis. Numerous proximal splinter haemorrhages are more likely to indicate systemic disease such as infective endocarditis.
- *Nail clubbing*: associated with systemic problems, including chronic lung disease, cyanotic heart disease, IBD, and thyroid disease, but may be idiopathic or familial.
- *Spoon-shaped nails* (koilonychia): the soft nail plate in iron deficiency becomes concave. Children have physiological koilonychia.
- *Abnormalities in nail fold* (see Box 4.11).

Box 4.10 Changes in nail colour

- Dark discoloration: diffuse darkening or longitudinal bands of pigment are common in individuals with dark skin and are caused by melanocytic naevi in the nail matrix.
- Addison disease and ectopic ACTH production may lead to dark nails or bands of melanonychia.
- Does pigment extend onto the skin of the proximal or lateral nail fold? Discoloration caused by subungual haematoma (e.g. after repetitive trauma such as running) or fungal infection never spreads onto surrounding skin, but pigmentation associated with subungual malignant melanoma may affect adjacent skin (Hutchinson sign).
- Onycholytic nails become dark green when the space beneath the nail plate is colonized by *Pseudomonas aeruginosa*.
- Drugs, e.g. antimalarials, can darken nails (see ➡ pp. 380–1).
- Acquired leuconychia: fungal infection, trauma (punctate leuconychia). Hypoalbuminaemia, e.g. chronic liver disease, and some drugs cause apparent leuconychia in all the nails, because of changes in the nail bed, but discoloration fades with pressure.
- Congenital leuconychia: rare, affects all nails.
- Transverse white lines may occur after trauma, systemic illness, poisoning with arsenic (Mee lines), or thallium.
- Half and half nails (white proximally and reddish brown distally) are a rare sign of chronic renal failure.
- Yellow nails. Nails grow slowly and become thick and greenish yellow in the yellow nail syndrome, which is associated with lymphatic hypoplasia, peripheral oedema, and pleural effusions (rare).
- Red and white horizontal bands in HIV infection.

Box 4.11 Abnormalities in nail fold

- Boggy, swollen erythematous nail fold: most likely to indicate chronic paronychia. The cuticle is missing; low-grade *Candida* infection beneath the nail fold leads to ridging and discoloration of the nail. *S. aureus* may cause episodes of tender acute paronychia, when beads of pus exude from the swollen nail fold.
- Dilated nail fold capillaries and periungual erythema are valuable signs of a connective tissue disease (see ➡ Fig. 19.9, p. 410).
- Digital mucous cyst: the smooth swelling in the nail fold produces a vertical furrow in the nail plate.
- Papules in nail fold:
  - Viral warts; periungual fibroma in tuberous sclerosis; beaded papules in multicentric reticulohistiocytosis (see ➡ p. 426).
- Pustules around the nail and beneath the nail plate: seen in reactive arthritis (see ➡ p. 208), as well as in acropustulosis and parakeratosis pustulosa (both rare and possible forms of psoriasis) (see ➡ Box 9.9, p. 199).

Skin failure and emergency dermatology

Contents

Relevant pages in other chapters

Acne fulminans ➔ p. 248
Anticoagulant-induced purpura fulminans ➔ p. 376.
For more information about angio-oedema and urticaria, see
➔ p. 22 and p. 228. Also see Red man syndrome, ➔ p. 372.

Rash in a sick adult with a fever

Ill patients with rash and fever pose an urgent diagnostic problem. Life-threatening causes include infections, severe drug reactions, and acute GVHD (see Boxes 5.1 and 5.2). Taking a systematic approach to history and examination will help to establish the cause.

What should I ask?

- Explore symptoms, e.g. rigors, sweats, headache, photophobia, arthralgia, myalgia, nausea, or diarrhoea. Any mucosal problems, e.g. conjunctivitis, sore throat, oral or genital ulcers?
- Is fever sustained, remittent (elevated each day and returns to baseline, but not normal), or intermittent (intermittently elevated but returns to normal)?
- When did the rash develop, and how has it evolved?
- Any history of contact with an infectious disease?
- Document a travel history (were any preventative measures taken, e.g. vaccines, avoiding mosquito bites?) and sexual history.
- Explore the drug history (including use of recreational drugs).
- Any past history of drug reaction, infectious disease, or skin disease?
- Might the patient be immunocompromised?

What should I look for?

- Cutaneous signs:
  - Does the rash blanch with light pressure (erythematous), or is it purpuric (non-blanching)? Purpura in a febrile patient raises the possibility of meningococcal septicaemia (see ➲ pp. 102–3).
  - Is the rash morbilliform (measles-like erythematous macules and papules)? Is there any desquamation?
  - Are there erosions (denuded areas where the epidermis has been lost), blisters, or pustules? (See Box 5.1.)
  - Is the skin scaly, or is there superficial peeling (desquamation)?
  - Are the palms and soles involved? Is there oedema?
- Examine the conjunctiva, buccal mucosa, throat, and tongue.
- Check for lymphadenopathy.
- Is the neck stiff, or are the muscles tender?
- Examine the joints for warmth, erythema, swelling, or tenderness.
- Examine the cardiovascular, respiratory, GI, genitourinary, and neurological systems for localizing signs.

What should I do?

Investigations will be guided by your findings, but consider:
- Full blood count (FBC) and erythrocyte sedimentation rate (ESR); C-reactive protein (CRP), clotting screen.
- Liver function and renal function; urinalysis.
- Blood cultures, wound swabs, lumbar puncture, skin biopsy.

Further reading

Low DE. *Crit Care Clin* 2013;**29**:651–75.
The RegiSCAR Project. Available at: ⏏ www.regiscar.org/ (severe cutaneous drug reactions).
Young AE and Thornton KL. *Arch Dis Child Educ Pract Ed* 2007;**92**:ep97–100.

Box 5.1 Causes of rash and fever in sick adult patient

- Infections, e.g.:
  - Severe bacteraemia, e.g. meningococcal, pneumococcal.
  - TSS (see Box 5.2).
  - Rickettsiosis, e.g. Rocky Mountain spotted fever.
  - Viral haemorrhagic fevers and dengue.
- Severe cutaneous adverse drug reactions, e.g.:
  - TEN.
  - DRESS.
- Acute GVHD.
- Rheumatological disease, e.g.:
  - SLE, systemic vasculitis.

Box 5.2 Toxic shock syndrome

❶ TSS is a multisystem disease, usually caused by an exotoxin produced by *Staphylococcus aureus* which acts as a superantigen, resulting in immune cell expansion and a cytokine storm. Predisposing factors include surgical packing, contraceptive sponges, post-partum infections, and deep abscesses. TSS is also a potentially fatal complication of small burns in young children.

TSS can be produced by other bacterial exotoxins, including group A *Streptococcus, Pseudomonas*, and *Klebsiella* strains. TSS may be mild or rapidly fatal. Mortality for streptococcal TSS is around 50%.

What to look for in TSS

- Sudden onset of high fever >39°C, with myalgia, vomiting, diarrhoea, and headache.
- Hypotension. Disorientation or altered consciousness.
- Diffuse macular erythematous (not purpuric) rash that starts on the trunk and spreads outwards. If you find vesicles or bullae, think of SSSS (see ➡ p. 112) or TEN (see ➡ p. 116). If purpuric, consider meningococcaemia (see ➡ pp. 102–3).
- Erythema and oedema of palms and soles.
- Erythema of mucous membranes with strawberry tongue and conjunctival hyperaemia. No ulceration, unlike TEN.
- Organ dysfunction: renal failure, abnormal liver function.
- Lymphopenia is common. DIC (if severe)—deranged clotting and low platelets.
- Blood cultures frequently negative, and diagnosis is clinical.

▶▶ Management of TSS

- Resuscitate with intravenous (IV) fluids and vasopressor agents, if required.
- Treat with IV antibiotics (suppress toxin production).
- Remove wound dressings; clean wounds, and remove any potential nidus of infection such as a foreign body.
- IV immunoglobulin has been used in severe TSS.
- Skin desquamates, particularly on the palms and soles, after 1–2 weeks.

Vasculitis and purpura fulminans

Palpable purpura is the hallmark of a small-vessel cutaneous vasculitis, such as IgA vasculitis (Henoch–Schönlein purpura), whereas flat (macular) purpura is associated with non-inflammatory pathology (see ➔ pp. 436–9). In purpura fulminans, fibrin thrombi occlude dermal vessels, as well as vessels in the subcutis, leading to haemorrhage, ischaemia, and infarction. Purpura fulminans most commonly occurs in meningococcal septicaemia (see Box 5.3).

Meningococcal septicaemia (*Neisseria meningitidis*)

❶ Meningococcal infection may cause devastating septicaemia (acute meningococcaemia) and death within hours of first symptoms. The non-specific flu-like presentation, with fever, vomiting, headache, abdominal pain, and muscle aches, may be misleading.

Although 80–90% of patients develop purpura within 12–36h of onset of infection, the rash may be subtle and lesions few in number. You should examine the skin in a good light.

What should I look for?
- Early: a transient erythematous, maculopapular rash (may simulate TSS (see ➔ Box 5.2, p. 101).
- After 12–36h: small purpuric lesions (petechiae) with an irregular outline and (usually) raised centres. You will find petechiae most often on the limbs and trunk, but examine the head, palms, soles, and mucous membranes. Also look for purpuric lesions in pressure areas, e.g. under the waistband, or at sites of friction.

▶▶ *What should I do?*
- Consider the diagnosis in any febrile patient with a petechial rash. Frequently, meningitis is not clinically apparent.
- Commence immediate treatment with intravenous (IV) antibiotics, e.g. ceftriaxone 2g, without waiting to confirm your suspicions.
- ❶ Call the critical care team urgently.
- If not in hospital, treat with IV or intramuscular (IM) benzylpenicillin 1.2g, and call an ambulance.

Complications
- DIC and purpura fulminans (see Box 5.3). Extensive irregular haemorrhagic areas (ecchymoses) become bullous and may progress to well-demarcated blue-black gangrene of digits or whole limbs.
- Limb compartment syndrome 2° to thrombosis, venous congestion, and oedema. Muscle infarction and rhabdomyolysis.
- Shock, hypotension (late sign in young), confusion, tachypnoea.
- Waterhouse–Friderichsen syndrome (caused by haemorrhage into the adrenal cortex).
- Coma and multi-organ failure.

❶Box 5.3 What is purpura fulminans?

The term purpura fulminans describes a devastating illness that is characterized by rapidly progressive and extensive purpura with dermal vascular thrombosis and haemorrhagic infarction, but without vasculitis (see Fig. 5.1). In severe cases, subcutaneous vessels or major veins are thrombosed. Patients have a consumptive coagulopathy. The mortality is high. Survivors may be left with extensive scarring, missing digits, or amputated limbs.

Causes include
- Acute bacterial infection (commonest cause), e.g. *Neisseria meningitidis* or, much less often, β-haemolytic *Streptococcus, Streptococcus pneumoniae, Staphylococcus aureus*, and other bacteria.
- After infection (usually children 1–3 weeks after varicella or streptococcal infection).
- Congenital deficiency of protein C or protein S (presents in neonates).
- Acquired deficiency of protein C or protein S associated with drugs (warfarin) (see ➔ p. 376) or disease (renal dialysis, nephrotic syndrome, cholestasis, bone marrow transplantation).
- Antiphospholipid syndrome (see ➔ Box 20.10, p. 453).
- Heparin-induced skin necrosis (antibody-mediated platelet aggregation usually seen at the injection site of subcutaneous heparin) (see ➔ p. 376).
- Toxins or poisons (spider bites, snake bites).

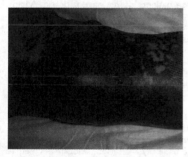

Fig. 5.1 Extensive purpura fulminans.

Further reading
Wada H et al. *J Thromb Haemost* 2013 Feb 4.

Anaphylaxis, angio-oedema, and urticaria

What is anaphylaxis?

❗ Anaphylaxis is a severe, generalized or systemic hypersensitivity reaction associated with release of histamine and capillary leak. Characterized by rapidly developing, life-threatening airway and/or breathing and/or circulatory collapse, usually associated with urticaria and mucosal swelling (angio-oedema).

Triggers include foods, drugs (see Box 5.4), and venoms (wasp, bee). Reaction develops within minutes of exposure to trigger, but often no cause identified (these are non-IgE-mediated) (see Box 5.5).

What should I look for?

- Sudden onset and rapid progression of symptoms.
- Life-threatening airway ± breathing ± circulatory collapse that may include stridor, hoarse voice, difficulty swallowing, wheeze, cyanosis, tachycardia, hypotension, reduced consciousness.
- Skin and/or mucosal changes (flushing, urticaria, angio-oedema)— signs may be subtle or absent in up to 20% of reactions.

What is angio-oedema?

Angio-oedema implies oedema of the deep dermis, subcutaneous tissues, mucosa, and/or submucosa. Laryngeal oedema, which may cause difficulty swallowing and respiratory obstruction, is life-threatening.

Angio-oedema occurs in anaphylactic reactions. ⚠ Rarely, angio-oedema is caused by C1 esterase inhibitor deficiency (inherited—AD inheritance or acquired). These patients do *not* have urticaria. Angio-oedema is usually triggered by mucosal trauma, e.g. dental procedures or, in ♀, sexual intercourse. Some patients complain of vomiting/abdominal pain. Prodromal features reported more commonly in women include fatigue, malaise, and short temper.

α-1-antitrypsin (AAT) deficiency is a rare cause (see ➜ p. 462).

Facial swelling in acute contact dermatitis (see ➜ pp. 214–16) or acute dermatomyositis (see ➜ pp. 408–9) may mimic angio-oedema (see ➜ Fig. 19.8, p. 409).

What is urticaria?

Urticaria (hives, wheals, welts) is a hypersensitivity reaction that may occur in isolation or associated with angio-oedema and/or anaphylaxis. Wheals are 2° to dermal oedema. They are raised, smooth, erythematous, and itchy. They come and go, leaving normal skin, but generally do not last >24h. Some patients provide a clear history of precipitants, such as drugs, latex, or foods (fruit, fish, peanuts), but many, especially with chronic urticaria, cannot identify a trigger. Many idiopathic (spontaneous) cases are not mediated by IgE. Allergy testing in chronic urticaria is unrewarding.

Urticaria may be acute or chronic, and often confused with EM (see Box 5.10). Most patients with urticaria do not develop anaphylaxis. Urticaria is a nuisance but, unless associated with airway problems (ask about throat swelling or wheeze), is not life-threatening (see ➔ p. 228). Non-sedating antihistamines are the mainstay of treatment (see ➔ pp. 232–3).

Box 5.4 Drugs linked to anaphylaxis

Virtually any class of drug can be implicated:
- Antibiotics, including penicillin and cephalosporin.
- Aspirin.
- NSAIDs.
- ACE inhibitors.
- Anaesthetic drugs, including suxamethonium, vecuronium, and atracurium.
- Contrast media, particularly iodinated media.

▶▶ Box 5.5 Management of anaphylaxis in adults

Use an ABCDE approach to assess and treat anaphylactic reactions:
- Place the patient in a comfortable position. Conscious patients with breathing difficulty may prefer to sit up.
- Remove the trigger, if possible.
- Adrenaline (epinephrine) 0.5mg IM (0.5mL of 1:1000)—repeat after 5min, if no better.
- Oxygen: 100% high flow as soon as possible.
- Rapid IV fluid challenge to restore tissue perfusion, e.g. 1L of warmed 0.9% saline infused in 5–10min. Monitor response, and give more fluids, if necessary, aiming to restore the patient's normal blood pressure.
- If wheeze persists, give bronchodilators.

After initial resuscitation:
- Chlorphenamine 10mg IM or IV slowly.
- Hydrocortisone 200mg IM or IV slowly.
- Ensure the patient is monitored.

❶ *Note that patients with angio-oedema 2° to C1 esterase inhibitor deficiency do not have urticaria and will not respond to adrenalin. They should be treated with C1 esterase inhibitor.*

Patients who have had an anaphylactic reaction should be referred to an allergy clinic both for further investigation and education, as these patients have a substantial risk of further reactions.

Adverse drug reactions should be reported to the Medicines and Healthcare products Regulatory Agency using the yellow card scheme.

Skin failure

What is skin failure?

Skin failure occurs following sudden onset of a widespread severe inflammatory dermatosis that impairs the normal physiological functions of the skin. The stratum corneum may be disrupted or the epidermis may be lost completely, leaving a denuded dermis.

Skin failure has a number of causes but is most often either 2° to deterioration of a pre-existing dermatosis or manifestation of a drug reaction (see Box 5.6).

What should I look for?

❶ Patients with skin failure have an inflammatory skin condition involving at least 90% of the BSA. Skin failure occurs in:
• Generalized scaly erythema (erythroderma, exfoliative dermatitis).
• Generalized erythema with pustules.
• Widespread blistering, with or without loss of epidermis.

The other features of skin failure may include:
• Cutaneous pain or widespread itching.
• Impaired temperature regulation: hypo- or hyperthermia. Heat is lost due to increased dermal blood flow. Patients feel cold and shiver to raise the temperature.
• Infection (the skin barrier is disrupted).
• Loss of fluid (4 or 5L of fluid are lost each day if 50% of the BSA is involved and the stratum corneum is destroyed).
• Loss of electrolytes and protein.
• Increased energy requirements.
• Oedema (vasodilated cutaneous blood vessels are more permeable).
• High-output cardiac failure (particularly in the elderly).
• Mucosal ulceration in some blistering disorders makes eating or drinking painful.
• Hair and nails may be lost acutely or 2–3 months later.

Causes of skin failure should be explored, and treatment directed towards treating the underlying disease and relieving discomfort (see Boxes 5.6 and 5.7). Skin failure may be life-threatening—patients may develop infection, hypothermia, or cardiac failure. Older patients, patients with extensive skin involvement, and those already taking corticosteroids/immunosuppressants are at risk of life-threatening complications.

Box 5.6 **Causes of skin failure**

- Erythroderma (generalized erythema and scale) 2° to eczema, psoriasis, or drugs.
- Cutaneous T-cell lymphoma (CTCL) is a rare cause.
- SSSS: causes very superficial blistering.
- Generalized pustular psoriasis.
- SJS/TEN caused by drugs.
- Widespread blistering:
  - Skin loss caused by thermal burns or phototoxicity.
  - Autoimmune bullous disorders, e.g. BP, pemphigus.
  - Inherited group of mechanobullous diseases, i.e. EB (rare).

Box 5.7 **General approach to managing acute skin failure**

- Search for the cause, and stop all unnecessary drugs.
- Record the evolution of the skin disease as objectively as possible—photographs may be helpful.
- Nurse patients with blistering disorders or denuded areas on a low-pressure (air) mattress.
- Minimize the risk of infection with reverse barrier nursing.
- Monitor fluid and electrolyte losses.
- Keep the patient (and room) warm, and monitor the core body temperature; the skin may look red and feel hot—this can be misleading, and the core temperature may be low. Hyperthermia is less common.
- Take skin swabs every 3–4 days.
- Take blood cultures; monitor for systemic infection, and limit indwelling lines to reduce the risk of infection.
- Ensure nutrition is adequate; protein and calorie requirements will increase, requiring high calorific food and protein supplements.
- Be alert for cardiac failure in the elderly with erythroderma.
- Apply bland emollients to soothe red scaly skin, e.g. 50% white soft paraffin (WSP) in liquid paraffin 3–4 times/day (you will need 500g tubs), or use Emollin® spray.
- Use an emollient as soap substitute.
- Ensure adequate pain relief.
- Prescribe sedating antihistamines, such as hydroxyzine 25–50mg four times a day (qds), to relieve intractable irritation.
- Consider low-dose heparin to reduce the risk of venous thrombosis—patients may be dehydrated and immobile.
- Contact a dermatologist urgently to discuss the diagnosis, investigation, and management.
- The disfigurement caused by widespread skin disease can be very distressing, and, as they recover, patients may need psychological support.

Erythroderma

What is erythroderma (also known as exfoliative dermatitis)?

Erythroderma is defined as erythema, with variable amounts of scale, affecting 90% or more of the body surface.

What causes erythroderma?

Search for the cause when you are taking the history, but remember the commonest cause is deterioration of a pre-existing skin disorder or drugs. Erythroderma may develop suddenly but, when associated with skin problems such as psoriasis, may evolve gradually. Causes include:

- Dermatitis of any type, e.g. atopic, seborrhoeic, contact, stasis, asteatotic (15–40% of cases).
- Psoriasis (8–25% of cases).
- Drugs (10–28% of cases)—numerous drugs have been implicated. Also see Red man syndrome, ➔ p. 372.
- Cutaneous T-cell lymphoma or leukaemia (15% of cases).
- Rare skin diseases, e.g. pityriasis rubra pilaris, pemphigus foliaceus, ichthyosiform erythroderma (<1% of cases).

In up to 30% of patients, erythroderma is classified as 'idiopathic', i.e. no cause found. Consider skin biopsy before prescribing treatments, such as topical or oral corticosteroids, which will reduce inflammation and mask signs. Skin biopsies may not reveal the underlying cause.

What should I look for?

- Itchy, erythematous scaly skin (see Fig. 5.2).
- Cutaneous oedema.
- Oozing of serous fluid.
- Pustules (suggesting infection or pustular psoriasis).
- Superficial blisters (suggesting acute dermatitis or, much less likely, pemphigus foliaceus).
- Keratoderma (thick skin on palms or soles).
- Ectropion if erythroderma affects the face.
- Hair loss.
- Thickened or ridged nails or loss of nails.
- Lymphadenopathy (dermatopathic lymphadenopathy is common in erythroderma and is not caused by lymphoma, but consider a biopsy if the nodes are large and rubbery).
- Evidence of a 1° skin disease, e.g. nail pitting suggesting psoriasis, psoriatic plaques on extensor surfaces or in flexures, stasis eczema around a leg ulcer.
- Non-specific symptoms and signs such as fever and malaise.

What should I do?

See Box 5.8 for immediate management.

Box 5.8 Immediate management of erythroderma

- Stop all non-essential systemic drugs.
- Take swabs for culture from oozing skin.
- Apply emollients such as Cetraben® cream or 50% WSP in liquid paraffin (prescribe 500g tubs) 3–4 times/day or Emollin® spray.
- Bath or shower daily, using a soap substitute such as Epaderm® ointment or Dermol® 500. A bath oil, such as Oilatum®, can be added to the bath.
- Prescribe a sedating antihistamine, e.g. hydroxyzine 25–50mg qds for severe itching.
- Treat 2° infection with oral antibiotics.
- Check fluid balance and body temperature, and monitor for other complications of skin failure (see Box 5.7).

❗ Moderately potent topical corticosteroids may be helpful, but do not prescribe very potent topical corticosteroids or oral corticosteroids, until the investigation and management have been discussed with a dermatologist. Corticosteroids are helpful in eczema but can make psoriasis much more unstable and difficult to manage.

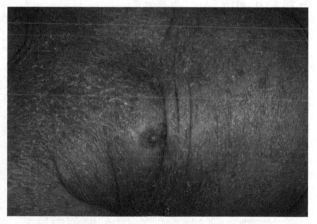

Fig. 5.2 Generalized erythema and scale in this patient with drug-induced erythroderma.

Localized blisters

What is a blister?

- A blister is a bump filled with clear fluid (serum).
- Small blisters, <1cm in diameter, are called vesicles; blisters >1cm in diameter are known as bullae.
- Blisters worry both patients and their doctors, but localized blisters are unlikely to be life-threatening. Always find out precisely what the patient or referring doctor means if they use the term blister.
- see ➲ Chapter 13, pp. 259–75 for details of blistering diseases.

Localized blistering that may present as an emergency

Acute contact dermatitis

(see ➲ Chapter 10, pp. 214–16.) The history may suggest the cause. The rash is itchy, rather than painful (as it is in cellulitis), and the skin is erythematous and oedematous. Scale takes time to develop and may not be apparent at presentation if the eruption is acute. A potent topical corticosteroid cream will act promptly. Patch testing is the investigation of choice if you suspect allergy, rather than irritancy.

Erythema multiforme

(see ➲ p. 111 and Fig. 5.3.)

Cutaneous infections

(see ➲ Chapter 6, pp. 129–48 and Chapter 7, pp. 149–69.)

- 1° herpes simplex infections may be oedematous and painful.
- Herpes zoster.
- Bullous impetigo.
- Blisters in association with cellulitis or erysipelas.
- Blisters associated with dermatophyte infection, usually on the feet.

Physical causes of blisters

- Insect bites: exclude 2° infections, and treat with a potent topical corticosteroid cream applied twice daily (bd).
- Sunburn and photosensitivity, including phytophotodermatitis (plant-induced photosensitivity) and drug-induced photosensitivity. Treat with a potent topical corticosteroid cream applied bd.
- Cold injury.
- Thermal burns: emergency care—remove burnt or hot wet clothes (unless stuck to skin), jewellery, etc. Cool the wound with running cold water for 20min—do not use ice, which causes vasoconstriction and more damage. Clinical findings indicate the depth of the burn:
  - Epidermal: painful, red, may be shiny and wet.
  - Superficial dermal: painful, pink, may have small blisters.
  - Mid-dermal: may lose sensation, slow capillary refill, dark pink, large blisters.
  - Deep dermal: absent sensation, absent capillary refill, blotchy red, may have blisters.
  - Full thickness: absent capillary refill and sensation, no blisters, thick white leathery appearance. Will heal with scarring.

Refer patients with burns to a plastic surgeon for definitive treatment.

Erythema multiforme

EM is an acute, self-limited illness triggered by infections, most often HSV. Other causes include orf, histoplasmosis, VZV, and cytomegalovirus (CMV). Drugs cause <10% of cases. EM resolves within 4 weeks, but some patients have recurrent episodes, usually triggered by herpes simplex infections. Persistent EM (rare) associated with atypical inflammatory lesions is caused by viruses (EBV, CMV, and HSV), IBD, and malignancy.

What should I look for?
(See Box 5.9.)
- Symmetrical, well-defined, round erythematous macules on knees, elbows ± palms; evolve into papules and target lesions, which may blister over days. Infrequently, the rash is widespread (see Fig. 5.3).
- Lesions are at different stages of development (multiform).
- Patients may have few ulcers on one mucosal surface—usually oral.
- EM can be often confused with urticaria (see Box 5.10).

What should I do?
- Take a skin biopsy to confirm the diagnosis.
- Take swabs from oral lesions for viral culture.
- Mouth ulcers: prescribe a mouthwash for pain relief, if required (see
 ➔ Box 14.4, p. 283).
- Cutaneous lesions: a potent topical corticosteroid cream applied bd may relieve discomfort but will probably not speed resolution.
- Recurrent disease: consider prophylaxis with aciclovir 400mg bd.

Box 5.9 Clinical criteria for diagnosing erythema multiforme

- Acute, self-limited illness with duration of <4 weeks.
- Symmetrical, discrete, round erythematous macules/papules that persist at the same site for at least 7 days.
- Some papules evolve into target lesions comprising two or three concentric zones of colour change. A central dusky purple zone is surrounded by an outer red zone and sometimes a white middle zone. The centre may blister or crust after several days.
- No mucosal involvement/one mucosal surface involved.

Box 5.10 Differences between erythema multiforme and urticaria

- Urticarial lesions resolve within 48h (usually much quicker) and disappear to leave normal skin; EM papules persist for ≥7 days.
- New crops of urticarial lesions continue to appear daily for weeks. All lesions of EM appear within the first 3 days.
- Urticarial papules may evolve into rings, but the central skin is normal. The central zone in the target lesions of EM is dusky, bullous, or crusted.
- Urticaria, unlike EM, may be associated with angio-oedema (deep swelling) of subcutaneous tissues or mucosa.
- EM, unlike urticaria, may be associated with mucosal ulcers.

Generalized blisters

❶ Generalized herpes simplex infection (eczema herpeticum)

A generalized infection commonly seen in children with atopic eczema. Eczema herpeticum is life-threatening, particularly in children, when it is generally a 1° infection (see ➲ pp. 152–5). Twenty percent of children will have localized recurrent infections. Generalized herpes simplex infection may also complicate burns and some rare skin diseases (pemphigus, Darier disease, ichthyosis).

What should I look for?
See Box 5.11.

What should I do?
See Box 5.12.

❶ Staphylococcal scalded skin syndrome

(see ➲ pp. 136–7.) SSSS occurs most often in infancy or children, and less often in the elderly or immunosuppressed. Patients have localized focus of staphylococcal infection, often in the nasopharynx. Staphylococci release epidermolytic toxins (ET) that cleave the skin high in the epidermis.

What should I look for?
- The skin is erythematous and tender. The erythema is accentuated in flexural and periorificial skin (see ➲ Fig. 6.2, p. 131).
- The thin-walled blisters rupture rapidly but are extremely superficial and, unlike the blisters of TEN, do not involve all the epidermis.
- Mucosal surfaces are never involved in SSSS. This and the superficial blistering help to distinguish SSSS from TEN.
- The diffusely erythematous rash in SSSS may resemble TSS in early stages, before blisters appear, but patients with TSS are more ill with high fever and hypotension (see ➲ Box 5.2, p. 101).

▶▶ *What should I do?*
- Culture swabs from possible foci of infection, e.g. nasopharynx. Culture of skin swabs from the blisters is negative in SSSS, because the condition is mediated by a toxin.
- If it is difficult to differentiate SSSS from TEN and if you want a rapid answer, gently peel the roof off a fresh blister; roll the fragment of tissue into a scroll, and take the fresh tissue to the pathology laboratory. Ask the pathologist to examine a frozen section. In SSSS, you will see the horny layer and very little else, whereas in TEN you will see full-thickness necrotic epidermis.
- Alternatively, you can make a Tzank preparation from the base of a fresh blister (see ➲ p. 647). In SSSS, there will be some keratinocytes in the smear, because the split is high within the epidermis. In TEN, the Tzank preparation from the base of a fresh blister has no keratinocytes, because the entire epidermis forms the blister roof.
- Treat with flucloxacillin—the prognosis is generally excellent.

ⓘBox 5.11 Signs of eczema herpeticum

(see ➲ Fig. 7.3, p. 155.)
- Sudden deterioration of atopic eczema.
- Pain as well as intense itching.
- Malaise, vomiting, anorexia, diarrhoea.
- Fever in variable number of cases.
- Vesicles (1° lesions), papules, and pustules (older lesions).
- Small punched-out ulcers, sometimes clustered, but these may coalesce into ulcers with irregular outlines.
- Oozing, sometimes haemorrhagic, and crusting.
- Lymphadenopathy.
- Signs may be difficult to differentiate from VZV (see ➲ pp. 156–7) or bacterial infection. 2° bacterial infection may complicate the picture.

▶▶Box 5.12 Management of eczema herpeticum

- Take swabs ideally from vesicles for both viral studies (polymerase chain reaction, PCR) and bacterial culture (see ➲ p. 644).
- A Tzank smear preparation can be used to confirm the diagnosis (see ➲ p. 647).
- Treat with an oral antiviral, e.g. aciclovir, as well as an antibiotic such as flucloxacillin. Severe cases will need IV aciclovir.
- Provide antipyretics, parenteral fluids, and pain relief.
- Eczema: in severe cases, all topical corticosteroids should be avoided until infection is controlled. In less severe cases, it may be reasonable to treat eczema with a mild topical corticosteroid ointment, once antivirals have been started.
- For less common causes of generalized blisters, see Box 5.13.

Box 5.13 Less common causes of generalized blisters that may present as an emergency

- Damage to basal cells (lichenoid reaction):
  - SJS (see ➲ p. 116).
  - TEN (full-thickness necrosis of epidermis) (see ➲ p. 116).
  - Acute GVHD (see ➲ pp. 532–3).
- Autoimmune blistering diseases (see ➲ pp. 264–5):
  - BP—the commonest.
  - Pemphigus foliaceus, pemphigus vulgaris.
  - Other rare autoimmune blistering diseases.
- Bullous cutaneous vasculitis (bullae will be haemorrhagic) (see ➲ p. 440).

Severe cutaneous adverse reactions

Cutaneous adverse drug reactions are common (2–3% of hospitalized patients). Most drug rashes are morbilliform and settle quickly when the drug is stopped (see ⊋ p. 372), but rarely a morbilliform rash is the first sign of a much more serious problem such as TEN (see ⊋ p. 370).

Life-threatening reactions that are discussed in this book include:
- Anaphylaxis, angio-oedema, and serum sickness (see ⊋ pp. 104–5 and p. 373).
- Erythroderma (see ⊋ p. 108).
- SJS (see ⊋ Fig. 5.4, pp. 116–20).
- TEN (see ⊋ Fig. 5.5, pp. 116–20).
- DRESS (see ⊋ pp. 122–3).
- Anticoagulant-induced purpura fulminans and skin necrosis (see ⊋ pp. 102–3).

What should I look for to help me to decide if this adverse drug reaction might be life-threatening?

see ⊋ Box 5.14 and Chapter 18, p. 370 for information about adverse drug reactions.

> **❶ Box 5.14 Indications of severe cutaneous adverse reactions**
>
> - General:
>   - Fever >40°C, hypotension, lymphadenopathy.
>   - Arthralgia, arthritis.
>   - Dyspnoea, wheeze.
> - Mucocutaneous:
>   - Erythroderma (generalized scaly erythema).
>   - Swollen face, swelling of tongue, urticaria (anaphylaxis).
>   - Skin pain or burning (TEN).
>   - Erosions; shearing stress detaches epidermis from dermis; bullae or mucosal erosions (TEN or SJS) (see Fig. 5.5).
>   - Vasculitis (palpable purpura) or extensive flat purpura.
> - Laboratory results:
>   - Eosinophilia >1000mm^3
>   - Lymphocytosis with abnormal lymphocytes
>   - Abnormal liver function tests (LFTs).

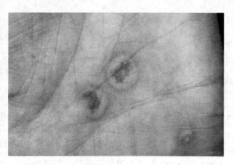

Fig. 5.3 Well-defined target lesions on the palms in erythema multiforme.

Stevens–Johnson syndrome and toxic epidermal necrolysis

These severe reactions with overlapping features (see Box 5.15) are commonly caused by drugs (see Box 5.16). Onset 2–3 weeks after commencing the drug. Patients often have underlying diseases, e.g. acquired immune deficiency syndrome (AIDS).

❶ If you see any patient with a painful erythematous 'drug rash' and mucosal signs, alarm bells should ring.

Stevens–Johnson syndrome

What should I look for?

- Vague upper respiratory tract symptoms (fever, cough, headache, sore throat, rhinorrhoea, and malaise) for 1–3 days prior to onset.
- Symmetrical, poorly defined painful erythematous macules evolving rapidly to papules and target lesions, with 2/3 concentric zones of colour change and dark purpuric centres.
- Large bullae rupture, leaving denuded skin, but typical SJS affects <10% of BSA (see Fig 5.4).
- The rash is usually maximal in 4 days.
- ❶ Severe mucosal ulceration with involvement of at least two mucosal surfaces (lip, oral cavity, conjunctiva, nasal, urethra, vagina, GI tract, respiratory tract). The lips become crusted and haemorrhagic. Painful stomatitis interferes with eating and drinking. Purulent conjunctivitis is associated with photophobia.
- Late ocular complications include dry eye, scarring, and loss of vision (see Box 5.20).

Toxic epidermal necrolysis

What should I look for?

- Flu-like symptoms may precede TEN. Fever is higher than in SJS.
- ❶ Complaints of painful skin or a burning discomfort should alert you to the possibility of TEN. These symptoms are not a feature of morbilliform drug reactions and are rare in other conditions.
- Tender, dusky erythema resembling SJS progressing to widespread subepidermal blistering (the roof of blisters is formed by dead epidermis). The flaccid, thin-walled blisters rupture easily (see Fig. 5.5). For differential diagnosis, see Box 5.17.
- Large sheets of necrotic epidermis that detach, leaving a painful denuded oozing dermis involving >30% of BSA.
- Gentle pressure extends the blisters, and the erythematous epidermis is detached from the underlying dermis by lateral pressure (Nikolsky sign).
- ❶ Inadvertent shearing pressure when handling the patient may cause further detachment.
- Examine the mouth, eyes, and genitalia. Mucosae usually involved (unlike SSSS). Ulceration causes dysphagia, photophobia, or painful micturition.
- Epithelia of the respiratory tract and GI tract may be involved.
- Sequelae may include scarring, irregular pigmentation, dry eye, corneal scarring, photophobia, visual impairment, phimosis, and vaginal synechiae (see Box 5.20).

Box 5.15 Classification of Stevens–Johnson syndrome and toxic epidermal necrolysis

The features in severe SJS overlap with those of TEN:
- SJS: <10% of BSA involved.
- Overlap SJS–TEN: 10–30% of BSA involved.
- TEN: >30% of BSA involved.

Box 5.16 Causes of Stevens–Johnson syndrome and toxic epidermal necrolysis

- Drugs (85%): sulfonamides, NSAIDs, antibiotics—penicillin-related and cephalosporin, anti-epileptics, barbiturates, allopurinol, tetracyclines.
- Viral infections: AIDS, HSV, EBV, influenza.
- Bacterial infections: *Mycoplasma pneumoniae*, typhoid, group A streptococci.
- Fungal infections: dermatophyte, histoplasmosis.
- Protozoal infections.
- Malignancy: Hodgkin lymphoma, leukaemia.
- GVHD.

Box 5.17 Toxic epidermal necrolysis: differential diagnosis

No mucosal signs
- TSS (no blisters, but may simulate early TEN) (see ➔ Box 5.2, p. 101).
- SSSS (also has blisters) (see ➔ p. 112, and Fig. 6.2, p. 131).
- Morbilliform drug rash (no blisters, but may simulate early TEN).
- DRESS (see ➔ pp. 122–3).
- Generalized herpes simplex infection: widespread vesicles (see ➔ p. 112).
- Varicella-zoster infection: widespread vesicles (see ➔ p. 156).

Mucosal involvement
- Acute GVHD.
- Pemphigus vulgaris (may be drug-induced).

Management

see ➔ Management in Stevens–Johnson syndrome or toxic epidermal necrolysis, pp. 118–20.

Further reading

Gueudry J et al. Arch Dermatol 2009;145:157–62 (ocular complications).
Koh MJA and Tay YK. Curr Opin Pediatr 2009;21:505–10.

Management in Stevens–Johnson syndrome or toxic epidermal necrolysis

▶▶ **What should I do?**

- Withdraw all drugs started in the last 4 weeks.
- Take a skin biopsy to confirm the diagnosis. Ensure the specimen includes the epidermis, which may detach during the procedure. The histology shows full-thickness epidermal necrosis in the roof of blisters.
- Rapid information about the level of blistering to differentiate TEN from SSSS may be obtained by detaching the roof of a blister, rolling this up gently, and freezing in liquid nitrogen. Frozen sections of the epidermis can be stained immediately. A Tzank preparation (see ➔ p. 647) can also be used to differentiate TEN from SSSS (see ➔ p. 112).
- Calculate the SCORTEN (see Box 5.19).
- ⚠ Involve a multidisciplinary team, and remind those caring for the patient that TEN is associated with less oedema, less fluid loss, and less vascular damage than a severe burn. Do not overload with fluids (see Box 5.18).

> **Box 5.18 Management—essentially supportive**
>
> - Admit to intensive care unit (ICU), high-dependency unit (HDU), or burn unit (familiar with TEN), particularly if significant skin loss.
> - Relieve pain with regular paracetamol and oral opiates—avoid NSAIDs. Use a VAS to assess pain in all conscious patients daily.
> - Establish peripheral venous access through non-affected skin, if possible, and change every 48h.
> - Central venous lines—risk of infection but can be useful for haemodynamic monitoring.
> - Nutrition: nasogastric (NG) tube (Dobhoff). Avoid total parenteral nutrition (TPN). Provide continuous enteral nutrition—deliver up to 25kcal/kg/day in early phase, and increase to 30kcal/kg/day in anabolic recovery phase.
> - Proton pump inhibitor in acute phase to protect GI mucosa.
> - Foley catheter: keep urine output at 40–60mL/h.
> - Fluids: do not overload. Pulmonary oedema is a frequent complication because of impaired alveolar barrier.
> - Nurse on an air mattress (air fluidized beds increase transepidermal loss of water and heat); use non-stick sheets and heating blankets; keep ambient room temperature at 30–32°C.
> - Skin: protect with 50% white soft paraffin in liquid paraffin, e.g. Emollin spray®, and non-adherent dressings, e.g. Mepitel®/ Mepilex®, or wrap the patient with Sofsorb™ impregnated with 0.5% silver nitrate solution.
> - Prevent infection: reverse barrier-nursing; culture multiple skin sites, sputum, blood, and urine. Repeat every 3 days to guide therapy in the event of sepsis. Avoid prophylactic antibiotics.
> - Eyes: 2-hourly application of lubricants, e.g. hypromellose eye drops; involve ophthalmologists to advise, e.g. use of topical corticosteroids,

Box 5.18 (Contd.)

gently separating synechiae to prevent scarring, corneal fluorescein examination for ulceration; for severe loss of ocular surface epithelia, consider amniotic membrane transplantation.

- Clean lips and oral mucosae with antiseptic mouthwashes/oral sponge.
- Use WSP 2-hourly on lips; protect oral mucosa with mucoprotectant mouthwash three times daily (tds)—e.g. Gelclair®.
- Provide local analgesia for oral mucosa, e.g. viscous lidocaine 2%.
- Consider potent topical steroid mouthwash qds.
- For urogenital skin, use white soft paraffin 4-hourly. Soft silicone dressing (e.g. Mepitel®) prevent adhesions and can be used on eroded vulval and vaginal areas. Dilators or tampon wrapped in soft silicone dressing e.g. Mepitel® should be inserted into the vagina to prevent synechiae.
- IV Ig (1g/kg) for 4 days is controversial. May not improve survival.
- Avoid systemic or potent topical corticosteroids (efficacy unproven, increased risk of infection).
- Subcutaneous heparin for DVT prophylaxis.
- Neutropenic patients may benefit from granulocyte colony-stimulating factor (G-CSF).

Box 5.19 Severity of illness score for Stevens–Johnson syndrome/toxic epidermal necrolysis: SCORTEN

- Rash usually maximal in 4 days, and the skin may start to re-epithelialize within days, but recovery is protracted.
- Sepsis and co-morbidities contribute to high mortality.
- Seven independent factors have been recognized as predictors of mortality. Allocate 1 point for each risk factor present at admission:
  - Age >40 years.
  - Malignancy.
  - Tachycardia >120bpm.
  - Initial percentage of epidermal detachment above 10%—use the rule of nines to calculate % of BSA affected (see ➔ Box 3.5, p. 51), or estimate using the patient's palms as a measure. Each palm without fingers = 0.5% of BSA.
  - Serum urea >10mmol/L.
  - Serum glucose >14mmol/L.
  - Bicarbonate <20mmol/L.

Predicted mortality
- 0–1:   4%
- 2:   12%
- 3:   32%
- 4:   62%
- 5:   85%
- 6:   95%
- 7:   99%

SCORTEN should be calculated in all patients with SJS/TEN within 24h of admission and re-measured at day 3/4.

Box 5.20 **Long-term sequelae of Stevens–Johnson syndrome/toxic epidermal necrolysis**

Chronic phase can develop insidiously over weeks/months.
- Fatigue—especially in early stage after discharge.
- Eyes: photophobia, pain, dryness, corneal scarring, and visual impairment.
- Skin dyspigmentation.
- Loss of nails/dystrophic growth.
- Urogenital dryness or scarring.
- Mouth dryness, scarring, or dental caries.
- Post-traumatic stress disorder, including nightmares, anxiety, and depression.
- Lungs: bronchiectasis.
- GIT—stenosis.
- Loss of muscle mass.

Further reading

Bastuji-Garin S et al. J Invest Dermatol 2000;**115**:149–53 (SCORTEN).
Harr T and French LE. Orphanet J Rare Dis 2010;**5**:39. Available at: ℘ www.ojrd.com/content/5/1/39.
Huang YC et al. Br J Dermatol 2012;**167**:424–32 (IVIg in TEN).
The RegiSCAR Project. Available at: ℘ www.regiscar.org/ (severe cutaneous adverse drug reactions).

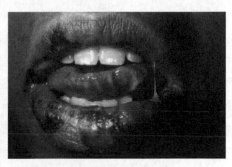

Fig. 5.4 Stevens–Johnson syndrome with crusted haemorrhagic lips and extensive mucosal ulceration in the oral cavity.

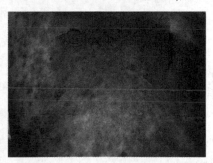

Fig. 5.5 The dusky erythema in toxic epidermal necrolysis progresses to widespread blistering, with loss of the full thickness of the epidermis. Even gentle pressure dislodges sheets of the necrotic epidermis.

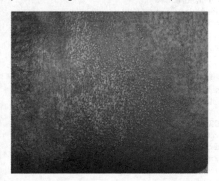

Fig. 5.6 Sheets of sterile non-follicular pustules on an erythematous background in acute generalized exanthematous pustulosis (AGEP). Generalized pustular psoriasis looks similar.

Drug rash, eosinophilia, and systemic symptoms (DRESS)

Synonym: drug-induced hypersensitivity syndrome.

DRESS is a life-threatening cutaneous drug reaction with systemic symptoms that is frequently misdiagnosed as infection. Reactivation of human herpesvirus may play a part in the pathogenesis. Diagnostic criteria are listed in Box 5.21. Commonly develops 1–2 months after the drug is started, but presentation is variable (see Boxes 5.22 and 5.23). The course may be protracted with major morbidity, including progression to liver failure. Mortality is 10%.

What should I look for?

- History of new drug started within prior 2 months (see Box 5.22).
- Flu-like symptoms, e.g. myalgia, arthralgia, headache, sore throat, abdominal pain.
- Fever.
- Sudden-onset diffuse erythematous morbilliform scaly rash with 'juicy' papules that coalesce to plaques (see Box 5.21 for clinical phenotypes). In some cases, onset subacute and protracted.
- Sometimes progresses to erythroderma.
- Pustules or vesicles or purpura.
- Facial oedema (simulates angio-oedema).
- Mild cheilitis/mucosal involvement.
- Lymphadenopathy.

What investigations should I do?

- FBC: eosinophilia common, less often lymphocytosis (sometimes atypical lymphocytes—check blood film), thrombocytopenia, neutrophilia/neutropenia.
- ESR and CRP (raised).
- Liver function tests (LFTs) (raised transaminases and γ glutamyl transferase): risk of liver failure.
- Immunoglobulins (risk of hypogammaglobulinaemia).
- Renal function tests and urinalysis: usually normal.
- Skin biopsy: lymphocytic infiltrate with few eosinophils; severe dyskeratosis may indicate greater systemic involvement.
- Blood cultures: sterile. EBV and CMV titres.

How should I manage DRESS?

- Stop suspected drugs.
- Manage temperature, fluid balance, etc., as for erythroderma (see ➔ Box 5.8, p. 109).
- Emollients, such as 50% WSP in liquid paraffin, to make the skin comfortable, e.g. Emollin® spray.
- Potent topical steroid ointment bd.
- Early treatment with oral prednisolone (0.8–1mg/kg body weight) or IV methylprednisolone recommended to prevent progression.

⚠ Box 5.21 Diagnostic criteria for DRESS

Three or more of the following:
- Acute drug rash (four recognized morphologies):
  - Urticated papular eruption.
  - EM-like (EM-like, atypical targets, often purpuric evolving into confluent areas of dusky erythema)—may be prognostic of more severe hepatic involvement.
  - Morbilliform erythema.
  - Exfoliative erythroderma.
- Fever >38°C.
- Lymphadenopathy.
- Systemic involvement variable; commonest hepatitis (↑ aspartate aminotransferase, AST), interstitial nephritis/pneumonitis, arthritis, and/or pericarditis.
- Blood anomalies: eosinophilia ± abnormal lymphocytes.

Box 5.22 Drugs associated with DRESS

Most frequent
- Anticonvulsants, dapsone, sulfonamides, including sulfasalazine.

Others
- Allopurinol.
- Antibiotics: vancomycin, minocycline, amoxicillin.
- Gold salts.
- Sorbinil.
- Calcium channel blockers.
- Ranitidine.
- Thalidomide.
- Mexiletine.
- Telaprevir (protease inhibitor to treat chronic hepatitis C).
- Imatinib.

Box 5.23 Differential diagnosis of DRESS

- Serum sickness or drug-induced vasculitis (see ➜ p. 373, p. 376).
- Infection: viral (HHV 6, CMV, EBV) or bacterial.
- Idiopathic hypereosinophilic syndrome.
- Lymphoma.
- Acute GVHD (lower T-regulatory cell levels)

Further reading

Husain Z et al. J Am Acad Dermatol 2013;68:693 and 709.
Kardaun SH et al. Br J Dermatol 2013;169:1071–80.

Generalized pustules

Introduction

Pustules are a focal accumulation of inflammatory cells and serum in skin. Pustules may indicate infection, e.g. staphylococcal folliculitis (pustules associated with hair follicles), but, in most infections, pustules are grouped, localized, and asymmetrical. For causes of widespread symmetrical pustular eruptions in sick patients, see Box 5.24.

What should I look for?
- Is the patient ill, e.g. high fever, malaise?
- What is the 1° lesion—is it really a pustule, i.e. a bump filled with creamy fluid, or is it a vesicle, i.e. a bump filled with clear serous fluid that evolves into a pustule (as in VZV infection)?
- Distribution: symmetrical (endogenous cause) or asymmetrical?
- How do pustules evolve? What is the time course?
- Are pustules associated with hair follicles, i.e. is it a folliculitis?
- Erythema, oedema, desquamation, or mucosal involvement.

Acute generalized exanthematous pustulosis (AGEP)

Over 90% of cases are drug-induced. Usually takes 1–3 weeks for rash to develop, but patients who are sensitized may develop AGEP within a few hours of exposure to the drug—for signs, see Box 5.25. May be difficult to distinguish from generalized pustular psoriasis (GPP).

What should I do?
- Reassure the patient and medical and nursing staff that this is a self-limiting condition and is not an infection.
- Culture blood and skin—these are sterile.
- Take a skin biopsy (shows subcorneal pustules).
- Stop the causative drug, most often an antibacterial.
- Prescribe an emollient, e.g. 50% WSP in liquid paraffin, a mild topical corticosteroid, and a sedating antihistamine to relieve discomfort.

Generalized pustular psoriasis

❶ Some patients have a history of psoriasis/psoriatic arthritis. Pustular psoriasis may be triggered by irritation of the skin, infections, withdrawal of systemic corticosteroids or drugs (lithium), but the trigger may not be identified. Lasts longer than AGEP (see earlier in this section and Box 5.26).

What should I do?
- Admit the patient, and manage skin failure (see ➔ Box 5.7, p. 107).
- Exclude an infection—cultures of blood and skin will be sterile. Reassure the patient and medical and nursing staff that this is not an infection.
- Check FBC, renal function, liver function, and serum calcium.
- Obtain a skin biopsy to confirm the diagnosis (subcorneal pustules).
- Avoid potential irritants. Prescribe an emollient, e.g. 50% WSP in liquid paraffin, a mild topical corticosteroid, and a sedating antihistamine to relieve discomfort.
- Continue to monitor for hypocalcaemia (rare complication).
- Consider acitretin or methotrexate—if not settling, see ➔ p. 668.

Box 5.24 **Causes of widespread pustular eruptions**

- Eczema herpeticum or varicella: the 1° lesion is actually a vesicle, but pustules with crusting occur as a 2° phenomenon—check for a history of atopic eczema (see ➜ p. 112 and p. 156).
- Pustular psoriasis: check for a history of psoriasis or arthritis.
- AGEP: ask about drugs started in previous 1–3 weeks.
- Acne fulminans: severe acne flare with haemorrhagic, crusted ulcers on the trunk and face and systemic symptoms (see ➜ p. 248).
- Subcorneal pustular dermatosis/IgA pemphigus (rare).

Box 5.25 **Acute generalized exanthematous pustulosis—what should I look for?**

(See Fig. 5.6.)
- Sudden onset of an oedematous erythema that burns or itches. Often begins on the face, axillae, and groins and spreads within hours.
- Flexural accentuation is a common feature.
- Soon followed by the appearance of hundreds of pinhead-sized, mostly non-follicular, pustules.
- Confluent pustules may produce superficial erosions.
- Some patients have marked facial swelling; few develop purpura, on legs. May also develop vesicles, bullae, and EM-like lesions.
- Over 20% have mild mucosal involvement (usually oral).
- Fever >38°C and neutrophilia (blood culture and swabs sterile).
- Systemic involvement unusual; liver, kidney, bone marrow, and lung involvement (associated with elevated CRP levels).
- Spontaneous resolution of pustules in <15 days (more rapid than in pustular psoriasis), followed by desquamation.

❶Box 5.26 **Generalized pustular psoriasis—what should I look for?**

- Evidence of psoriasis, e.g. nail pitting, psoriatic arthritis, but many patients report no prior history of psoriasis.
- Fever and neutrophilia (swabs and blood cultures sterile).
- Scaly, erythematous, tender skin.
- Sheets of sterile non-follicular pustules, particularly in flexures and genital skin, arising on a background of tender erythema.
- Pustules may coalesce into lakes of pus.
- Pustules dry and skin desquamates, leaving a shiny erythematous surface on which waves of pustules may continue to appear.
- Normal mucosal surfaces.
- The process may continue for weeks (unlike AGEP).
- Complications are those of skin failure (see ➜ p. 106).
- Hypocalcaemia is a rare complication.

Further reading

Sidoroff A *et al. J Cutan Pathol* 2001;**28**:113–19.

Necrotizing fasciitis

What is necrotizing fasciitis?

❶ Necrotizing fasciitis is a *life-threatening* soft tissue infection, characterized by rapidly progressive necrosis that spreads from subcutaneous tissue into the deep fascia. High mortality (25%) 2° to organ failure and to streptococcal TSS (see ➔ Box 5.2, p. 101 and Box 5.27).

Consider the diagnosis in any sick patient not responding to treatment for 'cellulitis' with pain that appears out of proportion to the signs. The depth and extent of necrosis may be much greater than the appearance of the skin suggests, and, in early stages, the condition is often misdiagnosed. Rarely can present at multiple sites.

What should I look for?

- History of recent trauma, e.g. insect bite, skin biopsy, chronic leg ulcer, surgery, IV drug abuse. Not all patients have an obvious portal of entry. For predisposing factors, see Box 5.28.
- Ill patient with high temperature, tachycardia, low blood pressure.
- Pain that is out of proportion to the signs in the skin.
- Altered level of consciousness—signs of shock are associated with 50% mortality.
- Rapidly spreading, poorly demarcated purplish erythema—commonly extremities > perineum, genitalia (Fournier gangrene—polymicrobial infection) > trunk.
- Oedema extending beyond erythema and tender induration/blisters.
- Malodorous serosanguineous exudate ('dishwater' pus).
- Crepitation in soft tissues (gas from aerobic and anaerobic bacteria).

In the later stages, you may see:
- Black necrotic plaques.
- Painless ulcers.
- Vascular occlusion and gangrene.

▶▶ What should I do?

- Request an urgent surgical opinion—immediate deep surgical debridement of all necrotic tissue is absolutely essential. The diagnosis is clinical—do not wait for results of investigations (see Box 5.29).
- Start a combination of IV broad-spectrum antibiotics immediately, and contact a microbiologist to discuss treatment (see Box 5.30).
- Gram stain and culture any blister fluid/fluid draining from the wound.
- Check FBC, electrolytes, and renal function.
- Arrange to take deep tissue at the time of surgery for histological examination and culture for aerobic and anaerobic bacteria.
- Magnetic resonance imaging (MRI) or computed tomography (CT) to identify subcutaneous air and define the extent of involvement.
- Admit to the intensive care unit (ICU) for resuscitation and monitoring.
- Consider IV Ig for streptococcal TSS.

Box 5.27 Classification of necrotizing fasciitis

- Type I: polymicrobial. Two or more pathogens. Obligate and facultative anaerobes. Trunk and perineum, older patients with co-morbidities, e.g. diabetes.
- Type II: group A β-haemolytic streptococci (50% occur in young healthy people) ± staphylococcal species (*Staphylococcus aureus*, including meticillin-resistant strains). Aggressive course. Associated with trauma, surgery, or IV drug use. Risk of TSS.
- Type III: *Clostridium* species (*C. perfringens* commonest—gas gangrene). Associated with trauma, e.g. surgery. Also seen with Gram-negative marine organisms, e.g. *Vibrio vulnificus* (commonest in Asia)—rapid progression.
- Type IV: fungal, e.g. *Candida* species, *Zygomycetes*. Limbs, trunk, perineum. Associated with immunosuppression.

Box 5.28 What factors predispose to necrotizing fasciitis?

- Diabetes, AIDS or other immune deficiency.
- Chronic alcohol or drug abuse, malnutrition.
- Surgery and other trauma.
- Obesity.
- Malignancy.
- Peripheral vascular disease.

Box 5.29 The finger test

The finger test may help to confirm the diagnosis. Can be performed at the bedside under local anaesthesia or during surgery.
- Make a 2cm vertical incision into the skin to the deep fascia.
- Push an index finger (or probe) gently into normal-appearing tissue at the junction of the subcutaneous tissue and fascia.
- If subcutaneous tissue easily dissected off underlying fascia, finger test is positive—confirming the diagnosis of necrotizing fasciitis. Necrotic tissue or 'dishwater' pus found between fascial planes.

Box 5.30 Choice of antibiotics in necrotizing fasciitis

- Initially, prescribe broad-spectrum antibiotic cover to treat Gram-positive and Gram-negative bacteria and anaerobes, e.g. vancomycin and meropenem.
- For those with penicillin allergy, use vancomycin plus clindamycin plus an aminoglycoside (or quinolone).
- Consult a microbiologist for advice on further treatment when the results of culture are known.

Further reading

Hakkarainen TW et al. Curr Probl Surg 2014;51:344–62.

Bacterial and spirochaetal infections

Contents

Relevant pages in other chapters

Chapter 5: Skin failure and emergency dermatology:
Rash in a sick adult with a fever ➜ p. 100
Box 5.2 Toxic shock syndrome ➜ p. 101
Meningococcal septicaemia ➜ pp. 102–3
Staphylococcal scalded skin syndrome ➜ pp. 136–7
Necrotizing fasciitis ➜ pp. 126–7
IgA vasculitis ➜ p. 442
Septic cutaneous vasculitis ➜ p. 448

Introduction

Skin flora

Skin creases, surface scale, and deep follicular orifices provide just what is needed for the survival of a wide variety of microflora. Conditions vary—the skin may be dry, greasy, or moist, the temperature warm or cool, the blood supply good or poor, and the surface intact or ulcerated. The environment and the host immune response modify the density and diversity of colonization in individuals.

Resident colonizing species include a mixture of staphylococci, micrococci, and diphtheroids, as well as yeasts. These maintain a viable reproducing population on the skin and help to defend the skin against pathogens. In some circumstances, overgrowth of the normal skin microflora is linked to problems, e.g. *Propionibacterium acnes* in the hair follicles in acne.

Some people carry *Staphylococcus aureus* in the nostrils, perineum, or axillae (see Box 6.1). Staphylococci also colonize the skin in diseases, such as atopic eczema, when large numbers of organisms may be shed with the scale. Methicillin-resistant *S. aureus* (MRSA) may be carried asymptomatically but, like methicillin-sensitive *S. aureus* (MSSA), may also cause cutaneous infections (impetigo—see Fig. 6.1, folliculitis, 'boils'). MRSA is resistant to β-lactam antibiotics, including penicillins and cephalosporins (see Box 6.2). MRSA decolonization aims to reduce risks of auto-infection and transmission.

Prescribe antimicrobials with care (Right Drug, Right Dose, Right Time, Right Duration) to limit the development of antimicrobial resistance (a global problem) and to reduce the threat of untreatable infections. Adhere to local evidence-based guidelines.

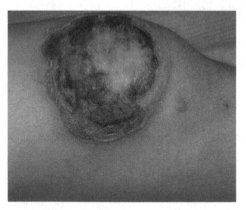

Fig. 6.1 Bullous impetigo with golden crusting (see ➔ p. 136).

Box 6.1 Nasal carriage of *Staphylococcus aureus*

- Nasal carriage of *S. aureus* is common, and some patients carry MRSA in the nose.
- There is no consensus about the best way of dealing with MRSA carriage.
- Mupirocin 2% ointment bd inside each nostril for no more than 7 days may eradicate nasal MRSA, but prolonged or repeated use will increase the risk of emergence of mupirocin-resistant strains.
- Chlorhexidine or neomycin creams may be helpful.

Box 6.2 MRSA and skin infections

- Community-associated and health care-associated strains of MRSA cause increasing numbers of skin infections.
- MRSA can survive for long periods in dust, furnishing, and clothing.
- Patients who have received fluoroquinolones and third-generation cephalosporins are more likely to be colonized with MRSA.
- MRSA is resistant to antibiotics such as penicillins and cephalosporins. Some strains are also resistant to erythromycin.
- Decolonize with antibacterial shampoo and a skin cleanser (triclosan, 4% chlorhexidine, or 7.5% povidone iodine), and tds antibacterial nasal cream (mupirocin 2%) for 5 days.
- Reinforce hygiene measures, and use alcohol-based hand rubs to prevent transfer of MRSA from patient to patient.
- Options for treatment of MRSA skin infections may include vancomycin, tetracyclines, trimoxazole, clindamycin, and linezolid.
- Some strains of MRSA also produce Panton–Valentine leukocidin (PVL), increasing virulence.

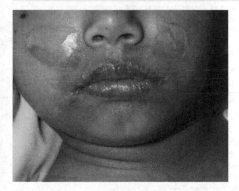

Fig. 6.2 Staphylococcal scalded skin syndrome (SSSS). Tender erythema and superficial desquamation caused by a circulating epidermolytic toxin (see ➲ pp. 136–7).

Further reading

Dixon J and Duncan CJA. *Infect Drug Resist* 2014;7:145–52.

Flexural bacterial infections

Erythrasma

Erythrasma is caused by overgrowth of *Corynebacterium minutissimum*, a skin commensal in the horny layer of the epidermis.

What predisposes to erythrasma?
- Warm humid climates, hyperhidrosis, obesity.
- Diabetes, immunosuppression, old age.

What should I look for?
- One or more asymptomatic, well-demarcated, slightly scaly, reddish brown patches in a moist flexure such as the axilla, under the breasts, in the groin, or between the toes.
- Erythrasma resembles a dermatophyte (tinea) infection, but skin fluoresces a striking coral pink under UV Wood light (see ➲ p. 640).

What should I do?
- Prescribe a topical antibiotic such as 2% fusidic acid (most effective), clindamycin, or tetracycline. A single dose of clarithromycin (1g/day) is also effective.

Pseudomonas and flexures

What should I look for?
- *Pseudomonas* infection of moist toe webs produces superficial erosions with a rather moth-eaten macerated border.
- *Pseudomonas aeruginosa* axillary infections are uncommon but may be potentiated by washes with antibacterial lotions that reduce colonization with Gram-positive commensals. The brownish grey, scaly rash fissures and is painful, unlike erythrasma.
- ⚠ *Pseudomonas* causes anogenital ecthyma gangrenosum in immunosuppressed patients. If untreated, pustules rapidly become bullous and necrotic (see ➲ p. 137).

What should I do?
- Axillary infection: stop antibacterial lotions; keep the skin dry.
- Biopsy and culture tissue from ecthyma gangrenosum. Treat promptly with IV antibiotics.

Perianal streptococcal dermatitis

Group A β-haemolytic *Streptococcus* causes perianal dermatitis in pre-pubertal children and, less often, in adults.

What should I look for?
- A history of an itchy, painful perianal rash unresponsive to topical antifungals or topical corticosteroids. Pain on defecation.
- Well-demarcated, bright red perianal erythema.
- Swelling, scale, and fissuring.

What should I do?
- Culture a skin swab.
- Treat with oral antibiotics, e.g. amoxicillin for 10 days.

Folliculitis and furunculosis

What is folliculitis?

Folliculitis is inflammation of hair follicles (see Box 6.3). *S. aureus* is the commonest cause of a bacterial folliculitis. *P. aeruginosa* may cause folliculitis after hot tubs or whirlpools. Superficial bacterial folliculitis is usually self-limiting but may be recurrent. Deeper folliculitis involving the entire follicle and surrounding tissues (furunculosis) heals with scarring or can progress to cellulitis. Community-acquired strains of *S. aureus* carrying genes that encode the neutrophil cytotoxin Panton–Valentine leukocidin (PVL) cause numerous deep furuncles, abscesses, cellulitis, and necrotizing pneumonia in healthy young adults and children. Severe and recurrent staphylococcal skin disease, which is difficult to treat, is leading to more hospital admissions.

What may predispose to bacterial folliculitis or furunculosis?

(The evidence is inconclusive.)
- Occlusion or maceration; tropical climates.
- Hot tubs or whirlpools (*P. aeruginosa* folliculitis).
- Crowded living conditions, poor hygiene, malnutrition.
- Diabetes, alcoholism, immunodeficiency, or oral corticosteroids.
- Blood dyscrasias and disorders of neutrophil function.

What should I look for?

- Superficial folliculitis may be itchy; deep folliculitis is tender.
- Perifollicular erythematous papules or small pustules—the pustule may be pierced by a hair.
- Crusting of follicular openings when pustules rupture.
- Tender, inflamed furuncles ('boils') with abscesses in deep infection.
- Furuncles may discharge and heal with scarring.
- A group of deeply infected follicles leading to a tender erythematous nodule—a carbuncle. Pus discharges from several points.
- Follicular pustules or papules 8–48h after exposure to hot tub or whirlpool at sites covered by bathing suit (*P. aeruginosa* folliculitis).

What should I do in bacterial folliculitis?

- Remove or minimize precipitating factors.
- Antiseptic washes are all that is needed in most superficial cases.
- If folliculitis does not settle, take swabs for culture from pustules.
- Alcohol-based washes or triclosan are effective against MRSA and strains of *Staphylococcus* producing PVL.
- Topical antibiotics, e.g. 2% mupirocin ointment, clindamycin lotion, or erythromycin lotion may be indicated.
- Deep infection requires oral anti-staphylococcal antibiotics.
- Carbuncles should be incised and drained surgically.

How should I manage recurrent cutaneous bacterial infections?

- Culture pus and swabs from potential carrier sites, e.g. nose, axilla, groin, and perineum, in the patient and the family.

- Exclude diabetes, and minimize other predisposing factors.
- Decolonize the skin with daily antimicrobial skin washes with triclosan, chlorhexidine, or benzalkonium chloride (Dermol 600®, Oilatum Plus®, or Aquasept®).
- Treat chronic *S. aureus* nasal carriage with short bursts of 2% mupirocin ointment.
- Benzoyl peroxide 5% gel applied bd may help to prevent recurrent staphylococcal folliculitis.
- Consider oral antibiotics, but check sensitivities, and choose wisely.
- Reinforce hygiene measures—recommend liquid antiseptic soap, instead of bars of soap, and separate towels for family members to reduce the risk of recolonization by household fomites.

Box 6.3 Differential diagnosis in patients with folliculitis

Mechanical folliculitis
- Waxing or plucking hairs.
- Ingrowing hairs, e.g. after close shave of curly hair (pseudofolliculitis) or close haircut 'grade 1'.
- Pulling back hair tightly (traction folliculitis).
- Friction caused by tight clothing.

Medicaments
- Topical preparations with high concentrations of tar.
- Occlusion of follicles with ointments.

Infections
- Bacterial: *S. aureus, Pseudomonas.*
- Dermatophyte (tinea) scalp: hair is lost, or beard (uncommon).
- Pityrosporum (a commensal yeast) folliculitis on the trunk (see ➔ p. 219).

Inflammatory skin diseases
- Acne: pustules on the face and sometimes trunk—look for comedones, nodules, and scars (see ➔ pp. 242–3).
- Rosacea: facial pustules, papules, erythema, but no comedones (see ➔ p. 254).
- Demodicosis in the immunocompromised (see also ➔ p. 178).
- Hidradenitis suppurativa: recurrent furunculosis in the groin and/or axilla. Look for groups of comedones, sinuses, and scars (see ➔ pp. 250–52).

Non-follicular pustules
- Pustular psoriasis (see ➔ pp. 124–5).
- Drug reactions (see ➔ p. 124).

Further reading

Fogo A et al. BMJ 2011;343:d5343 (PVL-positive *Staphylococcus aureus* infections).
Shallcross LJ et al. Epidemiol Infect 2015;143:2426–9.

Impetigo, toxin-mediated disease, and ecthyma

Impetigo

What is impetigo?
- Impetigo is a superficial skin infection that may develop on normal skin or may complicate eczema (impetiginized eczema).
- Crusted impetigo (impetigo contagiosa) is caused by *S. aureus*, *Streptococcus pyogenes*, or a combination of both.
- Bullous impetigo is mediated by epidermolytic toxins (ET) released by phage group II *S. aureus*. Toxins disrupt adhesion between keratinocytes in the superficial epidermis within an area of infection by cleaving a specific desmosomal cadherin, desmoglein 1. This enables S. *aureus* to penetrate the skin barrier, proliferate, and spread under the stratum corneum. (Also see ➔ Staphylococcal scalded skin syndrome (SSSS), p. 112.)
- Factors that predispose to impetigo include minor trauma, including insect bites, eczema, head lice, hot climates, crowded living conditions, poor hygiene, and immunodeficiency.

What should I look for?
- One or more areas of golden, honey-coloured crusting and oozing (see Fig. 6.1).
- Thin-walled, flaccid blisters that rupture rapidly, because epidermal cleavage is superficial, just below the stratum corneum.
- Patients with localized impetigo do not have systemic symptoms.
- Several members of the family may be affected.

What should I do?
- Take skin swabs from crusted skin for culture (in SSSS, swabs from the erythema and blisters will be sterile, as the signs are caused by the circulating toxin, and not local infection) (see ➔ p. 112).
- A topical antibiotic, such as fusidic acid or mupirocin, is sufficient in patients with a small focus of infection. In more widespread or recurrent infections, prescribe an oral antibiotic such as flucloxacillin or erythromycin—alter according to sensitivities.
- The focus of infection in SSSS (see ➔ pp. 136–7) should be treated with an oral antibiotic.
- Antiseptic wash may be helpful in patients with recurrent impetigo.

Toxin-mediated diseases

- ▶▶ *SSSS* (Ritter disease) presents in neonates, young children, adults with renal failure, and the immunosuppressed. Patients have a focus of impetigo caused by the strain of *Staphylococcus* that releases epidermolytic toxins. This focus may not be apparent. The circulating ET cause widespread erythema and superficial blistering (see ➔ p. 112 and Fig. 6.2).

- ▶▶ *TSS* is a multisystem disease caused by an exotoxin produced most often by *S. aureus*. TSS may be mild or rapidly fatal (see ➲ Box 5.2, p. 101).

Ecthyma

What is ecthyma?

- A deeper infection than impetigo that is caused by *S. pyogenes* or, less often, *S. aureus*.
- Commoner in the malnourished or immunosuppressed.
- Seen most often on the legs and usually preceded by a minor injury or insect bite.
- Starts as a blister with an erythematous border ('deep impetigo') but develops into a well-circumscribed 'punched-out' ulcer involving the full thickness of the epidermis. May enlarge to a diameter of 2–3cm, if untreated. Only a few lesions. Heals slowly with scarring.
- Systemic symptoms are uncommon.

What should I do?

- Take skin swabs for culture, and treat with oral antibiotics, e.g. flucloxacillin.

Ecthyma gangrenosum

What is ecthyma gangrenosum?

- ▶▶ This infection caused by *P. aeruginosa* is associated with debility and immunosuppression. Ecthyma gangrenosum is usually a manifestation of *Pseudomonas* septicaemia. It may not be possible to demonstrate a bacteraemia in the anogenital form in immunocompromised patients when *Pseudomonas* may enter the skin through a wound or hair follicle.
- Starts as a painless erythematous or purpuric macule on limbs or anogenital skin. Develops into a nodule with a central haemorrhagic vesicle that breaks down to form a large necrotic ulcer with a central dark eschar and an inflamed border. Several lesions may be present.
- Mortality is 10–20%.
- Differential includes PG, necrotizing vasculitis, cryoglobulinaemia, and septic emboli from other organisms.

What should I do?

- Take a skin biopsy for histology and culture (see ➲ Box 33.2, p. 645).
- Culture blood and urine.
- Treat with IV antibiotics.

Erysipelas and cellulitis

What are erysipelas and cellulitis?

These acute infections of the dermis and subcutaneous tissue are usually caused by *S. pyogenes*. Other bacteria, such as *S. aureus*, may be involved, particularly in the immunosuppressed or those with diabetes. Erysipelas involves the dermis, whereas cellulitis affects the deep dermis and subcutaneous tissues. Both are a common cause of hospital admission.

What predisposes to erysipelas/cellulitis?

- Defective skin barrier, e.g. eczema, tinea pedis, leg ulcers, wounds.
- Diabetes or immunosuppression.
- Chronic lymphoedema. Local immune deficiency predisposes to cellulitis, but each episode damages the lymphatics, which increases the predisposition to recurrence.
- Peripheral vascular disease.
- Previous episodes of cellulitis.

What should I look for?

- Sudden onset of pain.
- Malaise, fever, and rigors may precede a rash but may not be apparent in the elderly. Systemic symptoms are common in erysipelas.
- Asymmetrical, warm, tender spreading erythema that is particularly well demarcated in erysipelas; swelling sometimes with blisters.
- Examine both the unaffected and affected limbs for evidence of chronic lymphoedema, but signs may be subtle (see Box 6.4). 1° lymphoedema of the lower limb, 2° to aplasia or hypoplasia of lymphatic vessels, may be subclinical and bilateral.

What simulates erysipelas/cellulitis?

- Acute contact dermatitis: the patient usually complains of itch. Early in the presentation, the skin may not be particularly scaly but will be erythematous and oedematous. Blisters are common (see ➡ Fig. 10.1, p. 216).
- Dermatitis 2° to venous stasis or asteatotic dermatitis. Typically, cellulitis is asymmetrical. Reconsider your diagnosis if the patient seems to have 'cellulitis' affecting both legs. The redness, scaling, and swelling are much more likely to be a manifestation of dermatitis (see ➡ p. 220).
- Lipodermatosclerosis, a panniculitis associated with venous stasis (see Box 6.6; also see ➡ p. 308, and Fig. 15.6, p. 309).
- Herpes simplex infection, particularly a 1° infection (see ➡ p. 152).
- Erysipeloid (see ➡ p. 140).
- Eosinophilic fasciitis (see ➡ p. 421).
- Eosinophilic cellulitis (Wells syndrome) (see ➡ p. 68).
- ⚠ Autoinflammatory diseases (see ➡ pp. 234–5).

What should I do?

- Superficial skin swabs for culture are not helpful, unless there is an open wound or an exudate. Remember no chronic leg ulcer is sterile.
- Take blood for culture if the patient has systemic symptoms. Bacteraemia is common in erysipelas.
- Prescribe antibiotics, initially IV, e.g. ceftriaxone or flucloxacillin and penicillin (also see Box 6.5).
- Elevate the affected part.

Box 6.4 Signs of chronic lymphoedema

- Firm, non-pitting oedema (oedema may pit in the early stages).
- Stemmer sign is present—thickening of the skin in the interdigital web space between the second and third toes makes it impossible to pick up a fold of skin.
- Papillomatous thickening of the skin surface (elephantiasis nostra).
- Fluid-filled blebs (lymphoceles).

Box 6.5 Recurrent cellulitis in lymphoedema

- Advise on skin care: antiseptic washes, emollients to prevent skin cracking; treat any tinea pedis.
- Control limb swelling with compression hosiery.
- Prophylactic penicillin V 250mg bd for at least 6 months has been shown to reduce the frequency of recurrent episodes.

Box 6.6 Lipodermatosclerosis

This chronic panniculitis (inflammation in fat) is associated with venous disease. It may be misdiagnosed as cellulitis but is not associated with systemic upset and does not respond to antibiotics.

What should I look for?
- Check for a history of venous disease, leg ulcers, or limb swelling.
- Skin in the gaiter area is erythematous, indurated, and tight.
- The skin may be tender but is not hot.
- Look for other signs of venous stasis such as pigmentation.
- You may see varicose veins (stand the patient up).
- Peripheral pulses are normal.
- As the condition progresses, the leg adopts the shape of an inverted champagne bottle. Tissues above the ankle tighten.
- The other leg may be affected.

What should I do?
- Treat with compression bandaging/stockings, but you may have to increase compression gradually because of pain.

Further reading

Thomas KS et al. N Engl J Med 2013;**368**:1695–703.

Erysipeloid

What is erysipeloid?

This acute infection of skin and soft tissue is caused by *Erysipelothrix rhusiopathiae*. The organism is inoculated through broken skin, usually on the hand. The infection is seen most often in individuals who are in contact with poultry, fish, crabs, or pigs, e.g. fishermen, butchers, farmers, and vets. The organism remains viable for months in decomposing material and can survive smoking or pickling.

What should I look for?

- Local pain, itching, burning, and swelling, usually on the hand or finger.
- A purplish red plaque, with demarcated raised borders, that expands peripherally and clears centrally. Occasionally, you may find >1 lesion.
- You may see blistering.
- Some patients have regional lymphadenopathy.
- Systemic symptoms, such as fever and malaise, are uncommon in patients with localized cutaneous disease (unlike erysipelas).
- Rarely, erysipeloid presents as a systemic infection. In addition to skin lesions, patients may have septic arthritis, bacterial endocarditis, cerebral lesions, or pulmonary involvement. These patients have positive blood cultures.

How can I distinguish erysipeloid from erysipelas or cellulitis?

- The occupational history may provide a clue to the diagnosis.
- Erysipeloid tends to involve the hands or fingers, whereas the face and leg are affected more often by erysipelas or cellulitis.
- Patients with erysipelas or cellulitis are more likely to have systemic symptoms such as fever or rigors.

What should I do?

- The organism is difficult to culture.
- A skin biopsy may help to confirm the diagnosis.
- ❶ Incision and drainage are contraindicated, as these prolong the course.
- Although localized cutaneous disease is usually self-limiting, prescribe penicillin to prevent progression to systemic disease with the risk of endocarditis.

Cat-scratch disease

What is cat-scratch disease?

Bartonella henselae, a common infection in cats, causes localized cutaneous infection in humans. The organism is passed between cats by the bites of cat fleas and is transmitted to humans by cat scratches or the saliva in cat bites. Most patients are under 21 years of age.

What should I look for?

- A history of a cat bite or scratch (90% of patients).
- After 3–10 days, an erythematous papule, pustule, vesicle, or nodule develops at the site of inoculation. It may persist for several months.
- Tender regional lymphadenopathy develops about 2 weeks after the bite or scratch and may persist for 2–4 months. Cat-scratch disease is the commonest cause of chronic benign lymphadenopathy in children and adolescents.
- Mild fever.

What should I do?

- The disease is self-limiting, resolving within 2–6 months. No specific treatment is needed.

Bacillary angiomatosis

What is bacillary angiomatosis?

Bacillary angiomatosis is a life-threatening infection caused by *Bartonella henselae* (transmitted to humans by the scratches or saliva of infected cats) or *Bartonella quintana* (transmitted by the human body louse) that presents most often in immunosuppressed patients (HIV, organ transplantation, leukaemia, chemotherapy).

Skin, mucosal surfaces, bones, and viscera may be involved by tumour-like vascular masses.

What should I look for?

- Red or purplish cutaneous and/or subcutaneous vascular papules and tender nodules, ranging in diameter from a few mm to 10cm. The presentation may simulate Kaposi sarcoma (KS), but lesions are less common on soles or in the mouth than in KS (see ➡ pp. 362–3).
- Fever, nausea, vomiting, headache, malaise, and weight loss.
- Tender lymphadenopathy which may suppurate.
- Focal bone pain.

What should I do?

- Biopsy the skin, and take blood for cultures.
- Treat promptly with erythromycin 500mg qds (or doxycycline) for up to 4 months in immunocompromised patients.
- Provide analgesia for pain and fever.

Meningococcal infections

Meningococcal disease is caused by *Neisseria meningitidis*, a bacterium that is commonly carried in the nasopharynx. Disruption of nasal mucosal membranes, perhaps by viral infection, may facilitate the development of invasive disease. The severity of the disease is related, in part, to the virulence of the meningococcus and to the potential for release of endotoxin, which plays a key part in the pathogenesis of meningococcal septic shock.

Meningococcal septicaemia

▶▶ Fulminant meningococcal infection can cause septicaemia (acute meningococcaemia) and death within hours of the first symptoms. Early diagnosis may depend on the recognition of cutaneous signs that include:

- An erythematous maculopapular rash.
- Petechiae—usually palpable, but may be sparse in the early stages.
- Purpura fulminans with ecchymoses, large areas of haemorrhage, and haemorrhagic blistering.
- Gangrene and extensive skin infarction.

The condition is discussed on ⮕ pp. 102–3.

Chronic meningococcaemia

- This immune complex-mediated illness presents with a low-grade relapsing fever that is associated with a vasculitic rash and problems such as arthralgia, pneumonia, or ophthalmitis.
- Several blood cultures may be needed before the diagnosis is confirmed, but chronic meningococcaemia responds rapidly to systemic antibiotics.
- The differential diagnosis encompasses other causes of cutaneous vasculitis, including IgA vasculitis (Henoch–Schönlein purpura).

(See also ⮕ p. 442 and p. 448.)

Mycobacterial infections

Cutaneous tuberculosis

(See Box 6.7.)

Cutaneous TB is uncommon. *Mycobacterium tuberculosis* may be inoculated into the skin from an exogenous source or spread to the skin from an underlying infection or the bloodstream. Presentation is determined by the host immune response. Histology is granulomatous (see ➔ Box 33.5, p. 651). If suspected, send biopsy material for TB culture (see ➔ Box 33.2, p. 645). *M. tuberculosis* DNA may also be detected using PCR. Hypersensitivity reactions to 1° infection include EN (see ➔ pp. 458–9). Rarely, immunization with bacille Calmette–Guérin (BCG) (*M. bovis*) causes lupus vulgaris-like lesions, as well as cutaneous granulomas.

Non-tuberculous (atypical) mycobacterial infection

- *Mycobacterium marinum*: infection seen in owners of tropical fish who inoculate bacteria into the skin when cleaning the fish tank. Presents as an indolent reddish brown nodule (fish tank granuloma), usually on the finger or hand. May be self-limiting, but nodules may spread up the limb along lymphatic channels. Culture biopsy for mycobacteria at 30°C. Treat with antibiotics, e.g. tetracyclines, for ≥3 months.
- *Mycobacterium ulcerans*: tropical infection that causes progressive ulceration with destruction of the skin and subcutaneous tissue (Buruli ulcers).
- *Mycobacterium chelonae*: community-acquired infection of the skin and soft tissue. Bacteria are found in natural and processed water sources. Cutaneous infection is preceded by trauma, e.g. tattoos (non-sterile water used to clean needles and/or dilute ink), subcutaneous injections, lacerations, or fractures. Presents with non-tender brownish red subcutaneous nodules singly or in groups. Commoner in the immunosuppressed when may disseminate.
- *Mycobacterium kansasii* and *Mycobacterium fortuitum*: cutaneous infection may occur in the immunosuppressed. Localized infection has been described at sites of subcutaneous insulin infusion.

Leprosy (Hansen disease)

- Tropical infection caused by *Mycobacterium leprae*, seen outside the tropics as people migrate to other countries. Symptoms and signs determined predominantly by the host immune response, which may downgrade or upgrade. Bacteria have a predilection for cool skin, e.g. nose or ears, and for cutaneous nerves (see Box 6.8).
- Tuberculoid disease: high cell-mediated immunity, bacilli difficult to find in skin lesions, nerves damaged early by immune response.
- Lepromatous disease: poor cell-mediated immunity, widespread infection, numerous bacilli in the dermis.
- Borderline disease: intermediate immune response.
- Diagnosis is confirmed histologically.
- Drugs, e.g. rifampicin, dapsone, and clofazimine, are used in combination, according to World Health Organization (WHO) protocols.
- Surgeons and rehabilitation experts may be involved in the management of deformity or loss of function.

Box 6.7 Spectrum of cutaneous tuberculosis

- Chancres (indolent ulcers) after inoculation of the skin or mucosae.
- Scrofuloderma: direct extension of TB in underlying lymph nodes, bones/joints ('the King's evil'). Associated with pulmonary TB.
- Miliary TB: spread by bloodstream to a variety of organs, including the skin where TB presents as papules and pustules or purpura. This form is commoner in immunosuppressed patients. Painful eroded papules and plaques may develop on the tongue or palate.
- TB abscess (gumma): caused by extension of TB into the skin from an underlying focus such as the lung or bone.
- Tuberculosis verrucosa cutis: direct inoculation in patients who have some immunity. Hyperkeratotic warty plaques present on the knees, elbows, hands, feet, and buttocks.
- Lupus vulgaris: slow-growing destructive reddish brown plaque with scarring seen in patients with some immunity. Difficult to culture bacteria from skin biopsies. Caused by BCG rarely.
- Tuberculids: puzzling conditions in patients who have been exposed to TB but do not have clinically obvious infection. The tuberculids include erythema induratum (a nodular vasculitis on the back of the legs), papulonecrotic tuberculid (crusted papules that heal with scarring), and lichen scrofulosorum (small follicular papules on the trunk). Using PCR, mycobacterial DNA has been detected in biopsies taken from tuberculids.

Box 6.8 Signs in leprosy

Tuberculoid leprosy: mimics sarcoid and mycosis fungoides

- A few well-defined erythematous or hypopigmented macules or plaques with reduced sensation and loss of sweating—the skin feels dry and rough.
- Thickened, tender regional nerves near the skin lesions, muscle weakness, muscle atrophy, and neuropathic ('Charcot') joints.
- Perforating ulcers at pressure sites 2° to neuropathy.
- Mucous membranes are not affected.

Lepromatous leprosy: mimics mycosis fungoides

- Numerous symmetrical macules, papules, nodules, and plaques. Lesions are hypopigmented and erythematous, but poorly defined.
- Sensation is usually normal in the lesions. Spares warm skin such as flexures, scalp, palms, soles, midline of the back, and chest.
- Thickened skin on the face (leonine) in late disease. Eyebrows and eyelashes lost.
- Bilateral symmetrical peripheral neuropathy: 'glove and stocking'.
- Weakness and atrophy of muscles 2° to neuropathy.
- Ulceration, perforation, and destruction of the nasal septum, with nasal collapse and deformity (saddle nose).
- Ulceration of the nasopharynx, pharynx, palate, and larynx.

Syphilis

Syphilis (the 'Great pox'), a chronic infectious disease caused by *Treponema pallidum*, is increasing in incidence and is a great mimic. The skin is involved at all stages. Patients may not be aware of the 1° lesion. Atypical presentations may be a sign of HIV/AIDS (see ➜ p. 162). Syphilis may be transmitted to the fetus (see Box 6.9).

What should I look for?

1° syphilis
- A solitary, painless, well-demarcated, firm ulcer (chancre), ~1cm in diameter, about 3 weeks after sexual contact. The site of presentation (genitalia, anal, oral, face) depends on the contact.
- Regional lymphadenopathy.
- A depressed atrophic scar when healed (in around 8 weeks).

2° syphilis
Presents 1–6 months after 1° infection. Rash settles in 1–3 months.
- Non-itchy symmetrical rash on the face and trunk.
- Initially smooth red macules, then scaly copper-red papules. Scale develops later, and the rash may resemble psoriasis or cutaneous LE.
- Keratotic papules on the palms and soles.
- Scaly papules on the glans penis or shaft of the penis.
- Macerated hypertrophic flat-topped papules (condylomata lata) in moist skinfolds—perianal, inframammary, and vulva.
- 'Split papules' at the angle of the mouth.
- Patchy moth-eaten hair loss, loss of eyebrows and eyelashes.
- Mucous membranes: greyish white oval patches and erosion on the palate, buccal or labial mucosa, tongue ('snail track ulcers').
- Headache, low-grade fever, lymphadenopathy, and arthralgia.
- Lues maligna (rare): papulopustular rash that rapidly evolves into well-demarcated crusted ulcers. Seen with co-morbidities causing immunosuppression, e.g. HIV, chronic alcoholism.

Late (tertiary) syphilis
May develop years after untreated 1° infection. Presentations include neurosyphilis (tabes dorsalis, general paralysis) and cardiovascular syphilis (aortitis) and gummata. Gummata, painless rubbery nodules that ulcerate and scar, mainly involve the skin and bones.

What should I do?

- *1° syphilis*: spirochaetes can be isolated from the chancre. Treponemal tests (TTs): anti-treponemal IgM detected 2 weeks after infection, IgG detected by week 4/5. Non-treponemal tests (NTTs) react in about 21 days. (See Box 6.10.)
- *2° and late syphilis*: skin biopsy may be helpful. Serology positive. (See Box 6.10.)
- Discuss investigation with a genitourinary physician.
- If diagnosis confirmed, refer the patient to genitourinary medicine for screening for other STDs, treatment, and contact tracing.

Box 6.9 Some late signs of congenital syphilis

Hutchinson triad
- Interstitial keratitis.
- Abnormalities of the permanent upper central incisors.
- Deafness.

Other signs
- Abnormalities of 6-year molars (mulberry molars).
- Rhagades (radiating scars around the mouth).
- Frontal bossing, depressed saddle nose, shortened maxilla.
- High-arched palate.
- Perforation of the nasal septum and palate by gumma.
- Thickening and anterior bowing of tibia (sabre shins).
- Thickening of the sternoclavicular portion of the clavicle.
- Painless hydroarthrosis of the knees and sometimes elbows (Clutton joint).
- Hair loss.

Box 6.10 Serological tests for syphilis

- Non-treponemal tests (NTTs) detect IgG/IgM antibodies to (mostly) cardiolipin released from damaged host cells and spirochaetes. Include venereal disease research laboratory (VDRL) and rapid plasma reagin (RPR) tests (more sensitive).
- NTT-positive reaction: confirm the diagnosis with specific treponemal tests (TTs).
- Quantitative NTT used for monitoring response to treatment: titres decline after effective treatment.
- False-negative NTT: some previously treated, early untreated, and late latent cases. False-positive NTT: viral infections, pregnancy, autoimmune diseases, malignancy, very elderly.
- TTs: detect antibodies against *T. pallidum*. Include *T. pallidum* haemagglutination assay (TPHA), *T. pallidum* particle agglutination assay (TPPA), and fluorescent treponemal antibody absorption assay (FTA-ABS). New TTs use recombinant antigens derived from *T. pallidum*, e.g. treponemal enzyme immunoassays (EIAs), *T. pallidum* chemiluminescence assays (CIAs).
- TTs positive earlier than NTTs but remain positive, even after effective treatment. Confirm the diagnosis with quantitative NTT.
- False-positive TTs: other spirochaetal infections, e.g. *Borrelia*.
- Both NTTs and TTs are recommended for screening and diagnosis. Seek the advice of a genitourinary physician on the choice of tests and the interpretation of results, taking into account the medical/ sexual history and history of syphilis, including previous treatment history.

Further reading

Morshed MG and Singh AE. *Clin Vaccine Immunol* 2015;**22**:137–47.
Sena AC *et al*. *Clin Infect Dis* 2010;**51**:700–8.

Lyme disease

What is Lyme disease?

Lyme disease is an infection caused by spirochaetes of the group *Borrelia burgdorferi* sensu lato. The spirochaetes are transmitted by the bite of hard-bodied ixodid ticks. Birds, mice, deer, voles, and lizards are the main reservoirs of *Borrelia*. Infection is unlikely if the tick is attached for <48h. Lyme borreliosis occurs in forested areas throughout most of Europe, but particularly Germany (Black Forest), Austria, Slovenia, and Sweden, as well as the coastal areas of north-east USA, the upper Midwest of the USA, and the West coast of the USA.

How does Lyme disease present?

Erythema migrans is an early sign of localized disease. The rash usually resolves in days to weeks but may persist for a year. Disseminated Lyme disease may have cardiac (atrioventricular block, myopericarditis), rheumatological (monoarticular or oligoarticular arthritis), and/or neurological (meningitis, peripheral or cranial neuropathy, myelitis) manifestations. Late persistent manifestations include chronic arthritis and peripheral neuropathy. Late skin signs, acrodermatitis chronica atrophicans (bluish red atrophic skin on the hands, feet, and leg) and borrelia lymphocytoma (erythematous, dusky, or violaceous nodule, most often on the ear lobe, nipple, or scrotum), are seen predominantly in Europe.

What should I look for in early disease?

- Erythema migrans develops 7–10 days after the tick bite.
- The rash may be slightly itchy. Flu-like symptoms are common.
- A small erythematous macule/papule appears at the site of the bite.
- Erythema extends over days to weeks to produce an annular lesion with central clearing or a roundish smooth erythematous patch.
- Erythematous lesions range in size from 10cm to >50cm in diameter.
- Warm the skin to make the signs more obvious.

What should I do?

- Discuss how to reduce the likelihood of further tick bites.
- Take blood for serology if the patient has been infected for >6 weeks. Antibodies are not present in early infection. (Treated patients may remain seropositive for months to years.)
- Take a skin biopsy, if a rash is present.
- Prescribe amoxicillin 1500–2000mg/day in divided doses or doxycycline 100mg bd or cefuroxime 500mg bd for at least 4 weeks to treat erythema migrans.
- Some authorities recommend a single 200mg dose of doxycycline within 72h of a tick bite, and others doxycycline 100–200mg bd for at least 20 days, to prevent Lyme borreliosis after a tick bite.

Further reading

Aguero-Rosenfeld ME and Wormser GP. *Expert Rev Mol Diagn* 2015;15:1–4.
Cameron DJ et al. *Expert Rev Anti Infect Ther* 2014;12:1103–35.

Viral and fungal infections

Contents

Relevant pages in other chapters
Eczema herpeticum ➲ p. 112
Herpetic gingivostomatitis ➲ p. 280
Genital herpes simplex virus infection ➲ pp. 280–1

Viral exanthems

- Measles (rubeola): measles is becoming commoner in the UK, because parents have not immunized their children. The child is irritable with fever, cough, nasal congestion, photophobia, and conjunctivitis. The rash, which is preceded by Koplik spots on the buccal mucosa, develops about 14 days after exposure to the virus, starting on the forehead and then becoming widespread. Erythematous macules evolve into a red-brown maculopapular (morbilliform) eruption that is not itchy. Fades after 5 days, when the skin desquamates.
- Rubella: the child is usually well but may have mild fever. Erythematous macules and papules appear first on the face and neck and then generalize over 48h. Fades within 2–3 days without desquamation.
- Erythema infectiosum (fifth disease, slapped cheek syndrome): is caused by parvovirus B19 and occurs mainly in young children. Bright erythematous macules on the cheeks are followed by a lacy erythematous rash on the proximal limbs that fades within days but may recur with heat (exercise, bathing). Children are usually well.
- Gianotti–Crosti syndrome (papular acrodermatitis of childhood): is associated with infections with hepatitis B virus (HBV) or EBV. Discrete red-brown papules develop symmetrically first on limbs and buttocks, then the face. The trunk is spared. Papules may be purpuric. Fades in 3–4 weeks. The child is usually well but may have a mild fever. The prognosis is good, and liver involvement mild.
- Asymmetric periflexural exanthem of childhood: the cause is unknown. The child may have a mild fever and upper respiratory symptoms. The itchy erythematous papular or eczematous rash affects one flexure, often the axilla, from where it extends onto the trunk. It remains strikingly asymmetrical. Clears in 6–8 weeks.
- Kawasaki disease (mucocutaneous lymph node syndrome): mainly affects infants and small children. An infectious trigger is suspected. Children develop a persistent fever. Palms and soles become erythematous (within 5 days), and hands and feet oedematous. Children may also develop a widespread urticated or measles-like (morbilliform) erythematous rash or (uncommonly) an annular erythema. After 10–15 days, the skin peels (desquamates) around the tips of fingers and toes and sometimes the palm and wrist. Other signs include conjunctival injection (in 2–4 days), erythematous crusted cracked bleeding lips (may persist for 2–3 weeks), oropharyngeal erythema, strawberry tongue, and cervical lymphadenopathy. ⚠ Cardiovascular disease (pericarditis, myocarditis, endocarditis, coronary arteritis with aneurysms and stenosis) may cause sudden death. Treat early with aspirin and IV Ig to reduce the risk of coronary artery aneurysms.
- 1° HIV infection: morbilliform rash (see ➲ p. 162).

Pityriasis rosea

What is pityriasis rosea?

Pityriasis rosea is a common self-limited rash that presents in adolescents and young adults. It is thought to be caused by a viral infection (possibly HHV-6 or -7), but this has not been proven. The rash usually clears in around 8 weeks.

What should I look for?

- Some patients have a mild prodrome (headache, fever, malaise).
- A 'herald patch', usually on the trunk, preceding the onset of the rash by hours or a few days.
- A rash on the trunk and proximal extremities, usually sparing the face, palms, and soles. Oval to round thin, pink papules and plaques with overlying fine scale or a margin (collarette) of scale (see ➔ Fig. 18.7, p. 391).
- Papules and plaques distributed in a 'Christmas tree' pattern on the back, with long axes aligned along Langer lines of cleavage.
- Hyperpigmentation may be marked in darkly pigmented skin.
- Atypical presentations include flexural (inverse) pityriasis rosea, and vesicular, purpuric, and pustular variants.
- Most patients are asymptomatic. Itching is usually minimal.
- Signs suggesting another diagnosis:
  - 2° syphilis: copper-coloured macules on the palms and soles, split papules at the corner of the mouth, and condylomata lata, fever, and lymphadenopathy (see ➔ p. 146).
  - Guttate psoriasis: thicker silvery scale and plaques do not follow the 'Christmas tree' pattern. Did a sore throat precede the onset of the rash? Has the patient a personal or family history of psoriasis? (see ➔ p. 194.)

What should I do?

- Check the drug history to exclude a drug eruption (see ➔ p. 390).
- Reassure the patient, and wait!

Herpes simplex virus

HSV is a common cause of contagious infections. The virus causes intra-epidermal vesiculation and persists in the sensory ganglia. Lesions recur in the same site. HSV-1 causes skin infections and, less often, genital infection. HSV-2 is the 1° cause of genital herpes, a sexually transmitted infection. For oral and genital herpes, see ⮑ pp. 280–1. HSV can trigger EM (see ⮑ p. 111).

Patterns of herpes simplex virus 1 infection

- Recurrent 'cold sores' common in childhood and adolescence, most often on the lips or face, but may affect any skin surface. Recurrent infections (see Box 7.1) may cause recurrent EM (see ⮑ p. 111).
- Herpetic whitlows or 'felons' (painful erythematous vesicular swellings on the tips of fingers) in health-care workers, e.g. dentists, anaesthetists, nurses on ICU in contact with lips of patients shedding the virus (many are caused by HSV-2). Also in children who suck a digit.
- 'Scrum pox' on the face of rugby players and 'herpes gladiatorium' in wrestlers—caused by direct inoculation into grazed skin (see Fig. 7.1).
- Painful gingivostomatitis, lymphadenopathy, and fever in 1° HSV-1 infection (see ⮑ p. 280).
- ⚠ Widespread vesiculation (eczema herpeticum) in patients with atopic eczema, burns, and some rare skin problems. Life-threatening, particularly in children (see ⮑ p. 112).
- Immunocompromised: larger or deeper ulcers (see Fig. 7.2), satellite lesions, prolonged healing time, or systemic infection. May present as linear intertriginous ulcers or deep fissures (knife-cut sign).

What should I ask?

- Does the patient have warning of the onset? A tingling irritating prodrome of 4–6h is common.
- Does the lesion recur in the same place? This is very suggestive of HSV infection. The differential is fixed drug eruption, another blistering eruption that recurs in the same place, but without a prodrome.
- Does it scar? Uncomplicated cold sores heal without scarring within 7–10 days, but there may be a little residual erythema for some weeks.

What should I look for?

(See Fig. 7.1.)
- Vesicles that rupture and crust within 2–3 days and mild tender lymphadenopathy. For signs of eczema herpeticum, see Box 7.2.

What should I do?

For management, see Box 7.3.
- If you are not sure of the diagnosis, take a swab for virology. The swab must be put into a viral culture medium. Use a scalpel to get a little of the blister roof or base, as well as blister fluid, on the swab. PCR will give you a rapid result.
- A Tzank preparation (smear) for an immediate result (see Box 7.4).

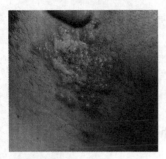

Fig. 7.1 Herpes simplex infection—fresh vesicles are obvious at the periphery of the plaque.

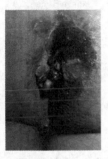

Fig. 7.2 Herpes simplex infection—presenting as a painful, persistent ulcer in an immunosuppressed patient.

Box 7.1 Factors that may trigger recurrences of herpes simplex virus 1 infection

- Sunshine.
- Menstruation.
- Local trauma, including dental procedures.
- Illness.
- Stress.

⚠ Box 7.2 Signs of eczema herpeticum

(See Fig. 7.3.)
- Sudden deterioration of eczema.
- Pain as well as intense itching.
- Malaise, vomiting, anorexia, diarrhoea.
- Fever in variable number of cases.
- Vesicles (1° lesions), pustules, and papules; small punched-out ulcers, sometimes clustered, but these may coalesce, producing widespread erosions.
- Oozing, sometimes haemorrhagic, and crusting.
- Lymphadenopathy.
- Signs may be difficult to differentiate from VZV or bacterial infection. 2° bacterial infection may complicate the picture.

Box 7.3 Management of cutaneous herpes simplex virus infection

- Localized recurrent disease only requires symptomatic treatment.
- Prescribe oral antivirals in patients at risk of developing widespread infection, e.g. immunosuppressed, atopic eczema, Darier disease—aciclovir 400mg ×5/day, valaciclovir 1g bd, or famciclovir 500mg bd for 7 days. (Also see ➲ Box 5.12, p. 113.)
- Surgery is contraindicated in herpetic whitlows.

Box 7.4 Tzank preparation (smear)

- You will need a glass slide and a No. 10 or 15 scalpel blade.
- De-roof a fresh vesicle, and gently scrape the base (you only need tissue fluid and keratinocytes—try not to contaminate the smear with blood).
- Smear the contents of your blade onto a glass slide.
- Air-dry; fix with methanol, and stain with Giemsa, toluidine blue, or Wright stain.
- Examine under a light microscope (×40). Multinucleated giant keratinocytes confirm the diagnosis of HSV or VZV infection.

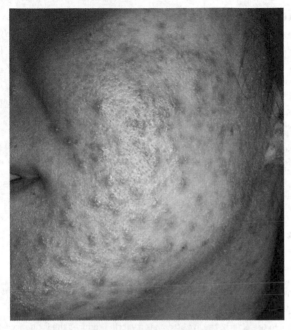

Fig. 7.3 Painful swelling and widespread vesicles in eczema herpeticum.

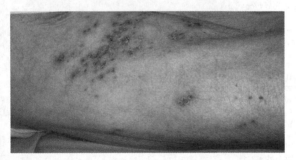

Fig. 7.4 Shingles: dried-up vesicles in the distribution of L2 and L3 dermatomes.

Further reading

Kuo T et al. Vaccine 2014;32:6733–45 (HSV vaccine).

Varicella (chickenpox)

A contagious infection spread by mucosal droplets. Patients are infectious from 2 days before until 5 days after the onset of the rash. VZV remains dormant in sensory ganglia after 1° infection. 1° VZV is a more severe infection in adults than children. Complications include pneumonitis and 2° bacterial infection. The live attenuated vaccine prevents severe infection in children.

What should I look for?

- Malaise, cough, coryza, sore throat.
- A rash that affects the trunk more than the limbs or face. Rarely may localize to sun-exposed skin.
- Crops of itchy, erythematous macules and papules that evolve into vesicles (may also be oral). After 2 days, pustules become crusted.
- Cropping that continues for 4–7 days.
- Healing, often with scarring, within 16 days.
- Haemorrhagic lesions in immunosuppressed patients (may be fatal).
- Respiratory symptoms in severe disease.

What should I do?

See Box 7.5.

Herpes zoster (shingles)

Commonest in the elderly. VZV in the sensory ganglia may be reactivated years after an episode of chickenpox. Herpes zoster in a young patient may indicate immunosuppression, e.g. lymphoma. VZV can be passed on to people who have not had varicella by direct contact with the rash. In the elderly, the live attenuated vaccine reduces the incidence of zoster and post-herpetic neuralgia (see Boxes 7.6 and 7.7).

What should I look for?

- Fever, malaise, and/or headache preceding the eruption by several days.
- Pain, burning, itching, or hypersensitivity often several days before the rash. Pain may simulate renal colic or myocardial infarction.
- Rash involving one or more dermatomes (may cross the midline).
- Clusters of erythematous papules evolving into vesicles and then pustules (see Fig. 7.4).
- Facial zoster: look for lesions on the sides/tip of the nose. These indicate involvement of the ophthalmic division of the trigeminal nerve, and the eye may be infected. ▶▶ Refer urgently to ophthalmology.
- Healing in 10–14 days, sometimes with scarring or pigment change.

What should I do?

- If the diagnosis is in doubt, take vesicular fluid for PCR (put into a viral culture medium), or examine a Tzank preparation (smear) (see ➲ Box 7.4 and p. 647).
- Consider starting antivirals (see Box 7.5).

Box 7.5 How should I treat varicella-zoster virus infection?

Children with varicella (chickenpox)
- Symptomatic treatment with antipyretics, calamine lotion, and tepid baths, provided the immune system is normal.

Adults with varicella (chickenpox) and herpes zoster (shingles)
- Varicella: valaciclovir 1g tds for 7 days (better drug levels than oral aciclovir).
- Shingles: treat if involves the eye or in the immunocompromised. No convincing evidence that antivirals reduce the incidence of post-herpetic neuralgia.

Immunocompromised or those at risk of severe disease
- Treat for 10–14 days, starting with IV aciclovir 10mg/kg every 8h for 7 days. Seek advice about treatment in pregnancy.

Box 7.6 Complications of herpes zoster

- 2° infection with staphylococci or streptococci.
- Ulceration in immunosuppressed patients.
- A generalized eruption in immunosuppressed patients.
- Corneal ulcers, corneal scarring, or blindness if the ophthalmic division of the trigeminal nerve is involved—refer to an ophthalmologist if the eye could be infected.
- Post-herpetic neuralgia; rarely motor paralysis or encephalitis.

Box 7.7 Post-herpetic neuralgia

This debilitating painful complication is commonest in patients aged >50. Pain may persist for many years and is often refractory to treatment. Patients may experience:
- Constant or paroxysmal pain.
- Burning, aching, stabbing, or electric shock pain.
- Allodynia (pain on stimulation of the skin).
- Severe pruritus, with or without pain.

Management
Seek the help of a pain clinic.
- Capsaicin cream (pretreatment with EMLA® may reduce the burning sensation felt when capsaicin is applied).
- Topical anaesthetics, e.g. EMLA®, 5% lidocaine patch.
- Local anaesthetics: subcutaneous, IV, epidural, intercostal.
- Other options: amitriptyline, opioid analgesia, gabapentin.

Further reading

Kawai K et al. BMJ Open 2014;4:e004833 (systematic review of incidence and complications).
Langan SM et al. PLoS Med 2013;10:e1001420 (efficacy of vaccine).

Molluscum contagiosum, orf, and milker's nodule

Molluscum contagiosum

Self-limiting skin infection, common in children, caused by a pox virus. Virus is transmitted by direct contact, including sexual contact.

What should I look for?

- Translucent, smooth, dome-shaped papules, up to 0.5cm in diameter, with a central umbilicated punctum, from which cheesy material can be expressed.
- Papules may become erythematous and swollen prior to resolution.
- Eczematous patches may develop around mollusca.
- Mollusca may leave small depressed scars.
- May be widespread in immunosuppressed or atopic patients. Many mollusca on the face of a young adult may indicate HIV infection.
- A solitary giant molluscum (1–2cm) in an adult may be misdiagnosed as a malignant skin tumour.

What should I do?

- The mean time to resolution is 13 months, but mollusca may persist much longer, particularly in atopics. Reassure anxious parents, and procrastinate if the child is not bothered.
- Disrupting papules with a cocktail stick may hasten resolution.
- Removal by curettage, after applying a topical anaesthetic, can be successful in stoical children.
- In adults, consider cryosurgery or curettage, but remind patients that mollusca may leave pox-like scars, or your surgery may be blamed for the scar.
- Topical 1% hydrogen peroxide cream or 5% potassium hydroxide solution may have a role in persistent disease.

Orf and milker's nodule

Orf is a self-limiting skin infection caused by a parapox virus that is transmitted by direct contact with infected sheep or goats. Milker's nodule is a self-limiting parapox virus infection that simulates orf but is acquired from cows' udders. Both can trigger EM (see p. 111).

What should I look for?

- A history of contact with infected animals (incubation period may be a few days or several weeks).
- One or more itchy or painful reddish blue papules, usually on a finger (see Box 7.8). May look vascular, like a pyogenic granuloma.

What should I do?

- No investigations are necessary, unless the diagnosis is in doubt, in which case take a skin biopsy for histology or arrange electron microscopy on the crust or biopsy material.
- Most lesions resolve spontaneously in 5–7 weeks.
- Treat 2° infection.

Box 7.8 Clinical features in orf and milker's nodule

Lesions progress through a number of stages:
- A 0.5–1.5cm macule that evolves into a dome-shaped papule.
- A target-like appearance, with a peripheral halo of erythema encircling a white ring that surrounds the central erythematous papule.
- A nodule that may ulcerate and weep.
- Spontaneous healing usually in 6 weeks but may take as long as 6 months.

Other features
- Lymphangitis and/or regional lymphadenopathy.
- Fever.

Further reading

Olsen JR et al. Lancet Infect Dis 2015;15:190–5 (molluscum).

Human papillomavirus

Human papillomavirus (HPV) infects epithelial cells of skin and mucous membranes; >150 types of HPV have been identified. These cause infections at different sites (see Box 7.9). Infections are transmitted by direct contact, which may be sexual, but the incubation time ranges from weeks to more than a year. HPV DNA is widely distributed on skin in the general population. Infection may be subclinical.

Human papillomavirus and cancer

HPV-16/18 are linked to the development of anogenital and cervical SCCs. Certain HPV types may play a part in the development of some cutaneous SCCs.

What should I look for?

- Common warts: papules or nodules with a hyperkeratotic surface, often at sites of trauma such as fingers, elbows, or knees. May coalesce into a plaque (mosaic warts). Filiform warts (tiny frond-like projections) are often perioral. Subungual warts lift the nail plate from the nail bed. Warts may be widespread in the immunocompromised.
- Plane (flat) warts: flat-topped skin-coloured papules. Side-lighting accentuates signs. Common on the face or other light-exposed sites. If widespread, consider HIV or epidermodysplasia verruciformis (very rare) (see Box 7.9).
- Common and plane warts may be linear (in scratches).
- Deep plantar warts: most frequent on weight-bearing skin and may simulate corns (see Box 7.10).
- Anogenital warts: perianal warts transmitted sexually or by auto-inoculation of cutaneous warts. Check children for signs that might suggest sexual abuse such as bruising, damage to the hymen, enlargement of the vaginal introitus, or thickening of the anal margin. Giant anogenital warts seen in the immunocompromised.

What should I do?

- Most viral warts will eventually disappear without treatment, but resolution may take time, particularly in immunosuppressed or atopic patients. Procrastinate, if at all possible. Explain that, when the wart goes, it will not leave a scar. Treatment is difficult, but treatment should not cause more problems than the wart itself (see Box 7.11).
- Immunostimulatory drugs, such as oral retinoids, have been advocated for widespread warts in adults, but results are variable. Sensitization with topical diphencyprone (contact immunotherapy) has also been tried.
- Anogenital warts: refer adults to a genitourinary physician for screening for other STDs. Women should have cervical smears. Children should see a paediatrician or genitourinary physician (most units will have agreed care paths for children). Topical 5% imiquimod cream or 10% podophylline paint can be very effective.
- Consider testing for HIV if widespread facial or perianal warts.

Box 7.9 Mucocutaneous infections and human papillomavirus type

- Common warts: HPV-1, -2, -4, -26, -27, -29, -57.
- Plane warts: HPV-3, -10, -28.
- Deep plantar warts: HPV-1, -63.
- Genital and anogenital warts: HPV-6 and -11 (low risk of SCC); HPV-16 and -18 (high risk of SCC).
- Oral mucous membranes: HPV-13 and -32.
- Epidermodysplasia verruciformis: rare. Autosomal recessive or acquired in immunosuppressed patients. Susceptibility to certain cutaneous HPV infections, mainly HPV-5, -8, and -14. Increased risk of Bowen disease and SCCs (UV is a co-carcinogen).

Box 7.10 Is it a plantar wart or a corn?

- Pinch the skin on each side of the wart or corn gently. Plantar warts are tender, unlike corns.
- Paring a wart will reveal bleeding or thrombosed capillaries (black dots). A corn has a uniform glassy appearance without capillaries.

Box 7.11 Treatment of common viral warts and plane warts

- Minimize trauma, e.g. advise patients to stop picking or nibbling at the skin around periungual warts.
- Common warts: regular application of a keratolytic containing 10–26% salicylic acid occupies the patient, until the wart disappears.
- Duct tape occlusion: apply tape to the wart, and leave in place for 6 days at a time for up to 8 weeks (probably a placebo, but painless, unlike cryosurgery, and does prevent trauma).
- Buying warts: another folk remedy, probably best practised by an elderly relative. At least the child profits from the wart!
- Plantar warts: keep flat to minimize discomfort. Pare warts when the skin is soft after bathing. Most children will not be bothered by a flat plantar wart (parents and teachers may take a different view).
- Cryosurgery is painful. Reserve for adults, unless the child is demanding treatment. Cryosurgery can be a good option for solitary filiform warts, which seem less likely to recur than other warts.
- Other surgical options (best for solitary warts) include electrocautery, hyfrecation, curettage, and laser surgery, but nothing guarantees cure because of latent virus in the skin.
- Intralesional bleomycin 0.5mg/mL is a painful option.
- Plane warts: try 0.025% tretinoin cream or 5% benzoyl peroxide cream ×1/day. Suggest stopping shaving if plane warts are in the beard area.

Further reading

Sterling J et al. Br J Dermatol 2014;171:696–712 (management guidelines).

HIV/AIDS and the skin

Over 30 million people are infected by the human immunodeficiency retroviruses HIV-1 or, in a minority, HIV-2, which cause AIDS by destroying or impairing the function of CD4+ cells. For risk factors, see Box 7.12. After infection, the CD4 count falls slowly, over 5–10 years, to <200 cells/mL, when patients develop overt AIDS, often complicated by opportunistic infections and/or tumours (see Box 7.15). Fifty percent of cases are diagnosed late, so always consider HIV testing (see Box 7.13).

HIV/AIDS is controlled by lifelong treatment with antiretroviral drugs which may trigger cutaneous manifestations of the immune reconstitution inflammatory syndrome (IRIS) (see Box 7.14).

How does 1° HIV infection present?

Onset 2–4 weeks after exposure, when HIV antibody tests are still negative. Diagnosis often missed. Features include:
- Transient glandular fever-like illness with malaise, fever, headache, sore throat, myalgia, arthralgia, and lymphadenopathy.
- Generalized morbilliform exanthem (spares the palms and soles).

What mucocutaneous infections/infestations suggest immunodeficiency?

Infections are often florid, recurrent, and atypical.
- Herpes simplex (chronic, non-healing ulcers), herpes zoster (severe, disseminated), molluscum contagiosum (many or large, face/flexures), viral warts (facial, genital, perianal), oral hairy leukoplakia on the sides of the tongue (EBV), CMV (perianal/genital ulcers, papules, purpuric macules, usually with visceral infection).
- Candidiasis (oropharyngeal, vaginal, cutaneous, nail), pityriasis versicolor. Dermatophytoses. Systemic fungal infections.
- Staphylococcal folliculitis/furunculosis (see ➲ pp. 134–5), atypical mycobacterial infection (see ➲ p. 144), bacillary angiomatosis (see ➲ p. 142).
- Syphilis: atypical 1°, 2°, and late (see ➲ pp. 146–7).
- Leishmaniasis, strongyloidiasis.
- Demodicosis (see ➲ p. 178), crusted scabies (see ➲ p. 173).

What other skin problems occur in HIV/AIDS?

- Seborrhoeic dermatitis: disseminated and atypical.
- Psoriasis: severe, atypical (flexural). Reiter syndrome.
- Atopic dermatitis in children (refractory to treatment).
- Pityriasis rubra pilaris (see ➲ p. 195), PCT (see ➲ p. 332).
- Drug reactions: including SJS and TEN (see ➲ pp. 116–21).
- Papular pruritic eruption: symmetrical, itchy, worst on extremities.
- Eosinophilic folliculitis: itchy follicular papules and pustules, usually on the face and trunk.
- Dry itchy skin, ichthyosis (scaly skin), keratoderma.
- Nail disease: hyperpigmentation, yellow nail syndrome.
- Lipodystrophy (with protease inhibitors) (see ➲ Box 22.4, p. 471).

Box 7.12 Risk factors for HIV/AIDS

- Sexual partner with HIV infection/AIDS.
- Unprotected homosexual or heterosexual intercourse.
- Multiple sexual partners, including one-night stands, holiday sex.
- Sexual partner from country with high prevalence of HIV/AIDS.
- IV drug abuse: sharing needles.
- Transfusion of blood products between 1977 and 1985, i.e. prior to screening. (Screening may not be rigorous in some countries.)
- Other sexually transmitted diseases.

Box 7.13 When should I test for HIV?

Consider HIV testing in all patients, but particularly if:
- Symptoms are more severe than usual.
- Symptoms are more long-lasting than usual.
- Inflammatory dermatosis has a widespread/atypical distribution.
- Response to standard treatments is poor.
- Relapses are frequent.

Box 7.14 Immune reconstitution inflammatory syndrome (IRIS) and skin

IRIS is characterized by an exacerbation of a pre-existing condition or the emergence of a previously unknown disease when the immune system is recovering in response to antiretroviral drugs. Increases in CD4/CD8 cell counts may contribute to inflammation. Presentations of IRIS described in the skin include:
- HSV and herpes zoster virus, viral warts, leprosy.
- Kaposi sarcoma.
- Eosinophilic folliculitis, seborrhoeic dermatitis, acne, psoriasis.
- Sarcoidosis, SLE.

Box 7.15 Cutaneous tumours in HIV/AIDS

- SCC, intraepithelial neoplasia (cervical, anal)—HPV-related.
- Melanoma.
- BCC.
- Merkel cell cancer (polyoma virus-related).
- Kaposi sarcoma (HHV-8) (see ➲ pp. 362–3).
- Cutaneous lymphoma; B-cell > T-cell (see ➲ pp. 358–9).
- Multiple dermatofibromas.

Dermatophyte infections (ringworm, 'tinea')

Dermatophytes infect skin, nails, or hair. Infections are transmitted indirectly through skin scales or shed hair. Fungi can be isolated from contaminated hairbrushes, clothing, carpets, or bed linen. (See Boxes 7.16 and 7.17.)

What should I look for?

- Asymmetrical, erythematous, scaly, well-demarcated patches that may be slightly itchy (see Fig. 7.5).
- Lesions expand slowly, often with some central clearing (ring-like). Scale is most marked on the outer edge of the ring.
- Anthropophilic fungal infections tend to be less inflamed than those caused by zoophilic fungi (see Box 7.16), which may have raised pustular borders. Check for a history of contact with animals.
- Scale is less obvious in fungal infections that have been misdiagnosed and treated with a topical corticosteroid, but treated patches will become more papular and pustular (tinea incognito). The active spreading edge is still well defined.
- One or more well-defined patches of hair loss and scale. Zoophilic scalp infections are inflamed, swollen, and pustular (kerion). A similar reaction may occur in the beard area. *Microsporum*-infected hairs fluoresce bright green under Wood lamp (see ⮕ p. 640).
- One or more thickened, crumbling discoloured nails. Dermatophytes are the commonest cause of onychomycosis. Moulds and *Candida* species may infect nails, particularly in the elderly or immunocompromised or if other nail damage or peripheral vascular disease. Many abnormal nails: consider an alternative diagnosis, e.g. psoriasis.
- Widespread or atypical patterns of infection may be a marker of immunodeficiency, e.g. HIV/AIDS (see ⮕ p. 162).

What should I do?

- Take a skin scraping, scalp brushing, or nail clipping (see ⮕ pp. 646–7). In children with *Trichophyton tonsurans* infection, take scalp brushings for culture from family members and close contacts.
- Treat localized skin infections with a topical antifungal, e.g. terbinafine cream or clotrimazole cream.
- Treat widespread skin infections or infections that have been misdiagnosed and treated with a topical steroid with an oral antifungal, e.g. terbinafine or griseofulvin.
- Treat tinea capitis with an oral antifungal in combination with ketoconazole shampoo. *Microsporum canis* responds to griseofulvin or itraconazole, but *T. tonsurans* responds better to oral terbinafine.
- Nail infection is difficult to eradicate, and, after long-standing infections, nail dystrophy may persist. Amorolfine or tioconazole paints may be effective in superficial moulds, but dermatophyte infections require an oral antifungal, such as terbinafine, for 3 months or pulsed oral therapy with terbinafine or itraconazole.

Further reading

Ammen M et al. Br J Dermatol 2014;**171**:937–58 (onychomycosis guidelines).
Fuller LC et al. Br J Dermatol 2014;**171**:454–63 (tinea capitis guidelines).

Box 7.16 Commonly encountered dermatophytes

Species that infect only humans (anthropophilic) are the commonest cause of skin and nail infections:
- *Trichophyton rubrum*: foot, nail, groin, body.
- *Trichophyton interdigitale*: foot, nail, groin.
- *Trichophyton tonsurans*: scalp, body.
- *Trichophyton schoenleinii*: scalp (favus).
- *Epidermophyton floccosum*: foot, nail, groin.

Species of fungus that infect animals (zoophilic) cause a more inflamed rash in humans than the anthropophilic species:
- *Microsporum canis* (cats, dogs): scalp, body.
- *Trichophyton mentagrophytes* (rodents): scalp, body.
- *Trichophyton verrucosum* (cattle): scalp, beard, body.

Ask the patient about contact with animals. Geophilic (soil) species of fungus rarely infect humans.

Box 7.17 Dermatophyte infections at different sites

- Tinea corporis = body—typically occurs in ring-like patterns.
- Tinea cruris = groin—common, usually spares the scrotum. May be unilateral.
- Tinea pedis = foot (athlete's foot)—macerated scale between fourth and fifth toes or diffuse dry scale of the soles (moccasin-like).
- Tinea manuum = hand—usually one palm. Dry scale with little inflammation.
- Tinea unguium = nail.
- Tinea capitis = scalp—primarily seen in children. Fungus causes hair loss, unlike psoriasis or eczema. Inflammatory lesions are known as kerions.
- Tinea facei = face—uncommon but may develop a kerion in the beard area.

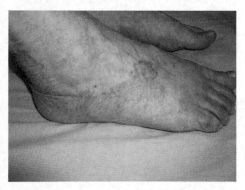

Fig. 7.5 Dermatophyte infection with a clearly demarcated scaly border.

Candida albicans

Candida albicans is a yeast that is a commensal in the mouth and GI tract. *C. albicans* may infect the skin or mucosae (mucocutaneous candidiasis), and the infection may be the presenting feature of an endocrine disease such as diabetes (see Box 7.18).

Invasive infections and candidaemia occur in immunosuppressed patients, e.g. HIV/AIDS. Rarely, severe and persistent infections may be linked to a specific T-cell deficiency (chronic mucocutaneous candidiasis).

What should I look for?

- Oral *Candida* (thrush): lacy white lines or whitish plaques on the buccal mucosa or tongue. These wipe off with a spatula, leaving an erythematous base (unlike LP; see ➲ p. 286).
- Angular cheilitis: most often in patients with ill-fitting dentures.
- Flexural, including interdigital, candidiasis (candidal intertrigo). Look for erythema with small superficial pustules on adjacent skin (satellite pustules).
- Vulvovaginal: whitish plaques, milky discharge.
- Balanitis.
- Chronic paronychia: boggy swelling of the proximal fingernail fold, with loss of cuticle and ridging of the nail. Pus may exude from under the nail fold. *Candida* species may invade the proximal nail plate which becomes friable and discoloured.
- Severe disease: erythematous nodules, pustules, vasculitis.

What should I do?

- Take swabs to confirm the diagnosis, if required.
- Minimize risk factors (exclude diabetes), and keep the skin dry.
- Prescribe antifungals (see Box 7.19). Remember that treatments, such as terbinafine and griseofulvin, that are used for dermatophyte infections are not effective in yeast infections.

Box 7.18 Risk factors for *Candida* infections

Mucocutaneous candidiasis
- Pregnancy.
- Occlusion and maceration, e.g. skinfolds, peristomal skin.
- Wet work or finger sucking—paronychia.
- Prolonged antibiotic therapy.
- Endocrine disease: diabetes, Cushing syndrome, hypoparathyroidism, hypothyroidism.
- Immune defects, including HIV/AIDS and immunosuppressive therapy.
- Iron and zinc deficiency.
- Inflammatory disease, e.g. oral GVHD (see ⮡ p. 535).

Invasive candidiasis
- Neutropenia.
- Prolonged antibiotic therapy.
- Indwelling catheters: urinary or IV.
- GI surgery.
- IV drug abuse.

Box 7.19 Treatment options for candidiasis

- Skin: imidazole creams.
- Oral: miconazole oral gel or nystatin suspension/drops.
- Vulvovaginal: itraconazole vaginal pessaries (200mg bd for 1 day) and antifungal creams.
- Severe disease requires systemic therapy with oral antifungal tablets, e.g. fluconazole.

Pityriasis (tinea) versicolor

This infection, common in young adults, is caused by *Malassezia* yeasts. These skin commensals proliferate in the stratum corneum, producing azelaic acid, which inhibits melanogenesis and prevents the skin in lesions from tanning (for risk factors, see Box 7.20).

What should I look for?

- Asymptomatic lesions predominantly on the trunk (see Fig. 7.6).
- Brownish red or pale (hypopigmented) macules of varying size, with a dusting of fine scale. Scrape the skin gently to see the scale.
- Lesions appear darker than surrounding untanned skin initially but, after sun exposure, appear paler than adjacent skin because the uninvolved skin tans.
- Pale lesions may be misdiagnosed as vitiligo, but vitiligo is not scaly and pigment loss in vitiligo is complete (depigmentation), not partial.
- *Malassezia* yeasts (also known as pityrosporum yeasts) may cause folliculitis on the trunk in patients with seborrhoeic dermatitis (see → p. 219).

What should I do?

- Examine under Wood light: infected skin fluoresces yellow (see → p. 640). (Not all *Malassezia* species fluoresce.)
- Take scrapes for microscopy: look for hyphae and spores ('spaghetti and meatballs') to confirm the diagnosis.
- Prescribe an antifungal (see Box 7.21).
- Explain that, once the scale has gone, so has the infection, but pale skin will continue to look paler than surrounding skin until exposed to sunlight.
- Warn that relapses are frequent (a sign of youth?).

Box 7.20 Risk factors for pityriasis versicolor

- Hot humid climates when the disease may be very extensive.
- Hyperhidrosis.
- Use of oily or greasy skincare products.
- Systemic and topical corticosteroids.
- Cushing syndrome.
- Immunosuppression.
- Malnutrition.
- Genetic susceptibility.

Box 7.21 Treatment options for pityriasis versicolor

- A topical imidazole, e.g. 2% miconazole nitrate, 2% ketoconazole cream, or 1% clotrimazole cream, for localized disease of a few lesions only.
- Ketoconazole 2% shampoo (preferable to 2.5% selenium sulfide) as a body wash daily for 5 days. Leave in contact with the skin for 5min. This can be very drying, and the patient may need a moisturizer.
- Ketoconazole 2% foam ×1/day for 7 days (not available in the UK).
- Oral itraconazole 200mg/day for 5–7 days for widespread disease.
- Relapses are frequent after any of these treatments.
- Prophylactic daily treatment with ketoconazole 2% shampoo for up to 3 days in the beginning of the hot summer has been recommended.

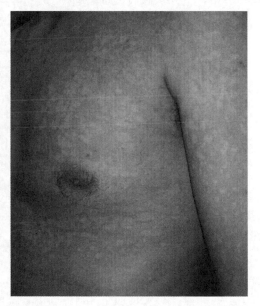

Fig. 7.6 Pityriasis versicolor with widespread scaly pale macules. Uninvolved skin has tanned.

Further reading

Hald M et al. Acta Derm Venereol 2015;95:12–19 (treatment guidelines).

Infestations and parasites

Contents

Relevant pages in other chapters
Erythema migrans ➲ p. 148

Scabies

What is scabies?

- Scabies is a common contagious and debilitating infestation in which allergy to the saliva, eggs, and excrement of the mite *Sarcoptes scabiei* var. *hominis* causes extraordinarily intense itching. Scabies may be an endemic problem in resource-poor settings.
- The mites mate on the skin surface, and the ♂ (0.2mm long) dies. The ♀ (0.4mm long) burrows into the epidermis and lays eggs (1–3/day) for 4–6 weeks (see Fig. 8.1). These hatch in 3–4 days and, within 10–15 days, reach adulthood.
- Although the patient may have only 10–12 adult mites, itch is widespread, severe, and distressing.
- Overwhelming infestation in a debilitated, old, or immunocompromised patient (>1000 mites per person) is known as crusted (Norwegian) scabies (see Box 8.1).
- Scabies is transmitted by close skin-to-skin contact (for at least 15–20min), e.g. sharing a bed, holding hands, sexual intercourse.
- The mites cannot jump or fly, but ♀ can burrow up to 2.5cm/min.
- The good news is that scabies can be cured—so it is a rewarding diagnosis to make.

What should I ask?

- Where is the itch? The head and neck are usually spared, except in the very young, the very old, or the immunosuppressed.
- What is the itch like? The itch is severe (some patients liken the itch to pain) and made worse by warmth, e.g. at night.
- Is anyone else itching? Carers, family contacts, including grandparents, and sexual contacts.
- Not everyone with an infestation will be itchy. Sensitization takes 2–6 weeks. Crusted scabies may not be very itchy.
- Is a close contact being treated for any skin complaint (scabies is often missed)? Granny with 'hand dermatitis' may be the index case.
- Enquire about other causes of itching, e.g. drugs (see ➲ pp. 60–1).
- What treatment has been provided? Treatment fails if all those infested (i.e. all close contacts) have not been treated at the same time.

Box 8.1 Crusted 'Norwegian' scabies

- The same mite as in ordinary scabies, but many thousands of them.
- Occurs in debilitated, elderly, or immunocompromised patients, including those with HIV/AIDS.
- Itching is often less marked than in normal scabies.
- The hands, elbows, knees, and ankles develop extensive thick crusts.
- The face, scalp, and nail beds are often involved.
- All the skin may be red and scaly.
- Crusts contain hundreds of live mites that can survive for a few days.
- Large number of mites may be found beneath the nails.
- This form of scabies is extremely contagious.

Female *Sarcoptes scabiei*

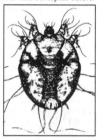

0.4 mm length

Fig. 8.1 ♀ scabies mite. Reproduced with permission from Eddleston M et al. *Oxford Handbook of Tropical Medicine*, 3rd edn, 2008. Oxford: Oxford University Press.

Management of scabies

What should I look for?

Search for proof—most signs are 2° to scratching (papules, erythema, and excoriation), but look for:

- Burrows (see Box 8.2).
- Finger web crusting.
- Nodules on the penis.
- Blisters or pustules on the palms and soles in infants.
- Mites either visualized with the dermatoscope as a tiny dark triangle just beyond the end of the burrow, extracted from a burrow using a needle (very satisfying), or found in scrapings from the roof of the burrow (you may see eggs as well as mites). Inspect your catch under a light microscope—the mite will walk around; do not lose it.
- Numerous mites in crusts and under the nails in Norwegian scabies.
- If you cannot find mites but still suspect scabies, either treat the patient and all close contacts for scabies or (preferred option) reduce the inflammation with a very potent topical corticosteroid, prescribe a sedating antihistamine, add an oral antibiotic (if required for 2° infection), and renew the search next week ... setting aside sufficient time to do a proper job. Ask the patient to bring close contacts with him/her to the clinic.

How should I manage scabies?

- Consider showing the mite to the patient, who may be interested to see the cause of the itch.
- Treat all members of the household and all close contacts (including sexual partners) at the same time, even if they do not have symptoms.
- Norwegian (crusted) scabies—treat all those in the nursing home or hospital ward if the patient has been there >24h, as well as other contacts. Use two treatments 3 days apart.
- Apply 5% permethrin cream to the whole body, except the head, including the fingers, toes, and skin under the nails. In a child <2 years or elderly or immunosuppressed patients, also apply the cream to the scalp, face, and ears. Leave the cream on for 8–14h, and then wash off. Repeat treatment after 7 days.
- Although the mites die rapidly once off the body, patients should either wash all clothes, bed linen, and towels in a hot wash and place items in a dryer for 10min on a high setting or isolate items that cannot be washed in a plastic bag for at least 72h.
- Itching may persist for 2–3 weeks after treatment. Prescribe calamine oily lotion or a moderately potent topical corticosteroid ointment. A sedating oral antihistamine (e.g. hydroxyzine 25–50mg at night) will help to relieve the itch.
- Ivermectin 200 micrograms/kg in a single dose, repeated in 7–14 days, has also been recommended for classic scabies.
- Crusted scabies: ivermectin 200 micrograms/kg on days 1, 2, 8, 9, and 15 plus permethrin 5% cream applied to all the body daily for 7 days, then ×2/week, until mites eradicated.

Box 8.2 Scabies burrows

(See Fig. 8.2.)

- Inspect the finger webs, flexural aspect of the wrists, elbows, and axillary folds, breasts (in women), genitalia (in men), and medial and lateral borders of the feet.
- Comma-shaped lines a few mm long are diagnostic. The narrow superficial curved lines are visible in the horny layer of the epidermis.
- Linear burrows on the creases of palms and soles may be followed by a V-shaped pattern of scale and inflammation that has been likened to the wake of a moving ship. The wake and associated burrow make a Y-shaped sign that points to the mite.
- In infants and young children, you may find burrows on the head and neck, as well as the palms and soles, often in association with pustules or blisters.
- The mite is visible to the naked eye as a pinpoint dark dot just beyond the end of the burrow. With a dermatoscope, you will see a small dark triangle. Sometimes a vesicle forms near the end of burrows—the mite is just beyond the vesicle.
- Burrows may be difficult to find if the skin is eczematous, scratched, and crusted.

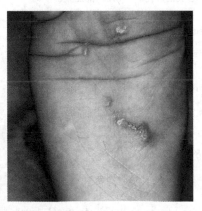

Fig. 8.2 Scabies burrow.

Further reading

Gunning K et al. Am Fam Physician 2012;**86**:535–41.

Lice

Lice suck blood. Itching, which may take 1–3 weeks to develop, is 2° to allergy to lice, not to bites. Heavy and long-standing infestation causes fatigue (incessant itching), anaemia (feeling lousy), and under-performance (nit-wit). For treatment, see Box 8.3.

Head louse (*Pediculus humanus capitis*)

- Head lice are almost ubiquitous in school-age children in the UK and sometimes infest their parents (and grandparents!) too. The elongated grey-brown lice, which are as fond of clean as dirty hair, are adapted to swing from hair to hair. Lice cannot jump or fly.
- Egg cases are cemented firmly to the base of hair shafts, but you will see them more easily once the louse has hatched, when they become white and the growing hair carries the empty case (nit) away from the surface of the scalp. Scalp scale, dandruff, or hair casts (pseudonits) may resemble nits but are easily removed from the hair, unlike nits which are firmly attached to the hair shaft.
- You may see elongated lice (2–4mm) moving in the scalp (in a bright light, look behind the ears or at the nape of the neck), or you may find lice by combing the hair over a piece of paper using a fine-toothed comb (also look at the comb) (see Fig. 8.3).
- Heavy infestations may become secondarily infected with bacteria.
- Examine all the family, and treat anyone with live head lice.

Pubic (crab) louse (*Pthirus pubis*)

- Pubic lice are transmitted by close contact, including sexual contact.
- The lice infest short, coarse body hair—pubic, perianal, axillary, moustache, beard, eyelash, eyebrow.
- The translucent lice, 2mm long, may be visible, crawling through the hair, or you may see the nits (empty egg cases) glued to the hair shafts. Look for louse droppings (dark brown or black powder) in underwear (see Fig. 8.4).
- Bites produce bluish macules (maculae cerulea) that may be mistaken for bruises.

Body louse (*Pediculus humanus humanus*)

- Infestations cause severe itching, especially at night.
- Look for bite reactions—small erythematous papules or wheals where the skin is covered by clothing—as well as evidence of scratching.
- 2° infection is common.
- Check the seams of clothing worn next to the skin for lice (2–4mm) and eggs.

Box 8.3 Treatment of lice

Head lice

- Treat all infested family members.
- Physically acting preparations may be the best option. Dimeticone 4% lotion coats head lice and interferes with water excretion. Spread onto dry hair over all scalp; allow to dry; shampoo after at least 8h. Repeat treatment after 7 days.
- Malathion 0.5% lotion may be effective, but head lice are becoming resistant to many insecticides. Apply until hair is thoroughly wet down to the roots. Allow hair to dry, and leave the lotion on the hair for 8–12h. Shampoo after 12h. Repeat treatment after 7 days.
- Regular wet combing ('bug-busting') with a fine-toothed nit comb for 30min, repeated every 4 days, for 2 weeks may reduce the population of lice but is less effective than dimeticone.

Pubic lice

- Aqueous 0.5% malathion lotion or 5% permethrin cream—wash off after 12h, and repeat application after 7 days.

Body lice

- Launder clothing and bedding. The lice are killed by extremes of temperature. A pediculicide may not be needed.
- Treat 2° cutaneous infection.
- Prescribe sedating antihistamines for itching.

Female *Pediculosis capitis*

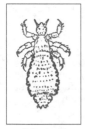

3 mm length

Fig. 8.3 Head louse, adapted to swing through hair. Reproduced with permission from Eddleston M et al. *Oxford Handbook of Tropical Medicine*, 3rd edn, 2008. Oxford: Oxford University Press.

Female *Phthirus pubis* with ovum within

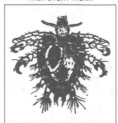

2 mm length

Fig. 8.4 Crab louse. Reproduced with permission from Eddleston M et al. *Oxford Handbook of Tropical Medicine*, 3rd edn, 2008. Oxford: Oxford University Press.

Further reading

Burgess IF et al. *BMC Dermatol* 2013;**13**:5.
Gunning K et al. *Am Fam Physician* 2012;**86**:535–41.

Demodicosis and other mites

What are Demodex?

- Demodex are mites, 0.1–0.4mm long, that live in or near normal hair follicles (*Demodex folliculorum*) and the ducts of sebaceous glands (*Demodex brevis*) predominantly on the scalp, eyelashes, external ear canals, forehead, sides of the nose, and cheeks. The tiny mites come out of follicles at night to walk around slowly (8–16cm/h) on the surface of the skin. They mate in the follicular openings.
- Demodex are rare in children <5 years old.
- Demodex are probably not pathogenic in immunocompetent humans. Increased numbers of mites are found in some papulopustular follicular eruptions, such as rosacea (see ➜ p. 254) and acne, but their role in pathogenesis is controversial, and it is not clear if eradication is helpful.
- Demodex infestation in immunocompromised patients with conditions, such as HIV/AIDS or acute lymphoblastic leukaemia, may cause inflamed papular eruptions (demodicosis).

What should I look for?

- Scaly erythematous papules or papulopustular lesions on the face, associated with variable swelling.
- No response to treatments for rosacea, e.g. oral tetracycline, topical metronidazole.
- Erythematous papules or papulopustular lesions on the scalp or chest.
- Blepharitis and pustules around the eyelids.
- Groups or clusters of erythematous papules, sometimes in annular patterns.
- Minimal itch.

What should I do?

- Take a skin scraping. Large numbers of mites will be visible in scale suspended in potassium hydroxide (see ➜ p. 646).
- Treat with 5% permethrin cream applied once a day for 3–5 days.
- Severe infestations can be treated with oral ivermectin.

Other mites

See Boxes 8.4 and 8.5.

Box 8.4 Harvest mites

- The larvae of these minute mites (*Trombicula autumnalis*) are found in grassy meadows, cornfields, and other herbage. The larvae are active during the day and can be a problem in dry sunny weather, especially in late summer and early autumn.
- The reddish larvae (0.2mm long) are just visible to the naked eye.
- The larvae congregate to feed on warm-blooded animals, including humans. The larvae hook onto exposed skin and repeatedly suck blood from the same site for 3 or 4 days, before dropping off the skin onto the ground to complete their life cycles.
- Bites cause intense irritation.
- Look for erythematous papules, 'heat spots', usually on the legs.
- Larvae are easily killed with an insecticide.
- A moderately potent topical corticosteroid will relieve irritation.
- Local names for the larvae include:
  - Harvest bugs.
  - Velvet mites.
  - Harvesters.
  - Berry bugs.
  - Bracken bugs.
  - Chiggers.
  - Orange-tawneys (in Ireland).
- The adult mites are harmless.
- The larvae of some related tropical species transmit a *Rickettsia* organism to humans, causing scrub typhus (mite typhus).

Box 8.5 Bird mite dermatitis (gamasoidosis)

- Pigeons are a well-known host for the blood-sucking bird mite *Dermanyssus gallinae* (the chicken mite). The mites are found where pigeons build their nests and can survive for 4–6 months without feeding on blood. The ♀ measures 0.7mm × 0.4mm, and the ♂ 0.6mm × 0.3mm.
- Humans working in buildings near the nesting sites of pigeons (window ledges, air conditioners) or patients lying beside open windows may become infested with mites looking for a meal. Bites may be painful, and the rash is extremely itchy.
- Look for an intensely itchy papulovesicular rash on exposed surfaces of the skin. The 1–2mm papules erupt in clusters or lines. The eruption resembles scabies, but you will not find burrows.
- The mites move extremely rapidly and leave the host, once they have fed, so they may be difficult to find. They hide in shady cracks and crevices during the day but emerge at night to 'bite and run'.
- The solution—get rid of the nests and the pigeons!
- Note: the mites infest other birds … and pet gerbils.

Fleas and bugs

Fleas are small (1.5–3.3mm), dark-coloured wingless insects adapted to feeding on the blood of warm-blooded vertebrates, including dogs, cats, pigs, chickens, and, unfortunately, humans. Most often, humans are bitten by animal fleas (usually cat or dog fleas), but these fleas do not live on humans and need access to their animal host to reproduce. Nowadays human fleas are found most often on farms. They live on pigs, which have similar skin to humans.

Fleas have extraordinarily hard shiny bodies that are virtually impossible to crush between the fingers or with a hard instrument. They are prodigious jumpers—their muscular legs can launch them vertically up to 18cm and horizontally up to 33cm (see Fig. 8.5).

Bedbugs are an increasing problem (see Box 8.6).

Papular urticaria

This eruption, frequent in children, is caused by an allergy to bites, usually those of cat fleas. The flea lays eggs on the cat, but these fall off into the bedding (or the sofa) where they pupate and then hatch in about 1 month. If the cat is not available, the flea is happy to bite another warm-blooded creature. Bites cause few symptoms, unless the patient is allergic to the flea's saliva. Fleas can survive for a year between meals, and pupae can remain dormant for 2 years or more. Presentation may be particularly dramatic if the house has been empty for a while, no cats have been in residence, and the fleas are hungry.

What should I look for?
- Clusters of itchy papules on the ankle and legs (the fleas jump up from the carpet to the nearest exposed skin). In crawling infants, the eruption may be more widespread.

What should I do?
- Try to convince the patient (or parent) that the problem lies with the cat (dog) and fleas. Explain that cat fleas are virtually impossible to eradicate, even though the pet has been treated, because the fleas are not living on the cat.
- Prescribe an antihistamine and a moderately potent topical steroid cream, such as clobetasone butyrate, to be applied to bites bd.
- Reassure everyone that the allergy will gradually become less of a problem.
- Recommend treating carpets, furnishings, pet bedding (and the cat) with appropriate insecticides and vacuuming frequently (but dispose of the vacuum bag afterwards).
- Recommend washing pet bedding every week, and consider moving the pet's bed to an area without carpets.

Human fleas (*Pulex irritans*)

- Itchy, dark red papules clustered in small groups ('breakfast, lunch, and tea') round the waist or abdomen suggest bites of human fleas.
- Hunt for the flea(s) to prove the diagnosis (see Box 8.7).

Box 8.6 Bedbugs

- Bedbugs thrive where standards of hygiene are poor and laundering is infrequent. The reddish brown bugs are 5mm long.
- Bugs bite exposed sites at night to feed on human blood. Bites irritate, and some people develop very brisk inflammatory reactions. Eyelid bites cause eyelid oedema ('eyelid sign').
- Bedbugs hide in a dark crevice during the day, e.g. in the mattress, within the bed frame or in the bed headboard, behind loose wallpaper or skirting boards, within paintings.
- Bedbugs can survive for a year without feeding.
- Look for spots of blood or brown excrement on bedding, or close to where the bedbugs are living, and a coriander-like sweet smell.
- Launder infested bedding in a hot wash.

Contact a pest control expert—heavily infested furnishings may have to be destroyed.

Box 8.7 Tracking down human fleas

Heavy infestation is no longer common. Most patients will have acquired just one or two human fleas. The fleas are found in the seams of clothing worn next to the skin, not on the patient, but they are difficult to see and even more difficult to catch and kill.

This technique has proved successful—advise the patient to:

- Prepare for action by dampening a bar of soap, which will be used to catch the flea(s).
- Stand fully clothed in a well-lit, pale-coloured bath tub (empty!).
- Take off each item of clothing; turn inside out, and shake thoroughly over the bath tub, paying particular attention to clothing next to the skin and the seams of the clothing.
- The flea or fleas will drop onto the shiny surface of the bath tub where it/they will be easy to see.
- Capture the flea using the sticky bar of soap (do not try to squash the flea—fleas are remarkably resilient, and they jump).
- Drown the flea by putting the bar of soap into water.
- Heavy infestation of the home by human fleas will need professional treatment.

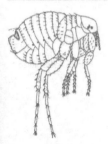

Fig. 8.5 Flea. Reproduced with permission from Collier J et al. *Oxford Handbook of Clinical Specialties* 8th edn, 2009. Oxford: Oxford University Press.

Tropical fleas, flies, and mosquitoes

Tunga penetrans

Synonyms: chigoe flea, sand flea, chigger, jigger.

Infestation with a flea (1mm long) endemic in Central America, the Caribbean, and sub-Saharan Africa causes tungiasis. The flea resides in warm, dry soil/sandy beaches. Usual hosts—pigs, cats, rodents. The ♀ burrows into the skin, feeding from dermal capillaries, enlarging, and breathing through a cutaneous punctum. After 2 days to 3 weeks, 150–200 eggs/day are released from the punctum. The flea dies *in situ* after 3–4 weeks and is eventually shed in a crust.

What should I look for?
- History of travel to an endemic area.
- An itchy, painful yellowish nodule with a central dark punctum on an exposed site, e.g. foot. Symptoms, caused by an immunological response, develop several days after the flea has penetrated the skin (see Fig. 8.6a).
- The punctum is easily visualized through a dermatoscope. After shaving the surrounding horny layer, it may be possible to see the tail of the flea in the punctum, or gentle compression may expel the white ovoid eggs (650 micrometres in length).

What should I do?
- Extract surgically after local anaesthetic (see Fig. 8.6b).
- Treat 2° infection.
- Advise patients travelling to endemic areas to cover exposed skin (socks, shoes) and to inspect the feet daily.

Furuncular myiasis

- Infestation with larvae of either *Dermatobia hominis*, the human botfly, or *Cordylobia anthropophaga*, the African tumbu fly. Human botflies, endemic in Central and South America, attach eggs to blood-sucking arthropods, e.g. mosquitoes. Mosquitoes leave eggs on the skin when having a blood meal. Tumbu flies, endemic in sub-Saharan Africa, lay eggs on shaded soil or clothing hung out to dry.
- Eggs hatch once in contact with warm skin. Larvae penetrate the skin and enlarge, while eating the tissue of the host. After 4–18 weeks, the larva emerges, falls to the ground, and pupates.

What should I look for?
- History of travel to an endemic area.
- Painful 'boil' with a central punctum and serosanguineous exudate. May itch or the patient may be aware of movement within it!
- The protruding respiratory spiracle in the punctum can be visualized through a dermatoscope.

What should I do?
- Occlude the punctum with white soft paraffin (e.g. Vaseline™), fat, or nail polish overnight to asphyxiate the larvae. Strip off the nail polish, if used. Remove protruding larvae with forceps, while squeezing the sides of the nodule gently.
- Treat 2° infection.

Tiger mosquitoes

Synonym: Forest day mosquitoes.

The tiger mosquito (*Aedes albopictus*) has spread to temperate regions, including Europe and the Americas, from tropical/subtropical countries. ♀ bites aggressively and repeatedly. Unlike other mosquitoes, this mosquito is active during the day and outdoors. In the tropics, mosquitoes are active all year, but, in temperate regions, they hibernate over winter. The eggs, laid on the inner sides of containers such as vases or old paint pots holding water, can survive freezing temperatures.

Bites may transmit viruses, including dengue and chikungunya.

What should I look for?
- History of aggressive daytime attacks by a small, dark mosquito with a white dorsal stripe and banded legs.
- Numerous intensely itchy or painful urticated papules, often on legs.
- Central punctum in papules.
- Papules may become purpuric or bullous.
- Allergy to mosquito saliva (Skeeter syndrome) causes a severe local reaction, simulating cellulitis with erythema and oedema, in addition to fever and vomiting.

What should I do?
- Treat bites with an ultra-potent topical steroid ×1/day.
- Prescribe an oral antihistamine.
- Treat 2° infection.
- Advise how to prevent further mosquito bites: repellents (applied after sunscreen), protective clothing.

(a)   (b)

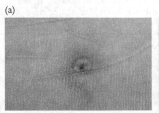 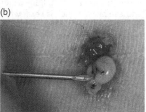

Fig. 8.6 Tunga penetrans. (a) Itchy papule with dark punctum on sole. (b) Flea extracted after shaving off the horny layer. (Images kindly provided by Dr Sam Gibbs.)

Cutaneous larva migrans

Synonym: creeping eruption

This parasitic skin disease is caused by hookworm larvae that usually infect domestic animals (see Box 8.8). In their animal hosts, the larvae penetrate the skin to reach the blood and lymphatic systems. They mature in the intestine. Eggs are excreted in faeces and take about 7 days to hatch. The larvae are found on beaches and moist soils that have been contaminated with animal faeces.

Cutaneous larva migrans presents in individuals whose skin has come into direct contact with the larvae, e.g. walking barefoot or lying on sandy beaches. The larvae tunnel through the stratum corneum into the epidermis but are unable to reach the dermis in humans, because they cannot penetrate the basement membrane. The disease is self-limiting, as humans are a 'dead-end' host.

Cutaneous larva migrans is usually acquired in tropical and subtropical regions, including the USA (south-eastern Atlantic and Gulf coastal regions), the Caribbean, South America, South East Asia, and East and West Africa.

What should I look for?

- The larvae migrate through the superficial epidermis, producing itchy, erythematous linear or serpiginous tracks (creeping eruption) (see Fig. 8.7).
- Tracks are often found on the feet but may be found on any skin surface that has been in direct contact with larvae.
- The track elongates 1–2cm per day.
- Sometimes blisters develop around or within the tracks.
- Most patients have one or two tracks, but heavy infestations, e.g. in HIV/AIDS, are associated with numerous itchy erythematous tracks, crusting, and 2° bacterial infection.

What should I do?

- The diagnosis is based on the history and clinical findings.
- A skin biopsy is not helpful, as it is difficult to predict exactly where to find the larva, which is somewhere just ahead of the leading edge of the track.
- Antihelminth treatment options include:
  - Ivermectin: a single dose of 12mg or 200 micrograms/kg (available on a named patient basis).
  - Albendazole: a single dose of 400mg or 400mg/day for 3–5 days for widespread infection (available on a named patient basis).
  - Topical 10–15% tiabendazole solution: applied qds for 1 week under an occlusive dressing (no commercial preparation available in the UK).
- Treat 2° bacterial infection.
- Prescribe a potent topical corticosteroid (apply bd) to reduce inflammation and relieve itching.

Box 8.8 Main causes of cutaneous larva migrans

- *Uncinaria stenocephala*: dog hookworm found in Europe.
- *Ancylostoma braziliense*: hookworm of wild and domestic dogs and cats found in central and southern USA, Central and South America, and the Caribbean.
- *Ancylostoma ceylonicum*: dog and cat hookworm found in Asia.
- *Ancylostoma caninum*: common dog and cat hookworm found in Australia.
- *Bunostomum phlebotomum*: cattle hookworm.

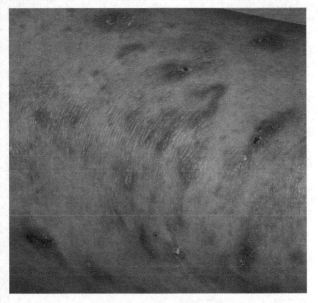

Fig. 8.7 Itchy serpiginous tracks in cutaneous larva migrans.

Cutaneous leishmaniasis

Synonyms: tropical sore, oriental sore, Baghdad sore, bouton d'Orient, Delhi boil, Aleppo boil, Chiclero ulcer.

Leishmaniasis is a vector-borne disease caused by obligate intramacrophage protozoa that belong to genus *Leishmania*. Twenty-one species of *Leishmania* can infect humans. The disease is endemic in tropical, subtropical, and southern European countries, including Central and South America, Asia, the Middle East, the Mediterranean, and East and North Africa. Animal reservoir hosts include rodents, bats, wolves, and foxes. Bites of ♀ sandflies transmit the parasite to humans.

Cutaneous leishmaniasis is the commonest type of leishmaniasis (see Box 8.9). Presentation is determined by infectivity and virulence of the parasite and the host response—some species induce a brisk inflammatory response, while others produce a more indolent disease.

What should I look for?

- A history of travel to an endemic region: the average incubation time is about 2 months, but cutaneous leishmaniasis may not present for more than a year after the sandfly bite.
- A history of sandfly bites (patients may not be aware of bites).
- Lesions on nocturnally exposed skin: face, neck, arms.
- One or more painless brownish nodules that may resemble bites, but usually do not itch, and slowly enlarge into plaques or warty lesions (Old World disease), or boil-like erythematous nodules that crust centrally and ulcerate in 1–3 months (New World disease). Ulcers may expand to a diameter of 3–6cm.
- Satellite nodules may develop around the 1° nodule. Nodules may spread along lymphatics ('sporotrichoid spread').
- Other members of the family may also have lesions, suggesting that the infection was acquired by bites at the same time.

What should I do?

- Take one or two full-thickness 4mm punch skin biopsies from the raised edge of a lesion or nodule for histological examination. Histology is granulomatous, but, even with a Giemsa stain, amastigote parasites may be difficult to find. Parasite DNA can be detected in lesional material by PCR, replacing culture in many centres.
- Make a smear from slit skin scrape, tissue, or aspirate (see Box 8.10). Parasites are easier to find in a smear than a biopsy.
- Culture material: first you will need to obtain the culture medium.
- Serology: usually unhelpful, because the antibody levels are low.
- Discuss management with an expert. Most lesions will heal without treatment in 3–18 months but leave a depressed scar which may be very disfiguring. Patients with New World leishmaniasis are at risk of developing mucosal disease. Intralesional, IM, or IV pentavalent antimony (sodium stibogluconate) is still the mainstay of treatment.

Box 8.9 Clinical types of leishmaniasis

- *Cutaneous leishmaniasis*: commonest form, Old World—caused by *Leishmaniasis tropica*, *L. major*, *L. aethiopica*. New World— *L. mexicana* species complex, *Viannia* subgenus, *L. major*-like organisms, and *L. chagasi*.
- *Leishmaniasis recidivans*: chronic destructive central facial lesion that enlarges over many years—seen in Iran and Iraq. Caused by *L. tropica*.
- *Mucosal leishmaniasis*: deep destructive mucosal ulceration (nose, pharynx, palate, lip) that occurs 1–5 years after cutaneous disease has healed. Occurs in South and Central America. Caused by *Viannia* subgenus (mainly *L. [V.] brasiliensis*, also *L. [V.] panamensis*, *L. [V.] guyanensis*, *L. amazonensis*).
- *Visceral leishmaniasis* (kala-azar, black sickness): caused by *L. donovani* complex, *L. tropica*, and *L. amazonensis*. Occurs in South America, Asia, the Mediterranean, and Africa. Patients are systemically unwell with a fever, sweats, weight loss, and massive splenomegaly. Skin is hyperpigmented. Intercurrent infections are common. Mortality, if untreated, is >80%. Visceral leishmaniasis may be an opportunistic infection in patients with HIV. Depigmented macules, nodules, and malar erythema are found in *post-kala-azar dermal leishmaniasis*.

Box 8.10 Investigations in cutaneous leishmaniasis (talk to an expert first)

- *PCR*: tissue the size of a rice grain should be placed in 300 microlitres of PCR buffer (Qiagen ATL).
- *Scrape*: pinch the skin around a nodule to exclude blood; slit the skin of the nodule with a scalpel blade to a depth of 1–2mm. Scrape the walls of incision, and smear the fluid thinly onto a clean microscope slide (the smear should not contain blood). Fix in methanol for 1min before staining.
- *Impression smear*: if you have taken a punch biopsy, remove excess blood by gently blotting on a towel, and then firmly press the cut surface of the tissue onto a clean glass slide several times. Fix in methanol for 1min before staining.
- *Aspirate smears*: sample three different areas from a nodule or the edge of a lesion. Attach a 0.5mm needle firmly to an empty 1–3mL syringe. Apply negative pressure, and advance the needle slowly in a straight line (to avoid blood contamination) along the edge of an ulcer or into the centre of a solid lesion. Withdraw in a straight line, but be careful not to draw any air into the syringe. Disconnect the needle; draw air into the syringe; reattach the needle, and blow out the contents rapidly onto a clean, polished, and alcohol-free microscope slide. Spread the aspirate gently on a slide using a needle tip. Fix in methanol for 1min before staining.

Further reading
de Vries HJC et al. Am J Clin Dermatol 2015;16:99–109.

Psoriasis

Contents

> **Relevant pages in other chapters**

What is psoriasis?

Derived from the Greek psor = itch or psorin = to have the itch.

Introduction

Psoriasis is a chronic inflammatory skin disease characterized by scaly, erythematous papules and plaques. The prevalence varies in different ethnic groups, but it affects around 2% of Northern Europeans. People of any age are affected, and the incidence is similar in men and women. Seventy-five percent of cases occur before the age of 46, but some studies have suggested two peaks of onset, between 16 and 22 years and 57 and 60 years. The disease remits spontaneously in 1/3 of patients, sometimes for 50 years, but the course is unpredictable.

Pathogenesis

The epidermis in psoriatic plaques is hyperproliferative, and the dermis contains tortuous, dilated small blood vessels, as well as an inflammatory infiltrate of CD4+ and CD8+ T-cells. Neutrophils are present in some forms of psoriasis. Dendritic cells contribute to pathogenesis.

It has been hypothesized that an antigen penetrating a defective epidermal barrier stimulates an immune response, but, although innate and adaptive immunity seem to be activated, no antigen has been identified. Cytokines released by epidermal keratinocytes and activated T-cells drive new vessel formation and proliferation of keratinocytes and T-cells. T-helper 1 (Th-1) cytokines (interferon (IFN) γ, IL-2, and IL-12) as well as tumour necrosis factor α (TNF-α), a pro-inflammatory cytokine, are present in psoriatic plaques. IL-22 and -23 (which activate Th-17 cells) also have a role in pathogenesis.

Genetic factors

Susceptibility to psoriasis is inherited—about 30% of patients with psoriasis have an affected first-degree relative. Linkage studies have shown that the genetics of psoriasis is complex (see Box 9.1). Environmental factors may trigger psoriasis in genetically predisposed individuals (see Box 9.3).

Psoriasis is more than skin deep

Patients with psoriasis have an increased risk of developing other inflammatory diseases that are immunologically mediated—seronegative arthritis (psoriatic arthritis—see ➔ p. 206) and Crohn disease. Case control studies have also shown an increased prevalence of the metabolic syndrome (see Box 9.2) in patients with psoriasis, possibly related to chronic inflammation and circulating inflammatory cytokines, including TNF-α. The psychosocial burden of psoriasis is considerable. Anxiety and depression are common, and patients tend to smoke and drink too much alcohol. Treat the whole patient, remembering associated co-morbidities, including coeliac disease, cardiovascular disease (see Box 9.2 p. 191), hypertension, obesity, type 2 diabetes, peptic ulcer, and liver disease.

Box 9.1 Genetics: psoriasis susceptibility loci

More than 40 gene loci have been identified to be associated with psoriasis susceptibility. Psoriasis risk genes or genes that modify the severity of disease may include:

- Genes for factors that control inflammation.
- Genes involved in keratinocyte signalling.
- Genes regulating vascular growth.

At least 13 chromosomal loci PSORS1–13 have been linked to psoriasis, but no single psoriasis gene has been identified. Loci of particular interest include:

- PSORS1: the major genetic determinant of psoriasis. Located in the major histocompatibility complex (MHC) on chromosome 6p, close to HLA-Cw6. Strongly linked to guttate psoriasis. HLA-Cw6 is a marker for early-onset psoriasis. Early reports suggest that this genetic polymorphism could predict the response to biological agents.
- PSORS4: within the epidermal differentiation complex on chromosome 1q.
- PSORS8: overlaps with the Crohn disease locus on chromosome 16q. The frequency of Crohn disease in patients with psoriasis is increased.

In addition, susceptibility genes for psoriasis and psoriatic arthritis have been reported in the late cornified envelope (LCE) gene cluster, in particular the *LCE3* genes. Deletion of *LCE3B* and *LCE3C* are significantly associated with both diseases. For other rare genetic associations see Chandra A et al. (see ➲ Further reading).

Box 9.2 Components of metabolic syndrome

- Elevated waist circumference: men >102cm; women >88cm.
- Elevated triglycerides.
- Reduced high-density lipoprotein (HDL) cholesterol.
- Elevated blood pressure >130/85mmHg.
- Elevated fasting glucose.

Metabolic syndrome is defined as the presence of three or more of these criteria. The syndrome produces a prothrombotic and proinflammatory state.

Further reading

Chandra A et al. Mol Immunol 2015;**64**:313–23.
Di Cesare A et al. J Invest Dermatol 2009;**129**:1339–50.
Menter MA and Griffiths CE. Dermatol Clin 2015;**33**:161–6.
Nijsten T and Wakkee M. J Invest Dermatol 2009;**129**:1601–3.

The history in psoriasis

The diagnosis may be obvious to you (and the patient) from the appearance of the skin, but listen to the patient's story to help you to assess the impact of the psoriasis and to plan management.

What should I ask?

- Invite the patient to tell you about his/her skin condition, and then ask specific questions, taking a history, as described in ➲ Chapter 2, p. 18, pp. 20–1, pp. 30–31, and pp. 32–4.
- Inquire about symptoms—in psoriasis, these may include itch, bleeding from the skin, scaling, showers of 'dandruff', or pain (fissures on the palms and soles may be very uncomfortable).
- Find out what helps or exacerbates the rash (see Box 9.3).
- Explore quality of life—how does psoriasis affect daily activities, work, or school? Is the patient prepared to go swimming/wear clothing that reveals affected skin? How does other people's attitude affect the patient? (See ➲ pp. 32–4.)
- Psoriasis fluctuates in severity. How bad is the rash today? Ask the patient to rate the severity on a scale of 0 to 10 (worst possible).
- Explore lifestyle—alcohol intake, physical activity, and diet.

Treatments/drug history

- What treatments are being used now or have been used in the past? How effective are these—why were they stopped? (See ➲ pp. 30–31.)
- Patients may have been treated with UVB or psoralen with UVA (PUVA) photochemotherapy. Was burning a problem? Did the psoriasis respond? How quickly did psoriasis recur? How long was each course, and how many courses has the patient had?
- Is the patient taking drugs that might worsen psoriasis? (See Box 9.3.)

Family history

Does anyone else in the family have a skin disease? Patients who have relatives with severe psoriasis may be particularly concerned about their own prognosis and the risk of their children developing psoriasis.

Past medical history

- Has the patient had any previous skin problems?
- Is there a history of skin cancer (a risk after excessive PUVA)?
- Is there a history of arthritis? (see ➲ p. 206.)
- Severe psoriasis is associated with co-morbidities, including the metabolic syndrome. Document cardiovascular risk factors—hyperlipidaemia, obesity, smoking, hypertension, and diabetes.
- Is there a history of depression?
- Does the patient have HIV? HIV/AIDS may trigger severe psoriasis.

Measuring the impact of the psoriasis

There is a temporal relationship between psychosocial stress and exacerbation of psoriasis. Ask the patient to complete the DLQI to obtain a validated measure of the impact of the skin disease (see ➲ pp. 32–34).

Box 9.3 Environmental factors that exacerbate psoriasis

- Infections: β-haemolytic streptococcal tonsillitis or pharyngitis, HIV.
- Drugs: β-blockers, antimalarials, lithium, interferon α (IFN-α), alcohol, TNF antagonists.
- Rebound is common after systemic steroids.
- Trauma to the skin (Koebner phenomenon).
- Hormones: may improve or deteriorate in pregnancy.
- Stress or emotional upset.
- Sunlight: usually improves but, in 10%, exacerbates psoriasis.

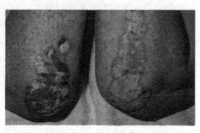

Fig. 9.1 Symmetrical plaque psoriasis on extensor surfaces.

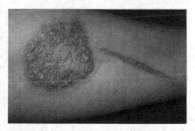

Fig. 9.2 Koebner phenomenon—psoriasis appearing in a scratch.

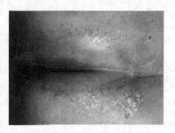

Fig. 9.3 Shiny, well-demarcated erythema in flexural psoriasis. Scaling is lost in the moist flexure.

Common clinical patterns

Psoriasis vulgaris (plaque psoriasis)

This is the commonest pattern of psoriasis (see Box 9.4). Onset may be gradual or sudden. The disease may be limited or widespread. Measure the extent of disease, and assess the severity (see ➲ PASI scoring, pp. 200–1).

What should I look for?

- Well-defined pinkish, scaly plaques of variable size, thickness, and shape in a symmetrical pattern, predominantly on extensor surfaces. Examine the elbows, knees, hairline (psoriasis is uncommon on the face but often involves the scalp margin), and trunk (see Fig. 9.1). Differentiate from pityriasis rubra pilaris (rare) (see Box 9.5 and Fig 9.4).
- Silvery scaling over the surface of the plaques: this may be thick in untreated disease or minimal if the patient is using topical steroids.
- Bleeding points where scale has been scratched off.
- Plaques in the scalp: ask about 'dandruff'; palpate to find plaques. Scalp psoriasis is not obvious on inspection, because hair is retained.
- The Koebner phenomenon: new psoriasis appearing at sites of cutaneous trauma, including excoriations or surgical scars (see Fig. 9.2).
- Post-inflammatory hypo- or hyperpigmentation, e.g. when psoriasis has improved after treatment or a sunny holiday.
- Nail involvement (50%) (see Box 9.5, and Figs. 9.5 and 9.6).
- Flexural psoriasis—see later in this section (see Fig. 9.3).

Guttate psoriasis

Gutta is Latin for droplet.

An acute form triggered by infection with group β-haemolytic *Streptococcus* (usually tonsillitis or pharyngitis) presents in children and adolescents. The rash erupts 2–3 weeks after infection and usually resolves within 3–4 months. Some patients progress to psoriasis vulgaris. Guttate psoriasis may recur after subsequent streptococcal infections.

What should I look for?

- A history of an infection preceding the eruption by 2–4 weeks.
- A history of the sudden onset of a widespread rash.
- Teardrop-sized erythematous, scaly papules, mainly on the trunk.

Flexural psoriasis and sebopsoriasis

Psoriasis in moist flexural sites is not scaly and often misdiagnosed as fungal infection, but symmetry suggests psoriasis (see Fig. 9.3).

What should I look for?

- Well-defined shiny, erythematous, minimally raised plaques in flexures, including inframammary skin, umbilicus, axillae, groins, and natal cleft.
- Ill-defined erythematous, greasy, slightly scaly skin in the central face (nasolabial folds), eyebrows, behind and within ears, and the scalp resembling seborrhoeic dermatitis (sebopsoriasis).
- Nail signs may help confirm a diagnosis of psoriasis (see Boxes 9.5 and 9.6).

Box 9.4 Clinical patterns of psoriasis

Patients may have >1 pattern of psoriasis:
- Psoriasis vulgaris (large plaque and/or small plaque) on extensor surfaces.
- Guttate psoriasis (sudden onset of widespread scaly papules triggered by a streptococcal tonsillitis or pharyngitis).
- Flexural (inverse) psoriasis, also known as sebopsoriasis, may be difficult to distinguish from seborrhoeic dermatitis (see ➔ p. 219).
- Palmoplantar pustulosis; generalized pustular psoriasis.
- Erythrodermic psoriasis.
- Nail psoriasis: may be the only sign of psoriasis (see Box 9.6).
- Napkin psoriasis (see ➔ Box 31.13, p. 605).

Box 9.5 What is pityriasis rubra pilaris?

- Pityriasis rubra pilaris (PRP) is a rare inflammatory papulosquamous disorder of unknown cause that may be misdiagnosed as psoriasis (much commoner) (see Fig. 9.4).
- Classical adult PRP presents with yellowish palmoplantar keratoderma and follicular hyperkeratotic papules. These coalesce into scaly, orange-red plaques with well-defined borders.
- Typically spares some patches of the skin—'islands of sparing'.
- PRP starts on the head, neck, and upper trunk and, over weeks, progresses downwards (cephalo-caudal progression).
- May eventually involve all body (erythroderma).
- Hair loss common (non-scarring) and thickened nails.
- The disease remits in 80% of patients within 3–5 years. Atypical adult PRP may persist for many years.
- May be associated with an underlying malignancy.
- Histopathology is characterized by alternating ortho- and parakeratosis rete ridges called the 'checkerboard pattern'.
- Treatment difficult—emollients important. Oral retinoids or methotrexate may have some impact.
- Most cases are sporadic. Familial PRP shows autosomal dominant inheritance. Both can be caused by gain-of-function mutations in the *CARD14* gene encoding the caspase recruitment domain family member 14 (CARD14) that is important in the activation of nuclear factor kappa B signalling.
- *CARD14* mutations and variants are also reported in familial plaque psoriasis and generalized pustular psoriasis, depending on the mutation or variant position of *CARD14*.
- Other types of PRP include juvenile forms (classical, atypical, circumscribed) and HIV-associated.

Nails in psoriasis

Nail signs may help to confirm the diagnosis of psoriasis. Signs depend on the location of the pathology—nail matrix or nail bed.

- Pits: usually small and shallow and irregularly scattered (likened to the surface of a thimble); some are deep—best seen with magnification and side-lighting. Psoriasis of the proximal matrix leads to a defective nail plate, which partially desquamates, leaving a depression on the nail surface (equivalent to scale on the surface of the skin) (see Fig. 9.5). Similar macropits are observed along the hair shafts of patients with scalp psoriasis.
- Onycholysis (separation of the free edge of the nail plate from the nail bed): the nail appears yellowish white with a proximal brownish red margin (see Fig. 9.6). Oval spots of salmon-coloured discoloration (oil spots). Both caused by psoriasis of the nail bed.
- Thickening and crumbling of the whole nail plate: caused by psoriasis of the entire nail matrix. (Asymmetrical nail dystrophy suggests fungal infection. In psoriasis, most nails are affected.)
- Subungual hyperkeratosis: caused by psoriasis of the nail bed.
- Splinter haemorrhages in fingernails.
- Soft tissue swelling of the proximal nail fold, with chronic paronychia and horizontal ridging of the nail plate.
- Acral pustulosis/parakeratosis pustulosa (see ➲ Box 9.9).
- Assess the severity using the Nail Psoriasis Severity Index (see Box 9.6).

Box 9.6 The Nail Psoriasis Severity Index (NAPSI)

NAPSI is used to assess the extent of severity of the nail bed involvement in psoriasis. NAPSI was developed to supplement PASI (see Fig. 9.7), which does not assess the impact of nail disease. NAPSI is particularly useful when nail disease has a major functional or cosmetic impact or for monitoring treatments initiated specifically for nail psoriasis.

- NAPSI assigns a score to each nail for nail bed/matrix psoriasis.
- The nail plate is divided into four quadrants; each one is scored.
- Nail matrix involvement is assessed by the presence of nail pitting, leuconychia, red spots in the lunula, and crumbling in each quadrant.
- Nail bed involvement is assessed by the presence of onycholysis, oil drop (salmon patch), splinter haemorrhages, and nail bed hyperkeratosis in each quadrant.
- Score 1 for involvement of each quadrant. Therefore, each nail has a matrix score (0–4) and a nail bed score (0–4), and the total is the sum of these two (0–8).

Further reading

Rich P and Scher RK. *J Am Acad Dermatol* 2003;**49**:206–12.

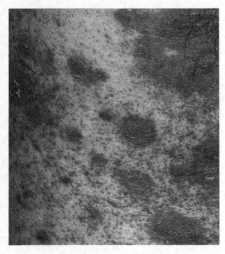

Fig. 9.4 Pityriasis rubra pilaris with follicular hyperkeratotic papules coalescing into orange-red scaly plaques.

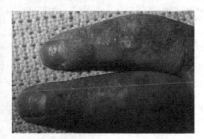

Fig. 9.5 Nail pitting and psoriatic arthropathy.

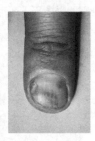

Fig. 9.6 Onycholysis.

Erythrodermic and pustular psoriasis

Erythrodermic psoriasis

Erythroderma is defined as redness and scaling affecting 90% of the BSA. Plaque psoriasis may evolve into erythroderma suddenly or gradually. Topical treatments that irritate the skin may precipitate erythroderma, as may some systemic drugs. Psoriasis may also flare after withdrawal of systemic corticosteroids. Less often, patients with no past history of psoriasis will present erythrodermic.

What should I do?
- Ask if the patient has any history of previous skin diseases (conditions such as atopic eczema may become erythrodermic) or has started any new drugs.
- Check the nails for signs of psoriasis.
- Seek expert help—erythroderma is a form of skin failure. The principles of management are discussed in ➲ Box 5.8, p. 109.
- ⚠ The skin is easily irritated—prescribe a bland emollient.
- Once the condition is stable, you may be able to introduce specific treatments, e.g. UVB, tar, methotrexate.

Palmoplantar pustulosis

Palmoplantar pustulosis is a chronic condition affecting the palms and soles (see Box 9.7) that is seen most often in middle-aged women who smoke cigarettes, but stopping smoking does not alleviate the problem. Genetic studies have shown that palmoplantar pustulosis is not linked to the same loci as psoriasis vulgaris. Most patients do not have any other psoriasis. For management, see Box 9.8.

Palmoplantar pustulosis is clinically and histologically identical to early keratoderma blenorrhagicum (see ➲ p. 208). Palmoplantar pustulosis is also triggered in some patients by treatment with anti-TNF drugs (see ➲ p. 389).

Generalized pustular psoriasis (GPP)

This rare life-threatening presentation is often misdiagnosed as infection, because patients have a fever, neutrophilia, and widespread superficial (subcorneal) pustules on a background of erythema. The clinical features are outlined in ➲ Box 5.25, p. 125. Familial GPP or GPP in the absence of chronic plaques is caused by homozygous or compound heterozygous mutations of IL-36RN (IL-36 receptor antagonist).

⚠ Pustular psoriasis may be precipitated by withdrawal of oral or very potent topical corticosteroids or may develop in some patients with plaque psoriasis treated with anti-TNF drugs (see ➲ p. 389).

What should I do?
See ➲ pp. 124–5.

Acropustulosis and parakeratosis pustulosa

Rarely, pustulosis may affect one or more digits in the absence of other forms of psoriasis (see ➲ Box 9.9 and p. 208).

Box 9.7 Palmoplantar pustulosis: what should I look for?

- Well-defined erythematous, scaly plaques on palms and/or soles are studded with pustules and/or vesicopustules.
- Dried-up pustules appear as yellowish brown, slightly scaly papules.
- The condition may be unilateral.
- Hyperkeratosis and fissuring complicate the picture.
- The condition may resemble infected chronic dermatitis, particularly if the vesicopustules and hyperkeratosis dominate the picture (vesicles without pustules suggest eczema).

Box 9.8 Palmoplantar pustulosis: what should I do?

- The diagnosis is clinical—a skin biopsy is not usually required.
- Take skin scrapes to exclude fungal infection, especially if unilateral.
- If hyperkeratosis with vesicopustules dominates the picture, it may be difficult to distinguish between infected dermatitis and psoriasis. Patch test to exclude an allergic contact dermatitis, if any doubt.
- Greasy emollients and soap substitutes reduce the tendency to fissuring.
- Potent or highly potent topical corticosteroid ointments applied bd will control inflammation and pustules. Skin on palms and soles are thick, so steroids can be used for a considerable time before producing atrophy. However, the disease tends to be chronic, and use of topical corticosteroids must be monitored. Consider alternative therapy if minimal improvement after 8–12 weeks.
- Keratolytics, e.g. salicylic acid, combined with a topical corticosteroid may control hyperkeratotic disease.
- Topical vitamin D$_3$ analogues or 0.1% tacrolimus ointment may help.
- Deep fissures—close with quick-drying glues such as superglue.
- Localized UV light treatment can be helpful (topical PUVA).
- Acitretin 20–30mg/day achieves control in some patients (see ➔ p. 669).

Box 9.9 Acropustulosis and parakeratosis pustulosa

- *Acrodermatitis continua/acrodermatitis of Hallopeau*: affects one or more digits. Sterile pustules form beneath and around the nail plate, which is lifted off by crust and lakes of pus. Nail loss may be permanent and associated with resorptive osteolysis. Very potent topical steroids or oral retinoids are indicated.
- *Parakeratosis pustulosa*: affects a single digit in young children—the skin is erythematous and scaly. Pustules/vesicles may be present early but do not persist, and changes look eczematous. The nail plate lifts up and becomes thickened. The condition is chronic but self-limiting. Topical steroids may be helpful. It is uncertain whether this condition is a form of eczema or psoriasis.

Assessing severity

Severity is a function of both the extent of the disease (impairment) and the impact on quality of life (disability). Impact should be assessed with a tool such as the DLQI (see ➔ p. 32).

Severity may be measured using a global rating (see Box 9.10) or with a disease-specific tool such as the PASI.

> **Box 9.10 Global assessment**
>
> - Mild <5% BSA.
> - Moderate 5–10% BSA.
> - Severe >10% BSA.
>
> Measure the BSA using the patient's hand. The palm and palmar surface of the digits = 1% of the BSA. But a simple assessment of the area of involvement does not take into account other problems such as itch, scale, redness, or thickness of plaques.

What is the PASI?

(See Fig. 9.7.) The PASI is a tool that was devised for assessing chronic plaque psoriasis. The PASI is a widely used outcome measure in clinical trials—a PASI 50 means that the patient shows a 50% improvement from the baseline PASI. The PASI can be used to record the progress of patients with chronic plaque poriasis. It is less useful in other forms of disease such as palmoplantar pustulosis and guttate psoriasis.

How do I interpret the PASI?

- Higher scores indicate more severe psoriasis.
- Although the PASI ranges from 0 (no psoriasis) to 72 (100% coverage in the worst possible psoriasis), in practice, a PASI of 12 or more indicates severe chronic plaque psoriasis, and a PASI of <7 indicates mild chronic plaque psoriasis.

How is the PASI calculated?

(See Fig. 9.7.)

- The body is divided into four anatomical regions (head, upper limbs, trunk, lower limbs).
- Redness (erythema), thickness (infiltration), and scaling in the psoriatic plaques in each region are each scored on a 5-point scale (0 = none; 1 = slight; 2 = moderate; 3 = severe; 4 = very severe).
- The area of skin affected in each region is estimated and given a numerical value.
- The final calculation uses a simple formula to adjust the score for each region, according to the proportion that the skin in each region is of all the skin.
- The PASI will only take a few minutes to complete, once you have had some practice. PASI scoring sheets, which will take you through the calculation, are widely available. Online calculators are also available, e.g. ℘ http://pasi.corti.li/ or ℘ www.pasitraining.com/calculator/step_1.php.
- Although the PASI is subjective, with experience, results are reproducible.

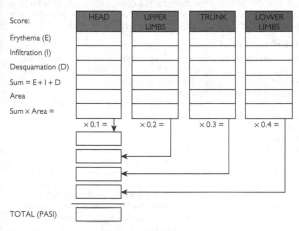

Score for symptom and area for
head, trunk, upper and lower limbs

Score	0	1	2	3	4	5	6
Erythema Infiltration Desquamation	None	Slight	Moderate	Severe	Very severe		
Area %	0	<10	10<30	30<50	50<70	70<90	90–100

Score:

Erythema (E)

Infiltration (I)

Desquamation (D)

Sum = E + I + D

Area

Sum × Area =

HEAD   × 0.1 =

UPPER LIMBS   × 0.2 =

TRUNK   × 0.3 =

LOWER LIMBS   × 0.4 =

TOTAL (PASI)

Fig. 9.7 Psoriasis Area and Severity Index (PASI). Adapted with permission of Salford Royal Hospital NHS Trust © 2002. See BAD website to download PASI scoring sheet ℛ http://www.bad.org.uk/healthcare-professionals/clinical-standards/clinical-guidelines.

Further reading

Feldman SR and Krueger G. *Ann Rheum Dis* 2005;**64**(Suppl II):ii65–ii68.
Schmitt J and Wozel G. *Dermatology* 2005;**210**:194–9.

Approach to management

Most psoriasis is not life-threatening, but living with psoriasis can ruin lives. You are breaking bad news when you explain to someone that he/she has psoriasis. Treatments offer control, rather than cure—psoriasis remits despite treatment, not because of treatment. Your assessment should establish the impact of the disease, efficacy of previous treatments, and the extent of the disease. Managing psoriasis is an art—help the patient to find a balance between living with psoriasis and living with problems caused by treatment. For investigations, see Box 9.11.

What should I do?

- Do not make any assumptions—explore the patient's expectations. Some patients are very bothered by limited disease. You will also meet patients with extensive disease who do not want systemic drugs. Using the DLQI can help.
- Address lifestyle. Lifestyle behaviour change, e.g. weight loss, exercise, reduced alcohol intake, can be helpful.
- Explain treatments control, but do not cure, psoriasis.
- Does the patient want treatment? No treatment is an option—psoriasis may scar the mind, but it does not scar the skin.
- Find out what the patient can manage to do to him/herself.
- Keep the treatment simple. Decide whether to recommend topical treatments, UV light, or a systemic drug, or to use a combination.
- Discuss the likely benefits (including how long it will take, before treatment has an effect), and explain the side effects of treatments.
- Negotiate a plan for management, provide a written management plan, and agree follow-up arrangements (see ➲ pp. 30–1).
- Provide information about psoriasis, including patient support groups such as the Psoriasis Association (UK)—available at ℜ https://www. psoriasis-association.org.uk/.

Topical treatment
see ➲ pp. 204–5.

Phototherapy (UVB)

Patients with widespread psoriasis, including guttate psoriasis, may benefit from a 6- to 8-week course of phototherapy with UVB ×3/week (narrow band 311nm). UVB may be combined with topical vitamin D_3 analogues, tazarotene, or systemic treatments (retinoids). Sunbeds emit UVA, which is much less effective than UVB and significantly increase the risk of melanoma and non-melanoma skin cancers.

Systemic treatment

(See Box 9.12.) Methotrexate (weekly dose), oral retinoids (acitretin), and ciclosporin are the most widely used drugs. In patients with psoriatic arthritis, the choice of systemic treatment should be made in collaboration with a rheumatologist. The new biological agents (e.g. anti-TNF-α) have revolutionized the treatment of severe psoriasis unresponsive to other treatments (see ➲ Chapter 34, and Box 34.5, p. 671).

Box 9.11 Investigations in psoriasis

- Diagnosis is not usually a problem, and skin biopsies are seldom required.
- If the disease is asymmetrical, take skin scrapings or nail clippings for fungal culture, as tinea is the differential diagnosis.
- If the patient is obese and at risk of the metabolic syndrome, check blood pressure, fasting glucose, cholesterol, and triglycerides.

Screening prior to systemic treatment

If you are considering prescribing systemic treatments, check:
- FBC.
- Liver function and renal function.
- Procollagen peptide 3 (prior to methotrexate—although this has poor clinical utility) (see ➔ Chapter 34, p. 668).
- Fasting cholesterol and triglycerides (prior to oral retinoids).

Box 9.12 Systemic treatments for psoriasis

Indications for systemic therapy include:
- Psoriasis poorly controlled by topical agents/UVB phototherapy.
- Psoriasis with a significant impact on physical, psychological, or social well-being (may be limited in extent).
- Extensive psoriasis (PASI score >10)
- Psoriasis in high-impact sites, e.g. severe nail psoriasis.

Systemic options include:
- PUVA photochemotherapy (oral psoralen plus UVA) ×2/week. More carcinogenic than phototherapy with UVB ×3/week. Limited lifetime dose. Contraindicated if high risk of skin cancers.
- Methotrexate—weekly dose. First-choice systemic drug. Takes time to work (see ➔ Chapter 34, p. 668).
- Ciclosporin—acts quickly (see ➔ Chapter 34, pp. 664–5).
- Acitretin—useful in palmoplantar pustular psoriasis (see ➔ Chapter 34, p. 669).
- Fumaric acid esters (see ➔ Chapter 34, p. 667).
- Mycophenolate mofetil (see ➔ Chapter 34, pp. 668–9).
- Biological therapy if other options fail:
  - Anti-TNF agents, e.g. infliximab, etanercept, and adalimumab.
  - IL inhibitors, e.g. ustekinumab (IL-12/23 inhibitor) see ➔ Box 34.5, p. 671.

Further reading

Menter A and Griffiths CE. *Lancet* 2007;**370**:272–84.

National Institute for Health and Care Excellence (NICE). *Psoriasis: the assessment and management of psoriasis*. Available at: ⚲ https://www.nice.org.uk/guidance/cg153.

Nelson PA et al. *Br J Dermatol* 2014;**171**:1116–22 (lifestyle behaviour change in psoriasis).

Topical treatments

General principles

- Topical treatment is a reasonable option for limited disease.
- Discuss the likely outcome—control, not cure. Explain that you are not aiming to clear, but to make the condition tolerable.
- Patients need time (and may need help) to apply treatments. If time is a problem, suggest concentrating on the most troublesome area.
- Demonstrate how to apply the treatment—ideally, you will have a specialist nurse to help you.
- Select the right base (usually the one the patient prefers) for each treatment—ointment, cream, lotion, gel, or foam.
- Keep the treatment plan simple—the patient is much more likely to adhere to treatment—and prescribe enough of the preparations.
- In patients with extensive disease, topical treatments can be combined with UV light or systemic treatment.

Emollients

- Emollient creams (moisturizers) reduce scale and may relieve itch partially, but are less effective in psoriasis than eczema.

Vitamin D$_3$ analogues: suitable for limited plaque psoriasis

- Vitamin D$_3$ analogues (e.g. calcitriol, calcipotriol, tacalcitol) are effective, if applied ×1–2/day for at least 3 months. Patients like these preparations, because they are colourless and odourless.
- Plaques eventually become erythematous smooth patches but do not disappear.
- Vitamin D$_3$ analogues may be used for short periods in combination with a potent topical corticosteroid to reduce the risk of irritation (combination preparations are available).
- Vitamin D$_3$ analogues are not suitable for extensive psoriasis, because treatment has to be limited to affected skin, and patients should not use >100g/week because of risk of hypercalcaemia.
- Some vitamin D$_3$ analogues may irritate and are not suitable for the face or flexures.

Tar lotion: suitable for limited or widespread plaque psoriasis

- Coal tar 1% lotion applied ×1–2/day is as effective as a topical vitamin D$_3$ analogue for the trunk and limbs and easier to use in widespread psoriasis, because application does not have to be limited to affected skin.
- The lotion can be applied quickly all over the skin.
- Coal tar lotion may irritate and is not suitable for the face or flexures.
- Patients may not like the smell, but applying an emollient over the lotion reduces this.
- Liquor picis carbonis (LPC) 10% in an emulsifying ointment is also suitable for home use, but it is messier to use than coal tar lotion.

Topical corticosteroids: most suitable for limited plaque psoriasis

- Potent and highly potent corticosteroid creams or ointments are clean and easy to use.
- Applied ×1–2/day daily, corticosteroids are very effective and work quickly.
- If used for prolonged periods, corticosteroids cause skin atrophy. Large amounts used for prolonged periods may also cause adrenal suppression.
- Psoriasis will rebound when corticosteroids are stopped abruptly.
- Patients should be reviewed 8-weekly if using potent topical corticosteroids, and usage kept to a minimum (<50g/week).

Topical retinoids: most suitable for limited plaque psoriasis

- Topical retinoid (tazarotene) may reduce thickness, scaling, and erythema, if applied ×1/day for 3 months, but can be an irritant.

Treatments for facial and flexural psoriasis

- Calcineurin inhibitor (tacrolimus, pimecrolimus) ointments can be very useful in facial and flexural psoriasis (sebopsoriasis).
- Moderately potent topical corticosteroids are suitable for facial and flexural psoriasis, including sebopsoriasis. Apply ×1–2/day. For flexures, the corticosteroid is usually combined with an antifungal agent such as miconazole. Stronger topical corticosteroids are more effective, but very likely to cause atrophy in thin flexural skin.
- Some vitamin D_3 analogues are suitable for the face or flexures, but others irritate the skin.

Treatments for the scalp

- Mild scale: control with potent or highly potent steroid lotions or foams applied at night, or use a vitamin D_3 analogue scalp preparation. Advise the patient not to let the steroid preparation drip onto the neck or forehead (risk of atrophy).
- Thick scale: remove with keratolytic scalp compound, e.g. Cocois® ointment, Sebco® (coal tar solution and salicylic acid in coconut oil with applicator nozzle). Apply to the scalp (part the hair) once weekly. If severe, use daily for first 3–7 days. Leave on overnight, and shampoo off next morning.
- Tar-based shampoos may be helpful.

Other treatments

- Crude coal tar preparations, once the mainstay of topical treatment, are no longer first-line therapies. They are messy and difficult to use.
- Dithranol (anthralin), also reserved for difficult cases of plaque psoriasis, is available in the form of Dithrocream® and Micanol® to be used at home. The main side effect is irritancy to normal skin.
- Both dithranol and tar may be used for inpatients or for day care and are often combined with UVB.

Psoriatic arthritis

Overall, 4–30% of patients with psoriasis have an associated arthritis. Seventy percent of these patients develop psoriasis before arthritis, 10–15% arthritis before psoriasis, and, in the rest, the two occur within 1 year of each other. For classification criteria, see Box 9.13.

Joint involvement is classified into five major clinical subtypes that overlap. Most present with monoarthritis or oligoarthritis, but more joints tend to be involved in long-standing disease. Erosive and deforming arthritis occur in 40–60% of patients. Simultaneous flares in skin and joint disease have been reported, but conflicting evidence about whether the severity of psoriasis is related to the severity of arthritis.

What should I look for?

- A history of joint stiffness in the morning that lasts >30min, suggesting inflammatory disease.
- Symmetrical polyarthritis that may be indistinguishable from RA (rheumatoid factor (RF) negative, no rheumatoid nodules). Look for boggy soft tissue swelling in the small joints of the hands, suggesting synovitis.
- Asymmetric oligoarthritis with <5 small or large joints affected in an asymmetrical pattern. Look for effusions in large joints, e.g. knees.
- Psoriatic nail changes are commoner and associated with distal interphalangeal (DIP) inflammation.
- Involvement of the spine (spondylitis) and sacroiliac joints (sacroiliitis). This pattern is associated with the MHC class I molecule HLA-B27, like the other seronegative spondyloarthropathies (see ➜ Reactive arthritis, p. 208, and SAPHO syndrome, p. 248).
- Arthritis mutilans—destruction of the small joints of the hand, especially the DIP joints. This is associated with prolonged disease.
- Dactylitis, i.e. swelling of a whole digit, producing a sausage-like appearance (seen in 1/3 of patients). Probably a combination of tenosynovitis and synovitis or diffuse digital oedema (see Fig. 9.5).
- Enthesopathy, i.e. pain at sites where ligaments, tendons, fascia, and the joint capsule are inserted into bone, e.g. at the heel (plantar fasciitis), elbow (golfer's elbow or tennis elbow), and the Achilles tendon.

What should I do?

- Investigations: FBC—normocytic anaemia; leucocytosis in acute inflammatory arthritis. CRP, ESR—raised in acute inflammatory arthritis. RF—usually negative in psoriatic arthritis.
- Radiographs of affected joints and sacroiliac joints if low back pain sounds inflammatory, i.e. stiffness improving with exercise and not relieved by rest.
- Refer to a rheumatologist if symptoms not controlled by anti-inflammatory agents or evidence of synovitis, joint effusion, or deformity. Several tools have been developed to screen psoriasis patients for psoriatic arthritis, e.g. Psoriasis Epidemiology Screening Tool (PEST) (see Box 9.14).
- Early treatment prevents joint destruction, deformity, and loss of function. For management options, see Box 9.15.

Box 9.13 CASPAR criteria for classifying psoriatic arthritis

Criteria developed in 2006 for classification in research, rather than for diagnostic purposes. Sensitivity 91%, specificity 98%.

Inflammatory musculoskeletal disease with features such as erythema, warmth, and swelling of joints; morning and rest stiffness; painful joints, spine, and/or enthesium; plus at least three points from the following features:
- Current psoriasis (score = 2).
- Past history of psoriasis (unless psoriasis is present) (score = 1).
- Family history of psoriasis (unless psoriasis is present or there is a history of psoriasis) (score = 1).
- Nail changes (score = 1); dactylitis (score = 1).
- Juxta-articular new bone formation on radiographs (score = 1).
- Negative RF (score = 1).

Box 9.14 Psoriasis Epidemiology Screening Tool (PEST)

Annual screening is recommended for patients with psoriasis who do not have a diagnosis of psoriatic arthritis. Sensitivity and specificity are around 76% and 37%, respectively. A score of 3 or more indicates a referral to rheumatology should be considered:
1. Have you ever had a swollen joint (or joints)?
2. Has a doctor ever told you that you have arthritis?
3. Do your fingernails or toenails have holes or pits?
4. Have you had pain in your heel?
5. Have you had a finger or toe that was completely swollen and painful for no apparent reason?

Box 9.15 Management of psoriatic arthritis

- Early treatment prevents joint destruction, deformity, and loss of function. Patients benefit from a multidisciplinary approach involving physiotherapists, occupational therapists, and podiatrists, as well as rheumatologists and orthopaedic surgeons.
- Mono- or oligoarticular disease may be managed with NSAIDs or intra-articular steroids (warn patients about potential flare of psoriasis, as the effect of intra-articular steroid wears off).
- More severe erosive or polyarticular disease is treated with disease-modifying antirheumatic drugs such as methotrexate, sulfasalazine, or leflunomide. Biologic agents may be indicated in severe disease unresponsive to other treatments.
- Patients with severe skin and joint disease requiring systemic therapy may be managed best by rheumatologists working with dermatologists in a combined clinic.

Reactive arthritis

What is reactive arthritis?

Reactive arthritis is a seronegative, HLA-B27-linked spondyloarthropathy that shares features with the other arthropathies in this group, including psoriatic arthritis (see ➜ p. 206). Typically, patients (usually men aged 20–40) have a mono- or oligoarthritis affecting the lower limbs. Mucocutaneous signs are common.

Arthritis develops several days to weeks after an extra-articular infection. Viable pathogen is not detected in the joint (though intra-articular bacteria or bacterial fragments have been identified). The common causes of reactive arthritis are genitourinary infections (e.g. *Chlamydia trachomatis*) and GI infections (e.g. *Yersinia, Shigella, Salmonella,* and *Campylobacter*). HIV infection is another cause.

The triad of arthritis, a sterile (aseptic) urethritis, and conjunctivitis in a patient with dysentery was described by Reiter as a syndrome in 1916, and the term Reiter syndrome is still used sometimes to describe this triad.

What mucocutaneous signs should I look for?

- Keratoderma blenorrhagicum: a pustular rash on palms and soles—clinically and pathologically indistinguishable from palmoplantar pustulosis. However, pustules are followed by gross conical hyperkeratosis, which is not usually seen in palmoplantar pustulosis or psoriasis (see ➜ p. 198).
- Nail changes tend to be more pustular than in psoriasis and include:
  - Onycholysis, ridging, and splitting.
  - Brownish red or greenish yellow discoloration of the nails.
  - Small yellow pustules under the nail, often near the lunula.
  - Subungual hyperkeratosis.
  - Nail pitting.
- Erythematous macules at the urethral meatus and on the glans penis. These may coalesce into a circinate scaly, erythematous patch (circinate balanitis) (see Fig. 9.8).
- Flaccid pustular lesions that develop thick horny scale.
- Well-demarcated erythematous, scaly psoriasiform plaques on the scrotum, buttocks, trunk, and limbs.
- Thick psoriasiform scale on the scalp.
- Asymptomatic superficial erosions in the oral mucosa.
- Patches of denuded papillae on the tongue.
- Bilateral mucopurulent conjunctivitis, acute anterior uveitis (photophobia, redness, watering, pain, decreased visual acuity), keratitis (corneal inflammation).

What should I do for cutaneous disease?

Manage as you would psoriasis or palmoplantar pustulosis (see Box 9.7). Treatment options include moderately potent topical corticosteroids and oral retinoids.

The condition is usually self-limiting, but steroids and disease-modifying antirheumatic drugs (DMARDs) are sometimes required for persistent disease.

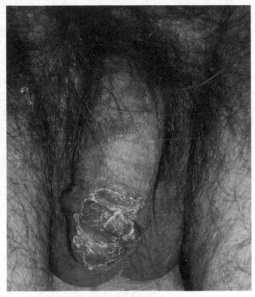

Fig. 9.8 Well-demarcated erythematous, scaly patch on the penis.

Eczema and lichen planus

Contents

Relevant pages in other chapters
Childhood eczema is discussed in ➲ Chapter 31,
pp. 604–11
Use of emollients and topical corticosteroids
➲ p. 655, pp. 656–7
Soaks and wet dressings ➲ p. 662
Mucosal lichen planus ➲ pp. 286–7
Photodermatitis ➲ pp. 326–7

What is eczema (dermatitis)?

The word eczema, derived from the Greek 'to break out or boil over', refers to the vesicles (bubbles) seen in acute eczema. Dermatitis means inflammation of the skin. The terms tend to be used synonymously. Eczema is a cutaneous reaction pattern that is poorly understood, and this is reflected by the confusing terminology used to describe different patterns (see Box 10.1). Oedema within and between keratinocytes (spongiosis) may produce weeping, with thin-walled vesicles (intraepidermal) that soon rupture. Eczema may be endogenous (commonest form—atopic eczema) or exogenous, but barrier function of the epidermis is abnormal in most forms of eczema, so the skin is easily irritated.

What should I look for?

Eczema is itchy. Patients with acutely inflamed eczema may also be very uncomfortable. Endogenous disease tends to be symmetrical, whereas the site of contact determines the distribution of a contact dermatitis. Signs depend on whether acute, subacute, or chronic but include combinations of:

- Erythema: often ill-defined (see ➡ Fig. 31.8, p. 611) (compare with psoriasis which is well defined (see ➡ Fig. 9.1, p. 193).
- Scaling, i.e. epidermal pathology: may not be present in the early stages of acute contact eczema in which the skin is erythematous and oedematous (see Figs. 10.1, 10.2, and 10.3,).
- Scratch marks (excoriations).
- Papules, oedema, and/or vesicles (occasionally bullae) in acute eczema.
- Exudation of serous fluid (weeping) and crusting in acute eczema (crusting may be a sign of 2° bacterial infection, as may pustules).
- Thickening of the skin, with increased skin markings (lichenification) 2° to chronic rubbing (see ➡ Fig. 31.9, p. 611).
- Prurigo (itchy, erythematous nodules): 2° to chronic rubbing (see Fig.10.6).
- Hyperkeratosis in chronic eczema.
- Hyperpigmentation 2° to chronic rubbing.
- Post-inflammatory hypo- or hyperpigmentation in dark skin.

What should I do?

- Generally, a skin biopsy is not required—the histology will not tell you the cause of the eczema, and the diagnosis is clinical.
- Take skin swabs from crusted weeping eczema for bacterial culture.
- In vesicular rashes, exclude herpes virus infection. Eczema herpeticum may complicate atopic eczema (see ➡ p. 112).
- Skin scrapes to exclude fungal (dermatophyte) infection in asymmetrical scaly rashes.
- Patch test if you suspect allergic contact dermatitis (see ➡ p. 214).
- Topical and systemic treatments (see ➡ Chapter 34, pp. 653–71).

Common patterns of eczema

Eczema is a cutaneous reaction pattern that is poorly understood. This is reflected by the complex terminology used (see Box 10.1). The name may imply the cause (contact dermatitis), links with other diseases (atopic), appearance of the skin (discoid eczema, pompholyx, asteatotic eczema), or distribution (varicose and seborrhoeic eczema). Patients may have >1 type of eczema, e.g. abnormal skin barrier function in atopic eczema predisposes to irritant contact dermatitis such as hand eczema (see Box 10.2); environmental irritants, such as soap, exacerbate asteatotic eczema; and allergic contact dermatitis may be superimposed on varicose eczema.

Box 10.1 Patterns of eczema (dermatitis)

Endogenous
- Atopic.
- Seborrhoeic.
- Discoid (nummular).
- Pompholyx (dyshidrotic).
- Varicose (gravitational, venous stasis).
- Asteatotic.
- Prurigo nodularis.
- Lichen simplex.

Exogenous
- Irritant contact/allergic contact.
- Photodermatitis/photo-aggravated.
- Drug-induced eczema.

Box 10.2 Hand eczema (dermatitis)

- In most cases, hand eczema is caused by irritant contact dermatitis and endogenous factors, e.g. atopy, but allergic contact dermatitis should be ruled out.
- Prompt intervention is recommended, because hand eczema can become chronic and significantly impacts on quality of life.
- Four main morphological subtypes are observed:
  - Recurrent microvesicular/pompholyx: classical presentation, palmar involvement, and lateral borders of fingers.
  - Hyperkeratotic eczema: well-demarcated thick, scaly plaques on palms (and soles), with painful fissures. Differential diagnosis: psoriasis, but less erythema and no nail changes in eczema.
  - Chronic fingertip dermatitis (pulpitis): dry fissured, scaling dermatitis of the fingertips, occasional vesicles. Can be debilitating, although appears mild.
  - Nummular hand eczema: coin-shaped patches (back of hands).
- Treatment options include potent and superpotent topical steroids, hand UVB or PUVA, oral retinoids (especially in hyperkeratotic eczema), e.g. alitretinoin (see ➲ Chapter 34, p. 669), and oral immunosuppressants.

Contact dermatitis

What is contact dermatitis?

Contact dermatitis is caused by exposure of the skin to an irritant or allergen. Irritancy is commoner than allergy. Impaired skin barrier function facilitates penetration of irritants and contact allergens into the epidermis, e.g. in atopic individuals, neonates, or older patients. Exposed body sites are often affected by contact dermatitis. Occupational contact dermatitis occurs more frequently in cleaners, hairdressers, nurses, homemakers, caterers, and builders (see Fig. 10.1).

Irritant contact dermatitis

Urine and faeces are irritants—the buttocks and perineum are affected in incontinent patients (see ➜ Chapter 31, p. 604). Detergents, alkalis, solvents, and cutting oils are also potential irritants. Some plants contain light-sensitizing furocoumarin chemicals that are phototoxic in the presence of sunlight (see ➜ Box 16.4, p. 327).

Allergic contact dermatitis

Pathogenesis: delayed (type 4) cell-mediated allergic reaction (see Box 10.3). The patient has to have prior exposure and sensitization before developing an allergic reaction characterized by itching, erythema, vesiculation, and scaling. For common cutaneous allergens, see Box 10.4. Always consider patch testing in chronic hand dermatitis, facial dermatitis, pruritus ani (when over-the-counter medicaments may have been used), and dermatitis associated with chronic leg ulcers. Patch tests are applied to the back on day 0, removed and read on day 2, and read again on day 4 or 5. An eczematous reaction indicates a positive result.

What should I ask?

- Take a history, as recommended in ➜ Chapter 2, pp. 20–3 and pp. 30–1. Ask about the occupation and hobbies; is the patient an obsessive handwasher? (see ➜ p. 566.)
- Find out what the patient uses—cosmetics, perfumes, hair dyes, over-the-counter medicaments, etc. Remember you can become allergic to a product that has been used for some time.
- Explore what provokes the rash. Does the problem improve when not in contact with the preparation, e.g. weekends, holidays?
- Is there a history of atopic eczema (irritant contact dermatitis is commoner than allergic contact dermatitis in atopics).

What should I do?

- Exclude 2° infection, particularly in genital dermatitis.
- Minimize contact with irritants, e.g. avoid soap, and use gloves.
- Prescribe emollients.
- Reduce inflammation with a potent corticosteroid ointment. A short course of prednisolone may be needed in severe blistering reactions.
- Refer for patch testing if you suspect an allergic contact dermatitis.
- If the patient is allergic to something, any contact with that allergen will produce a reaction, and complete avoidance is essential. An inevitable consequence of this diagnosis may be a change of occupation.

Box 10.3 Pathogenesis of allergic contact dermatitis

- Abnormalities in skin barrier function may facilitate the penetrance of an allergen and make some patients more prone to developing an allergic contact dermatitis (see ➜ Box 1.2, p. 6).
- Topical antigen penetrates the stratum cornea and enters the epidermis.
- The antigen is taken up by dendritic Langerhans cells within the epidermis and processed into small peptides. Peptides bound to class II MHC proteins are expressed on the surface of Langerhans cells. (Dermal dendritic cells may also process and present antigens.)
- Langerhans cells bearing the antigen migrate from the skin via lymphatics to the pancortical area of the draining lymph node where they activate CD4+ T-lymphocytes.
- IL-1 released by Langerhans cells triggers T-cells to release IL-2 and proliferate, with the generation of allergen-specific memory T-cells. These will recognize the antigen on re-exposure and migrate to the challenge site to produce cytokines and cytotoxic damage to the skin. This results in itch, erythema, and oedema.
- IL-5 and IL-13 cytokine production correlates with positive skin reactions, suggesting that Th-2, in addition to Th-1, cytokines play a role.

Box 10.4 Some common cutaneous allergens

- Nickel: in costume jewellery and jean studs.
- Chrome: in cement and leather.
- Fragrance mix: in perfumed cosmetics, soaps, air fresheners, household furniture spray polishes, etc.
- Balsam of Peru: fragrance and haemorrhoid creams.
- Methylisothiazolinone: preservative in cosmetics, wet wipes, and paints.
- Rubber accelerators (mercapto and thiuram mixes).
- Epoxy resin: in two part adhesive mixtures.
- Colophony: adhesive in adhesive plaster.
- Paraphenylene diamine (PPD): in hair dyes.
- Parabens: preservative in many creams and lotions.
- Wool alcohols (lanolin): lanolin in many creams.
- Medicaments such as benzocaine, neomycin, quinoline mix, and hydrocortisone.

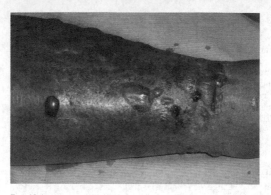

Fig. 10.1 Acute contact dermatitis simulating cellulitis with erythema and blistering.

Further reading

Schlapbach C, Simon D. *Allergy* 2014;**69**:1571–81.

Atopic eczema and seborrhoeic dermatitis in adults

Adult atopic eczema (dermatitis)

Atopic eczema is common in childhood. Eczema in 50–60% of children clears by puberty, but, in others, it is persistent or recurrent in adult life. In any adult with eczema, ask about personal or family history of atopic disease—infantile eczema, bronchial asthma, and/or allergic rhinitis. For more detailed discussion of the cause and management of atopic eczema in children, see ➜ Chapter 31, pp. 606–11.

What should I look for?
- Dry, scaly skin.
- A symmetrical erythematous, scaly rash, worse in flexures.
- Intense itch with excoriations, nodules (prurigo nodularis; see Fig. 10.6), and/or thickened (lichenified) skin 2° to scratching and rubbing (see ➜ Fig. 31.9, p. 611).
- Crusting, weeping, or vesicles suggesting 2° infection (bacterial or herpesvirus). Widespread vesicles and fever = eczema herpeticum, an emergency, most often seen in children (see ➜ p. 112).
- Atopic individuals have skin that is easily irritated, and adults may also have an irritant contact dermatitis, often on the hands or face.
- Erythroderma in severe disease (see ➜ p. 108).
- Thin skin (bruising, telangiectasia, striae) 2° to prolonged use of potent topical corticosteroids.

What should I do?
- Skin swabs for bacterial and viral culture if signs suggest infection.
- Soap substitutes (containing antibacterials) and emollients control dryness and reduce bacterial colonization of the skin. Even though the patient may have a long history of eczema, find out exactly how the skin is managed, and explain how to use emollients and to avoid irritants such as soap or shower gels (see ➜ pp. 30–1, p. 655, and p. 662).
- Prescribe a potent topical corticosteroid ointment to use once or twice daily (see ➜ pp. 654–8).
- Alternatively: tacrolimus ointment 0.1%, but avoid in infected skin.
- Oral antibiotics or antivirals to control infection, if required.
- A sedating antihistamine may relieve irritation, e.g. hydroxyzine.
- A short course of oral prednisolone (30mg/day, tailing off over 2–3 weeks) may be required for severe acute flares.
- Consider referral for patch tests to exclude an allergic contact dermatitis, particularly in patients with facial eczema or patients with no previous history of eczema.
- Consider skin biopsy to exclude CTCL if the patient does not have a personal or family history of atopic disease and this is a new presentation (see ➜ pp. 358–9).
- Courses of phototherapy or steroid-sparing agents (e.g. azathioprine, ciclosporin) may be indicated in severe chronic disease.
- Wet dressings can help (see ➜ p. 662).

Adult seborrhoeic dermatitis (eczema)

Pathogenesis is poorly understood. *Malassezia furfur* (*pityrosporum ovale*), a lipophilic yeast that is a skin commensal is found in large numbers in involved skin. Reaction to the yeasts may play some part in the pathogenesis. Adult seborrhoeic dermatitis is chronic and recurrent. Parkinson disease and epilepsy predispose to seborrhoeic dermatitis. Patients with HIV/AIDS may have very severe disease. Although seborrhoeic dermatitis is not particularly itchy, it is disfiguring. Infantile seborrhoeic dermatitis is unrelated to the disease in adults (see ➜ p. 602).

What should I look for?
One or more sites may be affected:
- Poorly defined scalp erythema and fine white scale (dandruff). Hair is retained.
- Poorly defined greasy, scaly erythema, affecting the nasolabial folds and central forehead.
- Fine scaling in the eyebrows, behind the ears, and within the ears (otitis externa), and/or blepharitis.
- Orangey, ill-defined erythema with fine scale in flexures (axillae, groin, umbilicus). May resemble flexural psoriasis (see ➜ Fig. 9.3, p. 193).
- Greasy, scaly, erythematous papules in the central chest and central back. May have an annular configuration.
- Follicular papules or pustules over the back and sometimes the chest (pityrosporum folliculitis) (see ➜ Box 6.3, p. 135).
- Normal nails—pitting suggests psoriasis.
- Erythroderma in severe disease (see ➜ p. 108).

What should I do?
It may be difficult to differentiate seborrhoeic dermatitis from flexural psoriasis (sebopsoriasis), but the approach to management is similar. Consider HIV/AIDS in patients with severe disease unresponsive to treatment. Treatment should tackle inflammation, scaling, and overgrowth of yeasts. Treatment options include:
- Greasy emollient to use as a soap substitute and skin moisturizer.
- Hydrocortisone 1% ointment, combined with an imidazole, applied ×1/day to the face and flexures—combinations of a corticosteroid with an antifungal are more effective than a corticosteroid alone.
- A moderately potent topical corticosteroid may be needed for a short time in the flexures, e.g. Trimovate® cream.
- Topical 0.1% tacrolimus ointment ×1/day is an alternative to a mild corticosteroid for facial or flexural seborrhoeic dermatitis.
- Ketoconazole shampoo for the scalp and as a body wash (useful in pityrosporum folliculitis)—perhaps ×2–3/week. Shampoo is drying and can irritate the skin—suggest the use of a moisturizer.
- Alternative shampoos include preparations with tar or salicylic acid, e.g. Capasal®, Polytar®, T-Gel®.
- A potent steroid lotion applied overnight may control scalp disease, e.g. Betnovate® lotion or Dermovate® scalp application.

Other common types of eczema

Asteatotic eczema

This pattern of mildly itchy eczema, common in the elderly, is often pre-cipitated by admission to hospital. Enthusiastic washing with soap, low humidity, and central heating dries out old skin. Also occurs in hypoaes-thetic skin (see ➜ p. 578).

What should I look for?
- Rash usually starts on the shins but may spread in a patchy fashion to the thighs and trunk (also see ➜ p. 578).
- A network of shallow erythematous fissures in the epidermis, giving the skin the appearance of 'crazy paving' (eczema craquelé) (see Fig. 10.2).

What should I do?
- Soap substitutes and emollients may be sufficient to settle irritation.
- Prescribe a mild topical corticosteroid ointment to use bd.

Varicose (stasis) eczema

What should I look for?
- Itching, erythema, scaling, and crusting (not pain) in the gaiter area.
- Signs of stasis—hyperpigmentation, oedema, atrophie blanche (see ➜ Box 15.4, p. 299), or venous leg ulcers (see Fig. 10.3).
- Usually bilateral and often mistaken for cellulitis. Ill-defined scaly erythema affecting both legs helps to differentiate from cellulitis which is unilateral and painful.
- Other differential diagnosis includes contact dermatitis (irritant or allergic).

What should I do?
- Check foot pulses, and measure the ankle–brachial pressure index (ABPI) to exclude arterial disease (see ➜ p. 300).
- Control oedema—ankle exercises, elevation, and compression.
- Prescribe emollients and moderately potent corticosteroid ointment.
- Consider ichthammol bandages or zinc-medicated bandages in combination with topical steroids and compression.
- Refer for patch testing if the rash does not settle promptly—patients with chronic leg ulcers become sensitized to constituents in topical preparations.

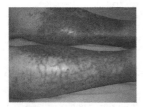

Fig. 10.2 Asteatotic eczema with a 'crazy paving' pattern of superficial cracking (eczema craquelé).

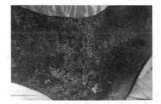

Fig. 10.3 Venous (stasis) eczema with erythema and scale in the gaiter area.

Discoid (nummular = coin-shaped) eczema

The pathogenesis is uncertain, but this chronic eczema is common in middle age. Atopic eczema may present in a discoid pattern in children. Differential diagnosis includes psoriasis and fungal infection.

What should I look for?
- A number of well-defined, extremely itchy, 'juicy', round or oval erythematous papules and plaques that may be scaly or vesicular (see Fig. 10.4). (Vesicles are not seen in psoriasis.)
- Golden crusting is a sign of 2° staphylococcal infection.
- Distribution tends to be symmetrical on the limbs and trunk.
- Check nails—they are normal in discoid eczema, unlike psoriasis.

What should I do?
- Take skin scrapings to exclude fungal (dermatophyte) infection.
- You may wish to take swabs for bacterial infection.
- Prescribe a soap substitute, an emollient, and a potent or very potent corticosteroid ointment to be applied ×1/day. Mild corticosteroid ointments are not sufficient to control irritation and inflammation.
- Treat infection with oral antibiotics.
- Sedating antihistamine in the evenings may relieve irritation at night.

Pompholyx (cheiropompholyx; dyshidrotic eczema)

Pompholyx (Greek for bubble) is a common recurring endogenous dermatitis that usually occurs in people aged 20–40 years.

What should I look for?
- An itchy rash on the sides of the fingers and centre of palms and soles.
- Erythema and pinhead-sized vesicles (not pustules) that may evolve into bullae (see Fig.10.5).
- Peeling, as the rash settles over 3–4 weeks.
- Exacerbations in hot weather.

What should I do?
- Exclude tinea pedis, which sometimes precipitates pompholyx.
- Soothe weeping eczematous skin with 0.01% potassium permanganate soaks (make a solution of rosé wine colour) or 0.65% aluminium acetate solution (Burow solution) (see ➋ p. 662).
- Prescribe a potent corticosteroid cream to be applied ×1/day.
- Consider referral for patch tests—usually negative.

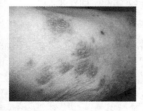

Fig. 10.4 Crusted itchy plaques in discoid eczema.

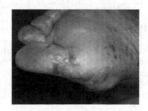

Fig. 10.5 Blisters in pompholyx eczema.

Chronic scratching and rubbing

Lichen simplex chronicus

Localized area of skin becomes thickened and leathery (lichenified) due to chronic rubbing, sometimes a stress-related habit (see Box 10.5). Tends to favour the calf, nape of the neck, vulva, and perianal skin.

What should I do?

• Take scrapes from scaly lesions to exclude a dermatophyte infection, and swab the genital skin to exclude candidiasis.
• Non-genital skin: apply a superpotent corticosteroid ointment bd, or use under occlusive hydrocolloid dressing, e.g. DuoDERM®. Dressings protect itchy skin from fingernails and can stay in place for 4/5 days, after which corticosteroid ointment is reapplied under a fresh dressing. Continue treatment, until the skin has flattened and the itch has settled (see ➡ p. 660).
• Genital skin: treat with potent corticosteroid–imidazole ointment for 2 weeks, and then step down to a weaker corticosteroid–imidazole combination to reduce the risk of atrophy. Use aqueous cream as soap substitute.
• Consider patch testing in genital lichen simplex.

Prurigo nodularis

Chronic form of eczema characterized by intensely itchy nodules. Pathogenesis poorly understood (see Box 10.5); 80% of patients have a personal or family history of atopy. Patients may report nodules appearing before the skin feels itchy, but, if the skin is occluded, nodules flatten.

What should I look for?

• Middle-aged or older patient with excoriated, firm, erythematous nodules, 1–2cm in diameter, usually symmetrically distributed on the extensor aspects of the limbs and the upper back. Numbers vary from a few to hundreds (see Fig.10.6).
• Post-inflammatory hyperpigmentation or scarring (see Fig. 10.7).
• Normal skin in the centre of the back (difficult to scratch).

What should I do?

• Explain that it is difficult to find the cause of itching ... and to treat.
• Explain that the changes are 2° to scratching.
• Exclude systemic causes of itch—renal failure, chronic liver disease, malignancies, psychological/psychiatric conditions, HIV, drugs.
• Exclude scabies.
• Attempt to break the itch–scratch cycle with a very potent corticosteroid ointment applied under occlusion (see ➡ p. 660).
• Recommend emollients and anti-itch creams such as crotamiton lotion or menthol 1% in aqueous cream.
• Consider a course of UV light (UVB).
• Consider sedating antihistamines or a small dose of amitriptyline (10mg) at night. (Also see ➡ Box 28.1, p. 567).

Quantifying itch

See ➡ pp. 32–4.

Box 10.5 What is itch?

- Itch is the commonest symptom in skin disorders, but the neurophysiology is poorly understood, and itch may be very difficult to control.
- The sensation of itch is transmitted by itch-dedicated afferent C neurons that are distinct from pain fibres.
- Itch causes a characteristic pattern of focal functional brain changes, which are different from changes associated with pain.
- Keratinocytes express neuropeptide mediators and receptors associated with itch. The epidermis with the associated fine intra-epidermal C-neuron filaments is the 'itch receptor'.
- Visual, auditory, and other stimuli that activate the reticular system lead to inhibition of itch pathways, so itch is less troublesome during waking hours than at night.
- Histamine and other mast cell mediators mediate itch by activating C neurons.
- Keratinocytes also release neurotrophins that may predispose to itch by causing proliferation of unmyelinated afferent nerve terminals, sensitization of afferent nerve terminals, and increased expression of neuropeptides.
- Sensory neuropathy may cause localized itch often associated with burning, tingling, stinging, hypoaesthesia, or hyperalgesia (neuropathic itch) (see ⊃ pp. 548–9).
- Localized itch, pain, or burning without any objective changes in the skin may be associated with psychological factors or stress (see ⊃ pp. 568–9, and Box 28.1, p. 567).

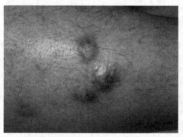

Fig. 10.6 Itchy nodules of prurigo nodularis.

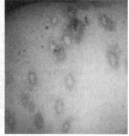

Fig. 10.7 Scarring 2° to picking and scratching in long-standing prurigo nodularis.

Further reading

Kremer AE et al. *Biochim Biophys Acta* 2014;**1842**:869–92.
Tey HL and Yosipovitch G. *Br J Dermatol* 2011;**165**:5–17 (reviews advances in the understanding of itch).

Lichen planus

LP is a chronic inflammatory condition of unknown cause that may affect the skin and/or mucosal surfaces (see ➜ pp. 286–7).

A band-like 'lichenoid' infiltrate of lymphocytes hugs the basal layer of the epidermis or epithelium. Apoptotic basal keratinocytes release melanin into the dermis where it is taken up by macrophages. The prevalence of autoimmune conditions, such as alopecia areata, vitiligo, and ulcerative colitis, is increased in LP. Some studies suggest an increased prevalence of infections with hepatitis B or C virus. LP can also be drug-induced (see ➜ p. 375). Many variants of cutaneous LP have been described. Itching is a common complaint. Lichen nitidus may be a variant of LP (see Box 10.6). For management, see Box 10.7.

What should I look for?

- Flat-topped, smooth, shiny, polygonal, purplish red, itchy papules (lichenoid papules) in a symmetrical distribution, often involving flexural aspects of the wrists, but the rash may be localized or generalized. Unlike eczema, the skin is not particularly scaly (see Fig. 10.8).
- Look closely to see the lacy white streaks (Wickham striae) that overlie the surface of the papules.
- Koebner phenomenon (papules arising in areas of trauma/scratching).
- Lacy white streaks on the buccal mucosa (cannot be scraped off, unlike mucosal candidiasis) and other oral and/or genital mucosal signs (see ➜ p. 286).
- Hypertrophic LP: itchy, hyperkeratotic, purplish nodules on the shins, resembling lichen simplex (see ➜ p. 222).
- Annular LP: often flexural. Look in axillae and on the shaft of the penis.
- Photoexacerbated LP: differentiate from cutaneous LE by checking antinuclear antibody (ANA) (often negative in cutaneous LE) and taking a skin biopsy (see ➜ p. 404).
- Nail dystrophy: longitudinal ridging, atrophy of the nail plate, irreversible scarring with pterygium, and loss of nails.
- Lichen planopilaris (LPP): patchy inflammation around hair follicles with destruction of follicles, eventually leading to scarring alopecia. Differentiate from cutaneous discoid LE. LPP may affect body hair and scalp—look for tiny purplish follicular papules, many of which contain a small central horn plugging the ostium of the follicle.
- Keratoderma: LP causing a well-demarcated thickening of the skin on palms and soles. Look around the edges of the inflamed skin to see the characteristic shiny papules.
- Painful erosive disease on the soles (see Fig. 10.9).
- LP pigmentosus (erythema dyschromicum perstans): seen in darker-skinned patients, usually from the Indian subcontinent. Disease causes long-standing disfiguring macular greyish hyperpigmentation. Inflammation is minimal, and treatments ineffective (see Fig. 10.10).
- Bullous LP: rarely, these patients have autoantibodies to the BP antigen BP180 (LP pemphigoides).

Box 10.6 What is lichen nitidus?

Lichen nitidus is an uncommon self-limiting eruption of unknown cause that occurs in children and adults. It is characterized by:

- Asymptomatic or mild itch.
- Shiny, discrete, flat-topped, pinhead-sized papules (not follicular).
- Predilection for flexural surfaces of upper extremities, anterior trunk, genitalia, and dorsa of hands.
- Rash may be generalized.
- Mucosal surfaces are not involved (unlike LP).
- Displays the Koebner phenomenon.
- Clears within a few years.
- Generally, no treatment is needed, except reassurance.

Box 10.7 Cutaneous lichen planus: what should I do?

- Take a careful history to ensure this is not a lichenoid drug reaction (see ⊃ p. 375).
- Confirm the diagnosis with a skin biopsy.
- The disease is generally self-limiting.
- Asymptomatic LP does not require treatment.
- A potent or very potent topical corticosteroid ointment ×1/day may reduce inflammation and itch.
- Topical 0.1% tacrolimus ointment ×1/day is worth trying if LP is unresponsive to topical corticosteroids.
- A sedating antihistamine may relieve night-time itch.
- Localized hypertrophic LP: apply very potent corticosteroids under occlusion (see ⊃ p. 660), or use intralesional corticosteroids.
- Severe cutaneous LP: short courses of oral corticosteroids will control itching, but unfortunately disease usually recurs on stopping corticosteroids. Other therapies that have been tried include UVB, oral retinoids, and oral ciclosporin.
- Mucosal LP: see ⊃ p. 286.

Fig. 10.8 Purplish (violaceous), smooth, shiny, flat-topped papules of lichen planus.

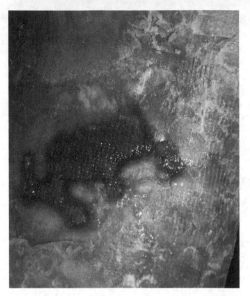

Fig. 10.9 Painful erosions on the sole of the foot are an uncommon manifestation of lichen planus.

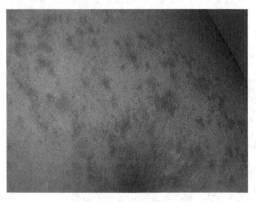

Fig. 10.10 Lichen planus pigmentosus with pigmented macules on the trunk.

Urticaria and erythema

Contents

Relevant pages in other chapters

Urticaria

Urticaria (hives, wheals, welts) is a hypersensitivity reaction that may occur in isolation or associated with angio-oedema and/or anaphylaxis (see ➋ pp. 104–5 and Box 11.1). Urticaria erupts spontaneously, and smooth, erythematous, itchy swellings (wheals) persist for 2–24h, before fading to leave normal skin (see Fig. 11.1). Some patients have wheals every day; in others, it is episodic. The condition may persist for <6 weeks (acute urticarial) and may be precipitated by insect bites, drugs, e.g. penicillin, infections, contact with latex, and food allergies (see ➋ pp. 104–5). It can last for months or years (chronic) (see Box 11.1). The underlying mechanism may be immunological or non-immunological, but the end result is the same—mast cell degranulation with release of histamine and inflammatory mediators, increased capillary permeability, and transient fluid leakage into the dermis, causing swelling.

What is chronic urticaria?

(See Box 11.1.) In most patients with chronic urticaria, a cause is not identified, and it is called spontaneous (previously referred to as ordinary). Helminth infections should be considered as a cause, and urticaria is also common in SLE. Children and adolescents with severe spontaneous urticaria have an increased prevalence of coeliac disease.

What should I ask?

- Exclude physical urticaria by asking about precipitating factors (pressure, sun, heat, cold) and how long it takes urticaria to appear. Patients who are dermographic may notice wheals appear immediately when the skin is rubbed/scratched—wheals last <1h (see Fig. 11.2).
- What are the symptoms—itch, burning, pain?
- How long do the marks last? Delayed pressure urticaria may last up to 72h. Urticarial vasculitis is also long-lasting (see ➋ p. 443).
- Is it precipitated by contact with latex or foods, e.g. fish, nuts?
- What does the skin look like when urticaria fades? Skin should appear normal in urticaria. Urticarial vasculitis leaves bruising.
- Ask about wheezing and angio-oedema: lip and throat swelling (see ➋ p. 104).
- Is the patient taking any drugs that may cause or worsen urticaria—opiates (direct mast cell-releasing agents), salicylates, non-steroidal anti-inflammatories, ACE inhibitors? (see ➋ p. 372.)
- Does the patient report symptoms suggesting an underlying systemic disease, e.g. fever, arthralgia, myalgia, diarrhoea, weight loss?
- Is there a family history of urticaria? (see ➋ pp. 234–5.)

What should I do?

see ➋ Management, pp. 232–3.
- Check the skin surface—smooth, not scaly, in urticaria (see Fig. 11.1).
- Confirm that the rash is erythematous (does it blanch?).
- Stroke the skin with a spatula to see if the patient is dermographic (a wheal and flare appear within 10min at the site of pressure).
- Check that the skin looks normal where wheals have faded.
- Are the lips or tongue swollen?
- Assess using the urticarial activity score (UAS) (see Box 11.2). This has been validated for use in follow-up and monitoring of urticaria. Due to daily variability, sum scores over 4 or 7 days to monitor.

Box 11.1 Clinical classification of chronic urticaria

A. Chronic spontaneous (ordinary) urticaria

- Unknown aetiology (idiopathic).
- Autoimmune aetiology (30%) caused by histamine-releasing autoantibodies (routine tests for these autoantibodies are not available). May be associated with thyroid autoimmunity.

B. Chronic inducible urticaria

1. *Physical urticaria*
   Reproducibly induced by the same physical stimulus (see ➡ p. 230).
   - Mechanical:
     - Delayed pressure urticaria (swelling may last up to 48h).
     - Symptomatic dermographism (see Fig. 11.2).
     - Vibratory angio-oedema.
   - Thermal:
     - Cold urticaria.
     - Localized heat urticaria.
   - Other:
     - Aquagenic urticaria.
     - Solar urticaria.
     - Exercise-induced anaphylaxis.

2. *Cholinergic urticaria*
   Mediated by acetylcholine liberated from sympathetic nerves. Stimuli that increase the core temperature, such as anxiety, exertion, hot baths, or sexual activity, precipitate a transient itching, stinging erythematous rash within 15min. Each small urticated papule is surrounded by a wide erythematous flare, and flares coalesce, resembling a flush. The rash can usually be provoked by asking the patient to exercise hard enough to induce sweating. Urticaria is caused by the release of acetylcholine from sympathetic nerves in the skin.

3. *Contact urticaria*
   Contact with allergens or chemicals, e.g. latex.

C. Other forms of urticaria

1. *Urticarial vasculitis*
   Long-lasting wheals with bruising—vasculitis on skin biopsy. May be a sign of SLE (see ➡ p. 443).

2. *Auto-inflammatory diseases*
   (see ➡ pp. 234–5.)
   - Hereditary: cryopyrin-associated periodic syndromes (*NLRP3* mutations) cause familial cold urticaria.
   - Acquired:
     - Schnitzler syndrome (non-itchy urticaria, intermittent fever, bone pain, arthritis or arthralgia, raised erythrocyte sedimentation rate (ESR), IgM gammopathy, neutrophils in skin biopsy). Possibly a variant of urticarial vasculitis (see ➡ p. 443).

Physical urticaria

Each physical urticaria is induced reproducibly by the same physical stimulus and may coexist with ordinary urticaria. Consider challenge testing to prove the diagnosis, but testing is not without risk in severely affected patients who may develop systemic symptoms, including hypotension, wheezing, and anaphylaxis.

Symptomatic dermographism

Dermographism is the commonest physical urticaria. An itchy wheal develops within 10min of rubbing the skin lightly and lasts about 1h. Patients may have normal-looking skin, and you will need to stroke the skin with a spatula to elicit dermographism (see Fig. 11.2).

Cold urticaria

Itchy wheals appear within minutes if the skin is exposed to cold. Angio-oedema and hypotension may complicate the picture and can be life-threatening. Common triggers include cold winds and swimming in cold water.

Diagnosis is confirmed by an ice cube test—an ice cube in a polythene bag (the skin must remain dry to exclude aquagenic urticaria) is held against the forearm skin for 20min. Wheals develop rapidly when the skin re-warms.

Cold urticaria is occasionally associated with cryoglobulins, cold agglutinins, or cryofibrinogens (see ➲ pp. 444–5). Familial cold urticaria is one of the rare autosomal dominant hereditary fever syndromes caused by mutations in the *NLRP3* gene (see ➲ p. 236).

Delayed pressure urticaria

Sustained pressure causes itchy or painful wheals after a delay of between 30min and 6h. Swellings last up to 72h. Pressure urticaria may affect any site, including the soles or palms (after carrying a heavy bag).

Solar urticaria

Itchy wheals develop within 10min of exposure of the skin to UV or visible radiation. Solar urticaria occurs in erythropoietic protoporphyria (EPP), but this is a rare cause (see ➲ p. 335).

Other physical urticarias

Water (aquagenic urticaria), heat (heat contact urticaria), or vibration (vibratory angio-oedema) trigger localized itchy urticarial reactions at the site of application of the stimulus.

Urticaria appears within 10min and resolves within 2h.

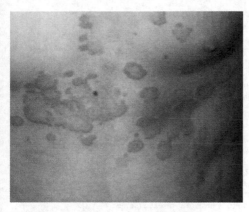

Fig. 11.1 Widespread chronic urticaria. The smooth erythematous papules and plaques may expand into annular shapes.

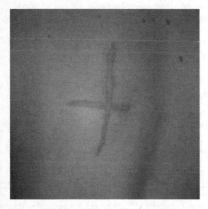

Fig. 11.2 Stroking the skin elicits wheals in patients who are dermographic.

Further reading

Systemic Autoinflammatory Disease (SAID) Support. Available at: ℛhttp://saidsupport.org/.

Management of urticaria

What should I do?

Investigations

Investigations should be guided by the history and clinical findings (see Box 11.3). If the history does not suggest an underlying cause, it is unlikely that investigations will be helpful in chronic urticaria.

General measures

- Explain the disease and the difficulty in pinning down the cause.
- Reassure the patient that urticaria can be controlled but that it may persist for some time. Fifty percent of patients with chronic spontaneous urticaria are clear within 6 months, but urticaria with angio-oedema may persist for years, as may physical urticarias.
- Offer written information about urticaria (British Association of Dermatologists; see ➋ Resources, p. 674).
- Assess and monitor persistent disease (see Box 11.2).
- Discuss how to minimize aggravating factors such as alcohol, overheating, pressure on the skin (tight clothes), or other physical triggers, if relevant. Warn patients with cold urticaria about the risk of immersion in cold water provoking anaphylaxis.
- Advise dermographic patients to try not to scratch.
- Minimize exposure to drugs that may exacerbate (see Box 11.4).
- Prescribe a soothing antipruritic topical preparation such as oily calamine lotion or aqueous cream with 1% menthol.

Specific measures

- Prescribe a non-sedating H1 antihistamine such as fexofenadine, cetirizine (works quickly but sedating in high doses), loratadine, or rupatadine. Patients may need to try several preparations before finding the optimal antihistamine and optimal dose. Forty percent of patients respond to antihistamines alone.
- Suggest taking the antihistamine so that the drug level is highest before the urticaria usually erupts, e.g. in the evenings if urticaria is worst at night. The dose may need to be above the manufacturer's recommended dose, provided potential benefits outweigh risks.
- Reassure that prolonged treatment with antihistamines is safe.
- Sedating H1 antihistamines, e.g. chlorphenamine 4–12mg, hydroxyzine 10–50mg, useful at night. Warn the patient about feeling drowsy in the morning. Avoid if driving, and caution in the elderly.
- Adding an H2 antihistamine (ranitidine) or anti-leukotriene (montelukast 10mg) may be helpful.
- Oral corticosteroids should generally be avoided but may shorten the duration of severe acute urticaria (prednisolone 20–30mg a day for 3 days in adults) and may be required in delayed pressure urticaria.
- Topical corticosteroids are not recommended.
- Cholinergic urticaria may improve with anticholinergics and anxiolytics, as well as antihistamines; use with caution in the elderly.
- Systemic treatments used include ciclosporin, methotrexate, and omalizumab (anti-IgE).

Box 11.2 Urticaria activity score

Score	Wheals	Itch
0	None	None
1	Mild (<20 wheals/24h)	Mild
2	Moderate (21–50 wheals/24h)	Moderate
3	Intense or severe (>50 wheals/24h or large confluent areas of wheals)	Intense or severe

Box 11.3 Investigations

Acute urticaria

Skin-prick testing (not patch testing) or specific IgE quantification indicated if immediate reactions suspected, e.g. to latex/foods.

Chronic urticaria

- Investigation is usually unrewarding but reassures the patient.
- FBC (eosinophilia may indicate bowel helminth infection).
- CRP/ESR (raised in hereditary fever syndromes).
- Thyroid autoantibodies and/or thyroid function tests.
- Skin biopsy if you suspect an urticarial vasculitis (see ➔ p. 443).

Box 11.4 Triggers for chronic urticaria

Infections and infestations

- Viral infections, e.g. hepatitis, infectious mononucleosis, seroconversion rash of HIV infection.
- Bacterial infections, including *Mycoplasma*.
- Intestinal parasites, including helminth infection.

Chemicals and venoms

- Drugs: opiates are direct mast cell-releasing agents. Salicylates, NSAIDs, and ACE inhibitors may aggravate (see ➔ p. 372).
- Foods, most often fish, nuts, or fruit (role of food additives?).
- Insect bites and venoms.

Systemic disease

- Connective tissue disorders such as SLE.
- Thyroid disease.
- Coeliac disease in children and adolescents.
- Lymphoma and other cancers.
- Hypereosinophilic syndrome—rare.
- Auto-inflammatory diseases—rare (see ➔ pp. 234–5).

Further reading

Greaves MW. *Immunol Allergy Clin North Am* 2014;**34**:1–9.

⚠ Auto-inflammatory diseases

These rare inherited diseases are characterized by unexplained bouts of fever and inflammation, mainly involving the abdomen, musculoskeletal system, and skin, that occur in the absence of infective causes, autoantibodies, or auto-reactive T-lymphocytes, and derive from defects in innate immunity. Symptoms are intermittent without true periodicity and with variable frequency (weekly to yearly). Amyloidosis is a life-threatening complication. For diagnosis, patients should be referred to a specialist centre.

Genetic basis

(see ➲ p. 236 and Box 11.5.)

The auto-inflammatory diseases also include the dominantly inherited pyogenic arthritis, PG, and acne syndrome (PAPA; see ➲ pp. 248–9), and PASH (the association of PG, severe acne, and hidradenitis suppurativa)—extremely rare. Schnitzler syndrome is an acquired auto-inflammatory disease (see ➲ Box 11.1, and p. 229).

Familial Mediterranean fever

- The most frequent type affecting populations of Mediterranean/ Middle Eastern descent.
- Inheritance autosomal dominant or recessive.
- Characterized by episodic fever, serositis (peritonitis, pleuritis, scrotitis, pericarditis), and large joint arthritis. Attacks are irregular and last hours to days.
- Erysipelas-like erythema of the legs or foot occurs in 1/3.
- Other cutaneous signs include urticaria, dermographism, and angio-oedema.
- Elevated inflammatory markers during acute phase, e.g. CRP, ESR, fibrinogen, C3, C4, serum amyloid A.
- Colchicine (1–2mg/day) is used for long-term prophylaxis.

Tumour necrosis factor receptor superfamily 1A-associated periodic fever syndrome (TRAPS; familial Hibernian fever)

- Inheritance AD or sporadic.
- Attacks last longer than in FMF, usually 5 days to 3 weeks.
- Patients may have myalgia, thoracic and scrotal pain, arthritis, periorbital oedema, and conjunctivitis.
- Skin affected in 75% of cases and may present as a pseudocellulitis— warm, erythematous, painful plaque of variable size on the limbs or torso—or urticaria-like patches and plaques.
- Colchicine is ineffective. Corticosteroids are the mainstay of treatment.
- Etanercept, which inhibits the action of TNF-α, may be helpful.

Hyperimmunoglobulin D syndrome (HIDS), also known as mevalonate kinase deficiency

- Inheritance autosomal recessive (AR).
- High serum levels of IgD distinguish HIDS from familial Mediterranean fever (FMF).
- Onset in infancy, characterized by attacks lasting 7 days and recurring every 4–8 weeks with fever, abdominal pain, diarrhoea, vomiting, arthritis, and cervical lymphadenopathy.
- Cutaneous signs include erythematous macules, papules, nodules, and urticarial lesions.
- Attacks precipitated by immunizations/infections.
- Corticosteroids are helpful. Anti-TNF agents may be effective.
- Bone marrow transplantation is the treatment of choice.

Cryopyrinopathies (cryopyrin-associated periodic syndromes, CAPS)

- Disease spectrum characterized by cold-induced neutrophilic urticaria (see → p. 230).
- Responds to IL-1 receptor antagonists (anakinra, rilonacept), and canakinumab (anti-IL-1β).
- Three separate diseases along this spectrum have been described:
  - *Familial cold auto-inflammatory syndrome 1* (FCAS1) (autosomal dominant): attacks of urticaria, fever and arthralgia lasting 2–10 days. Delayed onset, >1 hour after cold exposure.
  - *Muckle–Wells syndrome* (autosomal dominant): urticaria, renal amyloidosis, and sensorineural deafness. Sometimes conjunctivitis and arthritis.
  - *Neonatal-onset multisystem inflammatory disease* (NOMID), also known as chronic infantile neurological cutaneous and articular syndrome (CINCA) (sporadic or autosomal dominant): neonatal onset of a chronic urticarial eruption associated with neurological disease (meningoencephalitis, seizures, motor deficit, learning difficulties), hepatosplenomegaly, and articular disease with a disabling and deforming arthropathy. The facial appearance is characteristic.

Genetics of auto-inflammatory diseases

What is the genetic basis of auto-inflammatory diseases?

- NLRP3 is a NOD-like receptor, which is a pattern recognition receptor central to the innate immune response. It is part of the NLRP3 inflammasome, which is a molecular complex responsible for activation of caspase 1.
- Activation of caspase 1 through inflammasomes leads to the production of pro-inflammatory cytokines, e.g. IL-1β.
- Most auto-inflammatory diseases are monogenic diseases caused by mutations of genes that function in this system or in a related pathway (see Box 11.5).

> ### Box 11.5 Genetic basis of the auto-inflammatory diseases
>
> #### Classic periodic fever syndromes
> - FMF: mutations in *MEFV* gene that encodes pyrin. Pyrin and related proteins are involved in the regulation of apoptosis, inflammation, and processing of cytokines.
> - TRAPS: mutations in the *TNFRSF1A* gene that encodes the 55kDa TNF receptor TNFR1—abnormal protein trafficking in the endoplasmic reticulum.
> - HIDS: mutations in *MVK* gene cause mevalonate kinase deficiency—enzyme involved in cholesterol and isoprene synthesis (haem metabolism).
> - Cryopyrin-associated periodic syndromes (CAPS)—mutations in the *NLRP3* gene (→hyperactive inflammasome):
>   - FCAS2 (familial cold auto-inflammatory syndrome 2)—mutations in *NLRP12*.
>
> #### Disease with pustular/pyogenic lesions
> - PAPA (pyogenic arthritis, PG, and acne): mutations in *PSTPIP1/CD2BP1* gene encoding a protein that interacts with pyrin (see ➲ pp. 248–9).
> - DIRA: deficiency of IL-1 receptor antagonist. Pustular skin lesions and pyogenic bone lesions (osteomyelitis or periostitis).
> - DITRA: deficiency of IL-36 receptor antagonist (associated with generalized pustular psoriasis).
> - Majeed syndrome: mutations in gene encoding phosphatidate phosphatase LIPN2.
>
> #### Disease with granulomatous lesions
> - Blau syndrome: AD disease caused by mutations in gene encoding the NLR family protein NOD2 results in nuclear factor kappa B activation. Clinical triad of skin changes, granulomatous uveitis, and symmetrical arthritis.

Erythema annulare centrifugum

What is erythema annulare centrifugum?

This curious, but uncommon, condition is thought to be a 'hypersensitivity reaction' perhaps to drugs or infection, but, in most cases, a trigger is not identified. Small dermal blood vessels are cuffed by clusters of lymphocytes. Erythema annulare centrifugum (EAC) is commoner in adults than children. Do not confuse this with the other erythemas (see Box 11.6).

What should I look for?

- A history of recurring red marks that slowly expand by 2–3mm a day into annular or arcuate shapes that clear centrally and then fade over days to weeks to leave normal skin.
- The speed of evolution contrasts with the waves of rapidly expanding (1cm/day) erythematous concentric bands of erythema gyratum repens, a rare manifestation of internal malignancy (see ➔ p. 546).
- EAC tends to recur at the same site, i.e. trunk or proximal limbs.
- A seasonal EAC that recurs annually has been described (see Fig. 11.3).
- Sometimes patients complain the rash is itchy.
- One or more erythematous macules, papules, well-defined annular (ring-shaped) lesions or arcuate shapes. Lesions reach a maximum of 10cm in diameter.
- The trailing inner edge of the erythematous rings may be finely scaly in superficial EAC. Tinea corporis ('ringworm') is more scaly, and the scale is on the outer margin of the ring, rather than the inner edge.
- Sometimes EAC is oedematous and vesicular.

What should I do?

- Look for possible triggers—drugs, infections.
- Take a skin scrape for mycological culture to exclude fungal infection.
- Consider taking a skin biopsy if the diagnosis is in doubt.
- In widespread annular erythematous rashes, check the ANA and extractable nuclear antigen (ENA) to exclude subacute cutaneous LE (SCLE) (see ➔ p. 402).
- Explain that you are unlikely to be able to find the cause of the rash—'another of life's great mysteries'—but that it will not do the patient any harm. Most cases pursue a fluctuating course over many years but eventually regress spontaneously.
- Prescribe a moderately potent topical corticosteroid ointment to relieve irritation. Corticosteroids have no impact on the course of disease.

Box 11.6 'Erythemas'

Many skin conditions have descriptive names that include the word erythema. These are considered separately in different sections of the book:

- Erythema migrans (see ➔ p. 148).
- Erythema nodosum (see ➔ pp. 458–9).
- Erythema multiforme (see ➔ p. 111).
- Erythema marginatum—evanescent erythematous macules that spread into patches or may be polycyclic. Associated with acute rheumatic fever (fever, carditis, migratory polyarthritis) caused by group A β-haemolytic streptococcal infection.
- Erythema induratum (see ➔ pp. 460–1).
- Erythema gyratum repens (see ➔ p. 546).
- Erythema ab igne (see ➔ p. 452, and Fig. 20.5, p. 454).

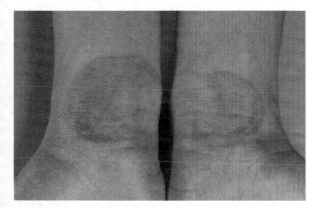

Fig. 11.3 Erythema annulare centrifugum was seasonal in this patient, appearing every summer. The scale follows the expanding erythematous ring.

Further reading

Berkun Y and Eisenstein EM. *Autoimmun Rev* 2014;**13**(4–5):388–90.
Broderick L et al. *Annu Rev Pathol* 2014;**10**:395–424.
Ozen S and Bilginer Y. *Nat Rev Rheumatol* 2014;**10**:135–47.

Pustular rashes

Contents

Acne: presentation

Acne is a disfiguring disorder of the pilosebaceous unit, usually starting between the ages of 12 and 14, that is experienced to some extent by almost all teenagers. Acne may persist into adult life, and we seem to be seeing more acne in older women. Pathogenesis is multifactorial (see Box 12.1).

What should I ask?

- When did the acne start? How bad is it today?
- What impact is the acne having on the patient's life? (see ➜ p. 32.) Acne may have a major psychosocial impact, eroding self-confidence and causing depression or even suicide.
- What treatment has the patient used and for how long? Most acne treatments take up to 4 months to have a maximal effect.
- How are topical preparations, such as benzoyl peroxide or topical retinoids, being applied—all over the face or trunk (as they should be) or just on 'spots'? Any adverse effects such as irritation of the skin?
- Oral antibiotics—most patients will need prolonged treatment for several years. What does the patient mean by 'taking a course'?
- What else is being applied to the skin—greasy cosmetics or pomades?
- What is the patient's occupation? Is he or she in a hot or humid environment, working with tars or oils, or wearing a cap that occludes the forehead?
- Is trauma irritating hair follicles (acne mechanica)—friction under chin straps, helmets, or shoulder pads (American footballers), or repeated rubbing of the face with exfoliative creams?
- Is the patient taking drugs that might exacerbate acne? (see ➜ Drugs and skin diseases, p. 384 and 388.)
- Refractory severe acne (see Box 12.4).

What should I look for?

(See Figs. 12.1 and 12.2.)
- Acne affects the face and/or upper trunk. If acne is in an unusual or asymmetrical distribution, could this be related to an external factor?
- More than one type of lesion: pustules, papules, comedones (blackhead = open comedone; whitehead = closed comedone), nodules, cysts, and scars (deep 'ice-pick' or flat).
- Record the types of lesions that are present, so you can monitor the outcome of treatment.
- Do comedones predominate? Suggests exposure to tar or chlorinated hydrocarbons. Could this be pomade acne on the forehead?
- Signs of virilization such as hirsutism. Check for cliteromegaly if you suspect virilization (see ➜ pp. 474–7).
- HAIR-AN syndrome (see ➜ p. 476).
- Even mild acne may cause acne keloids or, in dark skin, long-lasting hyperpigmentation. Prolonged courses of minocycline may cause hyperpigmentation in scars.
- See Box 12.2 for clinical variants.

Box 12.1 Pathogenesis of acne

The pathogenesis is not fully understood, but a number of factors play a part in triggering chronic inflammation around pilosebaceous units:
- Sebum excretion is increased (but may remain high when acne has cleared).
- Androgens stimulate sebum secretion by the sebaceous glands.
- Occlusion of follicular ducts by hyperkeratinization (may be exacerbated by application of some greasy topical preparations or tar).
- Bacterial colonization of follicular ducts by *Propionibacterium acnes*, a skin commensal. *P. acnes* breaks down triglycerides, releasing free fatty acids that trigger dermal inflammation. *P. acnes* may also activate Toll-like receptors on keratinocytes which induce inflammation.
- Increased fibroblast growth factor receptor 2 (FGFR2) signalling (mutations in FGFR2 leading to increased signalling cause acne in Apert syndrome; see Box 12.4). Androgens upregulate signalling.
- Genes: about 50% of patients have a family history of acne.
- Diet: a link between acne and dairy products has been suggested but needs more study.

Box 12.2 Variants of acne

- Acne 'excoriée de la jeune fille': young girls with mild acne, but obsessional picking scars the skin. Difficult to manage. Even mild disease may need systemic treatment (see ➋ p. 566).
- Neonatal and infantile acne: usually face. May persist until age 3 or 4. Consider inhaled corticosteroids as a cause (see ➋ p. 244).
- Acne conglobata: severe acne with grouped comedones, deep nodules, and abscesses with sinuses oozing pus (see ➋ p. 250).
- Acne fulminans: nodulocystic acne, fever, and joint pains (see ➋ p. 248).
- Synovitis, acne, pustulosis, hyperostosis, osteitis (SAPHO) syndrome (see ➋ p. 248).
- PAPA syndrome: rare AD auto-Inflammatory disease (see ➋ pp. 234–5 and pp. 248–9).
- PASH syndrome: rare auto-inflammatory syndrome (pyoderma gangrenosum, acne, hidradenitis suppurativa).
- Comedo-like acneiform lesions (chloracne) associated with exposure to dioxin.

Further reading

Bhate K and Williams H. *Clin Exp Dermatol* 2014;**39**:273–8.
Lwin SM et al. *Clin Exp Dermatol* 2014;**39**:162–7.
Melnik BC et al. *J Invest Dermatol* 2009;**129**:1868–77.

Acne caused by drugs

Drugs that cause or exacerbate acne

(see ⮞ p. 388.)

A number of drugs may induce acne-like eruptions or exacerbate pre-existing acne (acne medicamentosa). Consider this possibility in patients with atypical presentations.

What should I look for?

- Acneiform rash (erythematous follicular pustules and papules).
- Unusual distribution, predominantly on the trunk and upper outer arms.
- Absence of comedones (whiteheads, blackheads).

Which drugs may be implicated?

- Anti-epileptics (phenytoin, carbamazepine, gabapentin).
- Anabolic steroids—danazole, testosterone. Ask about these drugs in athletes or body builders with acne not responding to treatment.
- Antitubercular drugs (isoniazid).
- Ciclosporin.
- Corticosteroids, including corticosteroid inhalers or inhalation through a face mask, e.g. in young children.
- Epidermal growth factor receptor inhibitors (used for the treatment of some cancers).
- Growth hormone.
- Halogenated compounds (iodides, radio-opaque contrast materials, bromides in sedatives, analgesics).
- Lithium.
- Progestogens such as medroxyprogesterone.
- Vitamin B_{12} (cyanocobalamin).

Further reading

Dessinioti C et al. Clin Dermatol 2014;**32**:24–34.

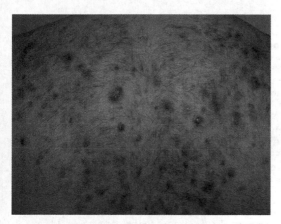

Fig. 12.1 Acne with papules, pustules, and nodules. Reproduced with permission from Warrell D *et al.* (eds) *Oxford Textbook of Medicine*, 5th edn, Layton A. Sebaceous and sweat gland disorders 2010. Oxford: Oxford University Press.

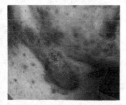

Fig. 12.2 Severe cystic acne for which isotretinoin is indicated.

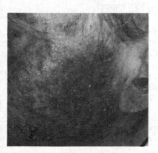

Fig. 12.3 Rosacea: erythema, papules, and pustules, but no comedones. A similar pustular rash may be induced by topical or oral corticosteroids.

Acne vulgaris: management

What should I do?

- Provide written information about acne—reassure that the skin is not dirty and that you can help.
- Explain that all treatments take 3–4 months to have a maximal effect and that acne may get a little worse before it gets better. Treatment may have to be continued for months or even years.
- If acne is not responding to treatment (and the patient is following your advice), have you made the right diagnosis? Is there an underlying systemic disease? (See Boxes 12.3 and 12.4.)

Mild acne

Start one or more topical preparations (combination more effective than monotherapy). Explain treatment should be applied to all the skin, not just 'spots'. Continue treatment for at least 4 months and usually longer. Topical preparations (cream, gel, or lotion) may include:

- Antibiotics, e.g. erythromycin or clindamycin lotion.
- Benzoyl peroxide 2.5% (as effective and less irritant than higher percentage, bleaches clothing; can combine with a topical retinoid).
- Topical retinoid (avoid in pregnancy), e.g. tretinoin, isotretinoin, or 0.1% adapalene (a retinoid-like drug). All are irritants and may cause post-inflammatory hyperpigmentation in dark skin. Increase contact time gradually, washing off after 30–60min at first.

Moderate acne

- Oral antibiotics for a 4-month course initially, e.g. oxytetracycline 500mg bd, lymecycline 408mg/day, or erythromycin 500mg bd, combined with topical benzoyl peroxide to reduce the incidence of bacterial resistance to antibiotics. Do not combine with a topical antibiotic. Avoid tetracyclines in children aged <12 years.
- ♀: oral contraceptive with anti-androgen activity such as co-cyprindiol (takes 6 months to have maximal effect). Avoid contraceptive pills containing norethisterone (androgenic properties).

Severe acne or acne with a major psychosocial impact
(See Fig. 12.2.)

- Refer to a specialist. The oral retinoid isotretinoin may be the best option (0.5–1.0mg/kg/day; cumulative dose 120–150mg/kg). Isotretinoin is teratogenic. Other adverse effects include mucosal dryness and, very rarely, depression. Contraception essential in women of childbearing age during treatment and for 1 month after stopping isotretinoin (see → Chapter 34, p. 669).
- Cysts: intralesional triamcinolone (0.1mL of 2.5–10mg/mL solution).

Scars

- Shallow scars become less obvious with time. Refer for cosmetic camouflage (see Changing Faces, available at: ℜ https://www.changingfaces.org.uk/Home).
- Surgical approaches (chemical peels, lasers, dermabrasion) may improve the appearance of deep scars but are not available through the National Health Service (NHS) and are not indicated until acne has been controlled.

Box 12.3 What is this pustular rash?

Papulopustular facial eruption, but no comedones
- Is this rosacea (see Fig 12.3)? Usually older patients (see ➔ pp. 254–5).
- Is the patient being treated with a systemic corticosteroid or another drug that may cause an acneiform rash? (see ➔ p. 244.)
- Is this perioral dermatitis (usually 2° to application of a topical corticosteroid)? (see ➔ pp. 256–7.)
- Could this be a bacterial folliculitis or fungal folliculitis, demodicosis, or pseudofolliculitis? (see ➔ pp. 134–5 and p. 178.)

Superficial small follicular pustules on back
- Is this pityrosporum folliculitis? (see ➔ p. 219.)
- ⚠ Could this be Behçet disease? (Rare; see ➔ pp. 284–5.)

Box 12.4 Why is severe acne not improving?

In patients with severe acne that is refractory to treatment, take the history again. Has anything been applied to the skin, or is the patient taking drugs such as anabolic steroids? Also consider:
- Polycystic ovary syndrome (obese ♀, oligomenorrhoea and/or infertility, hirsutism) (see ➔ pp. 476–7).
- Congenital adrenal hyperplasia (rare and caused by 21-hydroxylase deficiency) (see ➔ p. 474).
- An androgen-secreting tumour (adrenals, ovaries, or testes).
- XYY syndrome (tall ♂).
- Apert syndrome (low IQ, acrocephalosyndactyly) (see Box 12.1).

Further reading
Admani S and Barrio VR. *Dermatol Ther* 2013;**26**:462–6 (acne management).
Archer C et al. *Clin Exp Dermatol* 2012;**37** Suppl 1:1–6 (diagnosis and management of acne).
Dessinioti C et al. *Clin Dermatol* 2014;**32**:24–34 (reviews acneiform rashes).
Strauss JS et al. *J Am Acad Dermatol* 2007;**56**:651–63 (guidelines).

Acne with arthritis

⚠ Acne fulminans

This emergency affects adolescent boys who have previously had mild to moderate acne (see Boxes 12.5 and 12.6). Haemorrhagic, crusted, ulcerative skin lesions erupt on the back, chest, arms, and face. Systemic symptoms include fever, malaise, weight loss, myalgia, and arthralgia. Patients may have hepatosplenomegaly or erythema nodosum.

Radiographs show lytic bone lesions, most often affecting the sternum and clavicle, but osteolytic lesions have been seen in the hips, ankles, and humerus. Osteolytic lesions are sterile. Sternoclavicular hyperostosis and sacroiliitis have also been described. Periosteal formation of new bone, sclerosis, and thickening occur late. Bony changes are transient, and the prognosis is good. Findings may be consistent with SAPHO syndrome.

Acne conglobata

Seronegative spondyloarthropathy and SAPHO syndrome have also been described in patients with acne conglobata (see ➔ p. 250).

What is SAPHO syndrome?

SAPHO syndrome, an auto-inflammatory bone disease, may account for 4% of all patients with seronegative spondyloarthropathies. Inflammatory bowel disease is associated with SAPHO.

The syndrome is characterized by:

- Intermittent predominantly axial **S**ynovitis (sternum, clavicles, ribs, spine, pelvis).
- Aseptic **O**steitis and **H**yperostosis. Bony pain is common.
- CT scans show lytic bone lesions—these are sterile.
- Chronic (or relapsing) sterile pustular **A**cneiform eruptions or palmoplantar **P**ustulosis (for other skin diseases, see Box 12.7).
- Leucocytosis and anaemia.

Treatment is unsatisfactory. Tetracycline antibiotics or isotretinoin may control acne. Topical steroids and acitretin may control palmoplantar pustulosis. NSAIDs, prednisolone, and methotrexate have been used for synovitis. Infliximab (anti-TNF) and bisphosphonates (suppress osteoclasts) have also been recommended.

⚠ PAPA syndrome

Very rare AD auto-inflammatory syndrome caused by mutations in *PSTPIP1/CD2BP1* gene encoding a protein that interacts with pyrin. PAPA, like FMF, is associated with decreased apoptosis and high levels of IL-1B (see ➔ pp. 234–6). Patients have severe destructive sterile arthritis (often precipitated by minor trauma), as well as scarring cystic acne, sterile abscesses (often at injection sites), and PG-like ulcers (see ➔ p. 310). Treatments include corticosteroids, etanercept, infliximab, and anakinra.

Also see PASH (Pyoderma gangrenosum, Acne, Suppurative Hidradenitis)—another very rare auto-inflammatory syndrome (see ➔ p. 234).

⚠ Box 12.5 What is acne fulminans?

Acne fulminans is a severe variant of cystic acne, characterized by:
- Sudden onset of inflamed crusted haemorrhagic plaques and ulcers on the face, trunk, and arms (usually in an adolescent boy who has had mild to moderate acne).
- Systemic symptoms that may include fever, malaise, weight loss, myalgia, synovitis, and arthralgia.

Box 12.6 Acne fulminans: what should I do?

▶▶ Seek help from a dermatologist—acne fulminans is an emergency that needs immediate treatment.

Investigation
- Take skin swabs to exclude $2°$ staphylococcal infection.
- Check FBC (leucocytosis, anaemia), ESR (raised), and CRP (raised).
- Bone scans in areas of pain show increased uptake of radionuclide (not always required).

Immediate treatment
- Patients may need to be admitted, if very uncomfortable.
- Apply a potent topical corticosteroid bd to exuberant granulating ulcers. Antiseptic washes prevent $2°$ infection.
- Prescribe NSAID for arthralgia and myalgia.
- Start oral prednisolone 0.5–1.0mg/kg/day immediately. Continue for 4–8 weeks to control inflammation and prevent relapse.

Long-term treatment
- After 2–6 weeks of oral steroids, when the ulcerated lesions are beginning to settle, start isotretinoin, initially in a low dose (0.25–0.5mg/kg/day) to prevent a flare.
- After 4–6 weeks, provided acne has not deteriorated, gradually increase the dose of isotretinoin to 1.0mg/kg/day. Continue treatment for about 6 months.
- Tail off prednisolone, once the patient is established on treatment with isotretinoin.

Box 12.7 Skin diseases associated with SAPHO syndrome

- Acne fulminans.
- Acne conglobata and hidradenitis suppurativa.
- Palmoplantar pustulosis, GPP, plaque psoriasis.
- Other neutrophilic dermatoses, including PG, Sweet syndrome, and subcorneal pustular dermatosis.

Further reading
Hayem G. *Joint Bone Spine* 2007;**74**:123–6.

Follicular occlusion diseases: signs

Acne conglobata, hidradenitis suppurativa, and dissecting cellulitis of the scalp are diseases of adults in which follicular occlusion seems to play a part in pathogenesis. The conditions may coexist. Pilonidal cyst is another member of the 'folliculitis occlusion tetrad'. Seronegative spondyloarthropathy has been described in association with both acne conglobata and hidradenitis suppurativa, as has PG (see ➲ p. 310). ⚠ Rarely, SCC may complicate chronic disease.

Acne conglobata

What should I look for?
(See also Fig. 12.4.)

- Open comedones (blackheads) clustered into groups on the face and trunk. Papules, pustules, and nodules typical of acne.
- Fluctuant abscesses ('cysts') draining pus on the face, chest, and upper back, but also sometimes affecting the buttocks, groins, and axillae when signs overlap with those of hidradenitis suppurativa.
- Interconnecting sinus tracts linking adjacent abscesses.
- Large bowl-like scars, hypertrophic scars, or keloids.

Hidradenitis suppurativa

Hidradenitis suppurativa (acne inversa) is a chronic debilitating inflammation of the flexures, often misdiagnosed as staphylococcal furunculosis. Pathogenesis is uncertain, but follicular plugging may cause dilatation and rupture of follicles with 2° inflammation of apocrine glands. Hidradenitis is associated with obesity, polycystic ovary syndrome, and insulin resistance. Also associated with IBD, particularly Crohn disease. Cutaneous Crohn disease may simulate hidradenitis (see ➲ p. 508). Rarely associated with PG and acne (PASH syndrome) (see ➲ p. 234).

What should I look for?
(See also Figs. 12.5 and 12.6.)

- Recurrent 'boils' in axillae, breasts, groins, vulva, or perianal skin. Women tend to have involvement of the front of the body (groin, breasts), and men the back of the body (buttocks, perianal).
- Signs of insulin resistance: skin tags, acanthosis nigricans around the neck or flexures, obesity (flexural friction and sweating probably exacerbate follicular occlusion and the tendency to hidradenitis).
- Grouped open comedones (blackheads) in affected skin suggest hidradenitis—a useful sign in patients with recurrent flexural 'boils'.
- Tender nodules, abscesses, scars, and sinuses in flexures.

Dissecting cellulitis of the scalp

This rare condition, also known as 'perifolliculitis capitis abscedens et suffodiens', is commoner in black-skinned patients.

What should I look for?

- A history of recurrent and chronic painful abscesses in the scalp.
- Tender subcutaneous fluctuant scalp nodules, some of which drain pus, and intercommunicating sinuses.
- Patchy scarring with loss of hair (scarring alopecia).

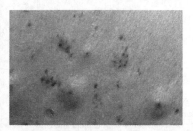

Fig. 12.4 Grouped comedones in acne conglobata.

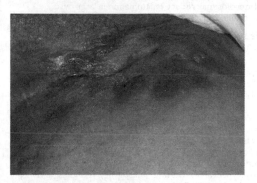

Fig. 12.5 Hidradenitis suppurativa with tender subcutaneous nodules, scars, and sinuses in the groin.

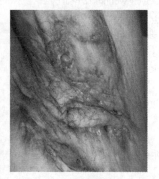

Fig. 12.6 Axillary hidradenitis suppurativa with scarring and deformity.

Follicular occlusion diseases: management

Management is difficult and at best control will be limited. Cultures of skin swabs may be negative or show a mixed growth, but *Staphylococcus aureus* may play some part in pathogenesis.

Acne conglobata

- Minimize exacerbating factors, e.g. drugs that may cause acne.
- The response to standard acne treatments with topical and oral antibiotics and topical retinoids is usually disappointing.
- Isotretinoin is worth trying, but disease can be very resistant.
- Intralesional steroids may reduce inflammation in large cysts.
- Cysts may be drained surgically.

Hidradenitis suppurativa

- Avoid smoking (some evidence nicotine exacerbates disease).
- Weight loss if obese (bariatric surgery was helpful in one case).
- Loose-fitting cotton clothing to reduce friction and sweating.
- Minimize follicular irritation by avoiding shaving and depilation.
- Antibacterial soaps and antiseptics (no evidence for efficacy).
- Topical 1% clindamycin lotion bd may control mild disease.
- Prolonged treatment (at least 6 months) with an oral tetracycline or erythromycin (as for acne) can be effective. Patients who do not respond may be treated with rifampicin 300mg bd in combination with clindamycin 300mg bd for 10 weeks.
- Anecdotal reports of therapies that may be helpful include antiandrogens (cyproterone acetate, finasteride), retinoids, and dapsone, as well as anti-TNF drugs, e.g. infliximab and etanercept.
- Severe disease requires a multidisciplinary approach—surgery or carbon dioxide laser surgery to remove scarred sinus tracts or marsupialize recurrent lesions. Leaving wounds to heal by 2° intention has been advocated, but grafts or flaps may be needed.
- Recurrence is common (less often in axillary disease), particularly after incision and drainage of abscesses, which is not recommended.

Dissecting cellulitis of the scalp

- Prolonged treatment with tetracycline antibiotics, as for acne, may be helpful. Combinations of rifampicin and clindamycin can be tried, as in hidradenitis.
- Isotretinoin has been tried (0.5–1.0mg/kg), with limited success, sometimes in combination with dapsone (50–100mg/day).

Further reading

Collier F et al. *BMJ* 2013;**346**:f2121 (hidradenitis review).
Gener G et al. *Dermatology* 2009;**219**:148–54 (hidradenitis treatment).

Rosacea

Rosacea is common in the third and fourth decades. Pathogenesis is uncertain, but genetic factors play a part. Rosacea has a particularly high prevalence in Ireland (Celts with fair skin).

What should I ask?

- Patients will often have had a long-standing tendency to flush or blush easily, now the face is permanently red (also see ➔ p. 520).
- What makes the redness worse? The skin is easily irritated by topical products. Alcohol, spicy foods, sudden temperature change, and hot drinks can all precipitate reddening. Sunlight may also exacerbate rosacea. The role of demodex is uncertain (see ➔ p. 178).
- What does the patient notice? Crops of red bumps (papules), 'yellow-heads' (pustules)? Is the skin rough or scaly? (Scale is seen more often in seborrhoeic dermatitis than rosacea, but the conditions may overlap; see Fig. 12.3).
- What medicaments is the patient using and for how long? Topical corticosteroids can cause a rosacea-like rash (perioral dermatitis; see ➔ p. 256). Oral corticosteroids cause a pustular rash and redness. Peripheral vasodilators may exacerbate redness (see ➔ p. 389).
- Patients may have noticed enlargement of the nose.
- Eye symptoms are common, e.g. burning, itching, redness, grittiness.

What should I look for?

(See Fig. 12.3.)

Signs vary. Rosacea may be predominantly erythematotelangiectatic (red), papulopustular, phymatous, or granulomatous. Look for:

- A rash affecting the central face, usually in a symmetrical pattern, but, on occasion, rosacea can be strikingly asymmetrical.
- Erythema and telangiectasia (see Fig. 12.3).
- Dome-shaped erythematous papules and pustules without comedones (see Fig. 12.3). Comedones suggest acne (see ➔ pp. 242–3), not rosacea. Facial angiofibromas in tuberous sclerosis may be misdiagnosed as rosacea (see ➔ pp. 556–7).
- Brownish yellow papules (granulomatous rosacea?) (see Box 12.9).
- Greasy skin, sometimes with diffuse fine scale. Prominent scaling suggests dermatitis (seborrhoeic or contact) or, if in a limited area, fungal infection. (Also see ➔ Demodicosis, p. 178.)
- Facial swelling (lymphoedema). Persistent erythema and solid oedema of upper 2/3 of the face (Morbihan disease) is a form of rosacea.
- A bulbous nose (rhinophyma) because of hypertrophic sebaceous glands and an overgrowth of soft tissues.
- Ocular rosacea—conjunctivitis, blepharitis, chalazion, hordeolum.
- Sparing of the trunk—unlike acne, rosacea does not affect the back or chest.
- Cutaneous B-cell lymphoma may simulate rosacea with firm erythematous papules on the forehead, cheeks, chin (rare).

Management

See Box 12.8.

Box 12.8 Rosacea: what should I do?

- Soap substitutes minimize irritation of the skin.
- A hat and sunblock creams will prevent photoexacerbation.
- Brimonidine tartrate gel ×1/day reduces redness (irritates; risk of rebound erythema and contact dermatitis).
- Mild papulopustular disease: 0.75% metronidazole cream or 15% azelaic acid gel applied bd for 3–4 months. Ivermectin 1% cream ×1/day may be more effective than metronidazole.
- Topical 1% pimecrolimus or 0.1% tacrolimus may have a role in papulopustular disease.
- An oral antibiotic (oxytetracycline 500mg bd, lymecycline 408mg/day, or erythromycin 500mg bd) taken for 4 months will control papulopustular disease but has little impact on redness. The dose can be reduced, once the disease is under control.
- Oral isotretinoin may reduce sebaceous gland overgrowth. In Morbihan variant, >6 months' treatment may reduce erythema/swelling.
- Rhinophyma can be pared down electrosurgically.
- Cosmetic camouflage or laser surgery may reduce redness.

Box 12.9 What is granulomatous rosacea?

Granulomatous rosacea is characterized by:
- Features of rosacea. Brownish yellow or red papules predominate.
- Granulomatous perifollicular inflammation without necrosis.
- Response to oral antibiotics, e.g. minocycline 100mg/day, lymecycline 408mg/day taken for 4–6 months.
- Isotretinoin is an alternative treatment.

Acne agminata (lupus miliaris disseminatus faciei) is probably a variant of granulomatous rosacea:
- Patients present with clusters of reddish brown or yellow papules, 1–3mm in diameter, distributed symmetrically around the eyes, including the eyelids, and sometimes elsewhere on the central face. Some patients have nodules in the axillae. Lesions last months, may become pustular and crusted, and eventually heal with pitted scarring.
- The histology shows superficial granulomatous inflammation with caseation necrosis, possibly a reaction to damaged pilosebaceous units. Acne agminata has no relationship to tuberculosis.
- The disease tends to regress spontaneously in 1–2 years.
- Tetracycline antibiotics, in acne doses, are usually effective in about 6 months.
- Isotretinoin and dapsone have also been effective.

Further reading

DelRosso JQ. Expert Opin Pharmacother 2014;14:2029–38.
Smith LA and Cohen DE. Arch Dermatol 2012;148:1395–8 (Morbihan disease).
Wilkin J et al. J Am Acad Dermatol 2002;46:584–7.

Perioral dermatitis (periorificial dermatitis)

Perioral dermatitis is an inflammatory condition that occurs in children and adults, usually young and middle-aged women. The cause is unknown, but exogenous factors, such as potent topical corticosteroids (see $\bigodot$ p. 657), inhaled corticosteroids, irritant cosmetics, fluorinated toothpastes, and occlusive emollients, have been implicated.

The name is misleading. Perioral skin is affected more often than other sites, but the condition may affect periocular and perinasal skin. It has also been reported on the trunk. Nor is perioral dermatitis a typical dermatitis; it is more akin to rosacea. Dermatitis is treated with a topical corticosteroid; yet topical corticosteroids are one of the causes of perioral dermatitis.

What should I look for?

- A history of a rash that burns, rather than itches.
- Explore what has been applied to the skin. Many (but not all) patients with perioral dermatitis will have been applying a potent topical corticosteroid to their face prior to the onset of the rash. The corticosteroid relieves burning and causes transient vasoconstriction, which reduces redness, so the patient continues to apply the cream in the mistaken belief that the corticosteroid is helping.
- Clusters of tiny (<2mm in diameter) erythematous papules and vesicopustules (the tiny vesicles rapidly evolve into pustules) around the mouth (see Fig. 12.7).
- The background skin is erythematous and may be scaly.
- The rash tends to spare the vermillion border of the lips.
- Periocular (usually below the eye) and perinasal lesions are probably commoner in children than adults.

What should I do?

- Try to identify the underlying cause—most often applications of a potent topical corticosteroid to the face—and advise avoidance of any potential skin irritant.
- Convince the patient that the topical corticosteroid (or other preparation) is the cause of the problem—this may be difficult. (Try to avoid blaming the doctor who prescribed the strong corticosteroid—it is quite possible that the patient has not followed the doctor's instructions or has obtained the corticosteroid from a well-meaning friend or relation.)
- Warn the patient that the skin is going to look worse, before it gets better, and to resist the temptation to restart the topical corticosteroid (the redness and irritation will be more obvious when the corticosteroid is withdrawn).
- Prescribe topical or oral therapy (see Box 12.10).
- Reassure the patient—the prognosis is good, and the rash generally clears in 8–12 weeks.

Box 12.10 Treatment of perioral dermatitis

- Withdraw potential irritants and potent corticosteroid preparations.
- Topical 1% pimecrolimus or 0.1% tacrolimus ointment may be effective in mild cases. Apply bd for 4 weeks.
- An oral tetracycline (e.g. oxytetracycline 250–500mg bd) will be required for 6–8 weeks in more severe cases.
- Avoid tetracyclines in children <12 years (they stain teeth), and use erythromycin instead, but this is not as effective as tetracycline.
- Prescribe a weak topical corticosteroid (1% hydrocortisone ointment), in combination with miconazole for any underlying eczematous skin problem (possibly seborrhoeic dermatitis), if required.

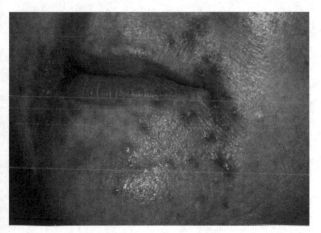

Fig. 12.7 Perioral dermatitis caused by very potent topical corticosteroid.

Further reading

Dessinioti C et al. *Clin Dermatol* 2014;**32**:24–34.

Blisters

Contents

Relevant pages in other chapters

Causes of blisters ➲ pp. 80–1
Emergency dermatology ➲ pp. 110–21
Photosensitivity ➲ pp. 324–6
Blisters in infants and children ➲ pp. 592–3
Epidermolysis bullosa ➲ pp. 624–5
Epidermolytic ichthyosis ➲ p. 627
Darier disease and Hailey-Hailey disease ➲ pp. 628–9
Incontinentia pigmenti ➲ p. 636

Introduction to blisters

What is a blister?

- A blister is a bump filled with clear fluid (serum).
- Small blisters, <0.5cm in diameter, are called vesicles.
- Larger blisters, >0.5cm in diameter, are known as bullae.

Why does the skin blister?

Blisters form, because adhesion fails, either between the keratinocytes just below the stratum corneum (subcorneal blisters), within the epidermis (intra-epidermal blisters), or within or below the dermo-epidermal junction (subepidermal blisters) (see Fig. 13.1).

Always exclude common (and often more easily treated) 2° causes of blisters, such as trauma, eczema, insect bites, or infection, before you diagnose a 1° bullous disease.

Common 2° causes of blisters are discussed in more detail elsewhere in the book. For the causes of blisters, see ➲ pp. 80–1.

Subcorneal blister

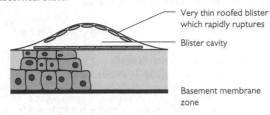

Very thin roofed blister which rapidly ruptures

Blister cavity

Basement membrane zone

Intra-epidermal blister

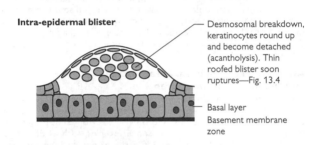

Desmosomal breakdown, keratinocytes round up and become detached (acantholysis). Thin roofed blister soon ruptures—Fig. 13.4

Basal layer
Basement membrane zone

Subepidermal blister

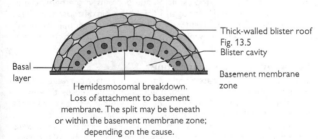

Thick-walled blister roof
Fig. 13.5
Blister cavity

Basement membrane zone

Basal layer

Hemidesmosomal breakdown. Loss of attachment to basement membrane. The split may be beneath or within the basement membrane zone; depending on the cause.

Fig. 13.1 Level of splits in blisters.

Adhesion in the epidermis

In order to understand the 1° bullous diseases, it will help to appreciate the interactions between structural proteins that provide the mechanical scaffolding of the skin.

Adhesion between keratinocytes

The main adhesion junctions between keratinocytes in the epidermis are desmosomes. Desmosomes contain transmembrane adhesion proteins (desmosomal cadherins) and cytoplasmic plaque proteins. Interactions between the extracellular portions of the transmembrane cadherins hold the keratinocytes together. The cytoplasmic portion of the cadherin inserts into the desmosomal plaque where it interacts with plaque proteins such as desmoplakin or plakoglobin. These plaque proteins link to keratins in the intermediate filament cytoskeleton, which are linked to the nucleus. Thus the whole network is stable, and signals can be transduced from the external surface of the cell through the desmosome to the nucleus (see Fig. 13.2a).

Adhesion between basal keratinocytes and the basement membrane

Hemidesmosomes at the base of basal keratinocytes attach keratinocytes to the basement membrane. Hemidesmosomes, like desmosomes, contain transmembrane adhesion proteins and cytoplasmic plaque proteins. Transmembrane hemidesmosomal proteins, such as BP antigen 2 BP180 (collagen XVII) and α6β4 integrin, extend into the basement membrane zone (BMZ) to interact with proteins, such as laminins, in anchoring filaments to bind the epidermis to the basement membrane. The cytoplasmic portions of these transmembrane hemidesmosomal proteins interact with cytoplasmic plaque proteins in the hemidesmosome such as plectin and BP antigen 1 (BP230). As in desmosomes, these plaque proteins link hemidesmosomes to the keratins of the intermediate filament cytoskeleton, which are, in turn, connected to the nucleus of the cell (see Fig. 13.2b).

The basement membrane zone

The surface area of the basement membrane interface between the epidermis and dermis is increased and adhesion enhanced by downward projections from the epidermis (epidermal rete pegs) that interdigitate with upward projections from the dermis (dermal papillae). Interactions between laminins, collagens, and non-collagenous proteins in the BMZ promote adhesion. The lamina lucida (electron-lucent zone) of the basement membrane, containing laminins, lies immediately beneath basal keratinocytes. Laminins attach to collagen IV in the underlying lamina densa. Fine anchoring filaments (laminin-332, laminin-311) bound to extracellular domains of the hemidesmosomal protein α6β4 integrin extend across the lamina lucida into the lamina densa where the filaments link to anchoring fibrils (collagen VII). The anchoring fibrils fasten the lamina densa to the underlying collagen bundles of the papillary dermis (see Fig. 13.2b).

(a)

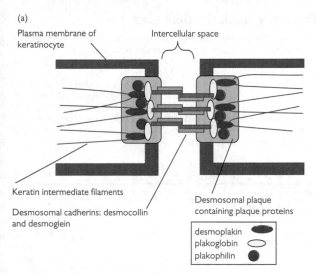

Plasma membrane of
keratinocyte

Intercellular space

Keratin intermediate filaments

Desmosomal cadherins: desmocollin
and desmoglein

Desmosomal plaque
containing plaque proteins

desmoplakin
plakoglobin
plakophilin

Fig. 13.2a Model of a desmosome, the main adhesion junction providing
adhesion between keratinocytes.

(b)

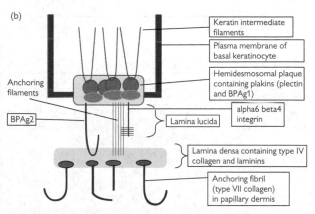

Keratin intermediate
filaments

Plasma membrane of
basal keratinocyte

Hemidesmosomal plaque
containing plakins (plectin
and BPAg1)

Anchoring
filaments

BPAg2

alpha6 beta4
integrin

Lamina lucida

Lamina densa containing type IV
collagen and laminins

Anchoring fibril
(type VII collagen)
in papillary dermis

Fig. 13.2b Model of the basement membrane zone, showing attachment of the
hemidesmosome of a basal keratinocyte to the underlying papillary dermis.

Primary bullous diseases

1° bullous diseases are caused by inherited defects in, or autoantibodies directed against, structural proteins in the skin—keratins, desmosomal proteins, hemidesmosomal proteins, or BMZ proteins (see Tables 13.1 and 13.2, and ➲ Chapter 32, pp. 624–5.

The level of the blister is determined by the structural protein that is either defective or targeted by the autoantibody. Intra-epidermal blisters are caused by problems with desmosomal components or the keratin intermediate filament cytoskeleton. Subepidermal blisters are caused by problems affecting hemidesmosomal components or components of the BMZ (see Figs. 13.2–13.5).

⚠ Table 13.1 Some inherited blistering diseases

Genetic disease	Defective protein	Level of split
Epidermolysis bullosa simplex	Keratin 5 or 14 (cytoskeleton)	Intra-epidermal
Epidermolysis bullosa simplex with pyloric atresia/muscular dystrophy	Plectin (hemidesmosome)	Intra-epidermal
Junctional epidermolysis bullosa: generalized severe, generalized intermediate	Laminin-332 or BP180 (anchoring filament or hemidesmosome)	Lamina lucida
Dystrophic epidermolysis bullosa (dominant and recessive forms)	Type VII collagen	Sublamina densa

see ➲ Chapter 32, Box 32.1, p. 625.

Table 13.2 Some autoimmune blistering diseases

Autoimmune disease	Major autoantigen (s)	Level of split
Pemphigus foliaceus	Dg 1 (desmosome)	Intra-epidermal
Pemphigus vulgaris	Dg 1 and 3 (desmosome)	Intra-epidermal
Bullous pemphigoid	BP230 and BP180 (collagen XVII) (hemidesmosome)	Subepidermal
Mucous membrane pemphigoid (cicatricial pemphigoid)	BP180 and α6β4 integrin (hemidesmosome) Laminin-332 and -311 (anchoring filaments) Type VII collagen (anchoring fibrils)	Subepidermal
Epidermolysis bullosa acquisita (see ➲ p. 272)	Type VII collagen (anchoring fibrils)	Subepidermal

Dg = desmoglein.

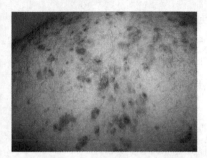

Fig. 13.3 Erythematous crusted papules on the trunk in pemphigus foliaceus resembling seborrhoeic dermatitis. The split is so superficial that blisters are uncommon.

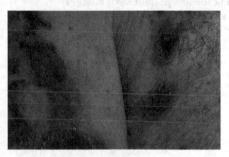

Fig. 13.4 Typical erosions in pemphigus vulgaris—the intra-epidermal blisters rupture easily.

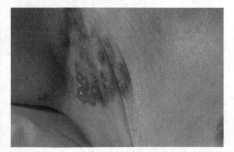

Fig. 13.5 Tense blisters, erosions, and urticated erythema (erythema without scale) in bullous pemphigoid.

Further reading

Turcan I and Jonkman MF. *Cell Tissue Res* 2015;**360**:545–69.

The approach to the patient

Blisters worry patients (and their doctors). ⚠ Extensive blistering with disruption of the epidermal barrier is potentially life-threatening and should be treated as a medical emergency (see ➔ pp. 112–9).

What should I ask a patient with blisters?

Take a full dermatological history (see ➔ p. 18 and pp. 80–1). Ask:
- Does a rash precede blistering?
- When did blistering start?
- Does the skin seem fragile or photosensitive?
- Are there mucosal symptoms—oral, conjunctival, or genital?
- What drugs or topical preparations are being used?
- Are there symptoms suggesting systemic disease?
- Does anyone else in the family have a blistering condition?

What should I look for in a patient with blisters?

- Is the patient ill, suggesting a systemic cause such as infection or drug?
- What is the distribution of the blistering?
    Localized and asymmetrical (suggesting an exogenous cause),
    e.g. at sites of pressure or in streaks, suggesting a reaction to
    something that has been in contact with the skin.
    - Generalized and symmetrical (suggesting endogenous disease).
    - On sun-exposed skin, suggesting photosensitivity.
- What precedes the blister, e.g. are there itchy, erythematous urticated papules or plaques (sometimes seen in BP)?
- Are the blisters intra-epidermal or subepidermal?
    - Blisters within the epidermis have a thin roof and rupture easily, leaving oozing crusted erosions or scaling (see Figs. 13.3 and 13.4).
    - Blisters that form at, or below, the basement membrane of the dermo-epidermal junction are tense, may contain blood, and are less likely to rupture, as the roof is formed by the whole of the epidermis (see Fig. 13.5).
- Are there ulcers? These form when the epidermis and superficial papillary dermis are lost. Ulcers suggest deep subepidermal blistering or 2° infection.
- Are the blisters umbilicated, i.e. do they have a central depression? Seen in some viral infections.
- Are there pustules? A secondary finding in a primary vesiculobullous disease.
- Are there mucosal blisters, erosions, or scarring? Check the eyes, mouth, and genitalia (see ➔ pp. 48–9).
- What is left when the blisters have healed—scars, post-inflammatory hyper- or hypopigmentation?
- Are there milia? These pinhead-sized firm white papules are tiny intradermal cysts that are left when some subepidermal blisters heal. Milia suggest that blistering was subepidermal.

Investigations

See Boxes 13.1 and 13.2.

Box 13.1 Investigations in patients with blisters

- Exclude infection by taking skin swabs from erosions for microbiological and/or viral culture (see ➔ p. 644).
- Take a 4mm punch biopsy that includes a small early intact blister to show the level at which the blister has arisen. If the biopsy is taken from an old or ruptured blister, the roof may be lost and the floor may be re-epithelializing, making it difficult to decide if the blister is intra-epidermal or subepidermal.
- Take a 3–4mm punch biopsy from perilesional (unaffected) skin for direct immunofluorescence microscopy to look for Ig and complement deposits within the epidermis or at the basement membrane zone. Either snap freeze the specimen in liquid nitrogen, fix in Michel medium, or transport in normal saline if processed within 2–3 days.
- Take a blood sample for indirect immunofluorescence microscopy to look for circulating autoantibodies to antigens in the epidermis or the basement membrane zone.
- In patients with a history of skin fragility, blistering at sites of trauma, or photosensitivity, check for porphyrins in urine, stool, and blood. Wrap the specimen pots in tinfoil to prevent exposure to UV light (see ➔ Box 16.1, p. 323 and pp. 330–4).

Box 13.2 Indirect immunofluorescence on salt-split skin

In subepidermal blistering diseases, the autoantigen may be associated with the hemidesmosomes of basal keratinocytes or a component of the basement membrane or dermis. Indirect immunofluorescence studies on intact skin will produce a bright linear subepidermal band that does not differentiate between these autoantigens. Salt-split skin helps to localize the autoantigen in subepidermal blistering diseases.

- The lamina lucida is the weakest part of the basement membrane. Skin that is stressed mechanically by suction or exposure to salt will always split through the lamina lucida.
- A biopsy of normal skin is immersed in 1M saline for 3 days, and the artificially split skin is used as the substrate in an indirect immunofluorescence reaction.
- The patient's serum containing the autoantibody is incubated with skin that has been fractured through the lamina lucida, and antibody binding detected in the usual way.
- Autoantibodies that bind to antigens associated with the hemidesmosomes of basal keratinocytes (e.g. in BP) will bind to the epidermal side (roof) of the artificial split, whereas autoantibodies that bind to antigens associated with the lamina densa or dermis (e.g. in EBA or bullous SLE) will bind to the dermal side (base) of the split.

Pemphigus

A group of rare intra-epidermal autoimmune blistering diseases that can be life-threatening and difficult to control. Widespread superficial blisters and painful erosions caused by circulating autoantibodies that disrupt the desmosomal attachments between keratinocytes (see Box 13.3). Occurs at a younger age than pemphigoid.

What should I look for?

Pemphigus vulgaris
(See Fig. 13.4.)
- Slow-healing irregularly shaped erosions in oral mucous membranes—it is rare to see intact bullae in the mouth. Painful oral ulceration may precede skin involvement by months.
- Involvement of conjunctiva, nasal mucosa, pharynx, larynx, oesophagus, urethra, vulva, and/or cervix.
- Flaccid blisters and painful slow-healing cutaneous erosions affecting the scalp, face, axillae, upper trunk, groins, and pressure points. May be heaped up and vegetating in flexures (pemphigus vegetans).
- Nikolsky sign—applying a firm sliding pressure to the skin with your finger will produce an erosion, because the epidermis separates from the dermis. The test is painful and rarely necessary (also positive in TEN; see ⊃ p. 116).

Pemphigus foliaceus
(See Fig. 13.3.)
- A slowly extending rash on the scalp, face, chest, and upper back.
- Scaly erythematous papules—may resemble seborrhoeic dermatitis.
- Flaccid vesicles that rupture easily, leaving crusted painful shallow erosions that may be malodorous.
- Mucosae are not affected.

What should I do?

- Check the drug history (see Box 13.4).
- Take biopsies of fresh lesions for histology, perilesional skin for direct immunofluorescence (IMF) microscopy, and blood for indirect IMF microscopy.
- Check FBC, and renal and liver function.
- Take skin swabs from erosions, and prevent sepsis by cleansing the eroded skin and mucous membranes (see ⊃ p. 662).
- Potent topical corticosteroids may be sufficient to control mild localized pemphigus, but most patients require oral treatment with systemic corticosteroids (prednisolone 1mg/kg/day). Side effects, including septicaemia, are a major cause of death.
- Topical steroids may help to suppress oral ulcers. Painful oral ulceration and oral *Candida* can be relieved with mouthwashes containing nystatin and 2% lidocaine (see ⊃ Box 14.4, p. 283).
- Other immunosuppressive agents include azathioprine, methotrexate, cyclophosphamide, and mycophenolate mofetil.
- Plasmapheresis, IV Ig, and, more recently, rituximab have been used, with some success, in resistant cases.

Box 13.3 Pathogenesis of pemphigus

Pemphigus vulgaris
- The main antigen is the desmosomal cadherin desmoglein 3, which is expressed in mucosae and predominantly in the lower epidermis. Antibodies may also develop to desmoglein 1 (not expressed in mucosae, present in the superficial epidermis).
- A biopsy taken from an early lesion will show intra-epidermal spongiosis (oedema between keratinocytes), sometimes with eosinophils (eosinophilic spongiosis).
- Biopsy from intact vesicles will show splitting just above the basal layer of the epidermis, forming intra-epidermal blisters. Keratinocytes round up and separate from each other (acantholysis), but the basal keratinocytes remain attached to the basement membrane by hemidesmosomes. Their appearance has been likened to a row of tombstones, because the cells stand up in a row without their lateral attachments to each other.
- Direct and indirect IMF microscopy—IgG and C3 between keratinocytes.

Pemphigus foliaceus
- The antigen is the desmosomal cadherin desmoglein 1, which is expressed most strongly in the upper parts of the epidermis and is absent in mucosae.
- The split is high in the epidermis, just below the stratum corneum, but splitting can be difficult to find. The blister may contain a few neutrophils and some acantholytic keratinocytes.
- Direct and indirect IMF microscopy—IgG and C3 between keratinocytes.

⚠ Box 13.4 Rare variants of pemphigus

- *Drug-induced pemphigus*: sulfhydryl drugs, such as captopril, enalapril, and penicillamine, may trigger pemphigus, most often pemphigus foliaceus.
- *Endemic or Brazilian pemphigus foliaceus* (fogo selvagem = 'wild fire' in Portuguese): clustered in certain states in Brazil and possibly precipitated by an environmental factor, e.g. a biting insect (the black fly has been postulated to be a vector).
- *Paraneoplastic pemphigus*: associated with B-cell lymphoma, thymoma, and Castleman disease (a rare lymphoproliferative disorder) (see ➔ p. 538). Some cases have been linked to treatment with fludarabine (see ➔ p. 386).
- *IgA pemphigus* (very rare!): with features that overlap those of subcorneal pustular dermatosis (Sneddon–Wilkinson disease).

Further reading

Harman KE et al. Br J Dermatol 2003;**149**:926–37. Available at: ℬ http://www.bad.org.uk/library-media%5Cdocuments%5CPemphigus_vulgaris_2003.pdf.

Bullous pemphigoid

Bullous pemphigoid

BP is the commonest autoimmune blistering disease seen in the West. Presents most often in older patients but can affect younger adults and rarely children. Autoantibodies to collagen XVII, a transmembrane component of the hemidesmosomes, may initiate disease (see Box 13.5). The course is punctuated by exacerbations and partial remissions, but the disease may remit in 3–7 years.

What should I look for?
- Evidence of common causes of blisters, e.g. eczema/infection (see ➔ pp. 80–1).
- Itchy urticated papules or plaques (this itchy rash may be present for up to a year, before the blisters appear).
- Numerous tense blisters, 1–3cm in diameter, on inflamed or normal-appearing skin. Blistering in BP tends to predominate on the lower trunk, flexural surfaces of the limbs, axillae, and groins (see Fig. 13.5).
- Crusted erosions.
- Healing without scarring, provided that the blisters have not been scratched or become secondarily infected.
- Oral blisters or erosions (present in about 1/3 of patients).
- Check the eyes—the conjunctivae are not affected in BP.

What should I do?
- Take a skin biopsy for histology and direct IMF microscopy (see Box 13.6).
- Take blood for indirect IMF microscopy.
- Aspirate fluid from any large uncomfortable blisters.
- Take swabs from eroded skin to exclude infection.
- Check for associated medical conditions (see Box 13.7).
- Treatments include:
  - Skin care to prevent infection (see ➔ p. 662).
  - Very potent topical corticosteroid, e.g. 0.05% clobetasol propionate cream applied liberally ×1/day to all erythematous, eroded, and blistering skin.
  - Oral corticosteroids 0.5mg/kg/day (and bone protection). May respond to low doses.
  - Oral tetracyclines, erythromycin, or nicotinamide as steroid-sparing agents or as sole agents.
  - Immunosuppressive drugs, such as azathioprine and methotrexate, as steroid-sparing agents if disease proves difficult to control.

Rare variants of bullous pemphigoid

- Pemphigoid gestationis occurs in pregnancy or the puerperium (see ➔ p. 584).
- Mucous membrane (cicatricial) pemphigoid (see ➔ p. 272).

Box 13.5 Antigens in bullous pemphigoid

- The 230kDa *bullous pemphigoid antigen 1* (BPAg1, BP230) is a member of the plakin protein family, a group of intracellular cytoplasmic proteins that link the intermediate filament cytoskeleton to adhesion plaques such as hemidesmosomes and desmosomes in plasma membranes. BP230 is not exposed on the cell surface, and the antibodies to BP230 may only develop after keratinocyte injury but probably enhance the immune response.
- The 180kDa *bullous pemphigoid antigen 2* (BPAg2, BP180), also called collagen XVII, is a transmembrane protein in the hemidesmosomes that anchors basal keratinocytes to the basement membrane. BP180 extends from the cytoplasm of basal keratinocytes into the lamina densa of the basement membrane zone. The autoantibodies bind to epitopes in the NC16A domain, which is part of the molecule that is outside the basal keratinocyte but close to the keratinocyte plasma membrane. Autoantibodies to *collagen XVII* may initiate disease.

Box 13.6 Histology and immunofluorescence in bullous pemphigoid

- A biopsy taken from an early urticated erythematous lesion will show subepidermal oedema with an eosinophilic infiltrate in the papillary dermis. The amount of inflammation varies.
- Blistering is subepidermal, and blisters usually contain eosinophils.
- Direct (skin sample) and indirect (serum sample) IMF microscopy shows a linear band of IgG and/or C3 at the dermo-epidermal junction.
- The autoantibodies are directed against antigens associated with hemidesmosomes and localize to the epidermal side (roof) of salt-split skin (see Box 13.2).

Box 13.7 Associations with bullous pemphigoid

- Neurological diseases, e.g. cerebrovascular disease, dementia, Parkinson disease, multiple sclerosis—predisposing factor and poor prognostic factor (functional impairment increases the risk of infectious complications).
- Chronic use of neuroleptics.
- Chronic use of spironolactone.
- Can be triggered by PUVA/UVB, e.g. for treatment of psoriasis.

Further reading

Venning V et al. Br J Dermatol 2012;**167**:1200–14. Available at: ℘ http://www.bad.org.uk/library-media/documents/Bullous_pemphigoid_2012.pdf.

Rare subepidermal blistering diseases

⚠ Mucous membrane (cicatricial) pemphigoid

A rare variant of pemphigoid, characterized by painful subepithelial blistering, ulceration, and scarring (see Box 13.8). All mucosal-dominant blistering disorders are diagnosed mucous membrane pemphigoid. Corticosteroids, dapsone, and other immunosuppressants are used, but this chronic, disabling disease is difficult to control.

What should I look for?
- Scattered tense blisters or ulcers on the scalp, face, or upper trunk—these heal with scarring.
- Oral blisters or ulcers (affecting the gingiva or buccal mucosa).
- Conjunctival inflammation, blisters, or erosions.
- Adhesions between the surfaces of bulbar and palpebral conjunctivae (best seen by gently pulling down the lower eyelid and asking the patient to look to the left and then to the right) (see ➔ p. 49).
- Involvement of other mucosal surfaces—nasopharynx, larynx, oesophagus, genitalia, and/or rectum.

⚠ Epidermolysis bullosa acquisita

Rare mechanobullous subepidermal blistering disease, associated with autoantibodies to type VII collagen (see Box 13.9). Sometimes associated with IBD or RA. Patients usually aged 40–60 years. Corticosteroids, dapsone, other immunosuppressants, IV Igs, plasmapheresis, and rituximab have demonstrated variable success.

What should I look for?
- Sudden onset of skin fragility or blistering in areas prone to trauma—knuckles, elbows, knees, sacrum, and toes (may resemble PCT, but patients are not photosensitive nor do they have hypertrichosis) (see ➔ p. 332).
- Tense blisters and ulcers affecting skin exposed to trauma.
- Blisters may be haemorrhagic, and the underlying skin inflamed or scarred.
- Healing with scarring and milia (tiny subepidermal white firm cysts).
- Nail dystrophy or loss of nails; scarring alopecia.
- Less often:
  - BP-like with no predilection for sites exposed to trauma, tense bullae on erythematous skin, and minimal scarring.
  - Predominantly mucosal involvement. Ulcers and scars may affect the conjunctiva, oral mucosa, upper oesophagus, anus, trachea, and/or vagina.

⚠ Other rare subepidermal blistering diseases

- Linear IgA disease—affects children (also known as chronic bullous disease of childhood) and adults.
- Bullous LE (see ➔ Box 19.9, p. 405).
- Dermatitis herpetiformis (see ➔ pp. 274–5).

Box 13.8 Antigens in mucous membrane pemphigoid

- The 180kDa BP antigen 2 (BPAg2, BP180) is also involved in mucous membrane pemphigoid, but the predominant epitope site is in the C-terminal portion, much deeper within the epidermal basement membrane zone than in BP.
- Mucous membrane pemphigoid sera also have autoantibodies to laminin-332, and sometimes to laminin-311, as well as type VII collagen.
- Binding to these deeper antigens may be relevant to the scarring pathology that is a feature of this form of pemphigoid.

Box 13.9 Antigens in epidermolysis bullosa acquisita

- Type VII collagen, a component of the anchoring fibrils that fasten the lamina densa of the basement membrane to the underlying papillary dermis, is the antigen in EBA.
- Blistering is subepidermal.
- Direct and indirect IMF microscopy shows a linear band of IgG and/or C3 at the dermo-epidermal junction.
- The autoantibodies are directed against antigens that are associated with anchoring fibrils and localizesd to the dermal side (base) of salt-split skin (see Box 13.2).

Dermatitis herpetiformis

Uncommon blistering disease presenting at any age and associated with a gluten-sensitive enteropathy (see ➔ Coeliac disease, p. 514). Epidermal transglutaminase 3 appears to be the dominant autoantigen in DH, but pathogenesis of the rash is uncertain. Patients also have circulating antibodies that bind to tissue transglutaminase in reticulin fibres such as endomysium—a component of smooth muscle. Associated with HLA-DQ2 and HLA-DQ8. Confers an increased incidence of other auto-immune diseases, including thyroid disease, pernicious anaemia, type 1 diabetes, SLE, and RA, and an increased risk of developing intestinal lymphoma.

What should I look for?
- Sudden onset of an extremely itchy rash exacerbated by oral gluten.
- Symptoms suggesting coeliac disease—fatigue, 'irritable bowel' symptoms, diarrhoea—but patchy enteropathy is often subclinical.
- Family history of DH or coeliac disease (10% of patients).
- Clusters of excoriated papules in a symmetrical distribution on extensor surfaces—elbows, knees, buttocks, and shoulders. Unusual to see intact vesicles, because the rash is so itchy ('herpetiformis', because vesicles erupt in groups like herpes simplex) (see Fig. 13.6).
- Excoriated papules on the scalp or chin.
- Palmoplantar petechiae or, less often, purpuric macules on fingertips, suggesting vasculitis.
- Another cause of itching such as eczema or scabies (burrows on the sides of fingers, wrists, sides of feet, genitalia)—*very* much more likely than DH! (see ➔ p. 60.)

What should I do?
- FBC, iron, vitamin B_{12}, and folate.
- LFT, serum calcium.
- Autoantibody screen, including IgA anti-endomysial and/or tissue transglutaminase antibodies.
- Take a biopsy of an intact vesicle or non-excoriated papule for histology (see Box 13.10).
- Take a 4mm punch biopsy from uninvolved buttock skin for direct IMF microscopy (this may need to be repeated).
- Refer to gastroenterology for investigation of the small intestine if diagnosis is confirmed.
- Treat with dapsone (1–2mg/kg/day)—itching will subside within 48–72h. Dapsone has no effect on the enteropathy.
- Arrange for the patient to see a dietician—a strict gluten-free diet will control the enteropathy and eventually the rash (may take 2 years). Dapsone requirements will fall slowly if the patient adheres to the diet.
- Encourage the patient to stick to a strict gluten-free diet, as this will protect against the increased risk of lymphoma.

Box 13.10 Histology and immunofluorescence in dermatitis herpetiformis

- A skin biopsy from an early lesion shows small neutrophil collections (microabscesses) at the tips of oedematous dermal papillae.
- In older lesions, you may see small subepidermal vesicles containing neutrophils and some eosinophils.
- Direct IMF microscopy of biopsies taken from uninvolved skin show granular deposits of IgA at the BMZ in the tips of dermal papillae.

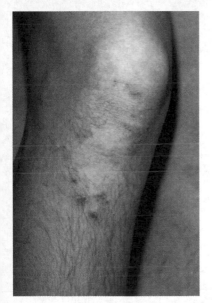

Fig. 13.6 Dermatitis herpetiformis: the itchy vesicles on extensor surfaces soon rupture, leaving small erosions and excoriated papules.

Further reading

Bolotin D and Petronic-Rosic V. J Am Acad Dermatol 2011;**64**:1017–24 and 1027–33.

Oral and genital mucosae

Contents

Relevant pages in other chapters
Examination of mucosae is discussed in detail in
➜ Chapter 3, pp. 48–9. Also see ➜ Chapter 4, pp. 86–7.
Extramammary Paget disease ➜ p. 361.

Oral and genital ulcers

Inflammation of the oral mucosa (stomatitis) may be caused by drugs, infections, skin diseases, or systemic diseases. Pain or burning are common presenting symptoms, and ulcers a frequent 2° finding. More than one mucosal surface may be affected, so, in any patient with stomatitis, it is important to ask about the eyes and genital symptoms.

Patients may be reluctant to volunteer anogenital symptoms. Genital ulceration may be 2° to trauma, infection, or inflammatory disease. *Pseudomonas aeruginosa* causes anogenital ecthyma in immunosuppressed patients (see ➡ p. 137). Disease may be localized or generalized, so examine skin and other mucosal surfaces.

❶ SCC may present as an 'ulcer' (see ➡ p. 350). Take a biopsy from any persistent ulcer (see Box 14.1).

Causes of oral and genital ulcers are discussed on ➡ pp. 86–7.

⚠ **Box 14.1 When to biopsy**
- Persistent ulcer (>2 weeks) of unknown cause.
- Ulcer unresponsive to treatment.
- Ulcer that persists despite removal of known precipitant.

Herpes simplex virus

Herpetic gingivostomatitis

1° infections with HSV (usually type 1, occasionally type 2) may be asymptomatic but can cause a painful ulcerative gingivostomatitis (most often in children) that resolves in 10–14 days. Recurrent herpes labialis is caused by reactivation of the latent virus (see ➲ p. 152). A tingling, burning, or itching prodrome is common. Erythema multiforme may be caused by herpes infections and may recur (see ➲ p. 111).

What should I look for in 1° infections?
- Malaise, headache, and fever; cervical lymphadenopathy.
- Well-defined vesicles, 2mm in diameter, on the dorsum of the tongue and hard palate, but vesicles may be scattered over the entire oral mucosa. Vesicles rupture rapidly to form very painful shallow ulcers with a yellowish grey floor and erythematous margins.
- Inflamed gingival margins.

What should I do?
Management is symptomatic with fluids and pain relief. Oral aciclovir, 200mg ×5/day for 5 days, is helpful in 1° attacks if vesicles are still present (within the first 3 days). Recurrent herpes labialis does not usually need treatment with aciclovir.

Genital herpes simplex virus infection

Genital infections are usually caused by HSV-2 and only occasionally by HSV-1. 1° attacks are more severe and long-lasting than subsequent attacks. Prevalence is highest in individuals adopting high-risk sexual behaviour, but viral carriage is often asymptomatic. Genital HSV increases the risk of acquiring and/or transmitting HIV.

What should I look for?
- Genital pain, itching, and/or burning.
- Erythematous vesicles that rapidly rupture, forming painful ulcers.
- Dysuria leading to urinary retention.

What should I do?
- Consider other causes of ulcers, including EBV (see Box 14.2).
- Bacterial and viral culture—use a viral culture medium.
- Biopsy may be indicated if diagnosis is uncertain.
- Prescribe oral analgesia and topical 2% lidocaine gel.
- Encourage high fluid intake.
- Recommend warm baths (easier to urinate in a bath).
- Prescribe oral antivirals in 1° disease.
- Oral prophylaxis with antivirals in severe recurrent disease.
- Genital HSV infection can be transmitted to the fetus or neonate.
- Prophylactic aciclovir from 36 weeks of gestation reduces the risk of HSV recurrence or HSV viral shedding at delivery.
- Refer for screening for other STDs.

Box 14.2 Epstein–Barr virus infection causing vulval ulcers

Clinical
- Age 10–30 years.
- Genital contact is not a prerequisite for EBV genital ulcers.
- Prodrome: fever and lymphadenopathy.
- Deep, painful, single or multiple vulval ulcers, 0.5–2cm in diameter.
- Irregular erythematous edges.
- Ulcer base: clean, seropurulent, or granulating.
- Heal within 2 weeks.

Investigations
- Monospot (heterophile antibody) test falsely negative during first 2 weeks of symptoms.
- Request IgM antiviral capsid antigen antibodies if you suspect EBV.

Management
- Avoid irritants, and use aqueous or Cetraben® cream as a soap substitute.
- Warm baths.
- Zinc oxide ointment.
- Pain relief.

Further reading

Sen P and Barton SE. *BMJ* 2007;**334**:1048–52.

Aphthous ulcers (canker sores)

These painful ulcers affect around 20% of the population and may occur in association with systemic disease (see Box 14.3), but most patients are healthy. Aphthous ulcers may be precipitated by stress, trauma, menstruation, or stopping smoking. Genetic factors may also be important.

Aphthous ulceration is divided into minor, major, and herpetiform subtypes. The diagnosis is clinical, and management symptomatic (see Box 14.4).

Minor aphthous ulcers (80% of cases)

Ulcers start in childhood or adolescence, are <10mm in diameter, and heal in 7–14 days. Crops of ulcers recur every 1–4 months. Ulcers become less frequent with age.

What should I look for?

* One to five shallow round or oval ulcers (<10mm in diameter) on non-keratinized mucosa—floor of the mouth, buccal or labial mucosa (vesicles in herpes simplex rupture to form ulcers, most often on the dorsum of the tongue and hard palate).
* Erythematous haloes.
* Grey-white slough on the base of the ulcer.
* Exclude other mucosal involvement, e.g. genital ulcers, ocular inflammation.

Major aphthous ulcers (10% of cases)

Ulcers usually start in childhood or adolescence, may be as much as 3cm in diameter, and heal over months, often with scarring. Ulcers recur at shorter intervals than minor aphthae. Major aphthae may be a sign of Behçet disease (see ⊃ p. 284).

What should I look for?

* Crops of 1–6 large ulcers (>10mm in diameter) with a firm raised margin in any part of the mouth.
* Considerable pain.
* Scarring and fibrosis (60%).
* Other mucosal involvement, e.g. genital ulcers, ocular inflammation.
* ❶ Palpate solitary long-standing non-healing ulcers to check for induration, and, if indurated, consider biopsy to exclude oral cancer.

Herpetiform ulcers (10% of cases)

These tend to occur in patients in their third decade. The ulcers, which resemble ulcers caused by herpesvirus, usually heal within 2 weeks and do not recur more frequently than monthly.

What should I look for?

* Many (up to 100) tiny ulcers (1–2mm in diameter) anywhere in the mouth.
* Scarring and fibrosis (30%).

Box 14.3 **Diseases associated with aphthous ulcers**

- Iron, folate, or vitamin B_{12} deficiency.
- Malabsorption: gluten-sensitive enteropathy, Crohn disease, ulcerative colitis (see ⮀ pp. 508–9).
- Behçet disease (see ⮀ p. 284).
- HIV infection (see ⮀ p. 162).
- Reiter syndrome (see ⮀ p. 208).
- Sweet syndrome (see ⮀ p. 518).
- Aplastic anaemia, neutropenia, and other immunodeficiencies.

Box 14.4 **Management of aphthous ulcers**

- Eliminate predisposing factors, and investigate for an underlying systemic disease, as indicated by the history and examination.
- Topical corticosteroids may speed ulcer healing, e.g.:
  - Hydrocortisone 2.5mg oral pellets placed on, or held next to, the ulcer ×3–4/day.
  - Fluticasone 400 micrograms (one Flixonase® nasule). Dissolve in 10mL of water. Hold in the mouth for as long as possible, and spit out. Use at night and after meals, if required.
  - Beclometasone dipropionate 50 or 100 inhaler sprayed onto the affected areas and held in the mouth for as long as possible ×4–6/day.
- Antiseptic mouthwashes:
  - Chlorhexidine 2.5% solution (dilute if it stings).
- Soothing oral preparations with local anaesthetic, e.g.:
  - 30mL of nystatin sugar-free mix plus 20mL of lidocaine 2% injection plus 10mL of a suspending agent such as mucilage; 5mL to be rinsed around the mouth before meals.
  - Benzydamine hydrochloride 0.15% (e.g. Difflam®) spray or oral rinse. Use 15min before eating or brushing teeth. Rinse with 15mL, and then spit out. Can be repeated 1.5- to 3-hourly.
- Major aphthous stomatitis may require treatment with systemic corticosteroids, prolonged courses of low-dose oral tetracyclines (e.g. minocycline 100mg/day or lymecycline 408mg/day for 6 months), or rarely thalidomide.
- NSAIDs for pain relief (more effective than opioids).

Further reading

Brocklehurst P et al. Cochrane Database Syst Rev 2012;9:CD005411 (recurrent aphthous stomatitis).
Cheng S and Murphy R. Br J Dermatol 2011;37:132–5.
Scully C and Felix DH. Br Dent J 2005;199:339–43.

Behçet disease

Behçet disease is rare, chronic, multisystem, and relapsing. The pathogenesis is not understood but involves immune complex-mediated vasculitis. Most commonly affects populations along the 'silk route' in Turkey, Iran, and Japan but is seen worldwide. Associated with HLA-B51. Diagnosis based on clinical criteria (see Box 14.5).

What should I look for?

Mucocutaneous lesions

- Oral ulceration (all patients): recurrent and painful; small ulcers heal without scarring, but larger ulcers may scar.
- Genital ulceration (85% of patients): usually scrotal or labial, may affect the vagina and cervix, usually leaves scars.
- Papulopustular lesions (85% of patients): resembling acne or folliculitis, appear as papules on an erythematous base, and develop into a pustule over 24–48h. Commonest on the trunk.
- EN-like lesions (50% of patients) on legs. Resolve, leaving pigmentation.
- Superficial thrombophlebitis (25% of patients): erythematous, tender, subcutaneous nodules in a line. May be confused with EN.
- Extragenital ulceration: uncommon but may occur at any site.
- History of pustules developing at sites of needle-prick (pathergy), e.g. 24–48h after venepuncture.

Eye disease (50% of patients)

- Chronic, relapsing anterior and posterior uveitis. Major cause of morbidity. May result in retinal haemorrhage, papilloedema, and macular disease, with loss of visual acuity and threat of blindness.

Musculoskeletal disease (50% of patients)

- Most often a non-deforming, non-erosive peripheral oligoarthritis, lasting a few weeks.
- Some patients have chronic arthritis, osteonecrosis, and myositis.

Neurological disease (5% of patients)

- Pyramidal, cerebellar, and sensory signs, sphincter disturbance, behavioural changes, and dural sinus thrombosis.
- Peripheral nerve lesions are unusual.

Vascular disease (5% of patients)

- Large-vessel vasculitis can result in thrombosis and occlusion.

Other systems (rare)

- GI mucosal ulceration, splenomegaly, glomerulonephritis, and cardiac involvement have been reported.

What should I do?

Investigations

- Pathergy test: hyper-reactivity of the skin to needle-prick (skin-prick of the forearm results in a papule or pustule in 24–48h). Sensitivity varies (~60%) and is highest in Japan and Mediterranean countries, but is highly specific for Behçet disease.

Recurrent oral ulceration

- Minor aphthous, major aphthous, or herpetiform ulceration observed by a physician or patient that recurred at least three times in one 12-month period.

Plus two of the following

- Genital ulcers (aphthous ulceration). Includes anal ulcers/swollen testicles or epididymitis observed by physician or patient.
- Eye inflammation (anterior uveitis, posterior uveitis, or cells in the vitreous on slit-lamp examination; or retinal vasculitis observed by an ophthalmologist).
- Cutaneous lesions (EN observed by a physician or patient; folliculitis or papulopustular lesions; or acneiform nodules observed by a physician in post-adolescent patients not receiving corticosteroids).
- Positive pathergy test (read by a physician at 24–48h).

International Study Group for Behçet's disease. *Br J Rheumatol* 1992;**31**:299–308.

Note: other classification criteria have been proposed, e.g. International Team for the Revision of the International Criteria for Behçet's Disease (ITR-ICBD). *J Eur Acad Dermatol Venereol* 2014;**28**:338–47.

- Biopsy: papulopustular lesions or pathergy reactions.
- Genital ulcers: exclude infection, e.g. herpesvirus, EBV (see ➔ pp. 280–1).
- FBC may show anaemia of chronic disease and leucocytosis.
- Inflammatory markers are not good indicators of disease activity.
- ANA, RF, and anti-neutrophil cytoplasmic antibody (ANCA) are negative.

Treatment

- A very potent topical corticosteroid ointment (clobetasol propionate) and topical 2% lidocaine gel may relieve pain in oral and genital ulcers (for treatment of oral ulcers, see Box 14.4).
- Refer to ophthalmology for eye symptoms or signs.
- Colchicine may reduce arthralgia and mucocutaneous lesions.
- The use of systemic corticosteroids is controversial.
- Other immunosuppressives used include azathioprine, ciclosporin, methotrexate, mycophenolate, and cyclophosphamide.
- Anti-TNF biologic agents infliximab, adalimumab, and etanercept may be effective in severe disease.
- Thalidomide can be effective for aphthous ulcers but has been replaced by the use of biologics.
- Interferon alfa may have a role in oral and genital ulcers.

Further reading

Ambrose N and Haskard D. *Nature Rev Rheumatol* 2013;**9**:79–89.
Hatemi G et al. *Ann Rheum Dis* 2009;**68**:1528–34.
Ozguler Y et al. *Curr Opin Rheumatol* 2014;**26**:285–91.

Mucosal lichen planus

LP is a chronic inflammatory condition of unknown cause that may affect mucosal surfaces and/or the skin (see ➲ p. 224). A band-like 'lichenoid' infiltrate of lymphocytes hugs the basal layer of the epidermis or epithelium.

LP can be drug-induced (see ➲ p. 375). Infrequently oral LP is caused by allergies to metals or flavourings in foods.

What should I look for?

- Asymptomatic lacy white streaks (Wickham striae), and white papules and plaques on the buccal mucosa, tongue, or genitalia (vulva, glans penis, shaft of the penis). These cannot be scraped off, unlike mucosal candidiasis (see Fig. 14.1).
- Erosive mucosal disease: glazed erythema, erosions with white lacy border, painful oral ulcers. May also have erosive genital disease—vulvovaginal–gingival syndrome, peno-gingival syndrome.
- Gingivitis (erythematous erosions, patchy hypopigmentation).
- Genital lesions may become hypertrophic.
- Annular LP on the shaft of the penis may be associated with flexural annular LP, e.g. in axillae.
- Erosive vulvovaginal LP (vulvar vestibule and vagina) with itch, dysuria, and/or dyspareunia. Associated with oral disease, especially gingival LP.
- Scarring in chronic erosive vulvovaginal disease, with atrophy and fusion of the labia and narrowing of the vaginal introitus.
- ❶ SCC is a rare complication in chronic erosive disease and may be asymptomatic—check for mucosal thickening, a nodule, or a persistent ulcer (see ➲ p. 350).
- Cutaneous disease: flat-topped, shiny polygonal purplish papules. Seen more often in oral and penile LP than vulval LP (see ➲ p. 224).
- Rarely, LP affects the oesophagus, larynx, bladder, and/or anus.

What should I do?

(See Box 14.6.)
- A biopsy may be required to confirm the diagnosis.
- Consider taking swabs for viral culture from painful erosions.
- Withdraw any potentially causative systemic drugs.
- Oral LP: consider patch testing to exclude allergy to metals or oral flavourings (rarely positive).
- ❶ Erosive mucosal disease may be chronic and persistent: patients should be counselled about the risk of SCC and reviewed regularly.

Differential diagnosis

- Chronic cutaneous GVHD shares many clinical and histological features with LP (see ➲ p. 534, and Figs. 26.2 and 26.4, p. 537).
- Oral DLE (see ➲ p. 404) can look similar to oral LP.
- Vulval LP may simulate lichen sclerosus (see ➲ p. 288).

Box 14.6 Management of mucosal lichen planus

- Avoid an irritant toothpaste.
- Dental hygiene (remove plaque).
- Chlorhexidine 2.5% solution as mouthwash (may need to be diluted).
- Asymptomatic mucosal disease does not require treatment.
- Potent or very potent corticosteroid ointments ×1/day or bd.
- Analgesia with topical 2% lidocaine gel and NSAIDs, as in aphthous stomatitis, if symptomatic or benzydamine hydrochloride spray or oral rinse (see Box 14.4).
- Topical 0.1% tacrolimus ointment bd for severe disease unresponsive to corticosteroids, but monitor erosive disease carefully because of the risk of malignancy.
- Genital LP: soap substitutes.
- Very severe cutaneous or mucosal LP: short courses of oral corticosteroids to control itching or pain, but unfortunately disease recurs on stopping corticosteroids. Other therapies that have been tried include UVB, oral retinoids, methotrexate, and ciclosporin.

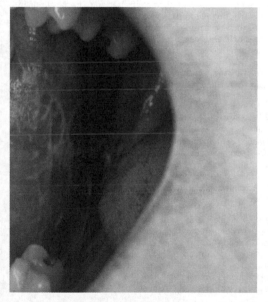

Fig. 14.1 Oral lichen planus with lacy white streaks on the buccal mucosa.

Further reading

Cheng S et al. *Cochrane Database Syst Rev* 2012;2:CD008092.
Scully C and Carrozzo M. *Br J Oral Maxillofac Surg* 2008;46:15–21.

Lichen sclerosus

This chronic inflammatory disease with a predilection for genital skin has two peaks of onset—childhood and post-menopausal. The cause is uncertain, but a lymphocyte-mediated autoimmune pathogenesis is suspected. Lichen sclerosus may occur in association with morphoea (see ➜ pp. 420–1) (with which extragenital lichen sclerosus shows considerable clinical and histological overlap), LP, and vitiligo.

Lichen sclerosus is commonest in adult ♀. It may be asymptomatic but usually presents with itch, pain, and/or dyspareunia. Perianal involvement with painful anal fissures may lead to constipation in young girls. Uncircumcised ♂ are affected. Lichen sclerosus of the foreskin (balanitis zerotica obliterans) is a major indication for circumcision. Lichen sclerosus may also develop around stomas, most often urostomies.

What should I look for?

- Pearly white papules and plaques on labia minora, clitoris, and interlabial sulci (see Fig. 14.2).
- Sparing of the vulvar vestibule (unlike LP).
- Signs may extend in a figure-of-eight configuration to perianal skin in ♀ (perianal skin is not affected in ♂).
- Atrophy gives the skin a shiny crinkled appearance (see Fig. 14.2).
- Discrete areas of haemorrhage (ecchymoses) within the white plaques (may be misdiagnosed as sexual abuse in young girls) (see Fig. 14.2).
- Loss of normal anatomy in chronic disease—resorption of the labia minora, fusion of the labia, and burying of the clitoris.
- Uncircumcised ♂—thickening and tightening of the foreskin, causing phimosis. White plaques on the glans penis, sometimes with scarring. Sometimes pearly white papules on the shaft of the penis.
- Extragenital lichen sclerosus is uncommon—the hypopigmented crinkled plaques contain follicular plugs (unlike morphoea; see ➜ pp. 420–1), ecchymoses, and rarely haemorrhagic blisters. Hypopigmented papules are sometimes seen in children.
- ❶ SCC is a rare complication in chronic genital disease in adults (around 5% of patients). Often presents with pain. Check for mucosal thickening, a nodule, or a persistent ulcer (see ➜ p. 350).

What should I do?

- Take a biopsy to confirm the diagnosis.
- Recommend a soap substitute for genital use, e.g. Cetraben® cream.
- A very potent topical corticosteroid (0.05% clobetasol propionate ointment), applied ×1/day for 4 weeks and then with gradually decreasing frequency for a further 8 weeks, usually controls disease and may even reverse the early changes (may also be effective in children).
- Counsel about the small risk of SCC; teach self-examination, and recommend annual reviews.

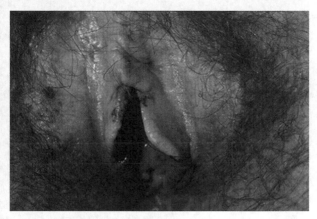

Fig. 14.2 Typical vulval lichen sclerosus with pallor and haemorrhage (courtesy of Dr Susan Cooper, Oxford).

Further reading

Cooper SM et al. Arch Dermatol 2004;**140**:702–6.
Edmonds EV et al. J Eur Acad Dermatol Venereol 2012;**26**:730–7.
Edwards SK et al. Int J STD AIDS 2015;**26**:611–24.
Virgili A et al. Br J Dermatol 2014;**171**:338–96.

Leg ulcers and lymphoedema

Contents

Relevant pages in other chapters

Introduction

You are likely to come across a patient with a chronic leg ulcer at some stage in most branches of adult medicine. One to 2% of people will develop a leg ulcer during their life, and chronic ulcers cause morbidity and disability, particularly in older people.

Traditionally, nurses care for leg ulcers, and doctors are asked to see the patient when complications ensue or the ulcer is not healing as expected. Many doctors feel poorly trained to deal with such patients, particularly because they have no experience of what is a 'normal' leg ulcer.

Learn from the expertise of the wound care nurses, and take an interest in patients' leg ulcers. Ulcers may be associated with systemic disease, as well as vascular problems, infections, and malignancy—you may be surprised what you find underneath the dressings!

The history

Take a full dermatological history (see ➲ p. 18, pp. 20–1), asking questions that will help you to pinpoint the likely cause of the ulcer, as well as looking for risk factors and factors that may delay healing (see Boxes 15.1 and 15.2).

What should I ask?

- When the ulcer developed and how it progressed. What preceded ulceration, e.g. trauma, pressure, tender pustule (may indicate PG), or blister?
- Explore concerns (patients may fear that they may lose the leg).
- Pain: character, how bad, what makes it worse or better? (see ➲ p. 304.)
- Does the patient sleep in a bed or in a chair at night?
- How much elevation is tolerated?
- Impact of ulcer on quality of life—use the DLQI (see ➲ p. 32).
- Mobility: how much exercise?
- Weight: obesity is common in venous disease.
- Problems with skin around the ulcer: redness, pain, itch?
- Swelling of limb: does it improve after elevation, e.g. overnight?
- Present management:
  - Dressings and bandages: how often is the ulcer dressed?
  - Any compression? How much elevation?
  - Pain relief: how much, how often is it taken?
- Any previous episodes of ulceration?
- Any history of cellulitis?
- Previous treatments for ulcer:
  - Dressings or bandages?
  - Topical treatments?
  - Surgical interventions, e.g. angioplasty, skin graft?
- Past medical history and functional inquiry, including:
  - Skin cancers and sun exposure? (see ➲ pp. 26–7.)
  - Hypertension, claudication, angina, myocardial infarction?
  - Cerebrovascular accident?
  - Diabetes, peripheral neuropathy?
  - Obesity?
  - Hypercholesterolaemia?
  - DVT or pulmonary emboli?
  - Varicose veins: varicosities in pregnancy, varicose vein surgery?
  - Major orthopaedic intervention, long bone fracture?
  - RA?
- Family history of varicose veins, leg ulcers, DVT, or pulmonary emboli?
- Social history: carers, home environment; job—prolonged standing?
- Drug history, e.g. nicorandil, prednisolone, hydroxycarbamide?
- Allergies: 'reactions' to dressings or bandages? Patch tested?
- Smoker?

Box 15.1 Common causes of leg or foot ulcers

(See Figs. 15.1, 15.2, 15.3, and 15.4,.)

- *Venous disease* (70%): venous hypertension, valvular incompetence, and venous reflux lead to inflammation and ulcers. Risk factors: genetic, ♀ sex, age, prolonged standing, obesity. Past medical history of pregnancy, DVT, trauma, operations to hips or knees.
- *Arterial disease* (5–10%): intermittent claudication, rest pain, night pain, pain worse when the leg is elevated. Smokers.
- *Mixed AV* (15%): venous and arterial disease.
- *Neuropathic*: sites of pressure—often asymptomatic. Blood on the floor may be the first indication of trouble to the patient. Commonest on the feet of diabetic patients when also associated with small-vessel disease (see ➡ pp. 550–1).

Box 15.2 Other causes of leg ulcers

- *Malignancy*: BCC commonest. Misdiagnosed as an 'ulcer' (see ➡ p. 350). Other malignancies that may cause chronic ulcers include SCC, metastases, and diffuse large B-cell lymphoma (leg type).
- *PG*: rapidly growing, very painful ulcer. Often preceded by a tender pustule. Associated with RA, IBD, and myeloproliferative disorders; 50% of patients have no underlying disease (see ➡ Fig. 15.5, and p. 310).
- *Vasculitic*: associated with connective tissue diseases, particularly RA, when immobility and coexisting AV disease often contribute to ulceration (see ➡ pp. 394–5).
- *Occlusive vasculopathy*, e.g. livedoid 'vasculitis' with atrophie blanche, sickle-cell disease, thalassaemia, thrombocythaemia, hypertensive ulcer (see Box 15.4), calciphylaxis, cryoglobulinaemia, antiphospholipid syndrome (see ➡ p. 444 and pp. 452–3).
- *Inherited disorders of coagulation*: mutations in protein C, protein S, antithrombin III, fibrinogen, or factor V genes.
- *Necrobiosis lipoidica*: associated with insulin-dependent diabetes.
- *Infection*: deep fungal, treponemal.
- *Drug-related*: hydroxycarbamide, nicorandil.
- *Trauma*: including IV drug abuse.
- *Dermatitis artefacta*: deliberate self-harm (see ➡ pp. 566–7).

Further reading

Bergan JJ et al. *N Engl J Med* 2006;**355**:488–98 (chronic venous disease).
White-Chu EF and Conner-Kerr TA. *J Multidiscip Healthc* 2014;**7**:111–17.

Preparing to examine the ulcer

The leg ulcer is likely to be hidden away under dressings and bandages. Many doctors are reluctant to remove bandages, perhaps for fear of what they might find underneath, but more often because they are pressed for time or feel ill-prepared to re-dress the leg, a task that may not be as easy as it sounds without the help of a skilled nurse. But it is important to inspect the limb beneath the bandages—try not to be put off.

Explain to the patient what you wish to do and why. Ask if any preparation is required, before the dressing is removed. Is analgesia required?

Try to find out what dressings or bandages are being used.

Discuss your plans with the nurses; arrange a suitable time; help the nurses to set up a dressing trolley … , and take the plunge.

What do I need?
- Plastic gloves (do not need to be sterile) and a plastic apron.
- A trolley with:
  - Gauze swabs, scissors, plastic forceps, and a sinus probe (if the ulcer might be deeply penetrating).
  - A bag for disposing of contaminated dressings.
- Water for washing the leg and the ulcer—a bucket may be useful.
- Cling film to cover the ulcer—exposing the ulcer to air may be painful.
- A sphygmomanometer, stethoscope, and Doppler ultrasound probe for checking the ABPI (see Box 15.6).
- A tendon hammer, tuning fork (128Hz), and disposable neurological pin if you suspect a neuropathic ulcer. (Ideally a Semmes–Weinstein 10g monofilament for evaluation of sensation if you know how to use it.)
- A tape measure.
- An acetate sheet (or the transparent cover of a dressing pack) and a pen for tracing the ulcer.
- A digital camera.
- Liquid paraffin 50% in WSP or a bland ointment, such as Hydromol®, to moisturize the skin.
- Dressings and bandages (see p. 306), including a viscose stockinette bandage, long enough to run from the toe to just below the knee to hold the dressing in place.
- Surgical adhesive tape for securing the end of the bandage—avoid safety pins.

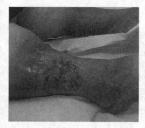

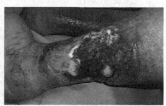

Fig. 15.1 Venous ulcer in the gaiter area in an obese woman.

Fig. 15.2 Ulceration in a patient with a combination of venous disease and lymphoedema (thick swollen folds of skin around the ankle, hyperkeratosis, and swelling of the dorsum of the foot, as well as the leg).

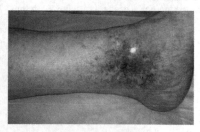

Fig. 15.3 Atrophie blanche (shiny white stellate scar with peripheral telangiectasia) in venous disease. Atrophie blanche may also be seen in occlusive vasculopathies such as livedoid vasculopathy or antiphospholipid syndrome (see ➔ pp. 314–15 and p. 452).

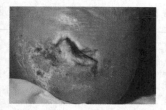

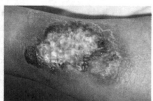

Fig. 15.4 Deeply penetrating neuropathic ulcer with surrounding callus and underlying osteomyelitis.

Fig. 15.5 Typical pyoderma gangrenosum with a purplish undermined border.

The examination

What should I do?

- Lay the patient comfortably on an examination couch.
- Adjust the lighting, so you can see the legs and ulcer.
- Protect the bedding beneath the legs with incontinence pads.
- Carry out a full physical examination that includes palpation of the abdomen to look for masses that might be causing external venous compression. Are the legs oedematous, or is there lymphoedema? (see ➲ pp. 316–17.)
- Check the blood pressure (see Box 15.3).
- Remove bandages to expose the leg. Gently peel off dressings, so that the ulcer is exposed. You may need to soak the dressing with normal saline prior to removal if it has stuck to the wound.
- Note the colour and quantity of the exudate on the dressing. Heavy exudate suggests heavy bacterial colonization. Green dressings indicate the presence of *Pseudomonas*.
- Remove loose crust, scab, or adherent dressing, and gently wash the ulcer with water, so you can see the base and wound edges.
- If the ulcer is painful when exposed to air, cover temporarily with cling film or a moist gauze swab.
- Assess the ulcer—site, wound edge, and wound bed (slough, granulation tissue, necrotic base) (see Box 15.4).
- Measure the ulcer (maximum diameters or trace onto an acetate sheet).
- Probe to assess the amount of undermining and depth of the ulcer.
- Record the appearance of the ulcer with photographs, if possible.
- Examine the surrounding skin, looking for signs that may be linked to the cause of the ulcer (see Boxes 15.3 and 15.4).
- Look for cellulitis—heat, swelling, tender erythema (this may be difficult to differentiate from lipodermatosclerosis (see ➲ p. 308).
- Assess the peripheral circulation, including the ABPI (see Box 15.6).
- Assess joint mobility at ankles and feet, and look for joint deformity.

Box 15.3 Hypertensive ulcer (Martorell ulcer)

- The existence of this entity is controversial, and these ulcers must be rare.
- Painful ulceration may be 2° to a thrombo-occlusive vasculopathy of cutaneous arterioles in long-standing hypertension.
- Patients present with an extremely painful superficial ulcer with an erythematous or purpuric rim, usually on the anterolateral aspect of the shin. Ulcers start as purpuric lesions which soon become necrotic.
- Management involves control of hypertension, pain relief, and compression bandaging.

Box 15.4 Signs in different types of ulcer

Venous (see Figs. 15.1 and 15.2)

- Gaiter area, just above the medial malleolus or (less often) lateral malleolus. Sloping, poorly defined wound edge. Shallow, but large, ulcer that may extend circumferentially around the limb. Pitting oedema.
- Varicose veins (assess standing): gently press any swelling to confirm it is a varicosity. The vein will empty and refill when you let go. Varicosities of the short saphenous vein are seen posterolaterally below the knee; varicosities of the long saphenous vein run more medially along the whole length of the limb.
- Venous flare (dilated superficial venules at the ankle), brownish pigmentation (haemosiderin and melanin), eczema in the gaiter area. Signs may be localized to the skin over varicosities—stand the patient up to see varicosities.
- Scar at sites of previous ulcer, atrophie blanche (see Fig. 15.3).
- Lipodermatosclerosis: erythematous, tight, indurated skin above the medial malleolus. May simulate cellulitis (see Fig. 15.6).

Arterial

- Peripheral on borders or sides of feet or initiated by trauma.
- Round ulcer, sharply demarcated with a punched-out appearance. Tendon may be exposed at the base.
- Cool, shiny, pale, or dusky skin with loss of hair. Peripheral gangrene. Reduced peripheral pulses, delayed capillary refill (for assessment of circulation, see ➲ p. 300).

Mixed AV Signs of arterial and venous disease.

Neuropathic (see Fig. 15.4)

- Pressure sites on the foot, most often under the second metatarsal head. Surrounded by callus. Limited joint mobility or deformity. (Charcot joints caused by impaired joint position sense and sensation).
- Check footwear for source of pressure or trauma. Osteomyelitis complicates deep neuropathic ulcers.
- Dry skin may indicate autonomic dysfunction (see ➲ p. 550).
- Assess vibration sense (128Hz tuning fork to the apex of the great toe), pinprick (just proximal to the great toenail), temperature (on the dorsum of the foot with tuning fork placed in iced or warm water), sensation with a 10g monofilament, and Achilles tendon reflex.

PG: bluish, undermined wound edge, base with slough (see Box 15.11 and Fig. 15.5).

Vasculitis: purpuric wound edges. Palpable purpura, nodules, livedo (see ➲ p. 440, pp. 440–7).

Occlusive vasculopathy: livedo, atrophie blanche (see ➲ pp. 312–5, pp. 444–5, p. 452, and Box 15.3).

Malignancy: non-healing ulcer. BCCs or SCCs may be misdiagnosed as 'leg ulcers'. Rarely, SCC arises within a chronic ulcer. Consider taking a biopsy in any chronic non-healing leg ulcer.

Assessing peripheral circulation

What should I do?

- Compare the signs in the legs.
- Check peripheral pulses (dorsalis pedis, posterior tibial, popliteal, femoral).
- Listen for bruits in the femoral arteries.
- Peripheral perfusion: push on the nail bed, until it turns white. Let go, and colour should return (capillary refill) in <2s—not a very reliable test.
- Buerger test: soles should be pink with the patient supine. Elevate both legs to 45° for 1–2min. Compare the soles. Marked pallor suggests ischaemia. Sit the patient up, and lower the legs over the side of the bed. Colour will return to the legs, but an ischaemic limb will become blue and then very red. Post-hypoxic vasodilatation causes hyperaemia.
- Assess the peripheral arterial circulation by measuring the ABPI using a handheld Doppler ultrasound probe (see Boxes 15.5 and 15.6).
- Pulse oximetry has been recommended as an alternative to the Doppler ABPI for assessing peripheral circulation, particularly if the leg is very oedematous, but not all vascular surgeons agree that relying on pulse oximetry is safe practice. More work is needed in this area.
- Consider referral to vascular surgeons for lower limb venous duplex scans to detect venous reflux in superficial and deep venous systems.
- Refer to vascular surgeons for arterial colour duplex scan if the ABPI is <0.8. ▶▶ Refer urgently if the ABPI is 0.5 or less.

Box 15.5 How to measure the ABPI

- Seek for permission for what you are going to do—'I would like to compare the blood pressures in your arm and in your leg. We will both be able to hear your pulse, because I am going to use this Doppler machine.' Warn that the cuff may feel uncomfortable for a short time when it is tightened on the leg.
- The patient should lie relatively flat for 20–30min, before commencing measurements. Ensure the patient is comfortable in that position.
- Apply a sphygmomanometer cuff to the arm.
- Inflate the cuff, while feeling the radial pulse to get a rough idea of the systolic pressure.
- Apply ultrasound gel to the skin over the brachial pulse.
- Angle the Doppler probe at 45–60°, and find the brachial pulse (adjust the position and angle of the probe, until the sound is maximal).
- Inflate the cuff, until the sound disappears.
- Slowly release the pressure, and record the pressure at which the sound of the brachial pulse reappears.
- Repeat in the other arm, and take the higher of the two readings.
- Place cling film around the leg, covering the surface of the ulcer.
- Place the cuff around the leg just above the medial malleolus.
- Palpate the dorsalis pedis pulse between the first and second metatarsals. Apply ultrasound gel to the skin over the pulse, and find the dorsalis pedis pulse using the probe. Angle the probe at 45–60° to the foot.
- Inflate the cuff, until the sound disappears; deflate slowly, and record the pressure at which the sound reappears.
- If possible, repeat at the posterior tibial pulse, and take the higher of the two readings—but some patients do find the tight cuff uncomfortable.
- Repeat in the other leg.
- Calculate the ABPI in each leg: ABPI = highest ankle pressure/ highest brachial pressure.

Box 15.6 Interpretation of the ABPI

- ABPI: 0.9–1.0 = safe to apply high compression.
- ABPI: 0.8 = excludes significant arterial disease. Probably safe to apply compression—start slowly.
- ABPI: 0.6–0.8 = moderate arterial disease. Very gentle compression may be tolerated, if required, to control venous incompetence and oedema, but bandages should only be applied by an expert, and the patient should be monitored. Pulse oximetry may be used to check the immediate impact of compression.
- ABPI: <0.5 = severe arterial disease. Do not use compression— refer for an urgent vascular opinion.

⚠ *Warning*: the arteries are calcified and cannot be compressed in some older patients and in some with diabetes. In this situation, the ABPI is falsely high. If the results do not fit with your clinical findings, review the patient and the test.

Investigation of leg ulcers

Investigations should be directed towards determining the underlying cause of ulceration and excluding factors that may delay healing (see Box 15.7).

Blood tests

- FBC, iron studies, ESR, CRP.
- Serum albumin (low in malnutrition) and vitamin C, if indicated (may be deficient in older patients with a poor diet).
- Random glucose.
- Clotting screen, including lupus anticoagulant, anticardiolipin antibody, factor V Leiden, protein C, and protein S levels if multiple DVTs or a family history of DVTs and leg ulcers.
- If signs suggest vasculitis—ANA, RF, hepatitis serology, and complement 4 (low C4 with raised RF may indicate type II or III mixed cryoglobulinaemia; see ➲ p. 444). Check ANCA if indications of a systemic vasculitis.
- Cryoglobulins (keep the sample at 37° in a Thermos™ flask—it may be easiest to send the patient to the laboratory)—check if you suspect ulceration is 2° to type I cryoglobulinaemia associated with a paraprotein, e.g. myeloma, lymphoma (see ➲ p. 444).

Microbiology

- Surface ulcer swabs for microbiological culture are of limited value— ulcers are always colonized with some bacteria. Only take swabs if you suspect heavy colonization (increasing pain, malodour, and large amounts of exudate) or if you detect signs of cellulitis—warmth, extending tender erythema, oedema (see ➲ p. 138).

Ulcer biopsy

- Histology of biopsies from the edge of most ulcers, including PG and many vasculitic ulcers, is not diagnostic.
- Biopsies may be indicated to exclude malignancy or for culture.
- To exclude fungal or treponemal infection, take a deep biopsy that extends into the base of the ulcer. Send for histological examination as well as for culture.

Radiology

- Radiograph, MRI, or CT may be used in chronic deep penetrating ulcers to exclude osteomyelitis, e.g. neuropathic foot ulcers in patients with diabetes.

Patch tests

- Allergic contact dermatitis can delay wound healing. Patients with leg ulcers may be sensitized to topical medicaments, including topical corticosteroids, neomycin, and Balsam of Peru (a fragrance in many creams), as well as constituents of dressings or bandages.
- All patients with chronic varicose eczema or chronic leg ulcers should be patch tested. Repeat tests every 2–3 years if the patient has persistent eczematous skin changes or non-healing ulcers.

Box 15.7 Factors that may delay healing

- *Oedema*: gravitational, congestive cardiac failure.
- *Immobility*: contributes to poor calf muscle pump and oedema.
- *Anaemia or malnutrition*: vitamin C deficiency may be a particular problem in older patients.
- *Corticosteroids* (impact of other immunosuppressive drugs is less certain).
- *Repetitive trauma*, including poor dressing technique.
- *Heavy colonization with bacteria* (suggested by increasing malodour, increasing pain, and heavy exudate). Paradoxically some bacteria may promote healing, but the role played by bacteria is not fully understood.
- *Allergic contact dermatitis*: patch test every 2–3 years.

Pain and leg ulcers

Severe pain is common in patients with arterial ulcers, but do not underestimate the pain suffered by patients with venous ulcers. The pathogenesis of pain is complex. Local dehydration caused by dressings, cutaneous ischaemia, and bacterial infection may play a part. Chronic pain demoralizes patients, limiting physical activity, but older patients may be reluctant to report pain (see Box 15.8).

What should I ask?

- Where is the pain? Ask the patient to point. Ensure the pain is caused by the ulcer—arthritis of the back, hip, or knee may cause leg pain.
- What is the pain like? (See Box 15.8.)
- How bad is the pain? Obtain a measure of the overall intensity of the pain by asking the patient to grade the pain (mild, moderate, or severe) or rate the pain on a scale of 0 (no pain) to 10 (most severe).
- When did the pain start, and how long does the pain last?
- Has the pain changed? Worsening may indicate ischaemia or cellulitis.
- What causes the pain? Typically, arterial ulcers cause severe pain at night, but many patients with venous ulcers also have pain that interferes with sleeping. Standing and walking cause pain in venous, as well as arterial, ulcers. Dressing changes may be very painful.
- What relieves the pain—elevation? Compression?
- What is the impact of the pain? Is the patient depressed or socially isolated?
- What analgesia is being taken and how often?

What should I do?

- Ensure the skin is not inflamed and there is no evidence of infection.
- Review dressings. Most 'non'-adherent dressings are drying, adhere to wounds (despite the name), and cause pain; hydrogels and hydrocolloids relieve pain.
- Review the dressing technique—use warm water for washing the ulcer; leave the ulcer uncovered for the minimum amount of time.
- Ensure that bandages are not compromising the vascular supply. Check with a pulse oximeter, if any doubt (see ➔ p. 300).
- Prescribe analgesia to be taken prior to dressing changes.
- A bed-cradle may help to relieve night pain, as may elevating the head of the bed by 12–15cm in patients with arterial disease.
- Elevation and compression bandages may alleviate much of the pain associated with venous ulcers, but not all patients tolerate this treatment, and some have neuropathic pain that does not respond to compression.
- Advise patients to avoid standing for prolonged periods.
- Refer for a vascular opinion if the Doppler ABPI is reduced to below 0.8.
- Prescribe analgesics, according to a pain ladder (see ➔ pp. 304–5).
- Reassure the patient that analgesia taken for pain is rarely addictive, and ensure the patient understands the importance of taking analgesia regularly to prevent the onset of pain.

Pain ladder

Nociceptive pain

Mild pain

Paracetamol 0.5–1g 4-hourly (max. = 4g/day).

Box 15.8 Descriptors from the short-form McGill Pain Questionnaire (SF-MPQ)

Pain is a complex sensation difficult to describe. Physical, psychological, and social factors influence the perception of pain. Patients may have a mix of nociceptive and neuropathic pain. SF-MPQ has 15 descriptors (11 sensory; 4 affective). Patients rate the intensity of each descriptor. Nociceptive pain associated with venous and arterial ulcers is usually throbbing or aching. Shooting, stabbing, or sharp pain suggests a neuropathic component. Burning may indicate damage to the skin.

- *Sensory descriptors*: throbbing, shooting, stabbing, sharp, cramping, gnawing, hot/burning, aching, heavy, tender, splitting.
- *Affective descriptors*: tiring/exhausting, sickening, fearful, punishing/cruel.

Reproduced with permission from Melzack R, The short-form McGill pain questionnaire, *Pain*, 30:2, 1987, Elsevier.

Moderate pain

- Try increasing strengths of codeine with paracetamol.
- Co-codamol weak (8mg of codeine phosphate plus 500mg of paracetamol) 1–2 tablets 4-hourly (max. = 8 tablets/day).
- Co-codamol medium (15mg of codeine phosphate plus 500mg of paracetamol) 1–2 tablets 4-hourly (max. = 8 tablets/day).
- Co-codamol strong (30mg of codeine phosphate plus 500mg of paracetamol) 1–2 tablets 4-hourly (max. = 8 tablets/day).
- If not controlled, try dihydrocodeine, 30mg every 4–6h (max. = 240mg/day). Stimulant laxatives may be required with these drugs.

Severe pain

- Day pain: short-acting morphine, 10mg 4-hourly (5mg in the elderly), and increase the dose by 50% incrementally.
- Night pain: twice 4-hourly dose, i.e. 10 or 20mg nocte. Incident or breakthrough pain 5–10mg of morphine PRN, i.e. the 4-hourly dose.
- An antiemetic may be used in conjunction with these initially, but, if still nauseated after 3 days, the dose should be reduced.
- Once pain control is stable, change from short-acting morphine to slow-release. Divide the total dose into two portions for 12-hourly administration. Ensure that the patient has an 'escape' dose of short-acting morphine for breakthrough pain. The escape dose should be 1/6 of the daily morphine dose in mg.

△ *Avoid NSAIDs in older patients (often used with paracetamol). Adverse effects include GI bleeding, duodenal or gastric ulceration, and renal failure.*

Neuropathic pain

Difficult to alleviate. Antidepressants, e.g. amitriptyline 25–50mg/day, may help. Increase the dose gradually. Anti-epileptic drugs, e.g. gabapentin, are also effective in some cases.

Management of ulcers

General advice

Correct factors such as oedema, iron or vitamin C deficiency, and pain (see ➋ p. 304). Wash ulcers and surrounding skin with tap water. Pick off loose scale, and moisturize the skin with 50% WSP in liquid paraffin or Hydromol® ointment. (Ointments are less likely to sensitize than creams.) Clean and dry the skin between the toes, and trim or file nails (a chiropodist may help).

Wound care

Reduce bacterial contamination with antiseptic soaks or wet dressings (see ➋ p. 662). Moist wounds heal more quickly than those exposed to air, but too much moisture irritates the skin and macerates wound edges which become friable and break down. Protect the edges with zinc oxide paste or Cavilon® (expensive).

Choice of dressing depends on the type and state of the ulcer (see Box 15.9).

Venous ulcers

- Graduated compression bandaging promotes healing. Bandages should extend from the base of toes to below the knee. Experts apply bandages with an even tension, so that the pressure steadily reduces from the ankle to the calf (see Box 15.10). △ *Check the ABPI before compressing the limb* (see Box 15.6).
- Avoid prolonged standing (stand on tiptoes at intervals to activate the leg muscle pump) or sitting with the feet dependent (elevate the legs with the feet at heart level, and dorsiflex the feet regularly to activate the muscle pump).
- Encourage mobility and weight loss.
- Aspirin and pentoxifylline have been advocated to promote healing of venous ulcers, but their role is unproven.
- Skin grafts (pinch, punch, or split-thickness) may hasten re-epithelialization of ulcers with granulating bases, once oedema is controlled. Refer to a vascular service if the ulcer is not healing. Also refer patients with healed venous ulcers to a vascular service. Vascular surgery to correct venous hypertension may prevent recurrence.
- Once the ulcer has healed, ensure that the patient has compression hosiery (ideally class II). The patient may need help to put on stockings.

Arterial ulcers

- Keep the limb warm. Advise patients to stop smoking and control other risk factors for arterial disease such as hypertension or diabetes.
- Encourage regular graded exercise to promote circulation.
- Protect bony prominences and pressure areas (heels) with padding.
- Vascular surgeons may be able to improve the blood supply with balloon angioplasty or a femoropopliteal bypass graft.
- Skin grafting may have a role, once underlying vascular problems have been corrected. Consider involving a plastic surgeon.

Further reading

Fonder MA *et al. J Am Acad Dermatol* 2008;**58**:185–206.

Box 15.9 Primary dressings and topical treatments

Note: there are many equivalent products. Determine what is available locally, before you choose dressings or bandages.

Pain Non-adherent dressings: Atrauman®/Mepitel®/Mepilex® (also useful as blister dressings). Hydrating dressings (also encourage granulation tissue): hydrogels or hydrocolloids. May overhydrate. Reduce bacterial colonization (see below).

Topical steroid (e.g. Trimovate® cream) or silver sulfadiazine cream for short periods may relieve pain (not evidence-based).

Bacterial colonization Antibacterial wash, e.g. Prontosan®. Dressings containing iodine (may be painful). A microorganism-binding dressing, e.g. Cutimed® Sorbact. Honey (may be painful) or silver sulfadiazine.

Moderate exudate Alginates or cellulose dressings e.g. Aquacel® Ag. Alginates may also be used for wound packing.

Heavy exudate Cellulose dressings, e.g. Aquacel® Ag, and absorbent pad, e.g. Sorbion® sana, Keramax®.

Odour Reduce bacterial load with topical metronidazole (eliminates anaerobes) or dressings containing silver. Absorb odour with Clinisorb® (cheap) or Carboflex® (expensive).

Adherent slough/necrotic tissue Larvae (maggots) remove necrotic tissue but do not damage healthy tissue. In the UK, sterile maggots may be ordered from the Biosurgical Research Unit, Princes of Wales Hospital, Bridgend, Wales CF31 1RQ. Surgical debridement (avoid in arterial ulcers) to cut away necrotic tissue. Autolysis promoted by softening tissues with hydrating dressings, e.g. hydrogels, hydrocolloids.

Change dressings if wound leaks, smells, or is painful. Dressings should always be changed within 7 days.

Venous eczema Moderately potent topical corticosteroid ointment under compression. Either use elasticated tubular bandage (see Box 15.10)—easy to remove if topical treatment required—or apply a paste bandage under compression (see ➜ Box 34.4, p. 661).

Box 15.10 Compression bandages for venous ulcers

Note: there are many equivalent products. Determine what is available locally, before you choose dressings or bandages.

Apply bandages evenly from the toe to below the knee, without ridges or folds. Applied correctly, the pressure steadily reduces from about 40mmHg at the ankle to 15–20mmHg at the calf. Do not tape anything directly to the skin.

Mobile patients Tubifast® (elasticated viscose stockinette) and Soffban® with Actico® short stretch (inelastic) bandages or long stretch (elastic) bandages or compression using a multicomponent system containing an elastic bandage.

Immobile patients Long stretch (elastic) bandages, e.g. Tensopress®, Setopress®, or short stretch (see above). Shaped elasticated tubular bandage provides some compression but is not available in the community. Some graduated compression can be provided by placing a layer of unshaped elasticated tubular bandage size D from the toe to mid calf ,with a 2nd layer size E from the ankle to the knee. Always use Tubifast® under elasticated tubular bandage. Hosiery (two-layer) designed for patients with ulcers made by Activa and Medi.

Lipodermatosclerosis (sclerosing panniculitis)

- Lipodermatosclerosis is a complication of venous stasis that is seen more often in women than in men. Chronic inflammation causes fibrosis with progressive induration.
- △ The diagnosis is clinical, but frequently pain and erythema in acute lipodermatosclerosis are misdiagnosed and mistreated as cellulitis (see ➡ p. 138).

What should I ask?

- Look for a history of long-standing painful 'cellulitis' that has not responded to repeated courses of antibiotics.
- Ask about factors suggesting venous insufficiency, e.g. chronic swelling, previous DVT, varicose veins, orthopaedic procedures (see ➡ pp. 294–5).
- What factors improve or exacerbate the pain? Pain in lipodermatosclerosis is worse on standing and may be relieved by elevation.

What should I look for?

- Acute lipodermatosclerosis: a well-defined, very tender, indurated, erythematous plaque in the gaiter area, usually on the medial side of the leg, with little or no swelling (see Fig.15.6).
- Chronic lipodermatosclerosis: a well-defined, slightly tender, indurated 'woody' plaque. Fibrosis tethers subcutaneous tissues (sclerosing panniculitis). Eventually, the leg adopts the shape of an inverted champagne bottle.
- Signs of venous insufficiency, including venous eczema, venous flare, pigmentation, and ulceration in the gaiter area (see Box 15.5).
- An absence of signs suggesting cellulitis: spreading erythema (the erythema is localized in lipodermatosclerosis), acute swelling (the skin is usually tight in lipodermatosclerosis), lymphangitis, systemic flu-like symptoms.

What should I do?

- Explain that lipodermatosclerosis is caused by venous disease and is not an infection. Stop antibiotics.
- Provide pain relief (see ➡ p. 304).
- Control venous hypertension with compression (first exclude peripheral arterial disease). A pressure of 30–40mmHg at the ankle may not be tolerated in acute lipodermatosclerosis. Start with less pressure, and try to increase compression gradually.
- Advise about weight loss (if indicated), elevation, and exercise, as for patients with venous leg ulcers (see ➡ p. 306).
- The role of systemic treatments, such as prednisolone (to reduce acute inflammation) or fibrinolytic agents, is unproven.
- Refer to a vascular service. Vascular surgery may be indicated to prevent venous reflux and reduce inflammation.

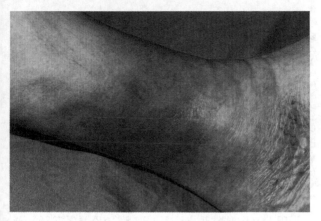

Fig. 15.6 Tender, indurated lipodermatosclerosis simulating cellulitis.

Pyoderma gangrenosum

❶ Pyoderma gangrenosum (PG) is a neutrophilic dermatosis character-ized by acutely painful, rapidly enlarging deep ulcers (see Box 15.11). PG is neither an infection nor gangrenous, but is probably an aberrant immune response. Clearance of inflammatory cells may be impaired by abnor-malities in, for example, neutrophil chemokines, integrins, or T-cells.

Ulcers can occur at any site, including the genitalia, but PG usually presents on the leg. It is seen most often in middle-aged adults but can affect any age. About 50% of patients have an underlying disease (see Box 15.12). Rarely, PG is triggered by surgery, often breast surgery. Diagnosis is clinical and may be difficult (see Box 15.12).

What should I ask?

(see ➋ pp. 294–5.)

- How did the ulcer start? (Was minor trauma involved?)
- Is the ulcer painful? How quickly is it enlarging?
- Has the patient another reason to have a leg ulcer (venous disease, arterial disease, infection), a past history of PG, or a systemic disease that might predispose to PG? (See Box 15.11.)

What should I do?

- Look for signs suggesting PG (see Box 15.12 and Fig. 15.5).
- Rule out common causes of ulceration, but venous or arterial disease may coexist with PG (see Box 15.12).
- FBC, ESR, CRP, protein electrophoresis, and Ig (20% have a benign monoclonal gammopathy), RF, antiphospholipid antibodies.
- Take a biopsy from the ulcer edge for histology (may be suggestive but is not diagnostic); culture (bacteria, fungi such as sporotrichosis) (see ➋ Box 33.2, p. 645).
- Prescribe analgesia.
- Dressings, such as hydrocolloids or alginates, may relieve pain.
- Try gentle compression to control oedema (if tolerated).
- Pustules, bullae, or small ulcers—a very potent topical corticosteroid ointment or 0.1% tacrolimus ointment may control pain, inflammation, and ulceration, but watch for 2° infection, e.g. *Pseudomonas aeruginosa*.
- ▶▶ Large ulcers—prompt treatment with prednisolone 40–60mg/day or pulse IV methylprednisolone is essential to minimize scarring. Steroid-sparing agents that may be tried include minocycline, ciclosporin, and dapsone.
- Anti-TNF agents may be effective, particularly in PG with IBD or RA.
- ⚠ Avoid surgery in active disease, as trauma will exacerbate ulceration. Skin grafting may be considered for large ulcers, but only when inflammation is controlled.

Further reading

Patel F et al. Acta Derm Venereol 2015;**95**:525–31.

Box 15.11 Systemic diseases and pyoderma gangrenosum

Fifty percent of patients with PG have an underlying condition:
- IBD (65%): PG may be peristomal (see ➲ Box 24.2, p. 509).
- RA and other inflammatory arthropathies, seropositive and seronegative (16%).
- Haematological disorders (12%), e.g. acute myeloid leukaemia, myelodysplastic syndromes—PG is often bullous (signs overlap with Sweet syndrome; see ➲ p. 518).
- Auto-inflammatory diseases, e.g. PAPA syndrome (pyogenic arthritis, PG, and acne), PASH (PG, acne, and suppurative hidradenitis)—vanishingly rare! (see ➲ p. 234 and pp. 248–9.)

Box 15.12 Diagnosis of pyoderma gangrenosum

Major features
(See Fig. 15.5.)
- Very painful necrotic cutaneous ulcer (pain is out of proportion to the appearance of the ulcer) with a purulent discharge.
- Rapid progression of the ulcer—may enlarge by 2cm/day.
- Irregular, violaceous, and undermined border—you may be able to insert a probe several mm under the edge.
- Rapid response to corticosteroids—sometimes one has to resort to a clinical trial if the diagnosis is not clear-cut.
- Post-surgical PG: presents in the immediate post-operative period with fever and wound dehiscence, progressing to painful ulcers with typical borders. Often misdiagnosed as wound infection.

Other suggestive features
- The ulcer was preceded by a sterile pustule or, less often, an erythematous nodule or a blister.
- History that minor trauma initiates ulcers, i.e. pathergy.
- Base with much slough or haemorrhagic base.
- Cribriform scarring (uneven sieve-like with perforations).
- Histology: follicular or perifollicular inflammation, intradermal abscesses, and/or sterile dermal neutrophilia without vasculitis. Findings are not specific.

Differential diagnosis
- Infection: deep fungal, atypical mycobacterial.
- Venous or arterial insufficiency: vasculitis or occlusive vasculopathy (see ➲ pp. 312–13, and p. 452).
- Granulomatosis with polyangiitis: ulcers affecting the limbs, perineum, or face may resemble PG (see ➲ pp. 446–7).
- Cutaneous malignancy.
- Bite of brown recluse spider.
- Dermatitis artefacta: well-defined, angular ulcers without undermined edges (see ➲ pp. 566–7).
- Drug-induced ulcers: nicorandil, hydroxyurea.

Calcific uraemic arteriolopathy

Synonym: calciphylaxis.

This life-threatening condition occurs most often in patients with chronic kidney disease on dialysis. Calcium deposited in the media of small cutaneous arteries leads to thrombosis and ischaemic necrosis with refractory ulcers often involving the lower extremity, abdomen, or buttocks. Deposition of metals (iron, aluminium) may play a part in the pathogenesis of endothelial injury and vascular calcification.

2° infection may lead to fatal sepsis, and mortality is high (60–80%). Incidence is increasing, and calciphylaxis may be seen in other situations (see Box 15.13) when it may be confused with cutaneous vasculitis or PG. Rarely, patients may have systemic problems such as proximal myopathy, aortic valve involvement, or pulmonary calciphylaxis.

What should I look for?

* A history of underlying risk factors (see Box 15.13).
* Sudden onset of painful mottled erythema on the thigh or leg, evolving to indurated plaques that eventually become necrotic and ulcerate. Initially may be misdiagnosed as cellulitis (see Fig. 15.7).
* Livedo reticularis: mottled, reddish purple, reticulated discoloration, reflecting a sluggish vascular flow in the superficial dermis (see ⟶ pp. 314–15 and p. 452).
* Ischaemic necrosis with black eschars (see Fig. 15.7).
* Other cutaneous signs may include:
  * Pathergy: minor trauma triggers ulceration.
  * Recurrent digital ischaemia with gangrene, necrosis of the penis.
  * Subcutaneous nodules on the breasts and abdomen.

What should I do?

* Check for cutaneous infection—take skin swabs (but surface swabs from ulcers are generally not very informative).
* Exclude peripheral vascular disease by clinical examination.
* Check renal function, serum calcium, serum phosphate, parathyroid hormone (PTH) level, and alkaline phosphatase.
* Check fasting glucose.
* Exclude other causes of an occlusive vasculopathy—check FBC and coagulation profile, including lupus anticoagulant, anticardiolipin antibody, protein C, and protein S (see ⟶ p. 452).
* Exclude cutaneous vasculitis—check complements (C3, C4), cryoglobulins, hepatitis B and C serologies.
* Consider taking a deep elliptical skin biopsy to demonstrate calcification in small arteries, vascular thrombosis, and intimal hyperplasia (endarteritis obliterans) … but the biopsy may not heal.
* Radiographs may show vessel calcification, including a net-like pattern of calcification extending beyond visible skin lesions.
* Management is difficult and requires a multidisciplinary approach (see Box 15.14) (no randomized controlled trials of therapy).

Box 15.13 Risk factors for calciphylaxis

Major risk factors
- End-stage renal disease.
- Elevated calcium phosphate product.
- Hyperparathyroidism—1° and 2°.

Non-uraemic risk factors
- ♀ gender.
- Obesity (rapid weight loss may induce calciphylaxis).
- Diabetes.
- Hypoalbuminaemia.
- Autoimmune diseases such as SLE, RA, and antiphospholipid syndrome.
- Warfarin.
- Protein C and protein S deficiency.
- Malignancy.
- Alcoholic liver disease.

Box 15.14 Management of calciphylaxis

- Pain relief and supportive care.
- Optimize wound dressings, e.g. hydrocolloid dressings.
- Avoid compression which may exacerbate cutaneous ischaemia and pain.
- Treat infections promptly with oral antibiotics, e.g. flucloxacillin.
- IV or intralesional sodium thiosulfate may promote healing.
- Attempt to normalize calcium and phosphate levels—discuss management with the renal physicians. The evidence base for management is weak, but strategies may include:
  - Discontinuing oral calcium supplements.
  - Lowering the calcium concentration in the dialysate.
  - More frequent dialysis.
  - Bisphosphonates such as IV pamidronate and oral etidronate.
  - Cinacalcet to downregulate PTH levels and correct elevated calcium phosphate products.
  - Parathyroidectomy.
- Control blood glucose.
- Hyperbaric oxygen has been suggested.
- ⚠ Avoid aggressive debridement—may trigger further ulceration.
- ⚠ Avoid immunosuppressive drugs—increase the risk of infection.
- The role of anticoagulation is controversial, but consider stopping warfarin, if relevant, and use another anticoagulant.

Further reading

Strazzula L et al. *JAMA Dermatol* 2013;**149**:946–9 (intralesional sodium thiosulfate).
Vedvyas C et al. *J Am Acad Dermatol* 2012;**67**:e253–60.

Livedoid vasculopathy

Synonyms: segmental hyalinizing vasculitis, livedo reticularis with summer/winter ulceration, livedoid vasculitis.

This painful thrombo-occlusive vasculopathy affects young to middle-aged women. Hyaline thrombi occlude small vessels in the upper and mid dermis. There is no vasculitis. The cause is unknown, but fibrinolytic and coagulation systems are usually normal. Ulceration may be chronic and recurrent. Pain reduces quality of life.

What should I look for?

- Focal purpuric lesions on the leg, usually around the ankle.
- Small, excruciatingly painful ulcers surrounded by a purpuric rim.
- Porcelain-white stellate scars with a rim of telangiectasia (atrophie blanche) (see Fig. 15.8).
- Livedo reticularis: mottled, reddish purple, reticulated discoloration, reflecting a sluggish vascular flow in the superficial dermis (see ➔ p. 452, and Fig. 20.4, p. 453).
- Signs of venous disease.
- Net-like hyperpigmentation on the leg at the site of previous livedo (differentiate from erythema ab igne, a reticulated brown staining that can develop if the skin is exposed chronically to heat from a radiator, open fire, or hot-water bottle (see ➔ Fig. 20.5, p. 454).

What should I do?

- Investigations (results usually unremarkable):
  - FBC to exclude thrombocythaemia.
  - Clotting screen, including antiphospholipid antibodies, protein S and C.
  - Protein electrophoresis to exclude paraproteinaemia.
  - ANA to exclude SLE (if indicated by the presentation).
  - Take a deep biopsy, including the edge of the ulcer, to demonstrate hyaline thrombi.
- Control pain (see ➔ p. 304).
- Venous disease: control oedema with compression, if possible.
- Try antiplatelet therapy, antithrombotic regimens, or fibrinolytic agents, but treatment is difficult, and there is no consensus about the best approach.
- Treatment with immunosuppression is ineffective.

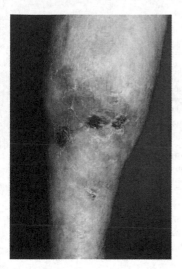

Fig. 15.7 Calciphylaxis: mottled erythema (livedo reticularis) and painful ulceration in a patient with diabetes.

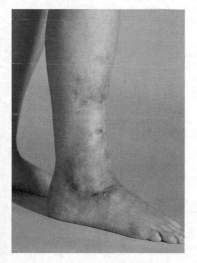

Fig. 15.8 Livedoid vasculopathy: atrophie blanche with painful ulceration around the ankles.

Further reading

Alavi A et al. J Am Acad Dermatol 2013;**69**:1033–42.

Lymphoedema

Lymphoedema causes unilateral (occasionally bilateral) chronic swelling, most often of the leg, that is associated with recurrent cellulitis and may occasionally be associated with leg ulcers. The lymphatic system is involved in immune surveillance, and all forms of lymphoedema predispose to recurrent cellulitis/erysipelas.

1° lymphoedema is caused by an intrinsic fault (structural or functional) in lymph drainage. Causal genes include *VEGFR3* (Milroy disease) and *FOXC2* (lymphoedema–distichiasis syndrome). Lymphoedema may not present until adolescence or adulthood.

2° lymphoedema is caused by lymphatic obstruction or damage to the lymphatic system, e.g. radiotherapy, lymph node dissection. Filaria parasites invade lymphatics, causing lymphoedema (40 million people affected—a huge disease burden). Rarely, pretibial myxoedema simulates lymphoedema (see ➲ Fig. 22.4, p. 473).

What should I ask?

- Where is the swelling? When did it commence, and how did it progress?
- Does the swelling change with the position of the limb, e.g. overnight? Unlike venous swelling, lymphoedema does not reduce with elevation.
- Any episodes of cellulitis? Flu-like symptoms with fevers, rigors, or vomiting precede blotchy redness. How often are these episodes?
- Any pain? (Usually not a problem in lymphoedema.)
- Any family history of lymphoedema (found in 20% of cases of lymphoedema; suggests 1° lymphoedema)?
- Past history of malignancy or surgery, e.g. lymph node dissection.
- Drug history—sirolimus is a rare cause of 2° lymphoedema.

What should I look for?

- Persistent swelling affecting the foot, as well as the leg (see Fig.15.2).
- Pitting oedema at the onset; non-pitting 'woody' swelling in chronic lymphoedema because of fibrosis.
- A warm leg and foot with thickening, fissuring, and hyperkeratosis, and papillomatous wart-like growths resembling 'elephant skin'.
- Bleb-like vesicles you can compress with your finger (lymphoceles).
- Stemmer's sign: it is not possible to pinch up a loose fold of skin on the dorsum of the foot at the base of the second toe, because the skin is thickened and fibrotic. Absence does not exclude lymphoedema.
- Ascites or pleural effusions in some 1° lymphoedemas.
- Chronic lymphoedema in obese euthyroid patients may be associated with a nodular dermal mucinosis (obesity-associated lymphoedematous mucinosis).
- Bluish nodules or plaques suggesting angiosarcoma or KS (rare) (see ➲ pp. 362–3).

- Differentiate lymphoedema of the leg from lipoedema (see Box 15.15 and Table 15.1).
- Although lymphoedema may appear to be unilateral, lymphoscintigraphy studies have shown that the contralateral limb is often also abnormal. Examine both legs.

What should I do?

- Advise on skin care to reduce the likelihood of infection. The patient should wash the skin daily, ensure that folds of skin and the skin between the toes are cleaned and dried, and use an emollient to prevent fissuring. Cuts or abrasions should be kept scrupulously clean.
- Ensure the patient can trim his/her toenails, or refer to a chiropodist.
- If cellulitis occurs more than ×2/year, prescribe prophylactic phenoxymethylpenicillin 500mg daily (clindamycin if allergic to penicillin) for at least 2 years to prevent further cellulitis and lymphatic damage with worsening swelling.
- Refer to a lymphoedema clinic for manual lymphatic drainage, advice about exercise, and compression bandaging.

Box 15.15 Swelling of the leg: differential diagnosis

Unilateral
- DVT.
- Ruptured Baker's cyst.
- Cellulitis.
- Chronic venous insufficiency.
- Lymphoedema, e.g. pelvic tumour or lymphatic damage.
- Immobility.

Bilateral
- Congestive cardiac failure, renal failure, or nephrotic syndrome.
- Liver failure and hypoalbuminaemia.
- Malnutrition.
- Drugs, NSAIDs, calcium channel blockers.
- Lipoedema (see ➔ p. 318).
- Immobility, e.g. sitting in a wheelchair.

Further reading

Mortimer PS and Rockson SG. *J Clin Invest* 2014;**124**:915–21.

Lipoedema

What is lipoedema?

- Lipoedema, also known as painful fat syndrome, affects women and starts around puberty.
- Lipoedema may be familial (40% of cases).
- Nodules containing 'wet' fat are deposited in subcutaneous tissues on the buttocks, hips, thighs, and legs. The feet are not affected.
- Treatment is unsatisfactory. Dieting does not alter lipoedema—the trunk may become slim, but the legs remain large.
- Exercise and surgical support stockings may help.
- For differentiating lipoedema from lymphedema, see Table 15.1.

Table 15.1 Lipoedema or lymphoedema?

Lipoedema	Lymphoedema
Swelling is bilateral.	Swelling is usually unilateral.
The legs are painful, and the skin is tender.	Lymphoedema is usually painless.
The fat on the ankles creates a ring of fatty tissue that overhangs normal-looking feet. Fat is deposited on the buttocks and lower limbs.	The foot is affected, as well as the leg.
Swelling increases during the day and reduces during the night when the leg is elevated.	Position does not influence the amount of swelling.
Swelling does not pit.	Swelling pits in early lymphoedema but is non-pitting in late disease.
The skin tends to be thin. Easy bruising and subcutaneous bleeding are common.	The skin is thickened, fissured, and hyperkeratotic.
Stemmer's sign is absent.	Stemmer's sign is usually present.

Sun and skin

Contents

Relevant pages in other chapters
For the history in suspected photosensitivity,
see ➔ Chapter 2, p. 28, and for the examination
findings that suggest photosensitivity, see ➔ Box 4.6, p. 73.
Skin cancer is discussed in ➔ Chapter 17, pp. 346–57.

Introduction

Life on earth depends on the sun's warmth and light. Our spirits rise in the sun, and sunny days evoke memories of long holidays (as well as revision for exams). But the sun has the potential to harm—there can be 'too much of a good thing'. Sunburn, skin cancer, and most photosensitivity disorders are caused by UVR.

How does ultraviolet radiation affect the skin?

The sun emits a broad and continuous spectrum of electromagnetic energy (the solar spectrum) (see Fig. 16.1). UVR is divided into short (UVC), medium (UVB), and long (UVA, 'black light') wavelength emissions. Ninety-eight percent of the UVR that reaches the earth's surface is UVA. All UVC and a little UVB are absorbed in the atmosphere by the ozone layer. UVB is absorbed by nucleic acids and proteins in the epidermis and stimulates the synthesis of vitamin D_3 (cholecalciferol). Some UVA is absorbed in the epidermis, but UVA penetrates into the dermis.

The damage caused by UVR depends on the duration of exposure, as well as the skin phototype (see Table 16.1).

- UVB causes immediate sunburn with painful erythema and, if severe, blistering. The UVB reaction peaks at 16–24h, then the skin desquamates over 2–3 days but becomes tanned and may develop solar lentigines (sunburn freckles).
- UVR, particularly UVB, damages DNA, and cumulative damage causes skin cancer (see → p. 346).
- Chronic UV exposure produces many of the signs we associate with ageing (photodamage)—wrinkling, blotchy pigmentation, telangiectasia, a sallow appearance—as well as skin cancer (see → Box 3.1, p. 43).
- UVR also causes local and systemic immunosuppression, which not only leads to problems, such as recurrent herpes simplex infection, but also contributes to the pathogenesis of skin cancer.

How is the skin protected from sun damage?

Nucleotide excision repair enzymes repair photodamaged DNA, but the capacity to repair declines with age (or may be abnormal in some rare photogenodermatoses; see → pp. 336–7). Epidermal melanin provides some UV protection by absorbing visible light, as well as UVR (see → pp. 12–3). Melanin also quenches oxygen free radicals.

Darkly pigmented skin has the same number of melanocytes as lightly pigmented skin, but more and slightly differently packaged melanin (melanosomes) within keratinocytes provides greater resistance to solar damage. However, even dark skin burns in the sun, if the dose of UVR is high enough.

UVA causes immediate darkening of the skin (oxidation of pre-existing melanin) that lasts a few hours and is not photoprotective. UVB is the main stimulus for the delayed tanning detectable 3–5 days after exposure (more melanocytes, synthesis of new melanin, redistribution of melanosomes). This provides some photoprotection and fades slowly.

Sun exposure also induces the injured epidermis to proliferate. Thickening of the horny layer (stratum corneum) supplies a little more protection from photodamage.

The solar spectrum

The solar spectrum ranges from cosmic rays, γ rays, and X-rays, through UVR (100–400nm), visible light (400–800nm), and infrared radiation (800–17 000nm), to radio waves (see Fig. 16.1). UVB and UVA contribute to tanning; UVB causes sunburn.

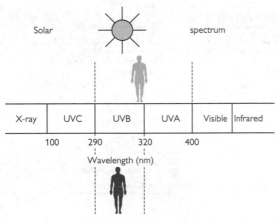

Fig. 16.1 Solar spectrum. UVA and visible light, unlike UVB, penetrate glass.

Skin phototype and photosensitivity

Skin phototype

Pale skins that burn easily and tan poorly, if at all, are most at risk of chronic photodamage and skin cancer, but it may be difficult to predict the phototype simply from the appearance of the skin. It is better to ask patients how quickly they burn and how easily they tan.

The Fitzpatrick classification (see Table 16.1) reflects the amount of melanin in the skin.

Table 16.1 Fitzpatrick classification

Skin type	Response of skin to sun	Appearance
I	Always burns, never tans	White or pale skin, many freckles, blond or red hair, blue or green eyes
II	Burns easily, tans poorly	Pale skin, possibly some freckles, blond hair, blue or green eyes
III	May burn, tans lightly	Darker white skin, dark hair, brown eyes
IV	Burns minimally, tans easily	Olive skin, brown or black hair, brown eyes—Mediterranean
V	Rarely burns, always tans deeply	Brown skin—Asian, Latin American, Middle Eastern
VI	Never burns, tans darkly	Black African

What is photosensitivity?

- Photosensitivity is defined as an abnormal cutaneous response to light/sunlight. It can be caused by a deficiency of photoimmunosuppression or as a result of an interaction between photosensitizing substances and sunlight or filtered or artificial light.
- People who are photosensitive burn easily in sunlight and may complain of reddening, swelling, blistering, itching, and/or painful skin after minimal sun exposure (see ➜ Box 4.6, p. 73).
  ❶ *Photosensitivity may lead to early skin cancers* (see ➜ p. 346).
- Photosensitivity may be 1° (i.e. idiopathic) but, more often, is acquired.

What should I do?

See Box 16.1.

Box 16.1 Photosensitivity: what should I do?

- Take a full medical history (see ➲ p. 28), and examine the patient (see ➲ Box 4.6, p. 73). Some skin diseases may be made worse by sunlight (photoaggravated) (see Box 16.2).
- Investigation of photosensitivity may include:
  - ANA, ENA (Ro antibodies are linked to photosensitivity).
  - Porphyrins in blood, urine, and stool (ensure the sample is not exposed to light by wrapping the specimen pot in tinfoil).
  - Skin biopsy for histology/fibroblasts for DNA repair disorders.
  - Patch testing and photopatch testing.
  - Phototesting to define the minimal erythema dose (MED) and action spectrum responsible. Skin can be exposed to light that simulates sunlight and also to specific wavebands by using a monochromator to fractionate the light.
  - Metabolic studies (aminoaciduria, hair analysis).
- Advise the patient how to protect the skin from UV light (see ➲ pp. 338–9).
- Manage the underlying problem.

Further reading

Hussein MR. *J Cutan Pathol* 2005;**32**:191–205.
Yashar SS and Lim HW. *Dermatol Ther* 2003;**16**:1–7.

Causes of photosensitivity

Photosensitivity in adults

Common causes
- Photoaggravated skin disease, e.g. cutaneous LE (see Box 16.2).
- Drug-induced photoallergy or phototoxicity (see ➔ p. 326 and Fig 16.2).
- Contact photosensitivity:
  - Soaps, tars, perfumes, drugs such as topical NSAIDs.
  - Plants: phytophotodermatitis (plants containing psoralen) (see Box 16.4).
- Polymorphic light eruption (PLE) (see ➔ pp. 328–9).

Uncommon or rare causes
- Cutaneous porphyrias, e.g. PCT (see ➔ p. 332).
- Pseudoporphyria (see ➔ p. 334).
- Idiopathic photodermatoses (see Box 16.5).
- DNA repair deficiencies (rare) (see ➔ pp. 336–7).
  - XP, trichothiodystrophy, Cockayne syndrome, Bloom syndrome, Rothmund–Thomson syndrome.
- Other very rare photogenodermatoses:
  - Kindler–Weary syndrome, Smith–Lemli–Opitz syndrome.

Photosensitivity in childhood

- Consider phytophotodermatitis, drug-induced photosensitivity, and PLE before porphyria or a rare genodermatosis.
- Remember that atopic eczema may be photoaggravated.

Box 16.2 Skin diseases that may be photoaggravated

Features of an underlying disease, but more severe on sun-exposed skin.
- Rosacea.
- Dermatitis—seborrhoeic, atopic.
- Psoriasis and pityriasis rubra pilaris (more often helped by sunlight).
- LP, EM.
- LE, especially subacute cutaneous LE.
- Dermatomyositis.
- Darier disease.
- Autoimmune blistering diseases—pemphigus, BP.
- Pellagra (niacin deficiency).

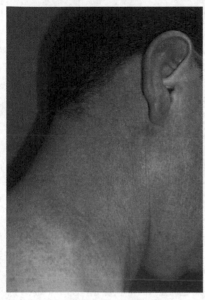

Fig. 16.2 Photosensitive patient with erythema of exposed skin, but with an abrupt cut-off where the skin is covered by clothing.

Drug-induced photosensitivity

Drugs are the commonest cause of photosensitivity (see Box 16.3). Photosensitivity is caused by phototoxicity more often than photoallergy, but the distinction is not always clear. Reactions may also be bullous or lichenoid. Other potential presentations of a drug-induced photosensitivity include pseudoporphyria (see ➲ p. 334) and LE (see ➲ p. 402).

What is phototoxicity?

Phototoxicity causes an exaggerated sunburn response with pain, erythema, oedema, and sometimes blistering of exposed skin. The action spectrum for phototoxins may be UVB, UVA, or visible solar radiation. The response depends on the amount of UVR (the patient may have no problems on a slightly cloudy day) and the dose of the drug but can occur on first exposure to the drug. The response is usually immediate but can be delayed. Reactions to amiodarone and chlorpromazine produce pigmentary changes. Chronic phototoxicity accelerates photoageing, e.g. patients taking voriconazole for antifungal prophylaxis. Examine the skin regularly.

Phytophotodermatitis is a phototoxic eruption caused by contact with plant juices containing light-sensitizing furocoumarin chemicals, e.g. psoralens (see Box 16.4).

What is photoallergy?

Photoallergic reactions are idiosyncratic delayed hypersensitivity reactions, similar to an allergic contact dermatitis, that do not develop, until the patient has been sensitized by prior exposure to the drug. The action spectrum for most photoallergens is in the UVA range (light coming through window glass causes problems). The response is not dose-dependent, and the reaction may spread to affect covered skin. Frequently, topical medicaments are implicated. Photopatch testing is positive.

What should I do?

- Withdraw the drug, if possible. Phototoxic reactions settle within a week. The signs of photoallergy (erythema) will also disappear within a week, but photosensitivity may persist for months after drug withdrawal (sometimes as long as 6 months).
- A potent topical steroid applied daily will help to settle the inflammation. Systemic steroids may be required in severe reactions.
- Sun protection with clothing, a hat, and a high-factor broad-spectrum UVA/UVB sunscreen is essential (see ➲ pp. 338–9).
- Photopatch testing may be helpful in suspected topical agent photoallergy, but less useful for systemic drug photosensitivity.
- ⚠ Chronic phototoxicity increases the risk of skin cancer.

Box 16.3 Drug-induced photosensitivity

- Phototoxicity: amiodarone, doxycycline, thiazides, phenothiazines, NSAIDs, quinolones, quinine, sulfonamides, retinoids, psoralens (in plants), coal tar, voriconazole, BRAF inhibitors.
- Photoallergy: topical antimicrobials, fragrances, sunscreens, angiotensin-converting agent inhibitors, non-steroidal anti-inflammatory agents, phenothiazines, sulfonamides, thiazides.
- Pseudoporphyria (a form of phototoxicity with blistering and skin fragility; see ➲ p. 334): nalidixic acid, furosemide, ciprofloxacin, bumetanide, NSAIDs.
- Lichenoid reactions resembling LP (see ➲ p. 224) (delayed in onset): hydrochlorothiazide, NSAIDs, quinidine-derived drugs.
- Photo-onycholysis (painful): tetracyclines, taxanes.

Box 16.4 What is phytophotodermatitis?

- Phototoxic reactions to light-sensitizing furocoumarin chemicals in plants can occur in anyone and are not an allergy.
- Causes of phytophotodermatitis include members of the *Apiaceae* family (previously *Umbelliferae*), e.g. Queen Anne's lace, giant hogweed, parsnip, celery; the *Rutaceae* family, e.g. garden rue (*Ruta graveolens*); and citrus fruit oils, e.g. lime juice.
- The patient, often a gardener wielding a strimmer or a child, is outside on a sunny day. Plant juice is deposited in a streaky linear fashion on exposed skin that has brushed against the plant or, with strimmers, the juice is sprayed over exposed skin.
- The psoralens in the plant juice cause a painful burning (rather than itching) erythema, often with blistering, about 24h after exposure to long-wave UVR (UVA).
- The reaction peaks at 48–72h and gradually settles over a few days.
- Linear streaks of hyperpigmentation persist at the site of inflammation and may take months to fade. These may be all you see when the patient presents (see ➲ Fig. 31.11, p. 615).
- The diagnosis depends upon the history and the bizarre linear pattern suggesting an external injury. Sometimes child abuse is suspected (see ➲ pp. 614–15).

Polymorphic light eruption

Polymorphic light eruption (PMLE, PLE) is the commonest of the idiopathic photodermatoses (see Box 16.5). It is sometimes known as 'sun allergy' or prickly heat. PLE affects about 15% of the young adult ♀ Caucasian population in northern Europe and may present in young adults or childhood. Genetic factors probably play some part in the pathogenesis. The abbreviation is confusing—PLE is not a form of cutaneous lupus erythematosus (LE).

UVR (mostly UVA; sometimes UVA and UVB) provokes a T-cell response. The mechanism is unclear. It may be caused by failure of normal photoimmunosuppression. Phototesting can be normal, but provocation testing (UVA or solar-simulated light) usually provokes a rash.

What should I look for?

- A story of an itching or burning rash that erupts within 2h of exposure to UVR but, in some patients, may not develop for 24–48h, or even longer. (The history is usually diagnostic.)
- A rash that fades within 1–6 days, leaving normal skin (no scars).
- Erythematous papules, plaques, vesicles, or, less often, haemorrhagic blisters. The rash is polymorphic in its presentation in populations, but individuals usually have one form of the disease.
- The problem usually presents in spring, but some patients only develop the rash when they go on holiday to a sunny climate on 'holiday-exposed sites'. Sunlight reflected from snow may provoke PLE.
- The rash may be triggered by as little as 10min of direct sunlight.
- Sunlight penetrating window glass (UVA) may cause the rash, as can unshielded fluorescent lights and UVA from sunbeds.
- Chronically exposed skin on the face and hands is usually spared.
- The rash usually erupts less frequently, as the summer progresses ('hardening'), provided exposure to sunlight continues.

What should I do?

- Exclude subacute cutaneous LE (see ⊃ p. 402), solar urticaria and oral contraceptive (oestrogen)-induced photosensitivity (rare).
- Management options include:
  - Potent topical corticosteroids for acute eruptions.
  - Gradual sunlight exposure to induce tolerance (may be difficult to achieve) and continued sun exposure to maintain tolerance.
  - Protective clothing: broad-brimmed hats, long sleeves (see ⊃ p. 338).
  - High-factor UVA/UVB sunscreens may prevent PLE. (UVB sunscreens may worsen PLE by allowing UVA through, but diminishing the protective immunosuppression produced by UVB).
  - Oral prednisolone 15–20mg/day for 2–3 days may be required to control an acute eruption, e.g. while on holiday.
  - Desensitization with UVB each spring. Treat ×2–3/week for 3–5 weeks. Patients must continue exposure to sunlight to maintain tolerance. Repeat annually if tolerance is not maintained.
  - Hydroxychloroquine can be helpful in some cases.

Box 16.5 The idiopathic photodermatoses

The pathogenesis of the idiopathic photodermatoses is incompletely understood. All are uncommon or rare, apart from PLE.

Common

- PLE: usually presents under age 30. Onset within hours of sun exposure, not minutes. Symmetrical rash (usually papulonodular or eczematous) that affects skin covered in winter. (Differential diagnosis: subacute cutaneous LE; see ➲ p. 402.)

Uncommon

- Juvenile spring eruption: mainly boys in spring/summer. Itching, uncomfortable papules and vesicles on exposed helices of the ears. Usually the rest of the skin is not affected. Generally, the rash spontaneously resolves within 1–2 weeks but can recur.
- Solar urticaria: may arise at any age. Itchy urticarial wheals appear within a few minutes of exposure to sunlight and last for <24h. (Differential diagnosis: drug-induced photosensitivity, erythropoietic protoporphyria.) Action spectra: UVA, UVB, and visible, including fluorescent, lights. Antihistamines and desensitization may be helpful.
- Chronic actinic dermatitis: most often elderly men (90%) with multiple contact allergies. Action spectra: UVB, UVA ± visible. Compositae (plants) commonest contact allergy. Potent immunosuppressants, such as azathioprine, are often required.

Rare

- Actinic prurigo: presents in childhood, commonest in American Indians/Mexicans. In the UK, strongly associated with HLA-DR4, in particular HLA-DRB1 0407. Itching papules evolve into chronic nodules and plaques. Rash is maximal in spring and summer. All exposed skin is affected but may involve covered sites (e.g. buttocks), so diagnosis often missed. May simulate atopic eczema. Solar cheilitis of the lower lip and conjunctivitis are common. Leaves pitted or linear scars. Usually resolves in early adulthood.
- Hydroa vacciniforme: presents in childhood, usually boys. Rash within minutes of exposure. Tender, itching, erythematous papules evolve into haemorrhagic vesicles that crust and heal, leaving chickenpox-like scars. Associated with EBV infection (Japanese). Usually spontaneous improvement by adulthood.
- Brachioradial pruritus: stinging or burning pain in the skin of forearms. Prevalence unknown. No rash. May be a form of light-induced chronic neuropathic damage (see ➲ Box 27.1, p. 548).

Further reading

Bylaite M et al. Br J Dermatol 2009;**161** Suppl 3:61–8.
Murphy GM. J Photochem Photobiol B: Biol 2001;**64**:93–8.

Porphyria

What is porphyria?

The porphyrias are a group of disorders caused by genetic or acquired partial deficiencies in one of the enzymes in the metabolic pathway for haem. Haem precursors accumulate in urine, faeces, plasma, and/or erythrocytes. Disease may be acute neurovisceral, non-acute cutaneous, or mixed (see Table 16.2).

Acute neurovisceral attacks are associated with a rise in 5-aminolevulinate and porphobilinogen. Blisters/skin fragility caused by accumulation of water-soluble porphyrins (uroporphyrin and coproporphyrin) in PCT, variegate porphyria, and hereditary coproporphyria. Painful photosensitivity is caused by raised protoporphyrin in EPP.

Although mutations reduce the activity of the enzymes by 50%, most (80%) of those who inherit an AD porphyria remain asymptomatic. Other factors that increase the demand for haem and/or decrease enzyme activity are required for the diseases to be expressed.

Acute porphyria: what should I look for?

* Episodic neurovisceral attacks that start between age 15 and 35.
* Commoner in ♀ (less likely after menopause).
* Severe pain (usually abdominal), nausea, vomiting, constipation.
* Hypertension, tachycardia, low sodium.
* Neurological/psychiatric signs: psychological upset, convulsions, muscle weakness.
* Trigger: e.g. drugs (oestrogens, progesterones, barbiturates, sulfonamides, tetracyclines, etc.), alcohol, infection, calorie restriction.
* Cutaneous involvement (none in acute intermittent porphyria but may be seen in some acute porphyrias, e.g. variegate porphyria). Skin fragility, blisters, milia, erosions, and/or scars on exposed sites such as dorsum of hands or face (like PCT; see ➲ p. 332).

Acute porphyria: what should I do?

* Remove precipitants, e.g. drugs, including recreational drugs.
* Treat symptoms—fluids (monitor sodium), analgesia, antiemetics.
* Collect a random fresh sample of urine during the attack to measure porphyrins. Protect the fresh specimen from light (see Box 16.4). Analyse faecal and plasma porphyrins to determine the type of acute porphyria. Urinary, faecal, and plasma porphyrin concentrations may return to normal during remission in all the AD acute porphyrias.
* Consider early administration of IV haem arginate to suppress the production of haem precursors.
* Screen family members.

Table 16.2 Classification of the porphyrias

Porphyria and inheritance	Enzyme deficiency	Clinical	Comment
Porphyria cutanea tarda (PCT) Sporadic (80%) = type I; AD (20%) = type 2	Uroporphyrinogen decarboxylase	Non-acute. *Skin only*. Blisters, skin fragility, erosions over photoexposed sites, pigmentation. Increased risk of hepatocellular carcinoma	*Common type* Acquired or inherited
Erythropoietic protoporphyria (EPP) AD	Ferrochelatase	Non-acute. *Skin only*. Burning, erythema/oedema of light-exposed skin. Baby cries on exposure to sun. Subtle scars on nose. Risk of cholestasis and liver failure	*Commonest AD type in children*
Congenital erythropoietic porphyria (Gunther disease). May have led to folklore of werewolves emerging at night to avoid sunlight AR	Uroporphyrinogen III	Non-acute. Severe photosensitivity, mutilating scarring, hypertrichosis, red teeth, haemolytic anaemia. Dark urine—stains napkin purplish red	Very rare. Presents in infancy.
Acute intermittent porphyria AD	Hydroxymethylbilane synthase	Acute neurovisceral attacks. *Skin unaffected*. Risk of liver cancer/renal failure	*Commonest acute porphyria*
Variegate porphyria AD; founder mutation explains prevalence in South Africa/Chile	Protoporphyrinogen oxidase	Acute neurovisceral attacks (20%) or blisters like PCT (60%) or both (20%)	Common in South Africa/Chile
Hereditary coproporphyria AD	Coproporphyrinogen oxidase	Acute neurovisceral attacks. Blisters like PCT (30%)	Very rare

Very rare variants have not been included, e.g. ALA dehydratase deficiency porphyria, homozygous variants of AD porphyrias.

Further reading

British Porphyria Association. Available at: ℗ http://www.porphyria.org.uk/.
Welsh Medicines Information Centre and Cardiff Porphyria Service. *Drugs that are considered to be SAFE for use in the acute porphyrias*. Available at: ℗ http://www.wmic.wales.nhs.uk/pdfs/porphyria/2015%20Porphyria%20safe%20list.pdf.

Porphyria cutanea tarda

PCT, the commonest porphyria, is the only type that may be either sporadic (80% of cases) or familial (AD). Reduced activity of uroporphyrinogen decarboxylase results in overproduction of photoactive porphyrins. Uroporphyrinogen decarboxylase is inactivated by an iron-dependent process that is not fully understood, but a variety of factors can initiate disease (see Box 16.6).

Water-soluble porphyrins cause skin fragility and blistering on exposed skin. Uroporphyrin also stimulates fibroblasts to produce collagen in the skin, and this may explain some of the cutaneous features.

What should I look for?

PCT only affects the skin and is commonest in men. The presentation is subacute, and the relationship to sun exposure may be missed.

- Skin fragility: minor knocks produce erosions on the dorsum of the hands.
- Itching or burning may precede blisters on sun-exposed skin.
- Haemorrhagic vesicles, bullae, and crusted erosions, most often affecting exposed skin on the dorsum of the hands, face, and upper chest (see Fig. 16.3).
- Superficial scars or milia (firm, white, pinhead-sized papules—sequelae of subepidermal blisters) (see → Epidermolysis bullosa acquisita, p. 272).
- Dystrophic calcification.
- Hypertrichosis usually starts on the temples and affects the cheeks and/or forehead.
- Blisters beneath the nail plate; painful discoloration (yellow, blue, or haemorrhagic) of the nail; loss of the lunula, onycholysis, or dystrophy.
- Diffuse or reticulated hyperpigmentation of sun-exposed skin.
- Waxy, yellowish thickening of sun-exposed skin ('sclerodermoid').
- Normal teeth (unlike congenital erythropoietic porphyria).
- Normal mucosa (involved in some autoimmune blistering diseases).

What should I do?

- Confirm the diagnosis, and exclude pseudoporphyria (see → p. 334) by measuring porphyrins in fresh samples of urine and stool (see → pp. 330–1). Fresh urine containing excess uroporphyrins is pink and fluoresces bright coral pink under UVA light (Wood light).
- Biopsy a fresh blister for histology: subepidermal cell-poor blister, periodic acid–Schiff (PAS)-positive glycoproteins at the BMZ and around blood vessels, and, for direct IMF, Igs deposited at the BMZ and around blood vessels.
- Exclude risk factors, including hepatitis C (see Box 16.6).
- Withdraw precipitating factors, including alcohol and oestrogens.
- Advise strict sun protection (see → pp. 338–9).
- Regular venesection (400–500mL every 2 weeks for 3–6 months) depletes iron stores. Alternatively, desferrioxamine can be helpful.
- Consider prescribing low-dose hydroxychloroquine (100–125mg ×2/week)—higher doses may cause hepatitis.
- Monitor for the development of hepatocellular carcinoma.

Box 16.6 Risk factors for adult porphyria cutanea tarda

Factors that reduce the activity of uroporphyrinogen decarboxylase in the liver can initiate disease in genetically susceptible individuals.
- Alcohol.
- Oral oestrogens: oral contraception and hormone replacement therapy.
- Oral iron.
- Mutations in the hereditary haemochromatosis (HFE) gene.
- Hepatitis C virus infection.
- HIV infection.
- Polychlorinated hydrocarbons.
- Chronic haemodialysis (azotaemia reduces the activity of uroporphyrinogen decarboxylase; porphyrins are inadequately cleared by haemodialysis). Check plasma and faecal porphyrins, as urinary testing is difficult to interpret if the patient is on dialysis. If porphyrins are normal, consider pseudoporphyria (see ➲ p. 334). Venesection is usually contraindicated in renal failure, and hydroxychloroquine is ineffective. Human erythropoietin reduces iron stores and may be an effective treatment.

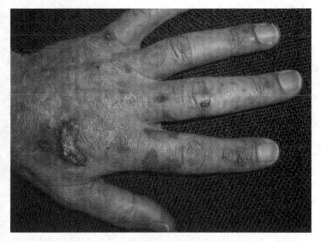

Fig. 16.3 Porphyria cutanea tarda: fragile skin on the back of the hand with crusted erosions and scars.

What is pseudoporphyria?

Pseudoporphyria is an acquired photosensitive blistering disease, with clinical and immunohistological features similar to PCT. The pathogenesis is uncertain, but porphyrins are normal.

Patients have PCT-like blistering, erosions, milia, and scars on sun-exposed skin (see Fig. 16.3), but, unlike PCT, patients rarely have hyperpigmentation, hypertrichosis, sclerodermoid changes, or dystrophic calcification.

Causes include:
- Chronic renal failure, haemodialysis, peritoneal dialysis (the antioxidant acetylcysteine may be an effective treatment) (see Box 16.6).
- UVA tanning beds, PUVA, excess sun exposure (generally women).
- A wide range of drugs, including:
  - NSAIDs (most frequent cause): naproxen and others (generally in women).
  - Antibiotics: nalidixic acid, tetracycline, ampicillin–sulbactam, cefepime, fluoroquinolones.
  - Antifungals: voriconazole.
  - Diuretics: furosemide, bumetanide.
  - Antiarrhythmics: amiodarone.
  - Sulfones: dapsone.
  - Vitamins: brewer's yeast, pyridoxine.
  - Retinoids: isotretinoin, etretinate.
  - Muscle relaxants: carisoprodol.
  - Anti-androgens: flutamide.

Further reading

Green JJ and Manders SM. *J Am Acad Dermatol* 2001;44:100–8.

Erythropoietic protoporphyria

EPP, caused by reduced activity of ferrochelatase, is a rare form of porphyria, presenting in childhood. Intense pain may cause infants to cry bitterly within minutes of sun exposure, but, as signs are subtle and the skin can look almost normal between episodes, the diagnosis is often missed. In 2% of cases, EPP is complicated by progressive liver failure.

What should I look for?

- Acute episodes of cutaneous photosensitivity that started in infancy. Window glass is not protective (sensitivity to UVA and visible light). Light reflected off snow, sand, or water may cause symptoms.
- Symptoms start in spring but reduce in autumn and winter.
- Burning, tingling, stinging, pain, and/or itching in light-exposed skin occurs within minutes of sun exposure. Children may try to relieve symptoms by plunging the hands into cold water.
- Erythema, urticaria, and/or swelling within minutes of sun exposure.
- Occasionally purpuric lesions, following sun exposure.
- Waxy skin thickening over the knuckles and on the nose.
- Subtle elliptical scars on the nose, cheeks, and/or dorsum of the hands.

What should I do?

- Check porphyrins: protoporphyrin is raised in erythrocytes and stool; urine porphyrins are not increased.
- Check FBC: some patients are anaemic.
- Advise on photoprotection (lifestyle, broad-spectrum sunscreens, clothing, UV-blocking films for window glass in home and car) (see ➔ pp. 338–9).
- Oral β-carotene taken from February until October may reduce photosensitivity, although efficacy variable. Patients may not tolerate the unsightly orange pigmentation.
- UVB phototherapy may improve tolerance to sunlight (probably the most effective treatment).
- Monitor for cholestasis and progressive liver damage.

⚠ Xeroderma pigmentosum

This rare AR photodermatosis affects all races and has an equal sex incidence (2.3 million cases/million live births in Western Europe). Patients develop premature photodamage, skin cancers, and ocular abnormalities. Thirty percent of patients develop progressive neurological disorders. The disease is devastating, and cutaneous malignancies cause early death (see Box 16.7). Normally, photodamaged DNA is excised and repaired with newly synthesized DNA (excision repair), but XP cells are unable to repair damaged DNA (see Box 16.7). The defect affects all cell types. Patients have an increased risk of cutaneous and ocular malignancy, as well as malignancy in other tissues, e.g. oral cavity, breast, lung, liver, gastric, renal, and brain.

Skin is normal at birth, but XP presents within the first few years and has a major impact on the lifestyle of the child and their family. Clinical features vary, but fair-skinned children are the most severely affected.

What should I look for?

- Easy sunburn that usually presents within the first 2 years of life.
- UVB-induced erythema that is delayed in onset and peaks in 2–3 days, rather than the usual 24h.
- A history of blistering or burning after very little sun exposure.
- Photophobia in young children.
- Dryness of sun-exposed skin (xeroderma).
- Irregular freckling appears in the first year of life on exposed skin.
- Scarring of exposed skin.
- Signs of premature photodamage—mottled hyperpigmented patches, hypopigmented macules, telangiectasia.
- Hyperkeratotic lower lip (solar cheilitis).
- Eyelid freckling, loss of lashes, ectropion, conjunctival telangiectasia, dry eyes, and corneal damage, leading to visual impairment.
- Solar keratoses (premalignant change).
- Skin cancers develop in all (median onset age 8 years)—BCC, SCC, melanoma.
- Parents with a history of skin cancers, but no other signs of XP.

Management

- The diagnosis is confirmed by skin biopsy and demonstration of the DNA repair defect in cultured fibroblasts.
- Care should be provided by a multidisciplinary team that may include paediatricians, dermatologists, ophthalmologists, neurologists, cancer specialist nurses, and plastic surgeons.
- ⚠ *It is crucial to protect the skin from photodamage* to slow the onset of life-threatening cutaneous malignancies (see ➲ pp. 338–9).
- Carers and/or patients should examine the skin regularly for signs of skin cancer. Cancers are treated surgically.
- Oral retinoids may reduce the incidence of skin cancer.
- Patients should be protected from cigarette smoke.
- Encourage patients to join XP Patient Support Group (see Box 16.8).

Box 16.7 What is xeroderma pigmentosum?

- XP is an AR disorder caused by defects in one of seven nuclear excision repair (*NER*) genes. Some XP genes are also involved in other processes, e.g. transcription and recombination.
- XP patients are photosensitive and prone to premature skin cancers, as well as internal malignancies, but patients are a clinically heterogeneous group.
- Patients were separated into different groups when it was found that the defect in excision repair in a cultured cell line from one XP patient could be corrected by fusion with a cell line from a different, unrelated XP patient. Patients whose cell lines failed to complement each other in culture were grouped together.
- Seven complementation groups have been identified (XP-A to XP-G).
- Wide variability in clinical features both between and within XP complementation groups, in part explained by the precise pathogenic mutation.
- XP-C is the commonest complementation group worldwide.
- Twenty percent of patients (mostly XP-A and XP-D) have progressive neurological abnormalities, e.g. hyporeflexia, intellectual disability, seizures, deafness, ataxia, quadriparesis. Accumulated DNA damage may cause degeneration of neural tissue, which cannot be replaced.
- Thirty percent of XP patients belong to a variant group (XP-V) with a less severe phenotype. XP-V patients have normal nuclear excision repair, but abnormal post-replicational DNA repair caused by defective DNA polymerase.
- Investigation into the genetic basis of XP has provided insights into DNA repair and the pathogenesis of cutaneous malignancy.

Box 16.8 XP Support Group

The XP Support Group is a UK charitable trust (available at: ℘ http://xpsupportgroup.org.uk/). The group supports patients and their families, keeps members up-to-date with the latest research, provides information on XP, and offers practical advice on a wide range of topics, including:

- How to deal with schools and education authorities.
- Where to obtain UV protective clothing and UV protective clear window film.
- Grants for UV protective products.
- Annual Owl Patrol night-time camps for children and their families.

Further reading

Daya-Grosjean L and Sarasin A. *Mutat Res* 2005;**571**:43–56.
DiGiovanna JJ and Kraemer KH. *J Invest Dermatol* 2012;**132**(3 Pt 2):785–96.
Fassihi H. *Br J Dermatol* 2015;**172**:859–60.

Photoprotection

Patients with photosensitivity disorders must protect their skin from the solar radiation that is responsible—UVA, UVB, visible light, or a combination. Severe photosensitivity can have a catastrophic impact on lifestyle—outdoor activities may be impossible. Sunscreens, clothing, hats, and shade (indoor activities when the sun is strongest between 11.00 a.m. and 3.00 p.m.) provide more effective photoprotection than sunscreens.

Clothing, hats, sunglasses, and windows

- Clothing and hats should have a tight weave, sufficiently thick to block transmission of visible light (check the transmission of visible light by trying to look through the item held up to the sun).
- Clothing should be loose-fitting (photoprotective fabrics are available). Patients should wear hats with broad brims (baseball caps do not protect the ears or neck), as well as a flap of cloth to cover the neck, shirts with long sleeves, trousers—not shorts, and shoes, rather than sandals. Some patients may need gloves for driving.
- UV-blocking films can be obtained for window glass, car windows, and fluorescent lights, if required.
- Sunglasses (wrap-around) to protect against UV radiation and blue light.

Sunscreens

(See Boxes 16.9 and 16.10.)
- Sunscreens may be physical or chemical.
- Physical sunscreens (sunblocks): opaque creams containing particles (titanium dioxide, zinc oxide) reflect and scatter UVR (UVB and UVA) and visible light. Physical sunscreens are less cosmetically acceptable than chemical sunscreens, but more effective and safer (see Box 16.10, **➔** Box 17.3, p. 347, and Box 17.4, p. 347).
- Chemical sunscreens absorb UVR of certain wavelengths, either UVB or UVA. UVB chemical sunscreens protect against UVB-induced sunburn by blocking UVB. They contain cinnamates and other agents. UVA chemical sunscreens provide limited protection and contain chemicals such as oxybenzone. New dual UVB/UVA filters and photon absorbers are being developed.
- Chemical sunscreens may cause contact dermatitis (irritant or allergic).
- Patients using a UVB-absorbing sunscreen that prevents immediate erythema or sunburn should be warned not to stay out longer in the sun, to prevent exposure to excessive UVA.
- Lips should be protected, as well as the skin.
- The potential of topical or oral antioxidants to reduce photodamage is being investigated.
- Patients avoiding UVB may become vitamin D-deficient (see Box 16.11).

Box 16.9 How much UV protection is provided by the sunscreen?

- The sun protection factor (SPF) indicates the UVB photoprotection provided by a sunscreen. An SPF of 10 means that it takes ten times longer for the skin to go red than unprotected skin exposed to the same amount of UVB. An SPF of 20–30 is adequate for most patients.
- The star rating (maximum 5) indicates the percentage of UVA absorbed in comparison to UVB. The UVA protection should be at least 1/3 of the labelled SPF.

Box 16.10 Why is the sunscreen ineffective?

- The sunscreen is not blocking the appropriate wavelengths. Broad-spectrum combination sunscreens with an SPF of at least 15 and a high UVA protection are the most effective.
- The sunscreen is not applied sufficiently thickly (at least six teaspoons of lotion are needed to cover the body of an average adult). Opaque sunblock creams do not have to be applied very thickly to be effective.
- The sunscreen is not applied evenly to the skin or to all exposed skin, including lips, sides of the neck, ears, and temples.
- The sunscreen is not reapplied every 2–3h or straight after swimming or activities causing sweating.
- Patient allergic to the sunscreen (refer for photopatch testing).
- Recommend physical barriers—sunglasses, clothing, hats, and shade—rather than encouraging patients to rely on sunscreens.

Box 16.11 Advice on optimal vitamin D synthesis

- UVB triggers conversion of 7-dehydrocholesterol in the skin to pre-vitamin D. Adequate levels of vitamin D are maintained if 15% of the body (face, arms, legs) receives about 1/3 of the minimal erythematogenic dose of UVB on most days of the week. In the UK, this equates to 15min of sun exposure on the arms, legs, and/or face ×3/week from May to September (during the rest of the year, sunlight at this latitude is insufficient for vitamin D synthesis).
- Patients who are very photosensitive and cannot tolerate any UVB radiation should take vitamin D supplements.
- Vitamin D supplements may also be needed by individuals living in countries with low levels of UV for much of the year.
- Vitamin D deficiency is common in the elderly, people with darker skin, or those who cover the skin when outdoors.

Further reading

González S et al. Clin Dermatol 2008;26:614–26.
Hollick F. Adv Exp Med Biol 2014;810:1–16.

Chapter 17

Tumours

Contents

> ### Relevant pages in other chapters
> The history and examination in patients with skin tumours are discussed on ➜ pp. 26–7 and p. 42. Also see ➜ Chapter 16, Sun and skin, pp. 319–39; Familial cancer syndromes, pp. 542–4; Tumours in childhood, pp. 594–99; Mastocytoma, Box 31.5, p. 593.

Common benign non-melanocytic tumours

Seborrhoeic wart

Also known as seborrhoeic keratosis or basal cell papilloma.

Benign epidermal tumours of unknown cause. Common in the elderly. They are commonest on the trunk but also affect the face and limbs. Patients may have one, several, or hundreds. Treatment is only required if the seborrhoeic wart is traumatized, when it may become inflamed or bleed, sometimes simulating a melanoma.

What should I look for?
- A well-defined oval, pigmented tumour, around 0.5–2cm in diameter, that appears stuck onto the surface of the skin.
- Rough surface that may feel slightly greasy. Dark pits studded over the surface—easier to see with magnification using dermoscopy.
- Colour can range from a pale pink-brown to dark brown or black.
- Seborrhoeic warts may be virtually flat or raised by several mm.

Chondrodermatitis nodularis helicis chronica

Nodules caused by prolonged pressure on the skin of the ear, but sun damage or cold may also play a part. The history is usually characteristic and differentiates this nodule from a skin cancer. The affected ear is generally the one on which the patient sleeps, and pain prevents from lying on that side. Apparently, nuns who wore wimples were affected by chondrodermatitis! Treatments include relieving pressure, topical or intralesional corticosteroids, cryotherapy and, surgery.

What should I look for?
- A tender nodule on the helix or, in women, the antihelix of the ear.
- A keratotic plug or a small ulcer in the centre of the nodule.

Dermatofibroma

Also known as fibrous histiocytoma or sclerosing haemangioma.

The localized proliferation of fibroblasts is probably triggered by minor trauma such as an insect bite. These benign growths are common in young women. If you can make a confident diagnosis, no treatment is required—excision will merely leave another scar. Multiple dermatofibromas have been reported in conditions such as HIV infection, SLE, and other diseases in which the immune state is altered.

What should I look for?
- A brownish red dermal nodule, 0.5–1cm in diameter, usually on the arm, shoulder, thigh, or leg.
- The overlying epidermis is usually smooth.
- The lesion is firm—this suggests the diagnosis.
- A central scar seen under dermoscopy with pseudo-pigmentation peripherally.
- Pinch the skin gently on each side of the tumour, and it will sink down into the dermis—the 'buttonhole sign' or 'dimple sign'.

Pyogenic granuloma

Typically, this vascular tumour presents at the site of a penetrating injury, e.g. rose thorn, usually on the fingers, lips, or face (see Fig. 17.1).

⚠ An amelanotic malignant melanoma or SCC may look like a pyogenic granuloma (see Fig. 17.11)—always ask the patient if anything preceded the development of the tumour. Was there a 'mole' at the site, or did it arise on normal skin? Always send excised lesions for histological examination.

What should I look for?

- A history of rapid growth: pyogenic granulomas grow on previously normal skin over a period of weeks to a size of 0.5–4cm.
- Fleshy vascular tumour composed of friable granulation tissue that bleeds readily on contact.
- Exclude any underlying pigmented lesion: inspect any 'pyogenic granuloma' at an atypical site particularly carefully, using a dermatoscope, if possible. Melanin can be mistaken for old haemorrhage.

Other common benign tumours or inflammatory nodules

Epidermal

- Viral infections, e.g. viral wart (see ➔ pp. 160–1) or molluscum contagiosum (see ➔ p. 158).
- Nodular prurigo (caused by chronic rubbing) (see ➔ Fig. 10.6, p. 223).
- Epidermal naevus (warty lesion, present since infancy) (see ➔ p. 560).

Dermal

- Epidermoid cyst or 'sebaceous' cyst: although not sebaceous at all, but arises from the upper part of the hair follicle. Has a punctum. Often becomes inflamed and ruptures.
- Pilar cyst: arises from the lower part of the follicle and usually found in the scalp—no punctum. Spontaneous rupture uncommon.
- Keloid: dense fibrous scar tissue spreading beyond the original wound.
- Spider naevus; Campbell de Morgan spot (cherry angioma).
- Infantile haemangioma (strawberry naevus) (see ➔ pp. 596–7).
- Neurofibroma (see ➔ Fig. 27.1, p. 555 and pp. 552–4).
- Xanthelasma or xanthoma (see ➔ p. 470).

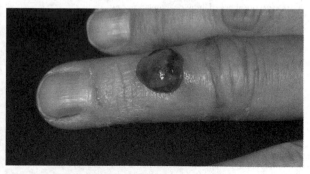

Fig. 17.1 Pyogenic granuloma—a friable vascular papule.

Common benign melanocytic tumours

Melanocytic naevus ('mole' or 'naevus')

(See Fig. 17.2.)

Melanocytic naevi present at birth, in childhood, or in young adults.

- Acquired melanocytic naevi start as flat, evenly pigmented (junctional) naevi in which melanocytes collect in small groups (nests) along the basal epidermal layer (see Figs. 17.3 and 17.4). As melanocytes migrate down into the dermis, flat moles evolve into raised, evenly pigmented, dome-shaped papules (compound melanocytic naevi, Fig. 17.4), sometimes hairy.
- Scalp naevi in children may be an early sign of being 'moley'. Patients with many moles tend to have a 'signature naevus', i.e. all their moles follow a pigmentation pattern that is characteristic for that patient. This is more easily visualized using dermoscopy.
- Over time, the epidermal component is lost, and moles change into flesh-coloured or pale brown papules (intradermal melanocytic naevi), before disappearing in old age. A new pigmented growth in an elderly patient is much more likely to be a seborrhoeic wart, solar lentigo (see next section), or melanoma than a melanocytic naevus.
- Congenital melanocytic naevi, usually >1cm in diameter (sometimes large and disfiguring = bathing trunk naevus) present at birth/early neonatal period. Large congenital melanocytic naevi >20cm and the presence of multiple satellite naevi are associated with an increased risk of malignant change and should be monitored.
- Halo naevi: a white ring develops around a benign melanocytic naevus which gradually disappears, leaving a depigmented macule that usually eventually repigments. Halo naevi are common in adolescence and of no significance. Halo naevi in adults (age 40–50 years) may indicate melanoma elsewhere—check the skin, eyes, and mucosal surfaces (see Fig. 17.5).

Lentigo (plural = lentigines)

- Simple lentigines are small, round, flat, evenly pigmented lesions that persist in winter, unlike freckles. The basal layer of the epidermis has increased numbers of individual melanocytes.
- Numerous simple lentigines are found in some genetic disorders, e.g. Multiple lentigines syndrome, Carney complex, Peutz–Jeghers syndrome (see ➲ p. 613).
- Solar (senile) lentigines, 3–12mm in diameter, are flat, brown marks present on sun-damaged skin in older patients.

Mongolian spot

- Slate-coloured macular areas of pigmentation are present in newborns—usually on the buttocks or sacrum where pigment may simulate a bruise and even be misdiagnosed as a sign of non-accidental injury (see ➲ Fig. 31.10, p. 615).
- Mongolian spots are commonest in black or Asian infants and gradually disappear with age.
- Melanocytes are deep within the dermis, and therefore pigment appears bluish, rather than brown.

Blue naevi

- Benign acquired small slate-blue to blue-black macules or papules that present most often on the dorsum of the hand or on the scalp.
- Melanocytes are present in the dermis, and tumours appear blue, rather than brown.

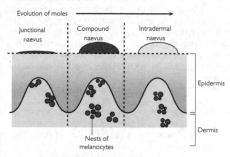

Fig. 17.2 Evolution of melanocytic naevi ('moles').

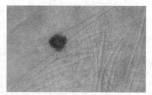

Fig. 17.3 Junctional melanocytic naevus. Flat and evenly pigmented. Reproduced with permission from Lewis-Jones, Sue (ed). Paediatric Dermatology, Oxford University Press 2010.

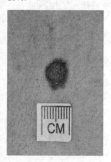

Fig. 17.4 Compound melanocytic naevus, with a central raised component and a flat rim of pigmentation. Reproduced with permission from Lewis-Jones, Sue (ed). Paediatric Dermatology, Oxford University Press 2010.

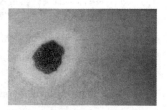

Fig. 17.5 Halo naevus. This mole has developed a rim of depigmentation. The mole will slowly disappear. Reproduced with permission from Lewis-Jones, Sue (ed). Paediatric Dermatology, Oxford University Press 2010.

Avoiding skin cancer

Excess UVR is the main cause of skin cancer (see Boxes 17.1 and 17.2). Encourage people to enjoy outdoor activities (some UVB maintains the levels of vitamin D), but those who have signs of sun damage, such as solar keratoses or skin cancers, or are taking immunosuppressive drugs should limit sun exposure (be sun-smart) and avoid sunburn. Spring and winter sunshine in the UK has insufficient UVB to promote much synthesis of vitamin D, but adequate levels of vitamin D will be maintained for most people through everyday exposure to the sun in the summer months, e.g. if the arms, legs, and/or face receive about 15min of sun exposure three times a week.

For more about the sun and skin, including information about vitamin D, photoprotection, and sunscreens, see ➜ Chapter 16, pp. 338–9.

A tan signals that the skin has been trying to protect itself from damage, while sunburn is foolish, unnecessary, and painful. Practical sun safety tips have been provided in the UK Shunburn campaign and Australian 'Slip–Slop–Slap–Seek–Slide' (see Boxes 17.3 and 17.4).

For signs of chronic sun damage (photoageing), see ➜ Box 3.1, p. 43.

Box 17.1 Ultraviolet radiation and skin cancer

- UVB is more photocarcinogenic than UVA, but both contribute to the pathogenesis of skin cancer by damaging DNA.
- Photodamaged DNA is usually repaired by nucleotide excision repair enzymes. Repair declines with age. Cumulative mutations lead to skin cancer by affecting the function of genes that regulate cell proliferation (oncogenes, e.g. *RAS*; tumour suppressor genes, e.g. *p53*) (see ➜ pp. 336–7).
- UV-induced immunosuppression may predispose to skin cancer by interfering with the recognition and elimination of abnormal cells.
- Fair skin types I and II with red or blond hair, and severe sunburn in childhood or adolescence, increase the risk of developing skin cancer.
- Chronic cumulative UVR, including PUVA (>200 treatments) and sunbeds, also predispose to skin cancer.
- Chronic photosensitivity (e.g. drug-induced) with accelerated photoageing increases the risk of skin cancer. Interactions between UVR and immunosuppressant drugs, e.g. azathioprine, photosensitize the skin to UVA, resulting in carcinogenesis.

Further reading

British Association of Dermatologists. *Sun awareness leaflets and posters.* Available at: ℰ http://www.bad.org.uk/for-the-public/sun-awareness-campaign/sun-awareness-leaflets-and-posters.
NHS UK. *Consensus vitamin D position statement.* Available at: ℰ http://www.nhs.uk/livewell/summerhealth/documents/concensus_statement%20_vitd_dec_2010.pdf.
UK SunSmart campaigns. Available at: ℰ http://www.sunsmart.org.uk/.
van Lümig PP et al. *J Eur Acad Dermatol Venereol* 2015;29:752–60.

Box 17.2 Other risk factors for skin cancer

- BCC: previous BCC, X-irradiation, immunosuppression (organ transplant, see ➲ pp. 500–1), HIV, chronic lymphocytic leukaemia, see ➲ Box 26.9, p. 541), chronic arsenic exposure, genetic conditions (Gorlin syndrome, see ➲ p. 542; albinism; XP).
- SCC: Bowen disease or solar keratosis, previous SCC, pipe smoker (lip), X-irradiation, thermal burns, immunosuppression (organ/bone marrow transplants, see ➲ pp. 500–1), HIV, chronic lymphocytic leukaemia, HPV infection, chronic wounds (sinuses, scars, or ulcers), tar, chronic arsenic exposure, *MC1R* gene variants (impaired UV protection responses), genetic conditions (albinism, XP), drugs (e.g. BRAF inhibitors), voriconazole.
- Melanoma: previous melanoma, >50 melanocytic naevi or many atypical (dysplastic) melanocytic naevi; giant 'bathing trunk' >20cm in diameter congenital melanocytic naevus (melanoma may develop early in childhood in large congenital lesions), *MC1R* gene variants (impaired UV protection responses), previous BCC/SCC, immunosuppression, family history of melanoma (mutations in *CDKN2A* and *CDK4* genes), genetic conditions (albinism, XP), drugs (e.g. BRAF inhibitors), other diseases (breast cancer, Parkinson disease, IBD).

(For XP, see ➲ pp. 336–7.)

Box 17.3 Slip–Slop–Slap–Seek–Slide (2007)

- Slip on a shirt: cover exposed skin with loose-fitting cotton clothing that has a tight weave.
- Slop on sunscreen cream (SPF30 or more) liberally and frequently to the face and other exposed skin, but creams are no substitute for hats, clothing, and a sensible lifestyle.
- Slap on a hat with a broad brim and tight weave (check how much light comes through the hat by holding it up to the sun). The neck should be protected, as well as the face and ears. Baseball caps do not provide adequate sun protection.
- Seek shade.
- Slide on wrap-around sunglasses to prevent sun damage.

Box 17.4 Shunburn Campaign 2014

- Cover up the skin—long-sleeved shirt, collar, long shorts/sarong.
- Slap on the sunscreens—use at least SPF30 generously.
- Wear a hat or cap; slip on the shades.
- Chill out in the shade. Reach for shade between 11 a.m. and 3 p.m.

Teenage Cancer Trust. *Shunburn: stay safe in the sun*. Available at: ℘ https://www.teenagecancertrust.org/what-we-do/education/shunburn/.

Premalignant epidermal lesions

Solar (actinic) keratosis

Solar keratoses are premalignant lesions (the epidermal basal cell layer is dysplastic) that indicate chronic sun damage and are a marker of the risk of developing skin cancer (see Fig. 17.6). About 20% regress spontaneously. Progression of single lesions to SCC is uncommon (<1 in 1000 per annum). Areas of coalescing solar keratoses on sun-damaged skin, i.e. 'actinic field change', have a higher risk of progression to SCC, particularly in the context of immunosuppression.

What should I look for?
- Asymptomatic or slightly itchy, brownish red, discrete scaly/keratotic patches on sun-exposed skin: bald scalp, face, helix of the ear, dorsum of the hands, and forearms (see Fig. 17.6).
- Some may be raised and warty: hypertrophic solar keratosis.
- Pain, induration, inflammation, or ulceration (suggests progression to SCC). Signs of chronic sun damage, including skin tumours: BCC, SCC, malignant melanoma.

What should I do?
- Advise patients to monitor their skin for development of skin cancers and to protect their skin from the sun (see ➲ p. 346).
- Treatment, e.g. cryosurgery, is only required if keratoses are troublesome. Topical treatments are effective for confluent areas of field change, e.g. topical diclofenac, fluorouracil, imiquimod, ingenol mebutate, or photodynamic therapy.

Bowen disease (SCC *in situ*)

Characterized by full-thickness epidermal dysplasia. Peak incidence in seventh decade. Only about 3–5% of plaques progress to SCC—but the risk of metastasis from SCC is increased. Aetiologies: chronic sun exposure (including sunbeds), radiation, oncogenic HPV (HPV-16 associated with anogenital, palmoplantar, and periungual SCC *in situ*), immunosuppression, and arsenic (lesions in sun-protected areas). Plaques are asymptomatic and enlarge slowly over years. Often misdiagnosed as 'discoid eczema' or 'ringworm' but fails to respond to treatment for these conditions.

What should I look for?
- A well-defined erythematous scaly or warty plaque (see Fig. 17.7).
- A flat edge: stretch the skin gently, and inspect the edge closely. A raised thready border suggests a superficial BCC, rather than Bowen disease.
- Dermoscopy shows glomerular vessels (focal nests of tortuous vessels resembling vessels in the renal glomerulus) with scaling.
- Nodularity or ulceration: this may indicate progression to SCC.

What should I do?
- Take a skin scrape to exclude a fungal infection, if indicated.
- Take a skin biopsy to confirm the diagnosis.

Treatment options include surgical removal (shave excision), topical fluorouracil, topical imiquimod, or photodynamic therapy. Patients should protect their skin from the sun (see ➡ p. 346).

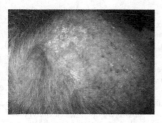

Fig. 17.6 Actinic field change: numerous solar keratoses arising in sun-damaged skin, with background solar lentigines (pigmented macules) and erythema.

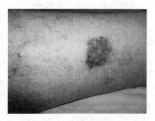

Fig. 17.7 Bowen disease: an asymptomatic scaly plaque on the leg. The differential includes tinea, eczema, and a superficial basal cell carcinoma.

Further reading

de Berker D et al. *Br J Dermatol* 2007;**56**:222–30. Available at: ℅ http://www.bad.org.uk/library-media/documents/Actinic_keratoses_guidelines_2007.pdf.

Morton CA et al. *Br J Dermatol* 2014;**170**:245–60. Available at: ℅ http://www.bad.org.uk/library-media/documents/SCC_in_situ_guidelines_2014.pdf.

Keratinocyte skin cancers (1)

Basal cell carcinoma (rodent ulcer, BCC)

BCC is the commonest skin cancer. BCCs grow slowly, virtually never metastasize, and are locally invasive. Some variants can be locally destructive. BCCs present predominantly in middle-aged Caucasians. (Also see ➲ Gorlin syndrome, p. 542.)

What should I look for?

- *Nodulocystic*: dome-shaped, pearly papule with telangiectasia coursing over the surface, more easily identified with dermoscopy, described as 'arborizing' vessels which are in focus when magnified. (Common on the face and neck.) Stretch the skin gently to accentuate the translucent appearance and borders. Older tumours may present as ulcerated nodules (rodent ulcers) with smooth rolled pearly edges and telangiectasia across the surface (see Fig. 17.8). Remove the loose crust, so you can see the granulating fleshy base.
- *Superficial*: one or more scaly erythematous plaques (most often on the trunk) with well-defined raised pearly edges. Stretch the skin gently to make the pearly border of superficial BCC more obvious, and differentiate from Bowen disease or fungal infection.
- *Pigmented*: any BCC may contain pigment flecks (seen as ovoid globules under dermoscopy), but heavily pigmented tumours can simulate melanoma. A pearly appearance provides clue to the correct diagnosis.
- *Morphoeic/infiltrative*: waxy, indurated plaque that may resemble a scar. The border may be difficult to define, even when the skin is stretched.

Squamous cell carcinoma

Cutaneous SCCs are the second commonest skin cancer (25% of all keratinocyte cancers). They usually present in elderly patients on sun-exposed sites and are three times commoner in men. Prognosis depends on the potential for metastasis, which is influenced by the anatomical site, pathological features of the tumour (rate of growth, depth, degree of differentiation), and host immune response (see Boxes 17.5 and 17.7).

What should I look for?

- A keratotic nodule or an ulcerated nodule with a granulating base and a rolled undermined border (see Fig. 17.9).
- Induration or ulceration of a solar keratosis or Bowen disease.
- Regional lymphadenopathy.

Keratoacanthoma

Perhaps best regarded as a well-differentiated SCC. These grow rapidly (<6 weeks), persist for 2–3 months, and then involute over 4–6 months, leaving a depressed scar. They are usually removed surgically for histological examination.

What should I look for?

- A history of rapid growth over <6 weeks.
- A pinkish symmetrical cup-shaped nodule, 1–2cm in diameter, on sun-damaged hair-bearing skin, usually the face or neck.
- Smooth rolled edges.
- A central keratin plug.

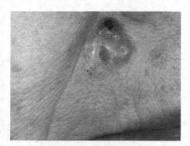

Fig. 17.8 Nodulocystic basal cell carcinoma with a pearly appearance.

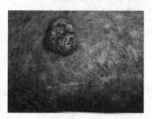

Fig. 17.9 Squamous cell carcinoma arising on severely sun-damaged skin, which is demonstrated by hypo- and hyperpigmentation.

Box 17.5 Prognostic 'high-risk' factors for squamous cell carcinoma

- High-risk anatomical sites:
  - Ear > nose = cutaneous lip = eyelid = scalp.
- Clinical diameter >20mm.
- Tumour depth >4mm (very high risk if >6mm).
- Histological features:
  - Perineural invasion.
  - Lymphovascular invasion.
  - Poorly differentiated.
  - Desmoplastic, adenosquamous, spindle cell, acantholytic, follicular subtypes.
- Squamous cell carcinoma arising within a site of:
  - Skin trauma, e.g. burns, scar tissue, or a radiotherapy field.
  - Pre-existing skin disease, e.g. venous leg ulceration or Bowen disease.
- Immunosuppression (see Box 17.7).
  - Increases the risk of multiple SCCs.
  - Increased the risk of metastases.

Keratinocyte skin cancers (2)

Treatment options for keratinocyte cancers
See Box 17.6.

Risk factors for skin cancer
see ➜ p. 346, and Box 17.7.

Box 17.6 Treatment options for keratinocyte cancers

Basal cell carcinoma

Choice of treatment depends on the age of the patient and the history, as well as the type and site of tumour, but options may include:

- Surgical excision (the gold standard); curettage and cautery.
- Mohs micrographic surgery: treatment of choice for locally recurrent skin cancers, cancers in sites where it is important to preserve tissue, e.g. adjacent to the eye/T-zone of the face, or cancers with ill-defined margins, e.g. morphoeic/infiltrative BCC.
- Topical imiquimod or topical fluorouracil: for superficial BCCs.
- Cryosurgery.
- Photodynamic therapy (PDT) (superficial BCC). Daylight PDT also demonstrated to be efficacious.
- Hedgehog signalling pathway inhibitors (Smoothened receptor inhibitors—vismodegib) (see ➜ p. 385).
  - Used to treat recurrent, locally invasive, or metastatic BCC.
  - Used to reduce the development of BCCs in Gorlin syndrome.
- Radiotherapy: second-line treatment for tumours not amenable to surgical intervention or as adjuvant therapy for keratinocyte tumours with perineural invasion.

Squamous cell carcinoma

- Surgical excision margins should aim to achieve complete histological clearance. For low-risk tumours, a clinical peripheral margin of 4mm is advised, and, in some situations, curettage and cautery is appropriate. For high-risk tumours (see Box 17.5), a peripheral margin of 6mm is advised.
- Mohs micrographic surgery can be considered in selected patients with high-risk tumours which might be at a critical anatomical site (as described for BCC).
- 1° radiotherapy can be used for tumours which are surgically challenging. Adjuvant radiotherapy should be considered for high-risk tumours or those with close or involved margins.

Box 17.7 Immunosuppression and skin cancer

- Immunosuppressed individuals are at significantly increased risk of developing skin cancers.
- This group includes, but is not limited to, solid organ transplant recipients, patients with haematological malignancies, e.g. chronic lymphocytic leukaemia and non-Hodgkin lymphoma, bone marrow transplant recipients, HIV-positive/AIDS patients, and individuals treated with prolonged immunosuppressant therapy, in particular azathioprine (which is a direct UV carcinogen), for any inflammatory condition, e.g. IBD.
- Skin cancer is the most frequent malignancy in organ transplant recipients and contributes to significant morbidity.
  - Non-melanoma skin cancers (SCC > BCC and other rare cancers, e.g. Merkel cell carcinoma, sebaceous tumours) are the commonest. Tumours tend to occur earlier, are multiple, behave more aggressively, and appear to have increased malignant potential. Early identification is essential, and these patients are best managed in a dedicated transplant dermatology clinic.
  - Melanoma is also increased in frequency, but prognosis only appears to be worse for thicker tumours.

Further reading

Cancer Research UK; *Skin cancer (non melanoma)*. Available at: ℅ http://www.cancerresearchuk.org/about-cancer/type/skin-cancer/.

Motley R et al. *Multi-professional guidelines for the management of the patient with primary cutaneous squamous cell carcinoma*. 2009. Available at: ℅ http://www.bad.org.uk/library-media/documents/SCC_2009.pdf.

Scottish Intercollegiate Guidelines Network. *SIGN 140: Management of primary cutaneous squamous cell carcinoma*. 2014. Available at: ℅ http://www.sign.ac.uk/pdf/QRG140.pdf.

Telfer NR et al. *Br J Dermatol* 2008;**159**:35–48. Available at: ℅ http://www.bad.org.uk/library-media/documents/BCC_2008.pdf.

Malignant melanoma

Malignant melanoma accounts for 5% of skin cancers, but incidence in the UK has quadrupled since the 1970s (>13 300 new cases in 2013). Melanoma is commoner in men than women, and almost 1/3 occur in people aged <50 (melanoma is the commonest cancer in young adults aged 15–34 years old). Superficial spreading melanoma (SSM) is the commonest type in Caucasians (see Box 17.8).

Most melanomas arise *de novo*; only 30–50% arise in pre-existing melanocytic naevi (usually SSM subtype). For risk factors, see ➔ pp. 346–7. Melanoma accounts for 75% of deaths associated with skin cancer.

What should I look for?

- Moles that are irregular in colour, outline, or shape (see Figs. 17.10, 17.11, and 17.12,).
- Use the ABCDE criteria to identify suspicious pigmented lesions:
  - Asymmetry in outline.
  - Border irregularity or blurring, sometimes with notching.
  - Colour variation (>3 colours) with shades of black, brown, and pink.
  - Diameter >6mm (cannot be covered by the end of a pencil).
  - Evolution: tumour that is changing in size, elevation, and/or colour.
- Moles that stand out or look different from the others, i.e. 'ugly duckling sign'. Better than ABCDE criteria for identifying nodular melanoma.
- New or changing longitudinal pigmented streaks in nails, especially if associated with damage to the nail.
- Pigment extending from the nail bed onto the skin of the nail fold (Hutchinson sign), suggesting melanoma, not subungual haematoma.
- Moles that are symptomatic (itching, swollen, tender), but, more often than not, these turn out to be irritated benign melanocytic naevi, rather than melanoma.
- Regional lymphadenopathy.

What should I do?

- Obtain a history of the tumour from the patient (see ➔ p. 26).
- Document risk factors (see Boxes 17.1 and 17.2).
- Record the findings, including the site and size of the lesion.
- Photography is helpful.
- Dermoscopy is a useful tool to monitor multiple atypical naevi.
- Refer any patient in whom you are concerned about a pigmented lesion for an urgent opinion. Prognosis is determined primarily by the Breslow thickness, and mortality increases significantly with increasing tumour thickness (see Tables 17.1 and 17.2).
- Dermoscopy, performed by an expert, may help with diagnosis (see ➔ p. 640).
- Excision is the treatment of choice for suspicious pigmented lesions.

Box 17.8 Types of cutaneous melanoma

- SSM (80–85%) is the commonest melanoma in Caucasians. Presents as a slowly enlarging, slightly raised, pigmented plaque with irregularity in colour and border. Eventually, a nodule appears within the plaque, indicating deep invasion. Most often on the trunk of men or legs of women (see Fig. 17.10).
- Nodular melanoma (10–15%) grows rapidly, invading deeply from the outset. If amelanotic (often some pigment can be seen using dermoscopy), may be misdiagnosed as a vascular tumour, e.g. pyogenic granuloma or SCC (see Fig. 17.11).
- Lentigo maligna melanoma (5%) arises within a slow-growing melanoma *in situ* known as lentigo maligna (Hutchinson's freckle). This type of melanoma is associated with chronic sun damage. It usually presents on the head or neck of an elderly patient (see Fig. 17.12).
- Acral lentiginous melanoma (2–8%): palms, soles, beneath the nail. Commonest in Chinese and Japanese. Commonest subtype in Fitzpatrick skin types IV/V.

Table 17.1 Prognosis of malignant melanoma

American Joint Committee on Cancer (AJCC) stage	5-year survival (overall >90%)
Stage 0 (melanoma *in situ*)	100%
Stage I (Breslow thickness <1mm)	92–97%
Stage II	53–81%
Stage III	40–78%
Stage IV (metastatic disease)	15–20%

Further reading

Cancer Research UK. Melanoma skin cancer. Available at: ℛ http://www.cancerresearchuk.org/about-cancer/type/melanoma/.

Marsden JR *et al*. *Br J Dermatol* 2010;**163**:238–56. Available at: ℛ http://www.bad.org.uk/library-media/documents/Melanoma_2010.pdf.

Management of melanoma

Management of cutaneous melanoma

- Surgery is the mainstay of treatment for 1° melanoma. Excision margin is determined according to the Breslow thickness (see Table 17.2).
- Sentinel lymph node biopsy can be used as a staging procedure but has no proven therapeutic value.
- Routine imaging is not warranted for melanoma. Extent of metastatic spread is assessed in patients with American Joint Committee on Cancer (AJCC) stage III or above, using whole-body CT or positron emission tomography (PET)-CT scans.
- Better understanding of molecular signalling and immunological responses in melanoma has led to targeted therapies and immunotherapies. Selection for targeted therapies is determined by molecular testing, e.g. BRAF V600E mutations, c-KIT mutations.

Table 17.2 Breslow thickness

Breslow thickness (mm)	Recommended lateral surgical excision margins (cm)
In situ	0.5
<1	1
1.01–2	1–2
2.01–4	2–3
>4	3

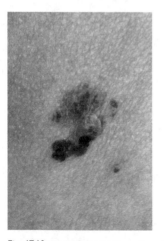

Fig. 17.10 Superficial spreading malignant melanoma with asymmetry in colour and outline. This melanoma did arise in a melanocytic naevus.

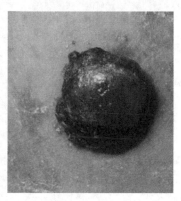

Fig. 17.11 Amelanotic nodular melanoma with a rim of pigmentation simulating haemorrhage. The tumour was misdiagnosed as a pyogenic granuloma.

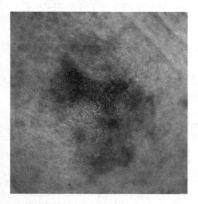

Fig. 17.12 Slow-growing lentigo maligna (melanoma *in situ*) on the cheek of an 80-year-old woman.

Cutaneous T-cell lymphoma

Clinical features, in combination with histological, immunophenotypic, and molecular studies, have helped to delineate subtypes and provide prognostic criteria in this heterogeneous group that includes:

- MF and Sézary syndrome.
- CD30-positive CTCLs, e.g. lymphomatoid papulosis—good prognosis. Anti-CD30 monoclonal antibodies (brentuximab) now available as a treatment option.
- CD30-negative CTCLs: poor prognosis.
- Adult T-cell leukaemia/lymphoma (ATLL).

Mycosis fungoides

MF, the commonest CTCL, is a malignancy of effector memory T-cells that responds well to skin-directed therapies. The aetiology is uncertain but may involve chronic antigenic stimulation (possibly viral) and mutations in oncogenes or DNA repair genes.

Disease is indolent, and the diagnosis often delayed (median age 55–60 years).

Prognosis is worse in patients aged >60 years and in late-stage disease.

MF progresses through three stages: patches, plaques, and tumours—which may overlap. MF variants include folliculotrophic, pagetoid reticulosis, and granulomatous slack skin. Early-stage disease (excellent prognosis) is managed conservatively. Options include emollients, potent topical corticosteroids, UVB, PUVA, topical nitrogen mustard, and bexarotene (retinoid that activates retinoid X receptors, causing T-cell apoptosis). Radiotherapy is effective for localized thick plaques or tumours. MF is relatively chemoresistant, and treatment of advanced disease is unsatisfactory. Sepsis is a common cause of death.

What should I look for?

- Symptoms: variable itch, ranging from minimal to intense.
- Early MF: one or more persistent and/or enlarging well-defined erythematous patches (flat) of variable size and shape with fine scale (compare with thick scale of psoriasis), often on covered sites—buttocks and breasts (see Fig. 17.13). Sparing of the elbows, knees, scalp, and nails in early MF (often involved in psoriasis). May be hypo- or hyperpigmented.
- Poikiloderma: mottled pigmentation, telangiectasia, and atrophy. Skin wrinkles like tissue paper, if pinched—not seen in psoriasis or eczema, unless ultrapotent topical steroids have been used for prolonged periods.
- First presentation of MF can be an erythrodermic emergency.
- Late MF: reddish brown, sharply demarcated, infiltrated plaques (elevated) that coalesce into annular or serpiginous shapes (see Fig. 17.13).
- Hair-bearing skin: follicular plugging and alopecia (hair is retained in psoriasis and eczema).
- Ulcerating mushroom-shaped tumours (late disease).
- Lymphadenopathy (may be 2° to inflammation in the skin and not malignant), enlarged liver, and/or spleen (late disease).

What should I do?

- Document the % of BSA involved and types of skin lesions.
- Exclude tinea (ringworm) by taking skin scrapes for mycology.

- Take two large elliptical skin biopsies for histology, immunophenotyping, and molecular studies, looking for T-cell receptor gene rearrangement. Repeated biopsies may be required, before the diagnosis is established.
- Check FBC, LFT, lactate dehydrogenase (LDH), and renal function.

Sézary syndrome

This form of CTCL accounts for about 5% of new cases. It is caused by malignant proliferation of central memory T-cells. Disease is character-ized by erythroderma (see **➲** p. 108 and Fig. 5.2), lymphadenopathy, and malignant circulating $CD4^+$ T-cells (Sézary cells) forming >5% of the total lymphocyte count. The CD4:CD8 ratio is high (≥10). As disease progresses, the malignant clone of cells expands, and the normal CD4 (T-helper) and CD8 (T-suppressor) populations decrease.

Prognosis is poor (median survival 32 months from diagnosis), and patients often die from infection as a result of a failing immune system. Treatment is unsatisfactory; PUVA is poorly tolerated. Options include extracorporeal photophoresis, multi-agent chemotherapy, immuno-therapy, and oral bexarotene, but prospective clinical trials are needed.

What should I look for?

- Generalized itching, often severe.
- Systemic symptoms such as fever, weight loss, and/or malaise.
- Erythroderma (generalized redness), with or without scale.
- Thickened erythematous skin on the face, with ectropion, thickening of skin on the palms and soles (keratoderma), hair loss, and nail dystrophy.
- Widespread lymphadenopathy.

What should I do?

- Carry out a full clinical examination.
- Check FBC, blood film, and count of Sézary cells (T-cells with hyperconvoluted cerebriform nuclei). Some circulating Sézary cells may be found in benign inflammatory skin conditions.
- Take an elliptical skin biopsy for histology.
- Look for T-cell monoclonal expansion in peripheral blood and skin by immunophenotyping and with molecular studies of T-cell receptor.
- Check LFT, LDH (for disease monitoring), and renal function.
- Check human T-lymphotropic virus (HTLV)-1 serology.
- Biopsy an enlarged lymph node (removal preferable to needle biopsy).
- If indicated, stage with chest X-ray (CXR), CT scan (chest, abdomen, pelvis) ± PET-CT scan, and bone marrow aspirate.

Adult T-cell leukaemia/lymphoma

This $CD4^+$ lymphoproliferative disorder, associated with infection with HTLV-1, is commonest in Japan and the Caribbean. Prognosis is poor, and opportunistic infection common.

What should I look for?

- Skin infiltration by ATLL cells leads to patches, plaques, papules, or tumours. Rarely erythroderma or purpuric rashes.
- Non-specific cutaneous inflammation (dermatitis) and infections, e.g. dermatophyte (tinea), *Candida*.
- Lymphadenopathy, hepatosplenomegaly.
- Raised LDH and hypercalcaemia.

Other malignancies and skin

Merkel cell carcinoma

This rare aggressive neuroendocrine skin cancer is associated with pathogenic factors such as UV exposure, immunosuppression, and/or Merkel cell polyomavirus. It presents as a rapidly growing bluish red or skin-coloured nodule, usually on a sun-exposed site, and spreads quickly to the lymph nodes, lungs, liver, or bone.

Dermatofibrosarcoma protuberans

A slow-growing, locally recurrent cutaneous soft tissue sarcoma caused by a chromosomal translocation t(17;22)(q22;q13) which results in a *COL1A1–PDGFB* fusion gene. Presents as an asymptomatic 'scar' or a violaceous, reddish brown, or skin-coloured nodule or plaque, which feels rubbery or firm. Has an infiltrative pattern, often with considerable subclinical and asymmetrical extension. Treatment: surgical excision (1–3cm peripheral margins) or Mohs micrographic surgery. Rarely metastasizes (<5%).

Paget disease

Paget disease is caused by direct extension of a mammary intraductal adenocarcinoma into the skin of the nipple or areola.

What should I look for?
- A weeping, erythematous, crusted eruption affecting one nipple.
- Is there a past history of atopic eczema? This is common on the nipple and sometimes is unilateral.
- Check the other nipple. Bilateral changes are much more likely to be eczema (atopic or contact) than cancer.
- Check for an associated breast lump.

What should I do?
- Biopsy any 'eczematous' nipple rash that persists despite potent topical corticosteroid ointments applied bd for 2 weeks.

Metastatic disease

Skin metastasis may be the first sign of an internal malignancy. The skin may be infiltrated by direct invasion of tumour cells or by spread from lymphatics or blood vessels. The tumour may also be implanted into surgical scars. Cancers most often associated with cutaneous metastasis are:
- Breast: skin of the chest, scalp, (rarely eyelid).
- Stomach, colon: skin of the abdominal wall, especially periumbilical.
- Lung: skin of the chest, scalp.
- Genitourinary system (uterus, ovary, kidney, bladder): skin of the scalp, lower abdomen, external genitalia.

What should I look for?
- Firm intradermal or subcutaneous nodules of varying colour.
- Scalp metastasis may cause a focal scarring alopecia.
- Cutaneous lymphatic invasion initially causes thickening and fibrosis and later firm pink papules or nodules.

- Carcinoma erysipeloides—most often associated with metastatic breast cancer. Lymphatic invasion produces a tender erythematous oedematous plaque, often initially misdiagnosed and treated as an infection (erysipelas or cellulitis), but antibiotics are ineffective.
- Extramammary Paget disease (EMPD)—a slow-growing, itchy, erythematous plaque in anogenital skin, especially the vulva. Biopsy shows mucin-containing tumour cells within the epidermis. EMPD is usually associated with an underlying adnexal carcinoma, often of apocrine origin, which may be difficult to localize, but 10–15% of patients have cancer of the rectum, prostate, bladder, cervix, or urethra.

Leukaemia cutis

Leukaemia cutis is rare but is seen most often with myeloid leukaemias, e.g. acute monocytic or myelomonocytic leukaemias. Cutaneous deposits may precede the transformation of myelodysplastic syndrome to leukaemia. It usually indicates a poor prognosis.

What should I look for?
- Firm purplish plaques or nodules.
- Infiltrates in scars or at injection sites.

Primary cutaneous B-cell lymphomas

Most B-cell lymphomas affecting the skin are systemic.
- Marginal zone lymphoma (mucosa-associated lymphoid tissue, MALT).
  - Dermal tumours in ♂ affecting the trunk and upper limbs.
  - Indolent and prone to recur.
  - Test for *Borrelia burgdorferi*.
  - Radiotherapy is the treatment of choice.
- Follicular lymphomas:
  - Multiple primaries, prominent plaques affect scalp and upper trunk.
  - Treat with radiotherapy or rituximab.
  - 95–100% 5-year survival.
- Diffuse large B-cell lymphoma:
  - Leg-type seen in older ♀.
  - Large, rapidly growing, bluish red tumours.
  - 50% 5-year survival.
  - Treatment is with radiotherapy/CHOP–rituximab.

Kaposi sarcoma (KS)

KS is a neoplasm caused by proliferation of the lymphatic endothelium, associated with HHV-8 infection of endothelial cells. May behave as a benign reactive process or pursue an aggressive life-threatening course (see Box 17.9). 2° skin infections and malignancies (lymphoma) may complicate KS. Pathogenesis is multifactorial. Chronic lymphoedema (see ➔ pp. 316–17) may predispose to KS, and HIV may exacerbate the pathogenicity of HHV-8. Circulating HHV-8-infected endothelial precursor cells localize to sites, such as the leg, where unregulated spindle cell proliferation is driven by interactions between activated CD8+ T-cells, HHV-8-induced intracellular signalling pathways, products of oncogenes (viral and host), and inflammatory cytokines, including HHV-8-encoded IL-6 and, in AIDS patients, the product of the HIV-1 *tat* gene.

If immunodeficiency is corrected, e.g. by withdrawing or reducing immunosuppression, KS may regress. KS lesions also shrink in HIV-positive patients treated with highly active antiretroviral therapy (HAART). Localized disease may be controlled with intralesional vinblastine, topical alitretinoin (9-cis-retinoic acid) gel, topical imiquimod, radiotherapy, laser surgery, or cryosurgery. Systemic options for widespread disease include IFN-α and multi-agent chemotherapy, e.g. anthracyclines (doxorubicin) or paclitaxel. The role of angiogenesis inhibitors and other drugs needs further investigation.

What should I look for?

(See Box 17.10.)

- KS has a predilection for the face, ears, lower limb, including the soles of feet, genitalia, and oral mucosa.
- Bruise-like purple or brownish red macules and patches which may be subtle in early disease. Consider the possibility of KS in any immunosuppressed patient with atypical 'bruises'.
- Blue, purple, red, brown, or brownish red elliptical vascular papules lying in parallel to the natural lines of cleavage in the skin (Langer lines). These may involve surgical scars.
- Dark blue or purple vascular nodules or indurated hyperkeratotic plaques that may ulcerate (see Fig. 17.14).
- Oral mucosal lesions (vascular patches, papules, or plaques) on the hard palate or, less often, gums, sometimes with overlying candidiasis. Trauma causes bleeding.
- Lymphadenopathy.
- Lymphoedema affecting the face, genitalia, and/or leg, caused by vascular obstruction, lymphadenopathy, and local cytokines (commoner in AIDS-related KS). Swelling out of proportion to cutaneous signs.

What should I do?

- Take a skin biopsy to confirm the diagnosis.
- Exclude immunosuppression, e.g. HIV infection.
- Investigate the GIT and/or respiratory tract, if indicated.

Box 17.9 Kaposi sarcoma: clinicopathological subtypes

- Classic: men, aged 40–70 years old, Mediterranean/central to eastern European (Ashkenazi) Jewish heritage. Affects the legs and feet. Indolent and pursues a chronic course. Countries bordering the Mediterranean basin have higher HHV-8 infection rates, compared with the rest of Europe.
- Endemic (African: sub-Saharan Africa): affects younger population than classic KS. ♂ predominance less marked in childhood. Not linked to AIDS. More aggressive than classic KS. Extensive skin infiltration, especially on the lower limbs. High rates of HHV-8 infection in the general population in this part of Africa.
- Iatrogenic: particularly in transplant recipients taking calcineurin inhibitors, e.g. ciclosporin, which inhibit T-cell function. Patients either have pre-existing HHV-8 infection or, less often, acquire HHV-8 when transplanted with an HHV-8-infected organ. KS has been described in patients taking other immunosuppressive drugs and may regress if immunosuppression is withdrawn.
- AIDS-related: predominantly in homosexual/bisexual men. The trunk, arms, head, and neck involved more frequently than in classic KS. Pursues an aggressive course, involving the mucosa, lymph nodes, and viscera (GIT, respiratory tract). Poor prognosis—death from opportunistic infection, GI haemorrhage, cardiac tamponade, or pulmonary obstruction. Treatment: HAART and liposomal anthracycline chemotherapy. Occasionally, IRIS seen after treatment with HAART can trigger a flare of KS.

Box 17.10 Kaposi sarcoma: differential diagnosis

- Melanocytic tumours: melanocytic naevi, melanoma—1° or metastatic (see ➡ pp. 354–5).
- Pyogenic granuloma, haemangiomas, or other vascular tumour.
- Pseudo-KS: vascular nodules seen in venous stasis or in association with AV malformations. Histology resembles KS.
- Metastatic renal cell carcinoma (also tends to be vascular) or another metastasis.
- Bacillary angiomatosis (see ➡ p. 142). Unlike KS, vascular lesions are uncommon on the soles or in the mouth.
- Reactive angioendotheliomatosis: Rare. Occurs distal to iatrogenic AV fistulae on upper limbs used for haemodialysis (see ➡ Box 23.1, p. 493), on the lower limbs of patients with severe peripheral vascular disease, and in systemic diseases.

Further reading
Bhutani M et al. Semin Oncol 2015;42:223–46.

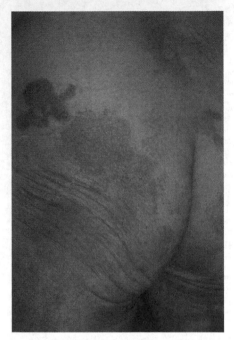

Fig. 17.13 Mycosis fungoides: fine scaly erythematous patch and a plaque with a serpiginous outline.

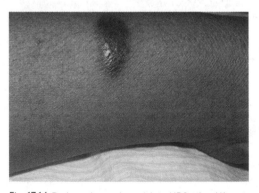

Fig. 17.14 Dark purple vascular nodule in AIDS-related Kaposi sarcoma.

Cutaneous reactions to drugs

Contents

Relevant pages in other chapters
Adverse effects of topical corticosteroids ➔ p. 657
Photosensitivity ➔ p. 326

Introduction

Cutaneous adverse drug reactions (see Box 18.1) are common (2–3% of hospitalized patients), the signs extraordinarily diverse, time courses variable, and, worryingly, some are life-threatening. Alternative therapies, including vitamin or herbal supplements, may also cause problems. Reactions may be pharmacological or idiosyncratic (see Box 18.2). Predisposition is probably multifactorial, involving genetic and environmental factors (see Box 18.3).

Advances in pharmacogenetics may help to predict which patients are likely to benefit from, or react adversely to, certain drugs. For example, *HLA-B*1502* allele in south-eastern Asian patients has been correlated with carbamazepine-induced SJS–TEN; *HLA-A*3101* allele is associated with carbamazepine-induced reactions in Europeans, and genotyping for *HLA-B*5701*, which is linked to abacavir hypersensitivity, is used to screen HIV-positive patients prior to starting treatment.

Cutaneous adverse reactions may not be recognized, if the reaction simulates a condition such as eczema or if the medication has been taken for months without problems. The exanthem of a viral infection looks like a morbilliform drug reaction, but exanthems are more likely in children than in adults. To compound diagnostic difficulties, reactions may not settle as soon as the drug is withdrawn—some persist for months—and generally there is no definitive test to confirm the diagnosis of 'drug reaction'.

These life-threatening or severe cutaneous adverse drug reactions are discussed in more detail elsewhere:
- Anaphylaxis and angio-oedema (see ➔ pp. 104–5).
- Erythroderma (see ➔ p. 108).
- Stevens Johnson syndrome (see ➔ pp. 116–17).
- Toxic epidermal necrolysis (see ➔ pp. 116–17).
- DRESS (see ➔ pp. 122–3).
- AGEP (see ➔ p. 124).
- Anticoagulant-induced purpura fulminans and skin necrosis (see ➔ pp. 102–3).
- Vasculitis (see ➔ pp. 436–9).

Box 18.1 What is an adverse drug reaction?

'An appreciably harmful or unpleasant reaction, resulting from an intervention related to the use of a medicinal product, which predicts hazard from future administration and warrants prevention or specific treatment, or alteration of the dosage regimen or withdrawal of the product'.
Edwards IR and Aronson JK. *Lancet* 2000;**356**:1255–9.

Box 18.2 Types of reaction

- Type A (80% of reactions)—pharmacological: augmentation of the known pharmacological actions of the drug. Predictable, dose-dependent. Reversed by reducing the dose or withdrawing the drug.
- Type B (20% of reactions)—idiosyncratic: not predictable and may be life-threatening. Mechanisms include pharmaceutical variation in drug formulation, receptor abnormalities, abnormalities in drug metabolism, and immune-mediated.

Box 18.3 Factors that predispose to drug reactions

- Adults, rather than children.
- ♀ gender.
- Polypharmacy: 50% chance of an adverse interaction if five or more drugs are taken concurrently.
- Abnormal drug metabolism, e.g. reduced in renal failure or liver disease; toxic metabolites produced by metabolizing enzymes.
- Genetic polymorphisms, e.g. receptor abnormalities or enzyme deficiencies may cause pharmacological or idiosyncratic reactions.
- Previous hypersensitivity to a related drug.
- Host disease, e.g. SLE, herpesvirus infection, HIV infection. (In HIV infection, the incidence of cutaneous adverse drug reactions, most often morbilliform or urticarial rashes, increases as immune function deteriorates. Trimethoprim–sulfonamides and aminopenicillins cause most reactions.)

Further reading

Kaniwa N and Saito Y. *Ther Adv Drug Saf* 2013;4:246–53.
Karlin E and Phillips E. *Curr Allergy Asthma Rep* 2014;14:418.
McCormack M et al. *N Engl J Med* 2011;364:1134–43.
National Institute for Health and Care Excellence (2014). *Drug allergy: diagnosis and management*. Available at: ℳ www.nice.org.uk/cg183.
Wu K and Reynolds NJ. *Br J Dermatol* 2012;166:7–11.

Mechanisms of idiosyncratic cutaneous adverse drug reactions

For mechanisms of cutaneous drug reactions, see Table 18.1.

Table 18.1 Mechanisms of cutaneous adverse drug reactions

Type of reaction	Mechanism	Clinical signs
Type I immediate	IgE-mediated involving release of histamine from mast cells	Urticaria, angio-oedema, anaphylaxis. Minutes to hours after exposure to drug
Type II antibody-mediated	Cytotoxic IgG or IgM antibodies	ANCA-mediated vasculitis, drug-induced thrombocytopenic purpura. Variable time of onset
Type III immune complex-mediated	Drug-antibody immune complexes (IgM, IgG and IgA)	Vasculitis, serum sickness 1–3 weeks after exposure to drug
Type IV delayed-type	T-cell mediated	
Type IVa	Th1 cells release IFN-γ	Allergic contact dermatitis 2–7 days after drug is in contact with skin
Type IVb	Th2 cells release IL-5, IL-4, IL-13, and eotaxin (recruits eosinophils)	DRESS
Type IVc	Cytotoxic CD4$^+$ or CD8$^+$ T-cells, IFN-γ, and TNF induce keratinocyte lysis via perforin/granzyme B, Fas/FasL, and granulysin	SJS, TEN, bullous drug reactions (Fig. 18.1)
Type IVd	Th17 cells release IL-17 and IL-22. Stimulated keratinocytes release IL-8 recruiting polymorphonuclear cells	AGEP
Pseudoallergic	Direct mast cell activation with histamine release or inhibition of kinin metabolism	Anaphylactoid reactions with angio-oedema
Autoimmune	ANAs	E.g. hydralazine-induced LE

Further reading

Harp J et al. Semin Cutan Med Surg 2014;33:17–27 (review).

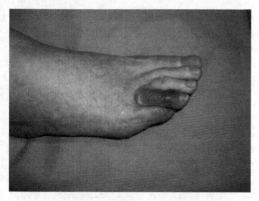

Fig. 18.1 Bullous fixed drug eruption. The blister recurs in the same place each time the patient takes the drug (type IV reaction).

Fig. 18.2 Purplish lichen planus-like eruption caused by ramipril (type IV reaction).

Clinical approach

In any patient with a rash, ask yourself if the problem might be a manifestation of an adverse drug reaction and if this could be serious. Exclude other causes, such as viral infection, but retain a high index of suspicion.

What should I ask?

- What medicaments is the patient taking or applying to the skin (including herbal or traditional remedies, recreational drugs including kava, long-term medications such as the contraceptive pill, contrast medium, and depot injections)?
- Has the patient been exposed to the medication before?
- When medications were started (dates), and what is the temporal relation to the onset of the rash? You may have to ask the GP. The interval between the start of therapy and onset of reaction is rarely <1 week, unless the patient has had the drug before, or >1 month.
- Is the reaction less severe if the drug dose is reduced, or does it settle if the drug is withdrawn? Pharmacological adverse reactions, unlike idiosyncratic reactions, are usually dose-dependent.
- Any predisposing factors? (See Box 18.3.)
- What are the symptoms—malaise, itch, mucosal swelling, cutaneous pain or burning (may indicate TEN), arthralgia, or wheeze?

What should I do?

- Full examination, including temperature and blood pressure.
- Document the cutaneous signs—erythema, scale, macules, papules, urticarial wheals (no scale), pustules, vesicles or bullae, purpura—and decide on the predominant pattern of reaction.
- Examine mucosae (mouth, conjunctiva, and genitalia).
- Assess the likelihood of this being a serious reaction (see Box 18.4).
- Consider how the adverse reaction is likely to evolve. Your next steps will be determined by the severity (see Box 18.5).
- Document the likelihood of an adverse drug reaction (certain, likely, possible, or unlikely) and which drug(s) is/are implicated.
- Contact pharmacy if you are not sure about the likelihood of a particular drug causing an adverse reaction.
- Report any possible reaction to the regulatory agency—in the UK, return a completed yellow card to the Medicines and Healthcare Products Regulatory Agency (MHRA). Local, national, and international registries also exist for monitoring cutaneous drug reactions—consult the local dermatology department.
- Ensure that the medical records state that the drug should be avoided in future (it may be possible to continue essential treatment, despite a morbilliform reaction), and notify the GP.
- Explain the likely cause to the patient.
- Arrange further investigations when resolved (see Box 18.6).

Further reading

Barbaud A et al. Br J Dermatol 2013;**168**:555–62 (utility of drug patch tests).
Polak ME et al. Br J Dermatol 2012;**168**:539–49 (potential of in vitro diagnostic assays).

⚠ **Box 18.4 Indications of severe cutaneous adverse drug reactions**

(see ➲ p. 114.)
- General:
  - Fever >40°C, hypotension, lymphadenopathy.
  - Arthralgia, arthritis, dyspnoea, wheeze.
- Mucocutaneous:
  - Generalized scaly erythema (erythroderma).
  - Swollen face, swelling of tongue, urticaria (anaphylaxis).
  - Skin pain or burning, erosions, shearing stress detaches epidermis from dermis, bullae, mucosal erosions (SJS, TEN) (see ➲ pp. 116–17, and Fig. 5.5, p. 121).
  - Purpura (vasculitis or anticoagulant-induced).
- Laboratory results:
  - Eosinophilia >1000mm³, lymphocytosis with abnormal lymphocytes, abnormal LFTs.

Box 18.5 Principles of management

- Withdraw non-essential medications, or reduce the dose (may help if the reaction is pharmacological). Drug withdrawal is not diagnostic immediately. Urticarial reactions settle in a few days, morbilliform rashes in 7–10 days. Other reactions may persist for >8 weeks.
- Manage life-threatening adverse reactions promptly, e.g. anaphylaxis, erythroderma, TEN, vasculitis (see ➲ p. 108, pp. 118–20).
- Exclude systemic involvement: FBC (may have eosinophilia or lymphocytosis), renal function, liver function, complement levels.
- Exclude infection with serological tests, if indicated, e.g. CMV, EBV, parvovirus B19 in patients with morbilliform rash; hepatitis B and C in urticaria; herpes simplex or mycoplasma in EM.
- Consider a skin biopsy (unhelpful in simple morbilliform reactions). The histological findings may not be conclusive.
- Emollients and soap substitutes relieve dryness (see ➲ p. 655).
- Moderately potent or potent topical corticosteroid ointments bd and sedating antihistamines reduce itch in morbilliform, eczematous, or lichenoid reactions (topical steroids are unhelpful in urticaria). (See Fig. 18.2.)
- Non-sedating antihistamines in urticaria (mediated by histamine).

Box 18.6 Further investigation of adverse drug reactions

- Once the reaction has resolved, patch testing with standardized dilutions of the suspected drug is helpful in allergic contact dermatitis and may sometimes be helpful in fixed drug eruptions, AGEP (see ➲ p. 124), and hypersensitivity syndrome (DRESS; see ➲ pp. 122–3).
- Unfortunately, skin testing (patch, prick, or intradermal) is rarely helpful in other forms of drug reaction.
- Oral re-challenge is usually inadvisable (except in fixed drug eruption).

Generally smooth erythematous drug reactions

Morbilliform (exanthematous)

- The commonest pattern of cutaneous drug reaction.
- Presents within 1–3 weeks of drug exposure.
- A symmetrical morbilliform rash (erythematous macules and papules of 2–10mm in diameter with a tendency to confluence) starts on the trunk. The rash spreads to the arms and legs and may become confluent.
- The rash may be itchy (not painful).
- The patient may have a slight (not high) temperature.
- Mucosae are normal.
- Settles with desquamation within 7–10 days of withdrawing the drug. Thick sheets of scale may detach from the palms or soles—do not confuse with the full-thickness loss of epidermis seen in TEN (see ➲ p. 116).
- Erythroderma is a rare complication (see ➲ p. 108).
- If the causative drug is essential, it may be possible to treat through a morbilliform reaction, but the patient may become erythrodermic.
- ⚠ Morbilliform reactions may resemble urticaria, but lesions are fixed, or (most often in children) a viral exanthem (take a thorough history).
- Morbilliform reactions may also precede a serious drug reaction such as TEN, hypersensitivity syndrome (DRESS), or serum sickness. Monitor for signs that suggest a serious reaction, e.g. facial swelling, mucosal involvement (see ➲ pp. 116–17 and Box 18.4).
- Common causes: ampicillin (particularly if the patient has glandular fever), sulfonamides, allopurinol, captopril, barbiturates, thiazides.

Urticaria and/or angio-oedema; anaphylactoid reactions

- IgE-mediated reactions may present within minutes of exposure, if previously sensitized. ACE inhibitors are the commonest cause of admission with angio-oedema.
- Urticaria: itchy erythematous wheals (no scale) that move around. Wheals fade within 24h to leave normal skin.
- Subcutaneous oedema (angio-oedema) affecting the lips, periorbital skin, tongue (when patient may have difficulty swallowing or breathing), external genitalia—an emergency (see ➲ p. 104).
- Common causes—penicillins, captopril, cephalosporins, thiazides, phenytoin, NSAIDs, ACE inhibitors (cause angio-oedema without urticaria and may not present until >4 weeks after the drug is started), aspirin, radiocontrast agents, opiates, quinine.
- Anaphylactoid reactions (not IgE-mediated) may present several weeks after the medication is started. Histamine is released directly from mast cells and basophils. Present as *red man syndrome* with flushing, erythema, and itching of the face and upper trunk, and sometimes angio-oedema, hypotension, dyspnoea, and chest pain. Caused by drugs such as vancomycin, ciprofloxacin, amphotericin, rifampicin, and teicoplanin.

⚠ **Drug rash, eosinophilia, systemic symptoms (DRESS)**
(see ➲ pp. 122–3.)
- DRESS is a life-threatening cutaneous drug reaction with systemic symptoms (high fever) that is frequently misdiagnosed as infection.
- DRESS may be associated with reactivation of HHV-6.
- The morbilliform rash is associated with facial oedema, simulating angio-oedema.
- Some patients progress to liver failure.
- Causes include allopurinol, anticonvulsants, minocycline, dapsone, sulfonamides, and other antibiotics.

Acute generalized exanthematous pustulosis (AGEP)
(see ➲ p. 124 and Fig. 5.6, p. 121.)
- Patients suddenly develop an uncomfortable oedematous erythema that burns or itches, and then becomes studded with tiny pustules.
- Caused by a wide range of drugs, including antibiotics such as penicillins, erythromycin, and tetracyclines.

Serum sickness
- Presents within 1–3 weeks of starting the medication.
- Erythema on the sides of fingers, toes, and hands progresses to a widespread morbilliform rash. Some patients also have urticaria.
- Malaise, fever, arthralgia, and arthritis are common.
- Causes include serum preparations and vaccines.

Interstitial granulomatous dermatitis
- Described in association with a range of drugs, including calcium channel blockers, β-blockers, lipid-lowering agents, ACE inhibitors, antihistamines, anticonvulsants, antidepressants, and TNF-α inhibitors. Also seen in association with connective tissue diseases, including RA, and lymphoproliferative disorders (see ➲ pp. 394).
- Presents months to years after initiation of treatment.
- Annular purplish red (violaceous) plaques on the arms, medial thighs, and flexures. May be mildly itchy.
- Histologically diffuse interstitial granulomatous infiltrate in the mid and deep dermis with lymphocytes, histiocytes, mucin deposition, and variable collagen necrosis.

Erythema nodosum
- Causes: oral contraceptive pill, sulfonamides, gold (but more often triggered by an infection (TB) or underlying systemic disease such as sarcoidosis or IBD) (see ➲ pp. 458–9).
- Tender erythematous subcutaneous nodules on the shins and sometimes forearms.
- Resolves in weeks, without loss of fat or scarring.
- NSAIDs relieve discomfort. Gentle compression with stockings that control swelling may speed resolution.

Also consider allergic contact dermatitis and SDRIFE
see ➲ p. 374.

More scaly erythematous drug reactions and pruritus

Allergic contact dermatitis (eczema)

- A localized allergic contact dermatitis is caused by topical preparations to which the patient has been sensitized by previous contact (see ➡ p. 214). The reaction appears within 48h of exposure.
- Skin is itchy, oedematous, erythematous, and scaly (may not be scaly if acute). It may blister if the reaction is severe (see ➡ Fig. 10.1, p. 216).
- Eczema may generalize if contact persists or if the patient takes a cross-reacting oral preparation.
- Consider allergic contact dermatitis in chronic leg ulcers, hand dermatitis, facial dermatitis, otitis externa, or pruritus ani. Causes include topical neomycin, benzocaine, incipients in topical medicaments, and topical hydrocortisone.
- Allergy to the constituents of subcutaneous heparin presents with well-demarcated infiltrated eczematous plaques at injection sites.
- Treat eczema with emollients and topical corticosteroid ointments.
- Investigate possible allergic contact dermatitis by patch testing.

SDRIFE: symmetrical drug-related intertriginous and flexural exanthema

- A distinctive erythematous flexural reaction to systemic drugs and iodinated contrast medium. Commonest cause: aminopenicillins.
- Latency hours to days. Occurs without prior exposure to the drug.
- Itchy, erythematous papules coalesce to produce a symmetrical, well-demarcated erythema on buttocks (baboon's bottom) and/or V-shaped erythema of the lower abdomen, groins, and thighs. Involves at least one other skinfold. May become bullous.
- No systemic symptoms or signs.
- Encompasses 'baboon syndrome', a distinct form of systemic contact dermatitis (sensitization by skin contact, and subsequently patient takes the agent by mouth).

Drug-induced photosensitivity

(see ➡ p. 326.)

- Drugs are the commonest cause of photosensitivity, more often phototoxicity than photoallergy.
- Look for an eczematous rash on exposed sites, sometimes with pigmentation (see ➡ Box 4.6, p. 73).
- Drugs may also cause photosensitivity by triggering PCT, pseudoporphyria (see ➡ p. 332, p. 334), or subacute cutaneous LE (SCLE) (see ➡ p. 402).

Lichenoid (lichen planus-like) reaction

- Very itchy, flat-topped, purplish red papules that may coalesce into erythematous plaques and become generalized. Often also an eczematous scaly component (see Fig. 18.2).
- Examine the buccal mucosa for reticulated white areas and erosions—found more often in LP than lichenoid drug reactions (see ➋ p. 224).
- Resolution is slow (months) after the drug is stopped.
- The papules fade to leave macular hyperpigmentation that persists for months, particularly in dark skin. Pigmentation tends to be more marked in lichenoid drug reactions than in LP.
- Very potent topical corticosteroid ointments may be required to relieve itch.
- Common causes: gold, antimalarials, penicillamine, β-blockers, thiazides, NSAIDs. Also reported with TNF-α antagonists.

△ Erythroderma (exfoliative dermatitis)

- Generalized scaly erythema—an emergency (see ➋ p. 108).
- Common causes: sulfonamides, carbamazepine, antimalarials, phenytoin, and gold.

Chronic eczematous eruptions

- Common in the elderly, but it may be difficult to identify the drug responsible.
- Calcium channel blockers (commonest cause).

Pruritus

- Itch without a 1° rash may be caused by a number of drugs, including statins (also dryness of the skin), ACE inhibitors, opiates, barbiturates, antidepressants, and oral retinoids (also dryness of the skin).
- Hydroxyethyl starch products (colloid volume expanders—in 2013, withdrawn in the UK because of risk of renal damage). Cause discrete attacks of severe intractable pruritus lasting for minutes up to an hour. Patients may have several episodes a day. Itch may persist for years.
- Signs are those of scratching sometimes superimposed on dry skin.
- Exclude other causes of itching, including urticaria (the rash is transient) (see ➋ p. 228), scabies (see ➋ p. 172), and renal, hepatic, thyroid, haematological, or neurological disease, including iron deficiency.
- Menthol 1% in aqueous cream is a soothing antipruritic. Sedating antihistamines may be helpful (ineffective in hydroxyethyl starch itch).
- Also see ➋ Eczematous reactions, p. 388.

Purpuric or pigmented drug reactions

Vasculitis (palpable purpura)
- Usually 1–3 weeks after starting drug, but interval may be longer.
- Palpable purpura (small-vessel cutaneous vasculitis) initially on legs but may become widespread. Purpuric papules may evolve into haemorrhagic blisters or purpuric plaques (see ➔ p. 440).
- Other signs may include urticaria, ulcers, and nodules.
- Vasculitis may affect the kidney, liver, GIT, and/or nervous system.
- Consider other causes of a small-vessel cutaneous vasculitis, including infection (see ➔ Box 20.3, p. 441).
- Common causes: penicillins and other antibiotics, allopurinol, phenytoin, thiazides, and thiouracils.
- Cocaine, adulterated by levamisole, may induce retiform purpura on the body and tender purpura of the ears, nose, cheeks, lips, and hard palate, sometimes with necrosis (vasculitis and/or occlusive vasculopathy).

Macular purpura: may be pigmented
- Aspirin, anticoagulants, calcium channel blockers, ACE inhibitors, analgesics.

Anticoagulant-induced purpura fulminans and skin necrosis
- Rare, but life-threatening, complication of treatment with warfarin.
- Risk greatest in obese ♀ patients with heterozygous deficiency of protein C or protein S. Warfarin inhibits protein C and protein S, inducing a hypercoagulable state.
- Three to 5 days after starting warfarin, painful, erythematous, indurated plaques develop on fatty areas—breasts, hips, and buttocks. The large, irregularly outlined plaques become haemorrhagic, bullous, and eventually necrotic. Biopsy shows microthrombi in capillaries, venules, and veins.
- ▶▶ Treatment: stop warfarin; administer vitamin K and/or fresh frozen plasma to restore levels of protein C/S. Use another anticoagulant, e.g. heparin.
- Heparin necrosis is rare. Presents 5–14 days after starting heparin. Erythema at injection sites (rarely distant sites) progresses to painful necrosis. Platelet aggregation is 2° to antibodies to heparin–platelet factor 4 complex. Platelets may fall. Stop heparin. Use non-heparin anticoagulant.

Cutaneous hyperpigmentation
- Mechanisms of hyperpigmentation include increased melanin synthesis and deposition of drug or drug metabolites in the skin.
- Photosensitivity may contribute to the colour change.
- Ask if the colour change was preceded by erythema or itching to differentiate drug-induced pigmentation from post-inflammatory hyperpigmentation, e.g. after dermatitis, lichenoid rashes, or fixed drug eruptions (see ➔ p. 378), particularly in individuals with dark skin.
- What is the colour and distribution of the change, e.g. is it predominantly in scars or on light-exposed skin?

- Increased melanin (brown pigmentation) may be caused by drugs such as cytotoxics, hydroxycarbamide (hydroxyurea), pegylated IFN (in chronic hepatitis C infection), ACTH, oral contraceptives (melasma on the face), and some antiretroviral agents (zidovudine and lamivudine).
- Flagellate brown hyperpigmentation is caused by bleomycin (see ➋ p. 383).
- Bluish grey pigmentation (may be worse on light-exposed skin) is caused by drugs such as minocycline (often in scars or on the shins) (see Fig. 18.3), phenothiazines, antimalarials, ezogabine (anti-epileptic), vandetanib, gold, and amiodarone (facial pigmentation with photosensitivity).
- Orange pigmentation is caused by the antimalarial mepacrine.
- Pink discoloration is caused by clofazimine.
- Facial hyperpigmentation caused by skin-lightening creams containing hydroquinone (acquired ochronosis).
- Resolution of pigmentation may be very slow (months or years) or pigment may persist, despite drug withdrawal. Photoprotection is often an important part of management.

Oral mucosal pigmentation

- Changes are often seen along the gingival margins but may develop on the lip, tongue, or palate.
- May be caused by drugs such as oral contraceptives (general darkening), minocycline (grey-blue), antimalarial drugs (grey-blue), phenothiazines (grey-blue), and ezogabine (blue-grey).
- Pigmented macules or patches may develop on the tongue in heroin addicts who inhale smoke.
- A black hairy tongue may be caused by drugs such as oral antibiotics (cephalosporins, chloramphenicol, clarithromycin, penicillins, sulfonamides), as well as corticosteroids and antidepressants.

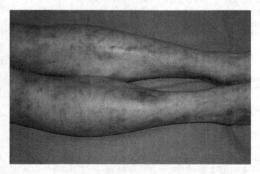

Fig. 18.3 Greyish pigmentation after prolonged treatment with minocycline.

Further reading

Magliocca KP et al. J Oral Maxillofac Surg 2013;**71**:487–92 (cocaine abuse).
Thornsberry LA et al. J Am Acad Dermatol 2013;**69**:450–62 (hypercoagulable states).

Drug-induced blisters or mucocutaneous ulcers

Blisters may be widespread or localized. Oral manifestations may be ery-thematous, vesicular, erosive, or ulcerative and can involve the tongue, as well as the buccal mucosa or gums. Blistering eruptions, such as TEN or SJS, may cause severe oral ulceration (see ➲ p. 116).

⚠ Any persistent oral ulcer should be biopsied to exclude malignancy.

Fixed drug eruption

- One or more well-defined circular, erythematous plaques that usually blister and then resolve over 7–10 days, leaving a hyperpigmented macule. Itching is uncommon (see Fig. 18.1).
- May also affect the oral mucosa, and, in severe cases, mucosal lesions may ulcerate.
- Each time the patient is exposed to the drug, the problem recurs within 24h in exactly the same place or places. Recurrent herpes simplex infection is the main differential diagnosis, but this does not usually leave macular pigmentation.
- Take a skin biopsy during the reaction to confirm the diagnosis.
- Causes: tetracycline, sulfonamides, allopurinol, aspirin (ask the patient what analgesic is taken for menstrual pain or headaches), phenolphthalein. Also consider herbal medicines and other over-the-counter preparations that are ingested sporadically.
- Oral challenge may help to confirm the diagnosis.

Aphthous ulcers

(see ➲ pp. 282–3.)
- Aphthous ulcers are caused by drugs such as azathioprine, captopril, ciclosporin, fluoxetine, sertraline, and sulfonamides.
- NSAIDs and nicorandil cause oral ulcers that may simulate giant aphthae, but the ulcers do not have the erythematous halo or yellow base of an aphthous ulcer.

Erythema multiforme

(see ➲ p. 111.)
- EM is an acute, self-limited illness. Infection (most often herpes simplex) is a much more likely trigger than a drug.

⚠ Stevens–Johnson syndrome and toxic epidermal necrolysis

(see ➲ pp. 116–17.) Life-threatening cutaneous reactions, with overlap-ping features, caused by drugs such as sulfonamides, aminopenicillins, anti-epileptics, barbiturates, NSAIDs, and allopurinol. Patients may have underlying diseases, particularly AIDS. Course protracted—at least 3 weeks.

- Tender EM-like rash, with severe mucosal involvement (oral, ocular, genital), blistering, and erosions that presents 2–3 weeks after drug is started.
- Epidermal involvement is more severe and widespread in TEN (>30% BSA) than in SJS (<10% BSA).

Coma-induced blisters

- Seen in association with decreased level of consciousness caused by overdose of agents such as barbiturates, benzodiazepines, heroin, methadone, imipramine, and alcohol. (Also reported in some neurological and metabolic causes of reduced levels of consciousness.)
- Blisters, preceded by erythematous plaques, are usually few in number, appear within 24h, and resolve in 10–14 days.
- Blisters are predominantly over bony prominences (pressure may cause hypoxic damage), but some may also be found elsewhere.
- Histologically: subepidermal bullae with sweat gland necrosis.

Chemotherapy agents

- Mucosal ulcers are common.

Contact stomatitis

- The patient may notice an oral burning sensation and xerostomia.
- Reactions develop after days or years of exposure.
- Patch testing will confirm the diagnosis.
- Caused by agents such as topical anaesthetics and antiseptic mouthwashes.

Cutaneous ulcers

- Nicorandil causes large, deep, painful persistent ulcers on perianal skin and other sites. Ulcers may resemble pyoderma gangrenosum (PG) or a cutaneous malignancy (see ➔ p. 310).
- Cocaine abuse may cause PG.

Other drug-induced blistering reactions

- Pseudoporphyria (see ➔ p. 334).
- Pemphigus, most often foliaceus-type with anti-dg1 autoantibodies, usually caused by thiol-containing drugs, e.g. D-penicillamine, captopril (see ➔ Box 13.4, p. 269).
- Paraneoplastic pemphigus caused by fludarabine (see ➔ Box 13.4, p. 269).
- Pompholyx caused by IV Ig. May evolve into a generalized eczematous rash.
- Linear IgA bullous dermatosis induced by vancomycin (most often) and other drugs, e.g. penicillin, ceftriaxone, metronidazole, moxifloxacin, diclofenac, phenytoin, amiodarone. Tends to be more severe than the spontaneous form and may mimic TEN.
- Iododerma (see ➔ p. 388).

Further reading

Chanal J et al. Br J Dermatol 2013;169:1041–8 (drug-induced linear IgA).

Drug-induced abnormalities of hair and nails

Diffuse non-scarring alopecia
- Exclude other causes, including iron deficiency, thyroid disease, and telogen effluvium after a severe illness.
- Diffuse alopecia caused by drugs such as cytotoxics, anticoagulants (heparin and warfarin), antithyroid drugs, and oral contraceptives.
- Temporary interruption of cell division may cause focal narrowing of hair shafts (Pohl–Pincus marks). If severe, hair shafts may fracture (correlates with Beau lines in nails—see later in this section).

Scarring alopecia
- Rare after chemotherapy with taxanes.

Increased hair growth
- Hirsutism = increased hair growth in ♀ in an androgen-dependent pattern (normal ♂ sexual pattern)—face, lips, chest, arms, thighs. Causes: oral contraceptive pill, other androgenic drugs.
- Hypertrichosis = increased hair growth at all body sites. Causes include: ciclosporin, corticosteroids, acetazolamide, phenytoin, IFN, minoxidil, and cetuximab.

Nail abnormalities
Common causes: tetracyclines, antimalarials, retinoids, antiretroviral agents, and chemotherapy agents. Drug-induced nail changes usually involve many or all of the nails and resolve when the drug is withdrawn. Drugs may affect the nail matrix, nail bed, periungual tissues, or blood vessels. Several mechanisms may be involved.
- Nail matrix damage:
  - Beau lines = transverse grooves in the nail plate caused by a temporary interruption of cell division in the nail matrix (common). If severe, nails may be shed (onychomadesis). (Correlates with Pohl–Pincus marks in hair shafts—see earlier in this section.)
  - Nail fragility, altered rate of nail growth, leuconychia.
  - Pigmentation: diffuse or in bands (longitudinal or transverse).
- Nail bed damage:
  - Separation of the nail plate from the nail bed = onycholysis (common) (see Fig. 18.4).
  - Photo-onycholysis (painful, may be pigmented).
  - Splinter haemorrhages.
  - Subungual hyperkeratosis or thickening of the nail bed.

- Proximal nail fold damage:
  - Periungual pyogenic granulomas (common).
  - Acute paronychia, sometimes with subungual abscess (unusual) (see Fig. 18.5).
- Nail blood flow alterations:
  - Ischaemic changes; subungual haemorrhages (purpura).
  - Nail atrophy.

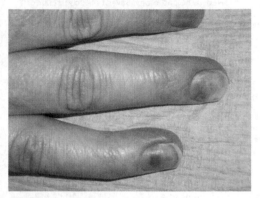

Fig. 18.4 Painful onycholysis caused by chemotherapy.

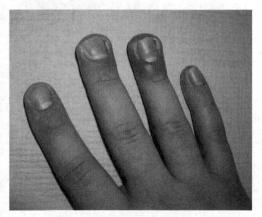

Fig. 18.5 Painful paronychia caused by tretinoin.

Reactions to chemotherapy agents: 1

Chemotherapy-induced hand–foot skin reaction

Synonyms: acral erythema or palmar–plantar erythrodysaesthesia.

- Occurs in association with systemic drugs such as cyclophosphamide, cytarabine, capecitabine, doxorubicin hydrochloride, fluorouracil, BRAF inhibitors (vemurafenib, dabrafenib), imatinib, and sunitinib. Eccrine glands involved in the pathology. Severity is dose-related. Occurs on skin exposed to friction or pressure.
- Causes paraesthesiae, tingling, burning, or pain predominantly of the palms and soles. Reduced tolerance to contact with hot objects.
- Symmetrical erythematous, oedematous papules develop on palms and soles. Skin may fissure, blister, and ulcerate. Sides of fingers and periungual skin may be erythematous.
- Erythema may extend to the dorsum of the hands and feet.
- Hyperkeratosis develops late (seen early with sorafenib). Tends to localize to pressure areas or areas of friction.
- Tenderness and pain may lead to withdrawal of treatment.
- Management:
  - Minimize pressure and friction: soft, loose-fitting shoes; cotton socks; padded gloves.
  - Pare hyperkeratotic areas gently—regular chiropody.
  - Keratolytic moisturizers with 10–25% urea or salicylic acid, topical anaesthetic creams (EMLA®), topical corticosteroids.
  - NSAIDs, pregabalin 50mg tds.

Neutrophilic eccrine hidradenitis

- Mainly in patients receiving chemotherapy for malignancy, most often haematological such as acute myelogenous leukaemia.
- Delay of about 10 days between start of chemotherapy and onset.
- Rash may be asymptomatic or painful.
- Presents with one or more erythematous, oedematous papules, nodules, or plaques. Sometimes pustular or purpuric centres to plaques.
- Lesions either grouped or disseminated widely in an asymmetrical distribution.
- Distribution is mainly proximal, affecting the upper trunk, upper limbs, and face, particularly periorbital skin, or distal involving the extremities.
- Usually spares groins and axillae.
- Mucosae are not affected.
- May show pathergy, i.e. lesions at sites of IV injections.
- Fever is common but may be linked to underlying neutropenia, rather than the rash.
- Skin biopsy shows neutrophilic infiltrate around degenerative eccrine glands.
- Lesions resolve without scarring in a few days or weeks. Some, but not all, patients relapse when re-exposed to the same drug regimen.

- Topical treatments are ineffective. The role of oral corticosteroids is unproven. NSAIDs may relieve pain and fever.
- Differential diagnosis includes cutaneous infection (culture tissue), leukaemia cutis, EM (symmetrical, target lesions, mucosal ulcers), and Sweet syndrome (see ➋ p. 111 and p. 518).

Eccrine squamous metaplasia

- Oedematous, erythematous plaques or macules that may become confluent. Sometimes vesicles. Typically affects the face, axillae, groins, and legs. May also have erythema and oedema on the palms and legs.
- Itchy or painful.
- Possibly a non-specific reaction to damaged eccrine ductal epithelium.
- Triggered by many chemotherapy drugs. Also seen with excessive sweating and in some skin diseases, e.g. infection (herpesvirus, CMV), inflammatory skin diseases, and skin tumours.
- Sometimes considered to be in the spectrum of neutrophilic eccrine hidradenitis.

Flagellate dermatitis

- Mainly seen in association with bleomycin.
- Appears 1 day to several months after administration of the drug.
- Intensely itchy, linear, erythematous, urticated plaques may affect the arms, back, and scalp, mimicking self-inflicted injury produced by a whip.
- Lesions fade, leaving post-inflammatory linear (flagellate) pigmentation.
- Treat with sedating antihistamines and potent topical corticosteroids.

Radiation recall dermatitis

(see ➋ Box 26.1, p. 531.)
- Well-defined cutaneous reaction at a previously irradiated site. Resembles an acute radiation reaction.
- Triggered most often by IV chemotherapy.

Nail changes are common

(see ➋ pp. 380–1 and Fig. 18.4.)

Reactions to chemotherapy agents: 2

BRAF inhibitors

Agents, e.g. vemurafenib, dabrafenib. Cutaneous toxicity, common, and dose-dependent. Regular skin monitoring recommended. Cutaneous toxicities may include:

- Itch and dry skin.
- Grover disease (itchy erythematous papules, acantholytic histology).
- Rashes, with or without itch—maculopapular, papulopustular, folliculocentric, seborrhoeic dermatitis-like, milia, keratosis pilaris-like.
- Hyperkeratotic hand–foot skin reaction (see ➔ p. 382).
- Photosensitivity (UVA-dependent) may cause painful blisters.
- Squamoproliferative tumours, e.g. papillomas, viral warts, seborrhoeic warts, warty dyskeratomas, palmar/plantar hyperkeratosis, solar keratoses, keratoacanthomas, SCCs. More at onset of treatment, then the rate of development of tumours levels off.
- Melanocytic proliferation, e.g. atypical melanocytic proliferation, second 1° melanomas, activated naevi, and lentigines. Monitor melanocytic lesions with a dermatoscope.
- Painful lobular panniculitis.
- Hair loss (non-scarring).
- Firm purplish papules with granulomatous histology.
- Pyogenic granuloma (vemurafenib).
- Radiation recall dermatitis (vemurafenib).

Epidermal growth factor receptor inhibitors

Agents, e.g. cetuximab, panitumumab, erlotinib, gefitinib. EGFR is expressed by basal keratinocytes and sebocytes, as well as the outer root sheath of hair follicles. Cutaneous adverse effects may include:

- Initial oedema, redness, and a burning sensation on the face and upper trunk. May be mildly itchy.
- Sterile itchy (unlike acne) papulopustular follicular eruption on the face and trunk 7–10 days after starting treatment (no comedones) (see Fig. 18.6). May spare skin previously treated by radiotherapy. Gradually crusts and resolves. Severity dose-related. Presence of rash may correlate with more effective treatment and increased survival time. Swab to exclude 2° staphylococcal infection. Treatment options: antihistamines (for itch), topical clindamycin, topical calcineurin inhibitors, oral tetracyclines, low-dose isotretinoin (20mg daily).
- Painful paronychia, periungual abscess, pyogenic granuloma of the nail fold.
- Brittle, curly scalp hair, increased facial hair, long eyelashes, scarring alopecia with pustules, i.e. follicultis decalvans (erlotinib).
- Mucosal ulcers, dry mouth.

Taxanes

Agents: docetaxel, paclitaxel. Cutaneous adverse effects include:
- Hand–foot skin reaction (common) (see ➲ p. 382).
- Radiation recall dermatitis (see ➲ Box 26.1, p. 531).
- Alopecia—usually regrows. Rarely scarring and permanent.
- Nail abnormalities:
  - Subungual haemorrhage leading to onycholysis (see Fig. 18.4).
  - Orange-brown discoloration.
  - Beau lines, transverse loss of the nail plate.
  - Acute paronychia and subungual abscess (see Fig. 18.5).
- AGEP.
- SCLE, photosensitivity, scleroderma-like changes of the legs, and erysipelas-like erythema.

Multikinase inhibitors

Agents, e.g. sorafenib, sunitinib, and vandetanib. Inhibit a variety of tyrosine kinase receptors, e.g. vasoactive endothelial growth factor receptor, platelet-derived growth factor receptor. Adverse effects may include:
- Hyperkeratotic hand–foot skin reaction (see ➲ p. 382).
- Morbilliform rashes, dry skin, itch.
- Comedonal acneiform eruptions, folliculitis.
- Alopecia, subungual splinter hemorrhages.
- Depigmentation hair/skin.
- Photosensitivity.
- AGEP, TEN.
- Sweet syndrome (nilotinib).
- Papillomas, BCCs, and SCCs.

Inhibitors of mitogen-activated protein kinase (MAPK) kinase (MEK inhibitors)

Agents, e.g. selumetinib, cobimetinib, trametinib. Adverse effects include.
- Morbilliform eruption.
- Papulopustular eruption (similar to EGFR inhibitors). 2° staphylococcal infection is common.
- Dry skin and itch.
- Paronychia, mild hair loss.
- Dusky erythema with urticated or targetoid patches.

Smoothened (Smo) receptor inhibitors

Agents: vismodegib (blocks hedgehog signalling pathway). Adverse effects include:
- Alopecia, taste disturbance.
- Possibly keratoacanthoma/eruptive SCCs (sun-damaged skin).

Mammalian target of rapamycin (mTOR) inhibitors

Agents: rapamycin, temsirolimus, everolimus. Mucocutaneous adverse effects are common and may include:

- Stomatitis—dose-related. Responds to potent topical corticosteroids.
- Morbilliform, eczematous, or acneiform eruptions on the trunk, spreading to the extremities, neck, face, and scalp.
- Paronychia, pyogenic granuloma-like lesions of the nail fold.
- Alopecia, itch, dry skin, vasculitis, poor wound healing.

Cytotoxic T-lymphocyte-associated protein 4 (CTLA-4) inhibitors

Agents: ipilimumab. Stimulates the immune system. Induces autoimmune adverse effects:

- Itch, morbilliform rash, vitiligo-like hypopigmentation.

Purine and pyrimidine analogues

Agents: fludarabine, cladribine, capecitabine, tegafur, gemcitabine. Cutaneous adverse effects include:

- Hand–foot skin reaction (see ➲ p. 382).
- Acral hyperpigmentation most marked in skin creases.
- Autoimmune phenomena, including paraneoplastic pemphigus (linked to fludarabine).
- Inflammation of actinic keratoses (caused by capecitabine which is a prodrug of 5-fluorouracil).

Hydroxycarbamide (hydroxyurea)

Cytostatic agent used in myeloproliferative disorders. Cutaneous adverse effects include:

- Diffuse hyperpigmentation and brown nails.
- Dermatomyositis-like eruption on the dorsum of hands (ANA-negative) (see ➲ Box 19.14, p. 411).
- Acral erythema and palmoplantar keratoderma (PPK).
- An atrophic poikilodermatous (see ➲ p. 410) appearance on the legs.
- One or more persistent, painful, well-defined shallow leg ulcers, usually over the malleoli, but may affect the calf, dorsal foot, or toes. Develop after an average of 5 years of treatment. Surrounding skin may be purpuric and atrophic. Heal when hydroxycarbamide is stopped.
- Oral mucosal ulcers.

Tretinoin

Acid form of vitamin A. Used in acute promyelocytic leukaemia. Cutaneous adverse effects include:

- Pruritus, erythema, and dry skin; dry mucosae and cheilitis.
- Alopecia, periungual pyogenic granulomas, acute paronychia (see Fig. 18.5).

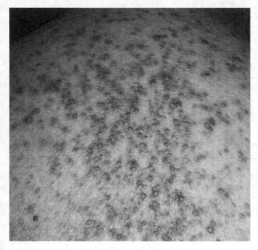

Fig. 18.6 Acne-like eruption caused by erlotinib (EGFR inhibitor).

Further reading

Belum VR et al. Curr Oncol Rep 2013;15:249–59.
Macdonald JB et al. J Am Acad Dermatol 2015;72:203–18.
Macdonald JB et al. J Am Acad Dermatol 2015;72:221–36.

Drugs and skin diseases

Acne or acne-like pustular eruptions
(see ➲ p. 244.)
- Causes include topical and oral corticosteroids; androgens, including anabolic steroids, phenytoin, phenobarbital, lithium, bromides, isoniazid, rifampicin, and EGFR inhibitors (see ➲ p. 384).
- A papulopustular rash develops within weeks of starting the drug. Comedones are unlikely, unless the reaction is caused by exogenous androgens. May take months to resolve, despite treatment for acne.
- Iododerma (rare, but commoner in renal failure when clearance of iodine in contrast medium is impaired). Acneiform papules/pustules, haemorrhagic bullae/pustules, plaques, or nodules.

Dermatomyositis-like
(see ➲ pp. 410–11.)
- Most often hydroxycarbamide (hydroxyurea) (see ➲ p. 386).
- Also reported with penicillamine, statins, IFN-β, anti-TNF agents, ipilimumab, and others.

Eczema
(see ➲ pp. 212–13.)
- Calcium channel blockers have been linked to generalized chronic eczematous eruptions in the elderly.
- IV Ig may precipitate pompholyx (vesicles on palms and soles) and eczema.

Elastosis perforans serpiginosa
(see ➲ Box 19.28, p. 431.)
- Penicillamine.

Erythema gyratum repens
- Azathioprine, pegylated IFN-α.

Halo naevi
- Multiple halo naevi (halo of hypopigmentation around regressing melanocytic naevi) may be induced by immune-modifying drugs, including infliximab, IFN-β1a, adalimumab, tocilizumab.

Ichthyosis
Kava dermopathy is a common reaction to heavy use of kava, a psychoactive drink prepared from *Piper methysticum*. Used recreationally throughout the Pacific and increasingly elsewhere. May be added to herbal remedies. Dermopathy is characterized by:
- Scaly skin (ichthyosiform dermatitis) that starts on the head, face, and neck, progresses to the body and feet, and becomes generalized.
- Sometimes facial oedema, alopecia, and hyperpigmentation of exposed skin.
- Resolves slowly when kava withdrawn.

Lichen planus-like

(see ⮞ p. 224.)

- Widespread lichenoid reactions may appear weeks or months after exposure to the drug (see ⮞ Fig. 18.2, p. 369, and p. 375).
- Discrete papules, resembling LP or plane warts, have been caused by palifermin, a recombinant human keratinocyte growth factor.

Neutrophilic dermatoses

- Pyoderma gangrenosum-like (see ⮞ p. 310). Nicorandil induces painful ulcers, as may cocaine.
- Azathioprine hypersensitivity syndrome resembles Sweet syndrome, with fever, neutrophilia, and papules/plaques with dense infiltrate of polymorphonuclear cells. Signs mainly on extremities, unlike Sweet syndrome (see ⮞ p. 518).
- Granulocyte colony-stimulating factor (G-CSF) is the commonest cause of drug-induced Sweet syndrome.

Psoriasis and palmoplantar pustulosis

(see ⮞ p. 196, p. 198.)

- Lithium exacerbates psoriasis more often than inducing disease.
- Antimalarials and IFNs may exacerbate psoriasis.
- β-adrenergic receptor-blocking agents may induce or exacerbate psoriasis.
- Systemic corticosteroids: an exacerbation of psoriasis, which may be pustular, can be triggered by withdrawal of systemic corticosteroids prescribed for an unrelated condition.
- NSAIDs, angiotensin receptor blockers, and ACE inhibitors possibly exacerbate psoriasis.
- Alcohol: psoriatic patients with a high alcohol intake tend to have more severe disease.
- TNF-α antagonists have been reported to induce plaque, guttate, erythrodermic, and pustular psoriasis, although these drugs are used to treat psoriasis. They also cause palmoplantar pustulosis.
- Ustekinumab (IL-12/23 inhibitor) may trigger pustular psoriasis.

Rosacea

(see ⮞ pp. 254–5.)

- Exacerbated by peripheral vasodilators, including glyceryl trinitrate, isosorbide, and alcohol (no increased risk found with calcium channel blockers in a study published in 2014).

Pigmented purpuric dermatoses

- A variety of drugs, including diuretics, NSAIDs, sedatives, antibiotics, cardiovascular drugs, isotretinoin, and vitamins.

Pityriasis rosea-like
(see ⬧ p. 151 and Fig. 18.7.)
- A mildly itchy rash, mainly on the trunk and proximal upper limbs. Papules and plaques are aligned in a 'Christmas tree' pattern with long axes parallel to the ribs (parallel to Langer's skin lines). Drugs that have been implicated include:
- Gold compounds, imatinib mesylate, barbiturates, D-penicillamine, captopril, terbinafine, isotretinoin, bismuth compounds, omeprazole, arsenicals.

Pemphigus
(see ⬧ pp. 268–9.)

Subacute cutaneous lupus erythematosus
(see ⬧ p. 402.)
   SCLE appears weeks to several years after starting the drug and resolves 1–24 weeks after stopping the drug. Anti-Ro antibodies may persist when the drug is withdrawn. Consider in older patients presenting with SCLE for the first time. A wide variety of drugs have been implicated, including:
- Diuretics (hydrochlorothiazide and spironolactone), calcium channel blockers, β-blockers, ACE inhibitors, proton pump inhibitors, antifungals (terbinafine and griseofulvin), chemotherapeutic agents, immunomodulators, biologics, NSAIDs, hormone-altering drugs, statins, and antihistamines

Porphyria cutanea tarda
(see ⬧ p. 332.)
- In genetically susceptible individuals, some drugs exacerbate PCT, including alcohol, oral oestrogens, oral contraception and hormone replacement therapy, oral iron, antimalarials, and griseofulvin.

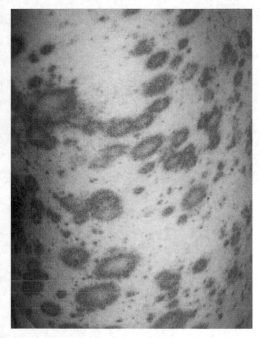

Fig. 18.7 Pityriasis rosea-like drug reaction with annular erythematous lesions.

Further reading

Ahronowitz I and Fox L. *Semin Cutan Med Surg* 2014;**33**:49–58 (drug-induced dermatoses).
Lowe G et al. *Br J Dermatol* 2011;**164**:465–72 (drug-induced SCLE).
Spoendlin J et al. *Br J Dermatol* 2014;**171**:130–6 (antihypertensive drugs and risk of rosacea).

Skin and rheumatology

Contents

Relevant pages in other chapters

Skin manifestations in spondyloarthropathies such as
Psoriatic arthritis ➔ p. 206, Reactive arthritis ➔ p. 208,
and SAPHO syndrome ➔ p. 248
Vasculitis ➔ Chapter 20, pp. 435–52
Autoinflammatory diseases ➔ pp. 234–6
Neutrophilic dermatoses ➔ pp. 518–19
Amyloidosis ➔ pp. 496–7
α-1-antitrypsin deficiency ➔ p. 462
Nephrogenic systemic fibrosis ➔ p. 498
Behçet disease ➔ pp. 284–5

Rheumatoid arthritis

RA is an autoimmune chronic inflammatory disease that may be complicated by a systemic vasculitis and extra-articular manifestations including pericarditis, pleurisy, interstitial lung disease, iritis, and neuropathy. Rheumatoid vasculitis is most common in seropositive (i.e. RF- or anti-CCP positive) patients with long-standing nodular disease.

Rheumatoid arthritis: what cutaneous signs should I look for?

- Pale, shiny, atrophic skin that is fragile and bruises easily.
- Palmar erythema.
- Bluish discoloration of fingertips and periungual erythema.
- Nails may be ridged longitudinally and may have red lunulae.
- Firm, skin-coloured, non-tender subcutaneous nodules, 5–40mm in diameter (20–30% of patients). Rheumatoid nodules are found most often on sites exposed to mild trauma or pressure, e.g. olecranon, knuckles (see Fig. 19.1), knees, and occiput (but may also be found in the lung). Nodules are linked to both seropositivity for RF and severe systemic manifestations. Nodules must be differentiated from tophi in chronic tophaceous gout (see Box 19.2).
- Rarely nodules ulcerate or become infected.
- Signs of small-vessel cutaneous vasculitis: palpable purpura, papulonecrotic lesions, or urticarial vasculitis (see ➋ pp. 440–3).
- Vasculitic lesions on the fingers, even in patients without systemic vasculitis, including papules, splinter haemorrhages, linear telangiectasia in the nail fold, petechiae, and brownish purpuric lesions of the nail fold or finger pulp (Bywater lesions) that may infarct and heal, leaving small scars. Painless, red-black lesions of the nail fold or finger pulp (microinfarcts of superficial dermal vessels) are also seen in SLE.
- Vasculitis involving medium-sized cutaneous vessels presents with livedo reticularis, nodules, and painful punched-out ulcers along the lateral malleoli or pre-tibial region. Twenty percent of patients with severe vasculitis have digital gangrene.
- Leg ulcers (10% of patients with RA) often multifactorial (see Box 19.1).
- Interstitial granulomatous dermatitis: an uncommon condition of unknown cause that may be associated with severe RA, as well as other systemic autoimmune diseases. Tender, linear, indurated bands arise symmetrically on the axilla, trunk, and inner portions of the thighs (see ➋ p. 373).
- Rheumatoid neutrophilic dermatitis, a condition of unknown cause associated with severe RA, characterized by papules, plaques, nodules, and urticarial wheals. Biopsy shows a dense dermal infiltrate of neutrophils. Neutrophilic dermatoses have also been described in SLE and dermatomyositis. May resemble Sweet syndrome (see ➋ p. 518).
- Blistering diseases, including mucous membrane pemphigoid, pemphigus, EBA, and subcorneal pustular dermatosis have been reported in association with RA (see ➋ pp. 264–72).

Box 19.1 Leg ulcers in rheumatoid arthritis

- Ten percent of patients with RA have leg ulcers.
- Pathogenesis is multifactorial, and management should address underlying causes, but always handle the skin gently.
- Trauma (beware the footrest of the wheelchair), skin fragility, and immobility with venous stasis are the commonest causes of ulcers (for advice on management, see ➔ p. 306).
- Systemic corticosteroids delay healing of ulcers and contribute to skin fragility, as well as complications such as 2° infection.
- Small-vessel cutaneous vasculitis presents with palpable purpura and, if severe, may lead to necrotic ulcers with purpuric rims (see ➔ p. 440).
- Deeper cutaneous ulcers may be produced by vasculitis involving medium-sized vessels. Look for livedo reticularis, nodules, and painful punched-out ulcers along the lateral malleoli or in the pre-tibial region.
- Painful, rapidly enlarging ulcers with undermined bluish red borders may be caused by PG (see ➔ p. 310).
- Patients with Felty syndrome (RA, leucopenia, and splenomegaly) may develop chronic leg ulcers that are refractory to treatment.

Box 19.2 Rheumatoid nodules or tophi?

- Tophi are nodules formed by deposits of urate crystals in cartilage, tendons, and soft tissues.
- Tophi tend to develop in patients with long-standing (>10y) polyarticular gout and severe hyperuricaemia.
- Tophi are often found along the helix of the ear. Other common sites include the great toe, fingers, wrist, hand, elbow (olecranon bursa, when tophi may resemble rheumatoid nodules), and Achilles tendon.
- Tophi, unlike rheumatoid nodules, may drain chalky material.
- In gout, uric acid is often raised, and RF is usually negative.
- Chronic tophaceous gout causes severe joint destruction, if not treated.

Further reading

Jorizzo JL and Daniels JC. J Am Acad Dermatol 1983;8:439–57.
Sayah A et al. J Am Acad Dermatol 2005;53:191–209.
Yamamoto T. Rheumatol Int 2009;29:979–88.

Lupus erythematosus

Systemic lupus erythematosus

- SLE is a chronic multisystem inflammatory disease with autoantibodies.
- The American College of Rheumatology (ACR) 1982 Classification Criteria for SLE (revised in 1997) are well known, but concerns about the shortcomings of these criteria (including lack of validation, duplication of terms relating to cutaneous lupus, omission of many cutaneous and neurological features of lupus) led to the development of new criteria in 2012 by the Systemic Lupus International Collaborating Clinics (SLICC) group (see Box 19.3). These are intended to be more clinically relevant and reflect new knowledge about lupus immunology.
- Cutaneous manifestations are the first sign of SLE in around 25% of patients, and eventually >90% will develop cutaneous features; 70% of patients are photosensitive.
- Patients with SLE may have cutaneous LE (see next section), as well as non-specific cutaneous signs, such as small-vessel cutaneous vasculitis, that may suggest SLE in the right setting. These non-specific signs are not diagnostic of SLE, and many may be seen in other connective tissue diseases (see ➋ Box 19.5, p. 401).

Cutaneous lupus erythematosus

- Cutaneous LE is an inflammatory skin disease that is a specific manifestation of LE. Some, but not all, patients with cutaneous LE may have SLE. Cutaneous LE is not a vasculitis, but a lichenoid reaction in the skin (see Box 19.4). Cutaneous LE is subdivided into:
  - Acute cutaneous LE (only seen in patients with active SLE) (see ➋ p. 402, and Fig 19.2).
  - SCLE (see ➋ p. 402, and Figs. 19.3, and 19.5,).
  - Chronic cutaneous LE (CCLE) (including DLE) (see ➋ p. 404 and Figs. 19.4 and 19.6).
- Patients may have >1 type of cutaneous LE, and all can occur in association with SLE.
- It is confusing, because the terms SCLE and DLE are used in two ways, either to describe a type of skin lesion or to refer to subsets of patients who share certain clinical and immunological features but do not meet the criteria for SLE.

Box 19.3 Systemic Lupus International Collaborating Clinics classification criteria for systemic lupus erythematosus

The patient must satisfy at least four criteria, including at least one clinical and one immunologic, OR the patient must have biopsy-proven lupus nephritis in the presence of ANA or anti-double-stranded (ds) DNA antibodies. Criteria do not need to be present concurrently.

Clinical criteria

1. *Acute cutaneous lupus*: lupus malar rash (do not count if malar discoid), bullous lupus, TEN variant of SLE, maculopapular lupus rash, photosensitive lupus rash, or subacute cutaneous lupus (non-indurated psoriaform and/or annular polycyclic lesions that resolve without scarring, although occasionally with post-inflammatory dyspigmentation or telangiectasias).
2. *Chronic cutaneous LE*: classical discoid rash (localized—above the neck; generalized—above and below the neck), hypertrophic (verrucous) lupus, lupus panniculitis (profundus), mucosal lupus, LE tumidus, chilblain lupus, discoid lupus/LP overlap.
3. *Oral ulcers*: palate (buccal, tongue) or nasal ulcers (in the absence of other causes).
4. *Non-scarring alopecia*.
5. *Synovitis*: ≥2 joints, characterized by swelling or effusion or tenderness in ≥2 joints and ≥30min of morning stiffness.
6. *Serositis*: typical pleurisy for >1 day, or pleural effusions, or pleural rub or typical pericardial pain for >1 day, or pericardial effusion, or pericardial rub, or pericarditis by ECG.
7. *Renal*: urine protein:creatinine ratio (or 24-h urine protein) representing 500mg of protein/24h or RBC casts.
8. *Neurological*: seizures, psychosis, mononeuritis multiplex, myelitis, peripheral or cranial neuropathy, acute confusional state (in the absence of other causes).
9. *Haemolytic anaemia*.
10. *Leucopenia* (<4000/mm³ at least once) or lymphopenia (<1000/mm³ at least once).
11. *Thrombocytopenia* (<100 000/mm³) at least once.

Immunological criteria

1. *ANA* above reference range.
2. *Anti-dsDNA* above reference range or ≥×2 above if enzyme-linked immunosorbent assay (ELISA).
3. *Anti-Smith* antibody.
4. *Antiphospholipid antibody*: lupus anticoagulant, false-positive rapid plasma reagin (RPR), medium- or high-titre anticardiolipin (IgA, IgG, or IgM), anti-β2-glycoprotein I (IgA, IgG, or IgM).
5. *Low complement*: low C3, C4, or CH50.
6. *Positive direct Coombs' test*: in the absence of haemolytic anaemia.

Petri M et al. Arthritis Rheum 2012 Aug;64(8):2677–86.

Box 19.4 Cutaneous lupus erythematosus: histological findings

- Skin biopsies from cutaneous LE show a lichenoid lymphocytic infiltrate (interface dermatitis), i.e. lymphocytic inflammation at the dermo-epidermal junction, with damage to the basal keratinocytes. This involves both the epidermis and hair follicles.
- Inflammation is most marked in chronic lesions.
- There is perivascular inflammation, but no vasculitis.

Further reading

Kuhn A and Landmann A. *J Autoimmun* 2014;**48–49**:14–19.
Lin JH et al. *Clin Rev Allerg Immunol* 2007;**33**:85–106.
Sontheimer RD. *Best Pract Res Clin Rheumatol* 2004;18:429–62.
Sontheimer RD. *Autoimmun Rev* 2005;4:253–63.

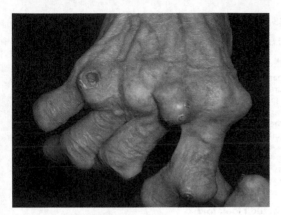

Fig. 19.1 Rheumatoid nodules.

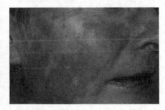

Fig. 19.2 Malar rash in systemic lupus erythematosus.

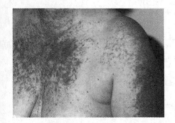

Fig. 19.3 Subacute cutaneous lupus erythematosus: scaly papules and plaques in a
photosensitive distribution.

Assessment of skin in systemic lupus erythematosus

What should I ask?

- Is the patient sensitive to sun—what happens and how long after exposure? (see ➜ p. 28.)
- Has the patient any skin problems or mouth ulcers (may be painless)?
- Is the rash leaving scars or pigment change?
- Does the patient notice pustules? (Seen in rosacea or acne, but not in cutaneous LE.)
- Is the scalp scaly or the hair changing? (Seborrhoeic dermatitis and psoriasis cause scale and erythema on the scalp but do not usually cause hair loss.)
- What drugs is the patient taking, and what is the relationship of starting drugs to the onset of any rash?

What should I look for?

- Signs suggesting photosensitivity, i.e. the rash is photoaggravated. Does the rash spare skin normally protected from sunlight such as under the chin, the eyelids (ask the patient to close his/her eyes), beneath hair, or behind ears? (For more information about signs of photosensitivity, see ➜ Box 4.6, p. 73.)
- Signs of cutaneous LE (acute, subacute, or chronic). (For more information, see ➜ p. 402 and pp. 404–5.)
  - Malar rash: erythematous plaques extending across the upper cheeks and bridge of the nose. Correlates with photosensitivity.
  - Scalp: perifollicular scale and erythema, hair loss, scarring (follicular orifices lost—may be easier to see with magnification, e.g. dermoscopy). Suggests DLE.
  - Ears (concha and helix): scars, follicular plugs (like 'blackheads'), pigment change. Suggests DLE (see Fig. 19.4).
  - Trunk, arms: erythematous scaly rash, annular scaly lesions, pigment change. Suggests SCLE (see Fig. 19.5).
  - Mucosal plaques: lips, hard palate, buccal mucosa.
  - Dorsum of hands and fingers: scaly erythematous plaques.
- Non-specific signs suggestive of SLE, including cutaneous vasculitis (see Box 19.5).
  - Look carefully at nail folds for periungual erythema or abnormal capillaries.
  - Check pulps of toes, as well as finger pulps, and palms for erythema, ulceration, and purpura.
  - Check limbs for livedo reticularis or palpable purpura.

Box 19.5 Non-specific cutaneous features that may be found in patients with systemic lupus erythematosus

- Urticaria (hives, wheals): itchy, smooth, erythematous bumps, lasting no more than 48h that fade to leave normal skin.
- Oral ulcers.
- Non-scarring alopecia 2° to:
  - Lupus hairs (hairs break off at the front of the scalp).
  - Telogen effluvium (shedding 8–12 weeks after severe illness).
  - Alopecia areata (autoimmune hair loss).
- Raynaud phenomenon.
- Vascular involvement: vasculitis or non-inflammatory occlusive vasculopathy (see ➲ p. 440 and p. 452):
  - Periungual erythema.
  - Linear telangiectasia on the posterior nail fold: a sign of a connective tissue disease also found in dermatomyositis, systemic sclerosis, and 5% of cases of RA.
  - Thrombosed nail fold vessels carried forward into a ragged cuticle.
  - Painless, red-black lesions of nail fold or finger pulp (microinfarcts of superficial dermal vessels)—also seen in RA.
  - Papular telangiectasia on the palms or fingertips.
  - Atrophie blanche (streaky telangiectasia interspersed with pale, scarred-looking skin) on plantar surface of toes or finger pulps.
  - Urticarial vasculitis: tender wheals lasting >48h and resolving to leave bruises; may indicate low complement (see ➲ p. 443).
  - Palpable purpura (i.e. non-blanching) at sites of stasis (legs), cooling (ear helix), or pressure (sacrum).
  - Livedo reticularis (discontinuous) that persists if skin is warm or retiform purpura: suggests the antiphospholipid syndrome which is associated with recurrent thromboses and neurological complications (see ➲ p. 452, and Box 20.10, p. 453).
- Neutrophilic Sweet-like dermatosis: also described in dermatomyositis and RA (see ➲ p. 518).

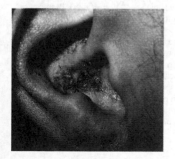

Fig. 19.4 Discoid lupus erythematosus scaly plaques in the ear.

Acute and subacute cutaneous lupus erythematosus

Acute cutaneous lupus erythematosus

Seen in patients with active SLE.

What should I look for?
- Erythematous, oedematous rash, with minimal scale spreading symmetrically across the upper cheeks (see Fig. 19.2).
- Rash is generally asymptomatic, unlike dermatomyositis which itches, burns, and is painful.
- No scarring and no pustules (pustules suggest rosacea or steroid-induced acne; see ➔ p. 244 and p. 254).
- Rash disappears quickly, once skin is protected from light.
- Erythema may be generalized in very ill patients.
- Rowell syndrome may occur in acute cutaneous LE or SCLE (see Box 19.6).
- Blisters are uncommon (see Box 19.9).

Subacute cutaneous lupus erythematosus

- Fifty percent of patients with SCLE fulfil the criteria for SLE, but only 10–15% will develop severe manifestations of SLE.
- SCLE may be drug-induced: hydrochlorothiazide, calcium channel blockers, NSAIDs, ACE inhibitors, griseofulvin, terbinafine, proton pump inhibitors, IFNs, and statins. The rash commences 4–20 weeks after starting the drug. Drug-induced SCLE does not always reverse, but most eruptions clear within 6–12 weeks after withdrawal of the triggering drug. Rarely, SCLE is paraneoplastic.
- In pregnant women, SCLE can affect the neonate (see Box 19.7).

What should I look for?
- Superficial scaly, annular lesions involving the V-area of the neck, upper trunk, upper limb, and dorsum of the hands (sparing the knuckles) (see Fig. 19.5). The rash may be slightly itchy but more often is asymptomatic, unlike dermatomyositis (see ➔ pp. 408–9). Blisters are unusual (see Box 19.9). Scaly, red papules resembling psoriasis are less common (see Fig. 19.3).
- Non-scarring, but post-inflammatory, hypopigmentation common.
- Although patients are photosensitive, the face is often spared.
- Differentiate the annular rash from fungal infection (ringworm, 'tinea') by checking the position of the scale. In SCLE, the scale appears after the erythema and on the inner aspect of the ring. In fungal infections, erythema follows the scale which is on the outer edge of the ring.
- Exclude psoriasis by checking for nail pitting, onycholysis, and well-demarcated plaques of psoriasis on the knees (sun-protected) or scalp (no hair loss in psoriasis).
- Immunology: anti-Ro antibodies.

What should I do?
For investigation and management, see ➔ pp. 406–7.

Box 19.6 What is Rowell syndrome?

Rowell syndrome is probably a severe variant of acute or subacute cutaneous LE. The three major diagnostic criteria are:
- Diagnosis of LE.
- EM-like erythematous target lesions or erosions simulating TEN, with or without mucosal involvement. Histology shows an interface dermatitis with features of both cutaneous LE and EM.
- Speckled ANA (usually anti-Ro or anti-La antibodies).

Common triggers
- UVR; drugs—furosemide, ACE inhibitors, doxycycline, aciclovir, naproxen, hydroxychloroquine, sodium valproate.

Also see: Zeitouni NC et al. Br J Dermatol 2000;142:343–6.

⚠ Box 19.7 Subacute cutaneous lupus erythematosus in pregnancy

Mothers with SCLE may have infants affected by neonatal LE, because anti-Ro antibodies cross the placenta. Rarely, these infants develop a connective tissue disease later in life. Affected infants may develop:
- Photosensitive cutaneous lupus (50% of infants) with scaly, erythematous papules and plaques that are aggravated by sun exposure. Less often annular patterns. The appearance of the periorbital erythema has been termed 'racoon eyes'. Rash usually resolves over 4–6 months but may leave atrophy with telangiectasia.
- Congenital heart block which is permanent (10% of infants). At 16–18 weeks' gestation, Ro-positive mothers should be referred for fetal echocardiogram and further monitoring. The risk of congenital heart block is greatest when a previous child has had neonatal lupus or congenital heart block (5–12% recurrence rate in subsequent pregnancies).
- Haemolytic anaemia, thrombocytopenia, leucopenia, elevated LFTs: all transient.

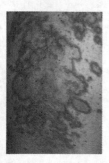

Fig. 19.5 Subacute cutaneous lupus erythematosus: annular scaling plaques.

Chronic cutaneous lupus erythematosus

Discoid lupus erythematosus

- The commonest form of CCLE. For less common forms of CCLE, see Box 19.8.
- Most patients with localized DLE (confined to the head and neck) do not develop significant systemic disease, and DLE remits eventually in about 50% of patients.
- SLE develops in 5–10% of patients, usually those with widespread DLE. The course of SLE in these patients is benign.

What should I look for?

- Erythematous, telangiectatic plaques or hyperkeratotic plaques, with adherent keratotic scale most often localized to the head and neck. These are usually asymptomatic (see Figs. 19.4 and 19.6).
- Chronic plaques cause scarring and deformity (lupus means wolf, and wolf bites are destructive).
- Plaques on the face tend to spare the nasolabial fold.
- Perifollicular inflammation in the scalp causes permanent hair loss (scarring alopecia).
- Acneiform plugged lesions (like blackheads) in the concha of the ears (see Fig. 19.4).
- Very hypertrophic lesions may resemble SCC.
- Plaques may involve the vermillion border of the lips or lower eyelids with loss of lashes and scarring.
- LP-like plaques may involve the buccal mucosa or palate (see ⮊ p. 286).
- Abnormal pigmentation (increased or decreased) is a common outcome in dark skin (see Fig. 19.4).
- Blisters are rare (see Box 19.9).
- Immunology: usually ANAs are not detected.

What should I do?

For investigation and management, see ⮊ pp. 406–7.

The Cutaneous Lupus Disease Area and Severity Index: the CLASI

The CLASI scores the severity of both disease activity (erythema, scale, mucous membrane involvement, hair loss, or non-scarring alopecia)

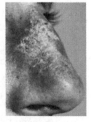

Fig. 19.6 Discoid lupus erythematosus: hyperkeratotic plaque.

and damage (dyspigmentation and scarring, including scarring alopecia). A revised score (RCLASI) has been developed to incorporate a wider range of subtypes of CCLE.

Box 19.8 Less common forms of chronic cutaneous lupus erythematosus

Lupus panniculitis (lupus profundus)
- Subcutaneous nodules on the shoulders, upper arm, face, and buttocks. Overlying skin may be affected by DLE. Fat loss is a disfiguring complication. Subcutaneous nodules may calcify and ulcerate. Skin biopsies may ulcerate and be slow to heal. SLE is unlikely.

Chilblain lupus
- Cold-induced purple plaques on the fingers or toes. Warty plaques if long-standing. May be associated with SLE.

Lupus erythematosus tumidus
- Smooth, erythematous, 'juicy' nodules on sun-exposed skin without scarring (Jessner lymphocytic infiltrate is probably the same disease). Photosensitive. May persist for weeks. Biopsy may not be diagnostic. SLE is unlikely.

Box 19.9 Vesiculobullous lupus erythematosus

Lupus erythematosus-specific vesiculobullous skin disease

Blistering may be a 2° phenomenon in severe cutaneous LE. If the interface dermatitis causes extensive damage to the basal keratinocytes, the epidermis detaches from the dermis. If the epidermal damage is full-thickness, the changes may even resemble TEN. The disease has been subdivided into:
- TEN-like acute cutaneous LE.
- TEN-like SCLE.
- TEN in SLE (patients without LE-specific skin lesions, in whom no drug-related cause for TEN can be identified).
- Vesiculobullous annular SCLE.
- Vesiculobullous DLE.

Lupus erythematosus-non-specific vesiculobullous skin disease

Blisters may develop in the context of a distinct autoantibody-mediated bullous disease. Histology does not show an interface dermatitis, but the features of the autoimmune blistering disease:
- DH-like vesiculobullous LE.
- EBA-like vesiculobullous LE.
- BP-like vesiculobullous LE.

Further reading

Albrecht J and Werth V. *Dermatol Ther* 2007;**20**:93–101 (discusses CLASI).
Bonilla-Martinez ZL et al. *Arch Dermatol* 2008;**144**:173–80 (discusses CLASI).
Klein R et al. *Arch Dermatol* 2011;**147**:203–8 (discusses CLASI).
Kuhn A et al. *Br J Dermatol* 2010;**163**:83e92 (discusses CLASI).
Ting W et al. *Lupus* 2004;**13**:941–50.

Management of cutaneous lupus erythematosus

What should I do?

- Investigate to confirm the diagnosis and exclude systemic disease (see Box 19.11).
- Advise the patient to stop smoking; more severe in smokers.
- Advise photoprotection (sun protection) to reduce the need for topical steroids or systemic treatment. Continue even when the disease is controlled (see ➜ pp. 338–9 and Box 19.12).
- Very potent topical corticosteroid (clobetasol propionate) ointment applied bd controls most localized cutaneous disease (use topical corticosteroids, even if the patient is also taking prednisolone for systemic disease). Apply before the application of sunscreen cream. Reduce the strength gradually to less potent preparations, such as mometasone furoate (potent—use ×1/day), as soon as inflammation is controlled and lesions have flattened. Gradually reduce the frequency of application.
- Scalp: clobetasol propionate scalp application at night.
- Intralesional triamcinolone (10mg/mL) may be effective in resistant plaques of DLE.
- Tacrolimus ointment 0.1% is worth trying, if facial DLE is not controlled by very potent topical corticosteroids.
- Most patients respond to oral hydroxychloroquine 200mg bd (<6.5mg/ kg/day) after 8–12 weeks. Combine with topical corticosteroids and photoprotection.
- If the rash gets worse, reconsider the diagnosis—has the patient also got psoriasis, which can be exacerbated by antimalarials? (See Box 19.10.)
- Check visual acuity if hydroxychloroquine is to be continued. Patients taking hydroxychloroquine should see an optician annually.

Box 19.10 Cutaneous lupus erythematosus is not responding to treatment

If cutaneous LE has not improved after 4 weeks of treatment:
- Ensure that the patient is using photoprotection.
- Ensure that the patient is applying a very potent topical corticosteroid (many patients have steroid phobia). Topical corticosteroids should be used, even if the patient is also taking oral prednisolone for systemic disease.
- Is the rash LE? Pustules suggest steroid-induced acne or rosacea, not LE; an asymmetrical facial scaling plaque may be caused by a fungal infection; might this be psoriasis triggered by antimalarials?
- Is the patient smoking?
- Is the patient allergic to the sunblock?

Box 19.11 Investigation of cutaneous lupus erythematosus

- SCLE: take a skin scrape from the edge of an annular lesion for mycological culture.
- Take a skin biopsy for histology from an active erythematous lesion, not a scar (generally not necessary in acute cutaneous LE).
- Direct IMF of involved skin for a 'lupus band' is not usually required to diagnose cutaneous LE.
- Detection of a 'lupus band' in a biopsy from sun-protected skin of the forearm has been used to predict the likelihood of renal involvement in SLE, but this test is not in widespread use.
- Anti-annexin 1 antibodies are associated with cutaneous LE.
- Does the patient have SLE? Check:
  - Urine RBC, protein, and microscopy—spin down for urinary casts.
  - FBC.
  - ESR: raised in both active SLE and in infection.
  - CRP: raised in infection, but not in active SLE.
  - Renal function.
  - ANA, anti-ds DNA.
  - ENA (anti-Sm, anti-La, anti-Ro, anti-RNP).
  - Anticardiolipin antibody.
  - Complements—C3, C4: may be low in patients with active SLE due to the presence of immune complexes. If C4 is low and the patient has cutaneous vasculitis, check for cryoglobulins.

Box 19.12 Photoprotection

(see → pp. 338–9.)
- Discuss lifestyle and the importance of limiting sun exposure, particularly between 11 a.m. and 2 p.m.
- Recommend wide-brimmed hats (hold up to sunlight to ensure that the weave is sufficient to block transmission of light).
- Recommend dark clothing with long sleeves and a tight weave.
- Prescribe high-factor (>20), broad-spectrum sunscreen creams containing the physical blocker titanium dioxide to block the entire UV and visible light spectrum.
- Patients should apply sunscreen creams liberally in the morning to all exposed sites, after application of topical corticosteroids to active cutaneous disease.
- Advise patients to reapply sunscreen creams 4-hourly during the hours of sunlight or after swimming.
- Vitamin D deficiency is common and has been proposed as a contributor to lupus disease activity. Measure and replace vitamin D in patients who avoid sun exposure.

Further reading

Callen JP. Br J Dermatol 2004;151:731–6.
Chang A. Curr Rheumatol Rep 2011;13:300–7.
Schneider L et al. Clin Rheumatol 2014;33:1033–8.

Dermatomyositis

Dermatomyositis is a multisystem autoimmune disease, in which inflammatory skin changes are associated with a polymyositis of skeletal muscle. Adults and children of all races are affected, but ♀ are affected more often than ♂.

The prognosis is variable and unpredictable. Interstitial lung disease or an underlying malignancy (20–25% of adult-onset patients; see Box 19.13) may be fatal. The disease spectrum encompasses:

- Cutaneous disease without muscle involvement—amyotrophic dermatomyositis. Muscle involvement may not develop until 20 years after the onset of cutaneous dermatomyositis.
- Cutaneous and systemic disease (skin and muscle problems present concurrently in 60% of patients).
- Polymyositis without skin changes (muscle involvement precedes inflammatory cutaneous disease in 10% of patients).

What should I ask?

- Ask about cutaneous symptoms; in dermatomyositis, the rash itches, burns, and is painful, unlike the rash of LE. Itch is worse in more severe disease.
- Is the face swollen, particularly around the eyes, and how long does the swelling last? Dermatomyositis may simulate angio-oedema, but angio-oedema is transient (see ➔ p. 104, and Figs. 19.7 and 19.8).
- Has the skin blistered (sometimes seen with intense oedema)?
- Is the skin sensitive to sun? UV light exacerbates the rash in up to 50% of patients, but many patients are not aware that the skin is sensitive to light.
- Is the scalp erythematous or scaly, or the hair thinning? Dermatomyositis, like LE, may cause hair loss and a scarring alopecia.
- Seek evidence of a proximal myopathy; ask about getting out of chairs, going up and down stairs, brushing teeth, or reaching up.
- Check for evidence of interstitial lung disease: dyspnoea, dry cough, and wheeze.
- Probe for symptoms that suggest an internal malignancy: weight loss, changes in bowel habit.
- Is the patient taking drugs such as hydroxycarbamide? Some drug-induced rashes may simulate dermatomyositis (see ➔ p. 388).

⚠ Box 19.13 Dermatomyositis and internal malignancy

- Twenty to 25% of adult-onset patients develop a malignancy within 2 years of diagnosis. History and examination should be directed towards identifying a malignancy.
- Risk is greatest in the first year and in women.
- Increased risk may persist for 5 years after diagnosis.
- Cutaneous signs linked to malignancy include corticosteroid resistance, intense erythematous flush on the shoulders, neck, face, and scalp (malignant suffusion), and ulceration.

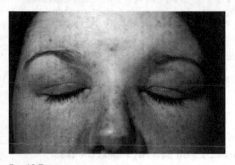

Fig. 19.7 Dermatomyositis with purplish (heliotrope) discoloration of eyelids. Reproduced from Harris A *et al. Dermatomyositis Presenting in Pregnancy, British Journal of Dermatology,* **133**:5, 1995.

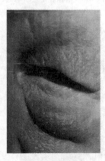

Fig. 19.8 Dermatomyositis: periorbital oedema simulating angio-oedema or an acute contact dermatitis.

Further reading

Santmyire-Rosenberger B and Dugan EM. *Curr Opin Rheumatol* 2003;15:714–22.
Sontheimer RD. *Curr Opin Rheumatol* 1999;11:475–82.
Vermaak E and McHugh N. *Int J Clin Rheumatol* 2012;7:197–215.

Dermatomyositis: the signs

What should I look for?

- Diagnostic signs in the hands, fingers, or nail folds (see Box 19.14).
- Assess the nail fold using an ophthalmoscope or dermatoscope.
- A symmetrical violaceous or heliotrope (violet-red) erythema of the eyelids and/or periorbital skin, associated with fine scale and periorbital oedema or facial swelling (see Figs. 19.7 and 19.8).
- Perifollicular scale in the scalp, with erythema ± diffuse hair loss.
- Erythema associated with fine scale affecting the upper chest, posterior neck, upper back and shoulders (shawl sign), arms, and/or forearms.
- Symmetrical erythematous, scaly papules or plaques over bony prominences of the elbows, knees, and/or greater trochanter of the hip (holster sign).
- Hypo- and hyperpigmentation, telangiectasia, and atrophy (as a result of chronic inflammation and known as poikiloderma).
- Necrosis and ulceration 2° to vascular damage.
- Calcinosis (commoner in children than adults).
- Signs suggesting an underlying internal malignancy in adult-onset disease (examine the abdomen, lymph nodes, breast, and pelvis in women, and the prostate in men).
- Signs of interstitial lung disease, e.g. fine inspiratory crackles.
- For differential diagnosis, see Box 19.15.

The Dermatomyositis Skin Severity Index: the DSSI

The DSSI is a measure of severity of skin disease in dermatomyositis. It takes into account the extent of disease (body surface area) and the amount of redness, induration, and scaling. The total DSSI can range from 0 to 72. However, the score does not take into account muscle disease or the impact of dermatomyositis on quality of life.

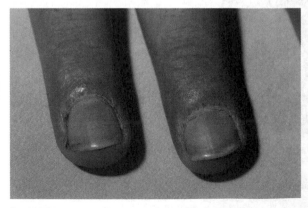

Fig. 19.9 Nail fold telangiectasia in dermatomyositis (also seen in systemic sclerosis and other connective tissue diseases).

Box 19.14 Diagnostic signs in the hands or fingers

(See Figs. 19.9 and 19.10.)

- Periungual erythema, tortuous nail fold capillaries and capillary dropout (avascular areas), thickened irregular cuticles with capillary haemorrhage.
- Gottron papules (flat-topped, violaceous, scaly papules over dorsal interphalangeal joints) are present in about 1/3 of patients and are pathognomonic of dermatomyositis. Gottron papules evolve into hypopigmented atrophic areas with irregular telangiectasia.
- Linear streaks of erythema over the extensor tendons of fingers.
- 'Mechanic's hands': hyperkeratosis, scaling, and fissuring on the lateral aspects of the thumb and fingers simulates contact dermatitis.

Box 19.15 Differential diagnosis

Cutaneous lupus erythematosus

Intense pruritus is not a feature of cutaneous LE. Cutaneous LE tends to spare the skin over joints on the hands and is hyperkeratotic, not oedematous.

Angio-oedema or urticaria

Oedema persists for 24–48h in angio-oedema but is long-lasting in dermatomyositis.

Seborrhoeic dermatitis

The greasy, ill-defined erythematous papular rash involves the central face but is not oedematous and spares the eyelids. The scalp may be erythematous and scaly, but hair is not usually affected. Seborrhoeic dermatitis may also involve the central chest, central back, and flexures.

Hand dermatitis

Nail fold capillaries are not involved in dermatitis.

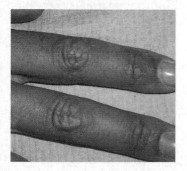

Fig. 19.10 Flat-topped, slightly scaly papules over the interphalangeal joints (Gottron papules).

Further reading

Carroll CL et al. Br J Dermatol 2008;158:345–50.

Dermatomyositis: investigation and management

What should I do?

- For investigation, see Box 19.16.
- Pruritus, skin pain, and burning are difficult to control; try sedating antihistamines such as hydroxyzine 25–50mg qds, cooling baths, aqueous cream with 1% menthol, and moisturizers or soap substitutes.
- Advise on photoprotection using clothing, wide-brimmed hats, and sunscreen creams (see **➲** pp. 338–9).
- Potent or very potent topical corticosteroid ointments or 0.1% tacrolimus ointment applied bd may control limited cutaneous disease.
- A potent steroid (betamethasone) lotion used at night may relieve scalp irritation.
- Hydroxychloroquine (<6.5mg/kg/day) takes 8–12 weeks to have an effect, and up to 6 months for maximal benefit, but is less effective in cutaneous dermatomyositis than in cutaneous LE.
- Oral prednisolone (0.5–1mg/kg/day) in reducing doses over 2–3 months may control symptomatic cutaneous disease, while hydroxychloroquine is taking effect.
- Other immunosuppressive drugs have been tried for cutaneous disease, with varying success.
- Management of calcinosis is difficult; sometimes painful deposits have to be removed surgically.
- Myositis may prove easier to control with oral prednisolone than cutaneous disease. Other steroid-sparing immunosuppressive drugs that have been recommended include methotrexate, azathioprine, ciclosporin, and mycophenolate mofetil.

Mixed connective tissue disease

Mixed connective tissue disease (MCTD) is an overlap syndrome associated with anti-U1-RNP antibodies. Clinical features usually emerge sequentially over several years and include:

- Raynaud phenomenon.
- Puffy fingers.
- Sclerodactyly.
- Myositis.
- Erosive arthritis.

Patients are at risk of developing pulmonary hypertension, which is the major cause of death in MCTD. Renal system and CNS diseases are uncommon.

Further reading

Sontheimer RD. *Expert Opin Pharmacother* 2004;5:1083–99.
Vermaak E and McHugh N. *Int J Clin Rheumatol* 2012;7:197–215.

Box 19.16 Investigations in dermatomyositis

Skin

- Biopsy-involved skin: skin biopsies show an interface dermatitis (vacuolar degeneration of basal keratinocytes and apoptosis), mild perivascular inflammation, oedema, and dermal mucin.
- These histological features are similar to those of cutaneous LE.

Muscles

- Inflammatory markers: ESR, CRP.
- Serum muscle enzymes, electromyography.
- Muscle biopsy or muscle MRI.

Autoantibodies

(see Box 19.17).

Lungs

- CXR, lung function tests. CT chest—interstitial lung disease. Exclude pulmonary hypertension with ECG and echocardiogram.

⚠ *Malignancy*

Most cancers present within 2 years of diagnosis. Frequently associated cancers are cervical, ovarian, lung, pancreatic, and GIT. Consider mammography, cervical smear, transvaginal ultrasonography, CT chest, abdomen, and pelvis, and tumour markers (CA125 and CA 19-9).

Box 19.17 Autoantibodies in myositis

ANA may be present in up to 80% of patients with dermatomyositis or polymyositis. There may be myositis-specific or myositis-associated autoantibodies.

- Myositis-specific autoantibodies are found in ~30% of patients and may be associated with particular clinical syndromes. They are usually mutually exclusive.
  - Antisynthetase antibodies (most commonly anti-Jo-1) are associated with interstitial lung disease, Raynaud phenomenon, arthritis, and mechanic's hands—the 'antisynthetase syndrome'. Other antisynthetase antibodies include anti-PL-12, OJ, EJ, PL-7, KS, Zo, and Ha.
  - Anti-SRP (signal recognition particle) antibodies are associated with a severe necrotizing myopathy.
  - Anti-Mi-2 antibodies are associated with acute onset of dermatomyositis and may respond well to therapy.
  - Other myositis-specific autoantibodies include anti-MDA5 (associated with rapidly progressive interstitial lung disease and amyopathic dermatomyositis) and anti-p140 (found in juvenile dermatomyositis).
- Myositis-associated autoantibodies (anti-Ro, anti-La, anti-RNP, anti-Sm, anti-PM/Scl, and anti-Ku) are found in other autoimmune diseases that may be associated with myositis such as SLE, Sjögren syndrome or scleroderma. Anti-U1-RNP is seen in MCTD.

Systemic sclerosis

Systemic sclerosis is a connective tissue disease characterized by collagen accumulation (fibrosis), associated with vascular injury and autoantibodies. Women, particularly black women, are most at risk. Average age of onset is 40–50 years. The disease is divided into two major subtypes: diffuse cutaneous systemic sclerosis (10-year survival 21%) and limited cutaneous systemic sclerosis (10-year survival 71%) (see Box 19.19).

Systemic sclerosis is also known as scleroderma, which can lead to confusion with localized scleroderma (morphoea), a self-limited, unrelated condition confined to skin and subcutaneous tissue (see ➔ pp. 420–1).

What should I ask?

- Any swelling of the hands, feet, or face? Develops acutely at onset of diffuse disease.
- Any skin tightness or itching?
- Raynaud phenomenon (see Box 19.18)?
- Joint pain or swelling (rheumatoid-like arthritis seen in diffuse disease)?
- Anorexia, fatigue, or weight loss (commoner in diffuse disease)?
- Dyspnoea on exertion or at rest?
- Muscle pain or weakness (common in diffuse disease)?
- Dysphagia or dyspepsia?
- Exposure to chemicals or drugs that may induce sclerodermoid changes (see Box 19.20)?
- Any features in the history suggesting other conditions that may have similar features (see Box 19.20)?
- Smoker?
- Assess functional impairment and impact on quality of life.

Box 19.18 Raynaud phenomenon

- Defined as episodic bilateral di- or triphasic (pallor, cyanosis, erythema) vascular reactions of the fingers, toes, ears, or nose that are provoked by cold or emotion.
- Occurs in 3–15% of the population.
- May be idiopathic (Raynaud disease).
- Associated with systemic sclerosis, SLE, and dermatomyositis.
- Also seen with cervical rib, emboli, and vascular trauma, including vibration injury.

Further reading

LeRoy C and Medsger TA. *J Rheumatol* 2001;**28**:1573–6.
Shah A and Wigley F. *Mayo Clin Proc* 2013;**88**:377–93.

Box 19.19 Subtypes of systemic sclerosis

Limited cutaneous systemic sclerosis

(Includes CREST: C = calcinosis cutis, R = Raynaud phenomenon,
E = oesophageal hypomotility, S = sclerodactyly, T = telangiectasia.)
- Occurs in older women more often than diffuse disease.
- Raynaud phenomenon may precede other features by 10–15 years.
- Skin sclerosis of the hands, forearms, face, or feet (i.e. distal to the elbows, knees, and clavicles), or absent.
- Cutaneous calcinosis and telangiectatic macules.
- Dilated nail fold capillary loops, usually without capillary dropout.
- Oesophageal dysmotility with reflux oesophagitis or dysphagia.
- Late incidence of pulmonary hypertension, with or without interstitial lung disease, biliary cirrhosis, and trigeminal neuralgia.
- Presence of anti-centromere antibodies.

Diffuse cutaneous systemic sclerosis
- Raynaud phenomenon within 1 year of onset of skin changes.
- Nail fold capillary dilatation and destruction (also seen in dermatomyositis and overlap syndromes).
- Truncal and acral skin involvement.
- Presence of tendon friction rubs.
- Early onset of interstitial lung disease, renal failure, GI disease, myocardial involvement.
- Presence of anti-Scl70 (anti-DNA topoisomerase I), anti-RNA polymerase III. Absence of anti-centromere antibodies.

Box 19.20 Differential diagnosis
- Morphoea: no Raynaud phenomenon, normal nail folds (see ➜ pp. 420–1).
- Some features of systemic sclerosis may be present in RA, SLE, dermatomyositis/polymyositis, and Sjögren syndrome.
- Chemicals (polyvinyl chloride, solvents, pesticides), drugs (bleomycin, pentazocine, ethosuximide, penicillamine), paraffin, aniline-contaminated rapeseed oil, salad oil (toxic oil syndrome), and *L*-tryptophan may induce a scleroderma-like disease.
- Scleredema: associated with infection, diabetes, and monoclonal gammopathy. Firm, non-pitting oedema of the face, neck, and upper back (see ➜ Box 22.2, p. 467).
- Scleromyxoedema: associated with paraproteinaemia, myeloma, lymphoma, and leukaemia (see ➜ Box 26.10, p. 541). Waxy, flesh-coloured papules on the face, trunk, and extremities. Eventually, stiffening of the skin causes sclerodactyly and reduced mouth opening. Patients do not have telangiectasia or calcinosis.
- Nephrogenic systemic fibrosis (see ➜ p. 498). Seen in patients with renal failure exposed to contrast medium containing gadolinium. Features similar to scleromyxoedema.
- PCT: waxy thickening of sun-exposed skin (see ➜ p. 332).
- Chronic GVHD: sclerodermoid form (see ➜ p. 534–6).

Systemic sclerosis: signs and investigation

Diffuse cutaneous disease: what should I look for?

- Non-pitting oedema of the hands, feet, and face.
- Distorted and irregular nail fold capillaries.
- Thickening of the skin proximal to the elbows (diagnostic of diffuse, rather than limited, disease). Palpate and pinch the skin to assess thickening. Sclerosis spreads to the proximal extremities, chest, face, scalp, and trunk over 3–12 months or may be present at onset.
- Facial sclerosis giving the face a mask-like stiffness with reduced mouth aperture, radial furrowing around the lips, and pinched nose.
- Neck sign: the skin of the neck skin is ridged and tightened when the head is extended. Positive in >90% of patients.
- Dusky cyanotic fingers and toes (see Fig. 19.11).
- Sclerodactyly and flexion contractures producing a claw-like deformity with painful ulcerations of the fingertips and knuckles (rat bite necroses).
- Prayer sign (see next section).
- Pigment change: generalized hyperpigmentation resembling Addison disease or focal hypo- or hyperpigmentation in areas of sclerosis.
- Tendon friction rubs.
- Swollen painful joints.
- ⚠ Evidence of systemic involvement, including hypertension, fine basal inspiratory crackles, right ventricular hypertrophy, heart failure, pericardial effusion, or malnutrition.

Limited cutaneous disease: what should I look for?

- Linear periungual nail fold telangiectasia without any irregularity.
- Atrophy of finger pulps with beaking of fingernails and resorption of bone in the terminal phalanges (also seen in association with Raynaud phenomenon in diffuse disease).
- Painful ischaemic ulceration of fingertips that heals, leaving pitted scarring (also seen in association with Raynaud phenomenon in diffuse disease; see Fig. 19.11).
- Thickening of skin, but limited to the hands, face, feet, and forearms.
- Prayer sign: symmetrical thickening and tightening of the skin distal to the metacarpophalangeal (MCP) joints (sclerodactyly) restricts opposition of the palms, when the wrists are extended. This sign indicates joint or skin pathology or shortening of the finger flexor muscles.
- Well-defined telangiectatic macules on the hands, tongue, lips, and face.
- Nodules of cutaneous calcinosis that may become inflamed and ulcerate, discharging chalky material. Cellulitis may complicate ulceration.
- ⚠ Evidence of pulmonary involvement: fine basal inspiratory crackles, right ventricular hypertrophy, heart failure.

What should I do?
See Box 19.21 and ➜ pp. 418–19.

Box 19.21 Investigations in systemic sclerosis

- FBC, ESR, renal and liver function tests, creatine kinase.
- Urinalysis and microscopy for casts.
- Igs and autoantibodies (see Box 19.22).
- Baseline CXR, ECG, and CT chest (interstitial lung disease).
- Annual lung function tests and echocardiogram (screening for pulmonary hypertension).
- Further investigations should be guided by clinical findings. May include GI endoscopy and barium studies.

Box 19.22 Autoantibodies in systemic sclerosis

- Ninety-five percent of patients have autoantibodies specific for systemic sclerosis or for overlap syndromes with other connective tissue diseases.
- Autoantibodies are usually present at the onset of disease and persist throughout the course of the disease.
- Less than 1% of patients have >1 systemic sclerosis-specific autoantibody.
- It is not clear if autoantibodies have a direct role in the pathogenesis, but autoantibodies predict different subtypes of systemic sclerosis.
- Anti-centromere antibodies: limited cutaneous disease and CREST. High risk for calcinosis, ischaemic digital loss, and pulmonary hypertension, but low risk of pulmonary fibrosis and low mortality.
- Anti-Scl70 (anti-DNA topoisomerase I): diffuse cutaneous disease, pulmonary fibrosis, high mortality from right ventricular failure 2° to pulmonary disease.
- Antinucleolar system antibodies, including:
  - Anti-PM-Scl: polymyositis–scleroderma overlap syndrome (benign and chronic course), limited cutaneous involvement.
  - Antifibrillarin (anti-U3-ribonucleoprotein): diffuse cutaneous systemic sclerosis and, in some populations, myositis, pulmonary hypertension, and renal disease.
  - Anti-Th/To: limited skin involvement, pulmonary hypertension, renal crisis.
  - Anti-RNA polymerase III: rapidly progressive skin involvement, scleroderma renal crisis (see Box 19.23), concomitant cancer.

Further reading

Hamaguchi Y. J Dermatol 2010;37:42–53.
Mehra S et al. Autoimmunity Rev 2013;12:340–54.

Systemic sclerosis: management

Cutaneous disease

- Moisturizers, aqueous cream with 1% menthol, soap substitutes, and sedating antihistamines may reduce pruritus.
- Fingertip ulceration: moisturizers (ointments) relieve dryness and cracking of the fingers. Topical antibiotics or antibiotic–steroid combinations may be helpful in superficial ulcers. Hydrocolloid dressings may relieve pain and promote healing.
- Prednisolone (low dose) and methotrexate or mycophenolate mofetil are sometimes used at onset of diffuse skin disease.
- Troublesome fingertip calcinosis may be removed surgically—curettage has been advocated.

Raynaud phenomenon and digital ischaemia

- Avoid nicotine—causes vasoconstriction.
- Keep peripheries warm using thermal underwear to raise core temperatures, as well as thermal gloves and/or socks.
- Heat pads (purchased in outdoor activity shops) may be used under gloves or socks. Thick-soled padded footwear is essential.
- Warming hands for 5min every 4h in a warm water bath may improve Raynaud phenomenon. Some patients find it helpful to warm their hands in water before going outdoors.
- Vasodilators, e.g. nifedipine 5–20mg bd, amlodipine 5–10mg daily, or losartan 25–50mg daily. ACE inhibitors and selective serotonin reuptake inhibitors (SSRIs) are also used.
- Glyceryl trinitrate (GTN) patches for acute digital ischaemia: 0.2mg/h (5mg patch) to start with, increasing to 0.4mg/h (10mg patch), if required, applied at the proximal end of the digit. There must be a 12-h 'off' period each day to prevent nitrate tolerance.
- Phosphodiesterase (PDE) 5 inhibitors (e.g. sildenafil 25mg tds), endothelin receptor antagonists (bosentan), and IV prostacyclin analogues (iloprost) are used in digital ulceration and active ischaemia.
- Digital sympathectomy or Botox® injections for severe disease.
- Rule out osteomyelitis in non-healing digital ulcers.

Box 19.23 Scleroderma renal crisis

- Typical presentation is with accelerated hypertension and progressive renal impairment.
- Patients with early diffuse cutaneous systemic sclerosis are at greatest risk.
- Scleroderma renal crisis has been associated with glucocorticoid use; therefore, glucocorticoids should be used with caution in systemic sclerosis and avoided where possible.
- ACE inhibitors are the first-line treatment.
- Approximately 2/3 of patients will require renal replacement therapy, of whom 1/2 may recover sufficiently to discontinue dialysis.

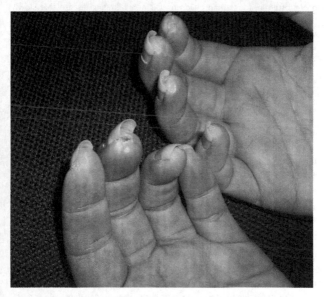

Fig. 19.11 Sclerodactyly with painful ulceration of the fingertips.

Further reading

Nihtyanova,SI et al. Clin Exp Rheumatol 2014;**32** (Suppl. **81**):S156–S164.
Sapadin AN and Fleishmajer R. Arch Dermatol 2002;**138**:99–105.

Localized scleroderma

Localized scleroderma (morphoea) refers to a group of conditions in which increased collagen deposition causes skin thickening. Internal organs are not involved, and localized scleroderma does not progress to systemic sclerosis. ♀ are affected more often than ♂. The frequency of the subtypes is different in adults and children. Some patients have >1 type of lesion.

Autoantibodies (ANAs, anti-Scl70, anti-centromere antibody, anticardiolipin antibody, RF) may be detected, but their role in pathogenesis is unclear. *Borrelia burgdorferi* has been implicated in the pathogenesis of some cases of morphoea, but these findings have not been substantiated.

Plaque morphoea

Plaque morphoea, the commonest type of localized scleroderma, occurs more often in adults than children. It is a self-limiting disease that slowly resolves over 3–5 years.

What should I look for?
- One or more smooth, erythematous patches, usually on the trunk.
- Patches progress to smooth, indurated, shiny, white or yellowish plaques with violet borders—the 'lilac ring' (see Fig. 19.12).
- Plaques hyperpigment, as they soften.

What should I do?
- Consider taking a deep elliptical skin biopsy that extends from normal into abnormal skin, but a biopsy is not always necessary.
- No treatment is required, but a very potent topical corticosteroid ointment may be applied, until the inflammatory ring has resolved.

Differential diagnosis
- Granuloma annulare: colour may be similar to morphoea, but look for a raised beaded margin in an annular configuration (see ➜ Box 22.3, p. 469).
- Erythema migrans (see ➜ p. 148). Subtle erythema but no thickening.
- Extragenital lichen sclerosus: resembles plaque morphoea, but the surface is slightly hyperkeratotic with follicular plugs. Lichen sclerosus (genital and extragenital) may occur with morphoea (see ➜ pp. 288–9).
- Dermatofibrosarcoma protuberans: a slow-growing fibrosing tumour that may present as a thickened plaque (see ➜ p. 360).

Generalized morphoea
- Much of the skin becomes sclerotic in this very rare variant.
- Involvement of the chest wall may cause disabling restrictive lung defects.
- Treatment is unsatisfactory, but phototherapy has been recommended.

Linear scleroderma

This uncommon type of scleroderma is seen more often in children than adults. Once the inflammatory stage has ended, linear scleroderma does not progress.

What should I look for?

- A unilateral sclerotic band, usually extending along a limb, following the lines of Blaschko (see ➜ p. 63 and Fig. 19.13).
- In the rare 'en coup de sabre' variant, an atrophic groove gradually extends from the anterior scalp, down one side of the face. Involvement of deeper tissues causes disfiguring hemifacial atrophy.
- Neurological complications (seizures, headache, hemiparesis), eye problems, and jaw malalignment in children with facial involvement.
- Hypo- or hyperpigmentation of affected skin (see Fig. 19.13).

What should I do?

- Assess limb length and diameter. Deep atrophy may affect subcutaneous tissues (fat, muscle, bone), so that the limb is short and wasted.
- ⚠ Complications, such as limb length discrepancy, joint contractures, or jaw malocclusion, should be managed by a multidisciplinary team.
- ⚠ If affecting the face, arrange an ophthalmological assessment, and consider MRI to detect CNS involvement.
- Placebo-controlled trials are needed to evaluate the impact of treatments such as phototherapy, oral prednisolone, intralesional triamcinolone, IV methylprednisolone, and/or methotrexate.
- Reconstructive surgery may reduce deformity, once disease is inactive.
- Cosmetic camouflage may be helpful.

Eosinophilic fasciitis (Shulman syndrome)

Vigorous exercise may trigger this variant of scleroderma, which involves deep fascia and initially may simulate cellulitis.

What should I look for?

- Symmetrical, non-tender, reddish brown, oedematous plaques, usually on the limbs, that develop into indurated, brawny plaques.
- Sclerosis extending into subcutaneous tissues restricts movement of tendons in the affected limb, e.g. patients are unable to extend the wrist and fingers simultaneously if flexor muscles of the forearm are involved.

What should I do?

- FBC, looking for a peripheral eosinophilia.
- Arrange a deep biopsy of fascia and muscle.
- Oral corticosteroids, methotrexate, and azathioprine have been advocated for treatment, but controlled trials are lacking, and disease remits spontaneously in about 1/3 patients.

Fig. 19.12 Morphoea: smooth, shiny, white plaque with a violet border.

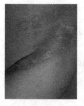

Fig. 19.13 Linear scleroderma with a mix of hypo- and hyperpigmentation.

Adult-onset Still disease

Adult-onset Still disease is a rare inflammatory disorder, characterized by fever, rash, and arthralgia or arthritis. Other common features are myalgia, pharyngitis, lymphadenopathy, and splenomegaly. Hepatomegaly and serositis occur less frequently.

What should I ask?

- Sore throat.
- Fever—usually quotidian (spiking daily) or twice a day. Pyrexia of unknown origin may be the presenting feature.
- Myalgia and arthralgia, with or without joint swelling.
- History to suggest serositis.

What should I look for?

- Rash is typically salmon-pink, evanescent (fleeting), macular, or maculopapular, and tends to occur with the fever, predominantly in the trunk and limbs. Koebner phenomenon may be present.
- Atypical skin lesions have been reported to include:
  - Dusky-red or brownish, pruritic, persistent erythematous or urticarial plaques.
  - Flat-topped lichenoid papules.
  - Linear urticarial lesions with scales or crusts.
  - Flagellate dermatitis.
- Synovitis.
- Lymphadenopathy, splenomegaly, hepatomegaly.

What should I do?

Investigations

- Marked acute phase response.
- Serum ferritin concentrations often exceeding 3000ng/mL, and sometimes 10 000ng/mL or higher.
- Leucocytosis.
- Elevated liver enzymes.
- ANA and RF are usually negative.
- Imaging later in the disease may demonstrate a destructive arthritis.
- Pancytopenia may represent the rare, but potentially fatal, complication of macrophage activation syndrome.

Management

Mild disease may respond to NSAIDs, but most patients require glucocorticoids. Methotrexate is used for joint involvement. Severe disease may require high-dose glucocorticoid therapy and biologic therapy (IL-1 or IL-6 inhibitors).

Further reading

Gerfaud-Valentin M et al. Autoimmun Rev 2014;13:708–22.
Yoshifuku A et al. Clin Exp Derm 2014;39:503–5.

Relapsing polychondritis

This rare disorder is characterized by episodes of inflammation of cartilage, leading to destruction with deformity. Relapsing polychondritis affects cartilage in the ear, nose, larynx, trachea, bronchi, and joints, as well as proteoglycan-rich tissues such as the skin, eyes, aorta, and heart. Antibodies to type II collagen have been found in cartilage. Onset is usually between the ages of 20 and 60 years. Relapsing polychondritis may be mild or rapidly progressive—about 25% of patients die of their disease after 5–7 years. Causes of death include pulmonary infection, systemic vasculitis, airway collapse, and renal failure.

What should I look for?

(See Box 19.24.)

- Fever, anorexia, weight loss, and/or myalgia.
- Erythema, tenderness, warmth, and swelling of the cartilaginous portion of the ear—usually both ears, and the non-cartilaginous ear lobe is always spared, unlike cellulitis (see Fig. 19.14) (85% of patients—a diagnostic sign). Episodes last from days to weeks. Repeated episodes may lead to a droopy pinna or cauliflower ear (destruction of cartilage).
- Asymmetric, usually migratory, non-erosive oligoarthritis or polyarthritis (50–75% of patients): most often MCP and proximal interphalangeal (PIP) joints and knees (may have RA).
- Episodic acute painful inflammation of the nasal cartilage, with rhinorrhoea, epistaxis, and eventually deformity (saddle nose) (54% of patients).
- Painful red eye: commonly episcleritis, scleritis, or keratitis (60% of patients).
- Laryngotracheobronchial disease (50% of patients): cough, hoarseness, dyspnoea, wheezing, choking. Tenderness over the thyroid cartilage and trachea. Airway obstruction or collapse. 2° chest infections.
- Narrowing of the external auditory meatus, with hearing loss. Vestibular dysfunction causes dizziness, ataxia, and nausea.
- Large-vessel vasculitis leads to aortic aneurysms.
- Aortic or mitral valve disease (5–10% of patients).
- Skin problems (50% of patients), including small-vessel cutaneous vasculitis (see → p. 440), livedo reticularis (see → p. 452), urticaria or angio-oedema (see → pp. 104–5), EN (see → pp. 458–9), and Sweet syndrome (see → p. 518).
- Migratory superficial thrombophlebitis.
- Neurological problems 2° to vasculitis.
- Renal disease (10% of patients)—may be fatal.
- Associated disease (25–35% of patients):
  - Connective tissue disease, e.g. RA, SLE.
  - Systemic vasculitides, e.g. granulomatosis with polyangiitis (GPA; Wegener granulomatosis). (See → p. 446).
  - Haematological disease, e.g. myelodysplastic syndrome, IgA myeloma, lymphoma.
  - GI disease, e.g. Crohn disease, ulcerative colitis.
  - Skin disease, e.g. vitiligo, psoriasis, LP.
  - Endocrine disease, e.g. autoimmune thyroid disease, diabetes, thymoma.
- For differential diagnoses, see Box 19.25.

What should I do?

- The diagnosis is based on clinical criteria (see Box 19.24).
- Biopsy of inflamed cartilage may be required to exclude other pathology.
- FBC (anaemia, leucocytosis, thrombocytosis).
- ESR (raised).
- Urinalysis and creatinine.
- ANA, RF (may be detected, but not helpful diagnostically).
- Further investigation should be guided by the clinical findings but may include CXR, pulmonary function tests, high-resolution laryngotracheal CT scans, ear, nose, and throat (ENT) assessment, and ophthalmological review.
- Recommended treatments include oral corticosteroids, NSAIDs, dapsone, and colchicine. Other steroid-sparing immunosuppressive agents that have been tried include methotrexate, hydroxychloroquine, cyclophosphamide, ciclosporin, and anti-TNF agents (infliximab).

Box 19.24 Relapsing polychondritis: diagnostic criteria

Three of these criteria should be present to make the diagnosis:
- Bilateral auricular chondritis (see Fig. 19.14).
- Non-erosive seronegative inflammatory polyarthritis.
- Nasal chondritis.
- Ocular inflammation, including keratitis, scleritis, episcleritis.
- Respiratory tract chondritis involving laryngeal and tracheal cartilages.
- Cochlear or vestibular damage manifested by neurosensory hearing loss, tinnitus, and vertigo.

Box 19.25 Relapsing polychondritis: differential diagnosis

- Ear: cellulitis or dermatitis. Sparing of the ear lobe rules out these diagnoses. Most cases of cellulitis are unilateral. Relapsing polychondritis is usually bilateral.
- GPA (Wegener granulomatosis) and polyarteritis nodosa do not cause chondritis of the ear or respiratory tract.
- Saddle nose: consider infection, including congenital syphilis, GPA (Wegener granulomatosis).

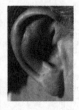

Fig. 19.14 Erythema and swelling in relapsing polychondritis do not affect the ear lobe.

Further reading

Arnaud L et al. Autoimmunity Rev 2014;13:90–5.
Mathew S et al. Semin Arthritis Rheum 2012;42:70–83.
Rapini RP and Warner NB. Clin Dermatol 2006;24:482–5.

Multicentric reticulohistiocytosis

If you recognize the cutaneous manifestations of this very rare disease, you will make the diagnosis. Patients, most often middle-aged women, present with systemic complaints, a destructive arthropathy, and, at some stage, a characteristic rash. Two-thirds of patients present with arthritis (skin signs appear within months or a few years), and about 1/5 with skin signs (arthritis appears at any time). Multicentric reticulohistiocytosis may be a paraneoplastic disorder.

What should I look for?

- Systemic symptoms: weight loss, weakness, and fever.
- A rapidly progressive, disabling, symmetrical arthritis, involving the DIP joints in 75% of patients (may be confused with Heberden nodes), sometimes with involvement of the PIP joints (producing an 'opera glass' deformity) and MCP joints, knees, shoulders, wrists, hips, ankles, feet, elbows, and vertebrae (see Box 19.26).
- Smooth, reddish brown papules and nodules, ranging in size from a few mm to 2cm in diameter on the ears, nose, dorsum, and lateral aspect of fingers, neck, and sometimes the trunk. Nodules over the PIP, MCP, and DIP joints may resemble Gottron papules seen in dermatomyositis (see ➲ Box 19.14, p. 411), but are not scaly or hyperkeratotic (see Fig. 19.15).
- Periungual nodules and papules with a 'coral bead' appearance (see Fig. 19.15).
- Papules and nodules on the lips, buccal mucosa, tongue, gingival, and nasal septum.
- Associated diseases:
  - Hyperlipidemia (30–58% of cases).
  - ⚠ Malignancy (25% of cases), most commonly breast or stomach, but also cervix, colon, lung, ovary, lymphoma, leukaemia, sarcoma, and melanoma.

What should I do?

- Skin biopsy shows characteristic lipid-laden multinucleated giant cells of a foreign-body type with 'ground glass' cytoplasm. Similar histiocytes also invade the synovium.
- Radiographs demonstrate a circumscribed erosive arthritis. Erosions advance from joint margins to involve the entire joint surface. The joint space is widened, with loss of cartilage and resorption of subchondral bone, but without osteopenia or periosteal new bone formation.
- Very potent topical corticosteroids may speed resolution of the cutaneous papules. Cutaneous signs resolve before the arthritis.
- Arthritis is difficult to control. Corticosteroids provide symptomatic relief, without inducing remission. Drugs, such as methotrexate, cyclophosphamide, alendronic acid, and anti-TNF agents, have been recommended, but controlled trials are lacking.

Box 19.26 Multicentric reticulohistiocytosis: differential diagnosis

The cutaneous signs are diagnostic but may not develop until some months or years after the arthritis. Consider:

- RA.
- Psoriatic arthritis.
- Reiter disease.
- Erosive osteoarthritis.
- Crystal-induced arthropathies.

(a)

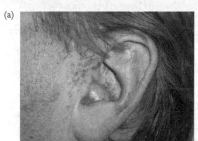

(b)

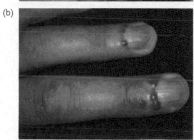

(c)

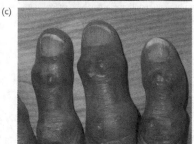

Fig. 19.15 Smooth, reddish brown papules and nodules on the ear (a) and fingers (b, c) in multicentric reticulohistiocytosis.

Ehlers–Danlos syndrome

Ehlers–Danlos syndrome (EDS) is a heterogeneous spectrum of inherited disorders with overlapping clinical features that may include hyperextensible skin, hypermobile joints, and generalized tissue fragility. ⚠ Vascular EDS carries a high risk of life-threatening uterine or vascular rupture. EDS is caused by mutations in genes that modify collagen proteins (see Table 19.1).

What should I ask?

- Skin: easy bruising or stretchy skin (apparent in early childhood).
- Joint hypermobility: pain, sprains, or dislocation.
- Surgical complications: delayed wound healing, post-operative hernia.
- Family history of similar problems or, in vascular EDS, sudden death.

What should I look for?

- Soft, doughy, velvety, hyperextensible skin that, once released, quickly snaps back to its original state (skin returns slowly to its former position in cutis laxa). Test at a site that is not subjected to mechanical forces or scarring, e.g. flexor surface of the forearm.
- Thin, transparent skin with easily visible vessels (chest, abdomen, limbs): seen in vascular EDS.
- Subcutaneous nodules on the forearms and shins. Nodules may calcify.
- Spontaneous bruising: bruises reappear in the same areas, often shins or knees, leaving hyperpigmentation.
- Wide atrophic 'cigarette paper' scars over pressure points.
- Molluscoid pseudotumours (small spongy tumours over scars and pressure points).
- Elastosis perforans serpiginosa (see Box 19.28 and Fig. 19.16) (a rare association).
- Joint hypermobility: influenced by age, sex, ethnicity, and family background. Do the little fingers dorsiflex passively to >90°? Do the elbows or knees hyperextend beyond 10°? Is it possible to flex the thumb down onto the flexor surface of the forearm? Hypermobility syndrome may be misdiagnosed as EDS.

What should I do?

- Confirm diagnosis with skin biopsy, biochemical analysis of collagen, and/or genetic testing. Refer to a clinical geneticist.
- Patients should be managed in a specialist centre by a multidisciplinary team.
- Echocardiography (mitral valve/tricuspid valve prolapse).
- Advise patients with easy bruising to avoid contact sports.
- Surgeons should take steps to minimize the risk of poor wound healing—avoid wound tension; use plentiful deep sutures; leave skin sutures in place for longer than usual; apply Steri-strip® to reduce stretching of scars.

Further reading

De Paepe A and Malfait F. *Clin Genet* 2012;**82**:1–11

Table 19.1 Some subtypes of Ehlers–Danlos syndrome. Many variants cannot be classified into one of the known subtypes

Subtype and inheritance	Major clinical features	Protein defect
Hypermobility AD (commonest subtype)	Marked joint hypermobility, joint pain, mild skin hyperextensibility	Unclear but may involve type V collagen or tenascin-X
Classic AD	Skin hyperextensibility Widened atrophic scarring Smooth and velvety skin Joint hypermobility Surgical complications	Genetic heterogeneity, type V collagen (50%), or unknown
Vascular AD	Easy bruising; thin, translucent skin (not hyperextensible); arterial/intestinal/uterine rupture—sudden death; characteristic facial appearance—acrogeria; hypermobility, tendon rupture; pneumothorax	Type III collagen
Kyphoscoliosis AR	Hypermobility, hypotonia, and kyphoscoliosis at birth, ocular fragility, rupture of globe	Lysyl hydroxylase-1 (responsible for cross-linking of collagen fibres to give tensile strength) or unknown
Arthrochalasia AD	Severe generalized joint hypermobility, congenital hip dislocation, skin hyperextensibility, wide atrophic scars	Type 1 collagen (loss of a procollagen-N proteinase cleavage site)
Dermatosparaxis AR	Skin fragility; sagging, redundant skin; excessive bruising Characteristic facies (oedema of eyelids, downslanting palpebral fissures, epicanthic folds, blue sclerae, gingival hyperplasia, micrognathia) Umbilical hernia	Procollagen-N-proteinase

Marfan syndrome

Marfan syndrome is an AD condition linked to mutations in the *FBNI* gene that encodes the extracellular matrix protein fibrillin-1. Fibrillin-1 deficiency may affect the development of tissues by dysregulating transforming growth factor (TGF)-β signalling pathways. Several hundred mutations have been described. Diagnostic criteria are shown in Box 19.27. ⚠ Aortic root dissection or ruptured aortic aneurysms may be fatal (also see ➜ Multiple endocrine neoplasia type 2B in Box 22.18, p. 483).

What should I look for?

- Skin: striae not associated with weight change, usually seen on the shoulders, back, or thighs (low specificity).
- Recurrent inguinal or incisional hernias.
- Musculoskeletal: limbs disproportionately long for the trunk, scoliosis, pectus excavatum or carinatum, arachnodactyly (fully flexed thumb extends beyond the ulnar border of the palm; distal phalanges of the thumb and fifth finger overlap fully when grasping the contralateral wrist), muscle hypoplasia, and myalgia.
- Facies: downslanting palpebral fissures, enophthalmia, and retrognathia.
- High arched palate with tooth crowding.
- Cardiovascular: mitral valve prolapse, dilatation of the ascending aorta with risk of fatal rupture or dissection, aortic regurgitation.
- Ocular: lens dislocation, myopia, retinal detachment, cataract, or glaucoma. May cause visual impairment or blindness. Slit-lamp examination is required to diagnose ectopia lentis.
- Pneumothorax and pulmonary emphysema (rare).
- Family history of marfanoid features or sudden death.
- Elastosis perforans serpiginosa—rare association (see Box 19.28).

What should I do?

- Diagnosis is clinical (see Box 19.27).
- Patients should be managed in a specialist centre by a multidisciplinary team.
- Refer for genetic counselling.
- Recommend that patients avoid competitive sport, straining, or isometric exercise that might raise the blood pressure.
- Avoid contact sports that might precipitate aortic dissection.
- β-adrenergic blockade is recommended to control blood pressure and slow the rate of aortic growth.
- Annual echocardiography is required to monitor the aortic root.
- Annual review by an ophthalmologist is recommended.
- Pregnancy carries a high risk of aortic complications.

Further reading

Callewaert B et al. *Best Pract Res Clin Rheumatol* 2008;22:165–89.

Box 19.27 Revised Ghent nosology of Marfan syndrome (MFS)

In the absence of a conclusive family history of MFS, the diagnosis can be established in four distinct scenarios:

- Aortic root dilatation (Z-score ≥2) or dissection and ectopia lentis.
- Aortic root dilatation (Z≥2) or dissection and the identification of a bona fide *FBN1* mutation.
- Where aortic root dilatation (Z ≥2) or dissection is present but ectopia lentis is absent and the *FBN1* status is either unknown or negative, an MFS diagnosis is confirmed by the presence of sufficient systemic findings (≥7 points).
- In the presence of ectopia lentis but absence of aortic root dilatation/ dissection, the identification of an *FBN1* mutation previously associated with aortic disease is required before making the diagnosis of MFS.

In an individual with a family history of MFS (a family member has been diagnosed using the above criteria), the diagnosis can be established in the presence of ectopia lentis, or a systemic score ≥7 points or aortic root dilatation with Z ≥2 in adults (≥20 years old) or Z ≥3 in individuals <20 years old.

The scoring of systemic features is explained in the reference below. Features include the wrist and thumb sign, pectus carinatum or excavatum, hindfoot deformity, pneumothorax, dural ectasia, protrusion acetabuli, scoliosis or kyphosis, reduced elbow extension, facial features, skin striae, myopia and mitral valve prolapse.

Loeys B et al. J Med Genet 2010;47:476–85.

Box 19.28 Elastosis perforans serpiginosa

- A rare disorder of elastic fibres. May be sporadic.
- Reported in association with disorders of connective tissue, including Marfan syndrome, EDS, pseudoxanthoma elasticum, and systemic sclerosis.
- Also seen in Down syndrome and in patients taking penicillamine.
- Most often affects the face, neck, and upper limbs.
- Abnormal dermal elastic fibres are eliminated through channels in the epidermis (transepidermal elimination), producing skin-coloured or erythematous keratotic papules with central plugs.
- Papules may erupt in annular or serpiginous patterns.

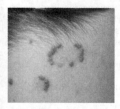

Fig. 19.16 Elastosis perforans serpiginosa: papules with central keratotic plugs.

Pseudoxanthoma elasticum

Pseudoxanthoma elasticum (PXE) is a rare inherited disorder in which elastic fibres become fragmented and calcified. PXE is caused by mutations in an ABC transporter gene encoding a transmembrane protein mainly found in the liver and kidney (multidrug resistance-associated protein 6, MRP6). PXE may be a systemic metabolic disorder with $2°$ mineralization of connective tissues.

The inheritance pattern is usually AR, and PXE is commoner in women. Clinical features, including age of onset, vary within and between families, but skin changes are not usually apparent until puberty (average age of onset = 13 years). For diagnostic criteria, see Box 19.29.

(△ Consider screening fundoscopies in young patients presenting with GI haemorrhage, macular degeneration, or unexplained claudication.)

What should I ask?

- Skin changes (mainly a cosmetic problem).
- Visual impairment (reduced visual acuity is a late problem).
- Cardiovascular disease: intermittent claudication (30% of patients), angina, and myocardial infarction (commences in third to fifth decades—caused by calcification of the internal elastic lamina of medium-sized arteries).
- Bleeding: GI (commonest). Other sites include subarachnoid, retinal, renal, uterine, bladder, nasal, and/or joints (spontaneous bleeding is seen in 10% of patients).
- Family history.

What should I look for?

- Asymptomatic yellowish, grouped 'cobblestone' papules, giving the appearance of 'plucked chicken' skin. Examine the sides of the neck, axillae, antecubital fossae, popliteal fossae, groins, and periumbilical skin. Yellowish plaques form when papules coalesce. For differential diagnosis, see Box 19.30.
- Redundant skinfolds or lax yellowish skin. The sagging skin gives a prematurely aged appearance (advanced disease).
- Yellowish papules on the mucosal surface of the lower lip (common).
- Calcium extruded from the skin in perforating PXE (advanced disease).
- Less common cutaneous manifestations include acneiform lesions, brown macules in a reticulate pattern, and EPS (see Box 19.28).
- Yellowish mottling 'peau d'orange' of the retina (may be the first ocular sign).
- Angioid streaks: present in >85% of patients. Breaks in the elastic lamina of the Bruch membrane produce single or multiple, dark red, brown or grey bands, usually radiating from the optic disc. Onset is between ages of 15 and 25 years, usually after the cutaneous signs.
- Reduced peripheral pulses.
- Hypertension (obstruction of calcified renal arteries causes renovascular hypertension in 25% of patients).
- Signs of mitral valve disease or restrictive cardiomyopathy caused by calcification of valves and/or endocardium.

What should I do?

- Take a skin biopsy from involved skin to confirm the diagnosis (wound healing may be slow). Consider biopsying a scar or flexural skin if no cutaneous signs.
- Eyes: refer for an ophthalmological assessment. Patients should be reviewed every 6–12 months—subretinal neovascularization and haemorrhages may result in loss of central vision.
- Refer for genetic counselling, and screen first-degree relatives by examining the skin and fundi.
- Arrange echocardiography to exclude mitral valve prolapse, mitral valve stenosis, and/or restrictive cardiomyopathy.
- Monitor blood pressure, peripheral pulses, and cardiac function.
- Minimize cardiovascular risk factors: control weight; advise patients to avoid nicotine and lower cholesterol; encourage regular exercise.
- Advise patients to avoid heavy straining, such as weightlifting, and contact sports with a risk of head trauma, e.g. football, wrestling.
- Avoid drugs, such as warfarin, aspirin, and NSAIDs, that may increase the risk of bleeding.

Box 19.29 Diagnostic criteria for pseudoxanthoma elasticum

Patients with three criteria definitely have PXE:
- Characteristic skin signs (yellow papules in flexural areas).
- Characteristic ophthalmologic features (angioid streaks, mottled 'peau d'orange' retinal pigmentation, maculopathy).
- Characteristic histological features in lesional skin: fragmentation, clumping, and calcification of dermal elastic fibres.

Box 19.30 Differential diagnosis

- Sun damage produces a waxy, yellowish appearance (solar elastosis) on chronically exposed skin (neck, face), associated with deep furrows (see ➲ Box 3.1, p. 43).
- Thalassaemia and sickle-cell syndromes: a PXE-like syndrome occurs with skin, ocular (angioid streaks), and vascular manifestations.
- PXE-like skin lesions may develop in chronic end-stage renal disease, L-tryptophan-induced eosinophilia myalgia syndrome, amyloid elastosis, and patients taking penicillamine.
- PXE-like papules occur in papillary dermal elastolysis (an acquired condition of older women).
- Angioid streaks may be seen in EDS, Marfan syndrome, Paget disease of the bone, and lead poisoning.

Further reading

Jiang Q et al. J Invest Dermatol 2009;**129**:348–54.
Le Saux et al. J Invest Dermatol 2006;**126**:1497–505.
Uitto J et al. Am J Med Genet 2011;**155**:1517–26.

Vasculitis

Contents

> **Relevant pages in other chapters**

Introduction

What is cutaneous vasculitis?

Vasculitis (angiitis) is a necrotizing inflammation of the blood vessels caused by various mechanisms (see Boxes 20.1 and 20.2). Necrosis of blood vessel walls leads to extravasation of RBCs (purpura), vascular obstruction, and tissue ischaemia or infarction. Vasculitis may affect vessels of different sizes in the skin, kidneys, gut, respiratory tract, peripheral nerves, and/or skeletal muscle.

The histological findings in vasculitis may include:
- Perivascular neutrophilic inflammation extending into vessel walls.
- Swelling and injury of endothelial cells.
- Necrosis of vessel walls.
- Fibrinoid deposition around vessels (fibrinoid necrosis).
- Extravasation of RBCs (clinically evident as purpura in the skin).
- Nuclear dust, indicative of leukocytoclasis (fragmentation of the nuclei of neutrophils).

Symptoms and signs vary, but palpable purpura is the hallmark of a small-vessel cutaneous vasculitis (see Box 20.2, and Figs. 20.1 and 20.2).

Clinical findings should be integrated with the results of serological, pathological, and imaging studies to reach a diagnosis. For classification criteria, see Box 20.1.

What is occlusive vasculopathy?

Vasculitis in the skin must be differentiated from an occlusive vasculopathy. Skin biopsy shows that the vessels are occluded, without significant vascular inflammation (see ➔ p. 452 and pp. 312–15).

Purpura: differential diagnosis

See ➔ p. 70.

Box 20.1 2012 Revised International Chapel Hill Consensus Conference Nomenclature of Vasculitides

This nomenclature system (it is not a classification or diagnostic system) was updated to improve the Chapel Hill Consensus Conference 1994 nomenclature, change names and definitions as appropriate, and add important categories of vasculitis that were not included in 1994. The names adopted are as follows:

- *Large-vessel vasculitis*:
  - Takayasu arteritis.
  - Giant cell arteritis.
- *Medium-vessel vasculitis*:
  - Polyarteritis nodosa.
  - Kawasaki disease.
- *Small-vessel vasculitis*:
  - ANCA-associated vasculitis:
    —Microscopic polyangiitis.
    —Granulomatosis with polyangiitis (Wegener) (GPA).
    —Eosinophilic granulomatosis with polyangiitis (Churg–Strauss) (EGPA).
  - Immune complex small-vessel vasculitis:
    —Anti-glomerular basement membrane (anti-GBM) disease.
    —Cryoglobulinaemic vasculitis.
    —IgA vasculitis (Henoch–Schönlein) (IgAV).
    —Hypocomplementaemic urticarial vasculitis (anti-C1q vasculitis).
- *Variable vessel vasculitis*:
  - Behçet disease.
  - Cogan syndrome.
- *Single-organ vasculitis*:
  - Cutaneous leukocytoclastic angiitis.
  - Cutaneous arteritis.
  - Primary CNS vasculitis.
  - Isolated aortitis.
  - Others.
- *Vasculitis associated with systemic disease*:
  - Lupus vasculitis.
  - Rheumatoid vasculitis.
  - Sarcoid vasculitis.
  - Others.
- *Vasculitis associated with probable aetiology*:
  - Hepatitis C virus-associated cryoglobulinaemic vasculitis.
  - HBV-associated vasculitis.
  - Syphilis-associated aortitis.
  - Drug-associated immune complex vasculitis.
  - Drug-associated ANCA-associated vasculitis.
  - Cancer-associated vasculitis.
  - Others.

Box 20.2 Vasculitic reaction patterns

Immunopathogenic mechanisms in vasculitis have traditionally been classified into four types (analogous to the types described for hypersensitivity reactions). More than one type of immune reaction may be involved during the course of a disease, and overlap syndromes may occur.

- Antibody-associated vasculitis (type II reaction), e.g. ANCA-mediated vasculitis in GPA (Wegener) and microscopic polyangiitis; antibodies binding to endothelial cell antigens, generating a thrombogenic vasculopathy in SLE, RA, or systemic sclerosis.
- Immune complex vasculitis (type III reaction), e.g. small-vessel cutaneous vasculitis such as IgA vasculitis (Henoch–Schönlein purpura) with complement activation, deposition of Ig in vessel walls, and release of Th2-type cytokines (IL-10, IL-6) (see Fig. 20.2). Circulating immune complexes are also present in urticarial vasculitis.
- T-cell-mediated hypersensitivity (type IV reaction), e.g. granulomatous large-vessel vasculitides such as giant cell arteritis. Lymphocytes and monocytes invade blood vessel walls, and CD4+ Th1-type cells produce IFN-γ.

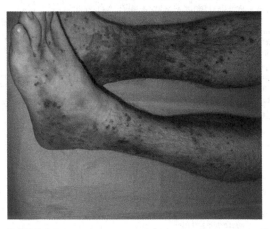

Fig. 20.1 Small-vessel cutaneous vasculitis with a symmetrical palpable purpuric rash and haemosiderin deposition.

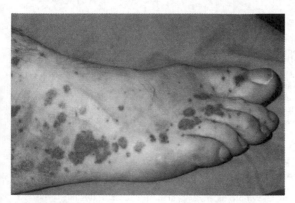

Fig. 20.2 Palpable purpura.

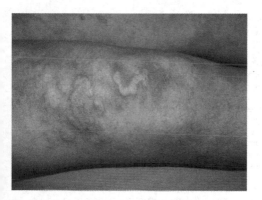

Fig. 20.3 Urticarial vasculitis and livedo reticularis.

Further reading
Marzano A et al. Autoimmunity Rev 2013;**12**:467–76.

Small-vessel cutaneous vasculitis

Synonyms: leukocytoclastic angiitis/vasculitis, cutaneous small-vessel necrotizing vasculitis, allergic vasculitis, hypersensitivity angiitis.

This is the commonest vasculitis affecting the skin. The vasculitic lesions in idiopathic small-vessel cutaneous vasculitis are identical to those in a small-vessel cutaneous vasculitis occurring as part of a systemic disease associated with circulating immune complexes (see Box 20.3). Idiopathic small-vessel cutaneous vasculitis confined to the skin usually resolves within a few weeks or months. Ten percent have recurrent disease lasting months or years.

What should I ask?
- Explore the distribution and evolution of the rash.
- Search for an underlying cause (see Box 20.3).
- Enquire about symptoms such as orogenital ulcers, dry eyes, dry mouth, GI symptoms, myalgia, arthralgia, or joint swelling.

What should I look for?
- Distribution:
  - Vasculitis involves dependent areas such as the leg, sites of trauma, pressure sites (elbows, sacrum, waist band), or cool skin (tip of the nose, ears, fingers) (see Fig. 20.1).
- Morphology:
  - Is the rash purpuric? Purpura, unlike erythema, does not blanch with light pressure (see Fig. 20.2).
  - Are the spots flat or raised (palpable)? Palpable purpura is the hallmark of small-vessel cutaneous vasculitis. Flat (macular) purpuric lesions are associated with non-inflammatory pathology (see ➲ p. 70 and p. 74).
  - How does the rash evolve? In small-vessel cutaneous vasculitis, small round or oval erythematous macules rapidly become raised and purpuric. Papules may coalesce into larger polycyclic or annular lesions.
  - Are there blisters, pustules, or ulcers 2° to inflammation?
  - What is left? Vasculitis fades gradually over 3 or 4 weeks, leaving macular pigmentation (haemosiderin) or atrophic scars.
- Note the position of leg ulcers, and check for signs of stasis or arterial disease (see ➲ Box 15.4, p. 299). Is there purpura around the edge of the ulcer (a feature of some vasculitic ulcers)?
- Look for livedo reticularis, retiform purpura, or ulcerated nodules indicating a necrotizing vasculitis affecting deeper vessels or an occlusive vasculopathy, e.g. cholesterol emboli (see ➲ p. 452).
- Is there evidence of a systemic disease (see Box 20.3)?

What should I do?
See Box 20.4.

Further reading
Goeser M et al. Am J Clin Dermatol 2014;15:299–306.
Tye Haeberle M et al. Arch Dermatol 2012;8:887–8.

Box 20.3 Causes of small-vessel cutaneous vasculitis

- Uncertain 'idiopathic': 50%.
- Infections: 15–20%. Remember hepatitis B or C in adults, IgA vasculitis (Henoch–Schönlein purpura) in children (see ➔ p. 442).
- Drugs: 10–15%; 7–21 days after commencing the drug.
- Connective tissue diseases: 15–20%. Rheumatoid vasculitis is commonest in seropositive patients with long-standing nodular disease.
- Malignancies: 5%. Most often lymphoproliferative disorders, e.g. Hodgkin disease, MF, lymphosarcoma, adult T-cell leukaemia, multiple myeloma.
- Inflammatory bowel disease.
- Others, e.g. prolonged exercise such as long-distance walks; marathons may trigger a cutaneous vasculitis on the leg—'exercise-induced purpura'. This fades within days.

Box 20.4 What should I do?

Investigations

- Guiac testing of stool (in children with IgA vasculitis).
- Urinalysis, including microscopy to check for cellular casts.
- FBC.
- Inflammatory markers (ESR, CRP).
- Renal function tests, LFTs, hepatitis B/C viral serologies.
- Complement levels (C3, C4), cryoglobulins if C4 is low.
- Igs, RF, and ANA.
- ANCA if evidence of systemic disease.
- CXR if concern about interstitial lung disease.
- Skin biopsy: cutaneous vasculitis can be diagnosed using standard histological techniques, but the histology is unlikely to reveal the cause, exclude systemic disease, or distinguish one form of systemic vasculitis from another. Take a biopsy from a purpuric papule about 12–24h old.
- Direct IMF of frozen tissue may be requested to look for deposits of Ig in vessel walls, e.g. IgA, but it is not necessary to demonstrate immune complexes to diagnose vasculitis. Immune complexes are not found in older lesions, so take a punch biopsy from the edge of a fresh lesion, and immediately freeze the specimen.

Management of small-vessel cutaneous vasculitis

- Eliminate precipitating agents (drugs or infections), but it may take several weeks for vasculitis to settle.
- Minimize local triggers by avoiding cooling or trauma and reducing stasis (elevate the legs; provide support stockings; encourage exercise).
- Most patients with small-vessel vasculitis limited to the skin do not require systemic corticosteroids or immunosuppressive agents.
- If cutaneous vasculitis is symptomatic, dapsone (50–200mg/day) may be helpful. Alternatives include colchicine (0.5mg bd) and low-dose methotrexate (10–25mg/week).
- Severe cutaneous vasculitis may require short courses of prednisolone or alternative immunosuppressants, e.g. mycophenolate mofetil (2–3g daily).

IgA vasculitis (Henoch–Schönlein purpura)

IgA vasculitis is the most common small-vessel systemic vasculitis in children but may also affect adults. It is triggered by infection, often in the upper respiratory tract. IgA immune complexes are present in the circulation and vessel walls.

Clinical features

- Palpable purpura (indicating a small-vessel cutaneous vasculitis) is present on extensor surfaces of the limbs, buttocks, and back. The distribution probably reflects stasis and pressure.
- In children, the purpura may be oedematous; early lesions may be urticarial (wheal-like), and the scalp, ears, hands, feet, and scrotum may be oedematous.
- Infantile acute haemorrhagic oedema of the skin is possibly a variant of IgA vasculitis, in which the oedematous component is particularly marked.

Features of systemic involvement in children include:
- Migratory arthralgia or arthritis, usually of the knees and ankles (60–90%).
- Colicky abdominal pain (50–70%), sometimes with blood in the stool or melaena.
- Haematuria, microscopic or gross, caused by glomerulonephritis (60%), but proteinuria, hypertension, and decreased renal function are less common.

What should I do?

- Direct the history, examination, and investigations towards confirming the diagnosis and determining the extent of systemic involvement (see ➲ Box 20.4, p. 441).
- Treat with:
  - Antibiotics, if indicated, for an underlying infection.
  - Paracetamol for pain control.
  - Fluids, bowel rest, and nutrition.
- The value of oral corticosteroids is controversial.

Prognosis

IgA vasculitis is self-limiting, but mild recurrences are common for a few months. Rapidly progressive renal failure is rare, and the prognosis is excellent.

Further reading

Yang Y et al. Autoimmunity Rev 2014;13:355–8.

Urticarial vasculitis

Patients with urticarial vasculitis have signs that indicate a mix of dermal oedema (urticarial wheals) and small-vessel cutaneous vasculitis (palpable purpura) (see Fig. 20.3). The smooth, erythematous papules (wheals) are uncomfortable (tender or burn) but may also itch; individual wheals last up to 72h, and wheals resolve, leaving bruising. Some patients have angio-oedema-like lesions. Simple urticaria is itchy; individual wheals last around 24h, and wheals fade to leave normal skin (see ➔ p. 228). Also see Schnitzler syndrome, ➔ Box 11.1, p. 229.

Associations

- Connective tissue diseases: some patients with low complement levels have anti-C1q antibodies and overlapping features with SLE, including pleuritis, glomerulonephritis, eye symptoms, and positive ANAs.
- Serum sickness (10 days after the administration of drugs or vaccines).
- Infections, including hepatitis C virus (HCV) infection.
- Haematological malignancies; IgM or IgG gammapathy.

What should I ask?

- Document the evolution of individual lesions. If the duration is uncertain, ask the patient to draw around fresh lesions, and note how long they last.
- Does the wheal blanch, or is it purpuric? Patients may have a mix of urticarial and purpuric lesions, as well as angio-oedema-like swellings. Is there residual bruising when lesions resolve?
- Ask about musculoskeletal symptoms (common: 50–75% of patients) or GI symptoms (less common).

What should I do?

- Search for an underlying cause, and check FBC (anaemia is common), ESR (often raised), complement (low complement, detected in 18% of patients, suggests an underlying systemic disease), and autoantibodies, including anti-C1q antibodies.
- Exclude systemic vasculitis (see Box 20.4, p. 441).
- Take a skin biopsy from a purpuric lesion to confirm the presence of a leukocytoclastic vasculitis.

Treatment options

- Antihistamines.
- Dapsone, colchicine, or hydroxychloroquine.
- NSAIDs.
- Severe disease: prednisolone or steroid-sparing agents (azathioprine, cyclophosphamide, ciclosporin, mycophenolate mofetil).

Further reading

Jara L et al. Curr Rheumatol Rep 2009;**11**:410–15.
Marzano A et al. Autoimmunity Rev 2013;**12**:467–76.
Zuberbier T and Maurer M. Immunol Allergy Clin North Am 2014;**34**:141–7.

Cryobulinaemic vasculitis and occlusive vasculopathy

Cryoglobulins are Igs that precipitate at low temperatures.

Type I cryoglobulinaemia

- Type I: monoclonal IgG or IgM (25% of cases).
- The cryoglobulins obstruct vessels (occlusive vasculopathy), causing RBC extravasation without inflammation (no vasculitis).
- *Associations*: chronic lymphatic leukaemia, multiple myeloma, Waldenström macroglobulinaemia.

What should I look for?
- Patients are sensitive to cold and complain of Raynaud phenomenon.
- Mottling of the skin or blotchy cyanosis of the helix of the ears, as well as fingers and toes.
- Initially, cold-induced lesions may be urticarial (see ➋ p. 230) but then become purpuric and blister or ulcerate.

Type II and type III mixed cryoglobulinaemia

- Type II: monoclonal and polyclonal Igs (25% of cases).
- Type III: polyclonal Igs (50% of cases).
- Immune complexes precipitated in vessel walls induce a small-vessel vasculitis that can affect many organs.
- *Associations*: connective tissue diseases, e.g. RA or SLE; infections, especially HCV infection in type II mixed cryoglobulinaemia. HCV infection triggers B-cell clonal expansions that may be associated with monoclonal gammopathy or, rarely, non-Hodgkin B-cell lymphoma.

What should I look for?
- Palpable purpura: the first sign in most patients.
- Arthralgia (70%).
- Sensorimotor neuropathy (60%).
- Raynaud phenomenon (30%).
- Renal involvement (20–30%).
- Chronic leg ulcers (15%), usually above the malleoli, surrounded by purpura, but without signs of venous stasis.

What should I do?

For investigation and management, see Boxes 20.5, 20.6, and 20.7,.

Box 20.5 Investigation of cryoglobulinaemia

- Type II or III mixed cryoglobulinaemia: measure complement C4, which is low in mixed cryoglobulinaemia and is easier to measure than cryoglobulins, as the blood does not have to be kept warm. If C4 is low, measure cryoglobulins (see Box 20.6).
- Type I cryoglobulinaemia: measure cryoglobulins and RF.
- Take a skin biopsy from a purpuric lesion or the edge of an ulcer. Dermal blood vessels are plugged by homogeneous eosinophilic material in monoclonal cryoglobulinaemia. You will see a vasculitis in mixed cryoglobulinaemia.

Box 20.6 Measuring cryoglobulins

- The clotted blood specimen must be kept warm (37°C).
- Place the container in a Thermos™ flask for transportation to the laboratory.
- It may be easier to send the patient to the laboratory for venesection.

Box 20.7 Management of cryoglobulinaemia

- Treat the underlying disease.
- Warmth:
  - Keep the trunk warm with thermal underwear.
  - Recommend thermal gloves and thermal socks.
  - Footwear should have thick soles.
- Control venous stasis with compression bandaging to promote healing of leg ulcers. Badly applied ridged bandages with uneven skin pressure may exacerbate cutaneous vasculitis (see ➔ Box 15.10, p. 307).
- Consider corticosteroids in combination with cytotoxic agents, but the response is variable.
- Plasmapheresis has been used to treat progressive vasculitis.

Further reading

Giuggioli D et al. *Semin Arthritis Rheum* 2015;**44**:518–26.
Skellet A et al. *Clin Exp Dermatol* 2013;**39**:250–2.
Yang C et al. *JAMA Dermatol* 2014;**150**:426–8.

ANCA-associated vasculitis

ANCA-associated vasculitis is rare but is the commonest 1° systemic vasculitis affecting adults. The vasculitis involves both small and medium-sized vessels.

Cutaneous findings are not specific. The diagnosis is based on the evidence of systemic vasculitis, which may be life-threatening, and not the cutaneous findings.

Subtypes

The three major subtypes have overlapping features:
- Granulomatosis with polyangiitis (GPA) (Wegener granulomatosis): granulomatous inflammation of the upper and lower airways, necrotizing small-vessel vasculitis, and necrotizing glomerulonephritis. Patients may have ENT symptoms such as nasal stuffiness, nose bleeds, sinus pain, ear pain, hearing loss, or red eye (uveitis).
- Microscopic polyangiitis: necrotizing glomerulonephritis, pulmonary capillaritis without asthma, necrotizing small-vessel vasculitis.
- Eosinophilic granulomatosis with polyangiitis (EGPA) (Churg–Strauss syndrome): allergic rhinitis and asthma, eosinophilia, necrotizing small-vessel vasculitis, and eosinophil-rich and granulomatous inflammation involving the respiratory tract.

What should I look for?

- Evidence of systemic disease: take a thorough history, and perform a full physical examination, including fundoscopy and a neurological examination.
- Systemic symptoms such as fever, malaise, arthralgia, and myalgia.
- A palpable purpuric rash on the legs 2° to small-vessel cutaneous vasculitis is common in all types of ANCA-associated vasculitis.
- Livedo reticularis, ulcers, or subcutaneous nodules indicate involvement of larger cutaneous vessels (see → p. 452).
- Progressive painful ulceration of the face, neck, or perianal skin, resembling pyoderma gangrenosum, is associated with GPA.
- Ulcerated papules on the limbs, particularly the elbows (like rheumatoid nodules), but also on the face and scalp, may occur in GPA and EGPA.
- 'Strawberry gingivitis' in GPA—swollen, erythematous gums covered with granular exophytic lesions with petechial haemorrhages.
- An underlying cause, e.g. infection, including HIV, autoimmune disease, drugs, malignancy.

What should I do?

- Baseline investigations to assess disease activity and organ involvement (see Box 20.8).
- Further investigation will be guided by the findings, e.g. patients with nodules on the chest radiograph may need high-resolution CT.
- Biopsy of internal organs is usually required to confirm the diagnosis.
- Biopsy of cutaneous lesions may show a vasculitis but will not distinguish between different forms of ANCA-associated vasculitis.

- ANCA-associated vasculitides are managed using immunosuppressive drugs such as prednisolone, azathioprine, and cyclophosphamide. There may be a role for drugs, such as rituximab, which depletes B-cells. Advise about sun protection (see Box 20.9).

Box 20.8 Baseline investigations in systemic vasculitis

- Urine dipstick: if proteinuria is detected, quantify the protein loss with a 24-h urine or protein:creatinine ratio.
- Urine microscopy to look for cellular casts.
- FBC.
- ESR, CRP.
- Renal function.
- Complement levels.
- ANA, RF, ANCA.
- Antiphospholipid antibodies and lupus anticoagulant, when indicated, e.g. in patients with SLE who have recurrent venous/arterial thrombosis, cerebral thrombosis, recurrent fetal loss, pulmonary hypertension, and/or livedo reticularis.
- CXR.
- Cutaneous nodules: take a deep incisional biopsy, extending down to fat, to detect pathology in arterioles or small arteries. The pathology will not distinguish between different forms of ANCA-associated vasculitis.

Box 20.9 Sun protection and vasculitis

Patients with ANCA-associated vasculitis are at increased risk of non-melanoma skin cancer. Patients on long-term immunosuppressants should be educated about sun protection and skin surveillance (see ➜ p. 346 and pp. 338–9).

Further reading
Ali FR et al. Br J Dermatol 2014;**171**:190–203.
Kallenberg C. Nat Rev Rheumatol 2014;**10**:484–93.
Mahr A et al. Best Pract Res Clin Rheumatol 2013;**27**:45–56.

Septic cutaneous vasculitis

Vascular damage may occur in infective endocarditis, meningococcae-mia, chronic gonococcaemia, Gram-negative septicaemia, and rickettsial infections. Septic vasculitis can also follow any intravascular procedure.

The vasculitis tends to involve both small and medium-sized vessels. Organisms damage blood vessels by direct invasion, release of endo-toxins that provoke thrombosis (DIC), and immune complex-mediated vasculitis.

⚠ Infective endocarditis

Signs include splinter haemorrhages in nails, mucosal petechiae, Osler nodes (tender, erythematous spots on the pulps of fingertips and toes), and Janeway lesions (non-tender red or haemorrhagic macules or nod-ules on the palms and soles). Skin manifestations are associated with a high risk of complications, e.g. cerebral emboli.

▶▶ Acute meningococcaemia

A life-threatening illness that must be treated immediately with IV antibi-otics, e.g. cefotaxime 2g. Purpuric lesions develop on the limbs or trunk within 12–36h of the onset of infection. These may be small and few in number. Purpura fulminans with DIC is a devastating complication (see ➜ pp. 102–3).

Fibrin thrombi occlude capillaries, venules, and vessels in the deeper dermis and subcutis, leading to ischaemia and infarction. Persistent cyanosis of the extremities is an early warning sign. Large, irregular, indurated ecchymoses become necrotic, blister, and may progress to extensive gangrene.

⚠ Gram-negative septicaemia (*Escherichia coli*, *Pseudomonas*, or *Klebsiella*)

Septic emboli produce erythematous wheals and papules that become irregularly purpuric and necrotic.

Chronic meningococcaemia and chronic disseminated gonococcaemia

Rare immune complex-mediated illnesses associated with fever, arthral-gia, arthritis, and a cutaneous vasculitis. Look for scattered purpuric papules and vesicopustules on the trunk and extremities (meningococ-caemia) or the palms, fingers, and toes (gonococcaemia). These may be few in number.

⚠ Rocky Mountain spotted fever

Rickettsia rickettsii invades the walls of small cutaneous vessels, inducing a focal lymphocytic vasculitis. Look for an erythematous maculopapular rash that becomes petechial and purpuric within 24–48h.

⚠ Septic vasculitis after percutaneous arterial puncture

Signs suggest unilateral cutaneous emboli: local infarction, livedo, and/ or retiform purpura.

Further reading
Servy A et al. *JAMA Dermatol* 2014;**150**:494–500.

Cutaneous involvement in medium-sized and large-vessel vasculitis

Polyarteritis nodosa

Polyarteritis nodosa (PAN) is a life-threatening systemic necrotizing segmental vasculitis that involves vessels ranging in size from arterioles to medium-sized arteries.

Cutaneous manifestations are infrequent but may include palpable purpura (small-vessel cutaneous vasculitis) or, less often, livedo reticularis, cutaneous nodules, ulcers, and peripheral gangrene (medium- to large-vessel vasculitis).

Cutaneous polyarteritis nodosa

A necrotizing vasculitis affects small and medium-sized muscular wall arteries in the deep dermis and subcutis. Major organs are not involved, but the disease is chronic and recurrent.

What should I look for?

- Painful cutaneous nodules, palpable purpura, ulceration, and livedo reticularis on the legs.
- Fever, malaise, arthralgia, and myalgia.
- Peripheral neuropathy.

What should I do?

- Screen for systemic vasculitis. Laboratory findings are unremarkable, except for leucocytosis and an elevated ESR.
- Ensure the patient is not hypertensive.
- Take a deep incisional biopsy to demonstrate vascular pathology in arterioles or small arteries.
- Control pain with NSAIDs, paracetamol, morphine, or amitriptyline.
- Try compression bandaging (may not be tolerated).
- Consider pentoxifylline or low-dose methotrexate (evidence lacking for efficacy).

Nodular vasculitis

see ➲ pp. 460–1.

⚠ Giant cell arteritis (temporal arteritis)

This granulomatous panarteritis of the large and medium-sized arteries, particularly those of the head and neck, generally affects patients >60 years of age. Some patients also have polymyalgia rheumatica. Both conditions are commoner in women.

Complications include retinal artery inflammation with sudden irreversible blindness or, less often, stroke.

What should I look for?
- A history of recent severe headache, scalp tenderness (noticed when combing hair or lying on a pillow), jaw claudication, and/or visual disturbance (transient loss, diplopia, ptosis).
- Systemic symptoms such as fever, malaise, or weight loss.
- Rarely, a tender non-pulsatile temporal artery or a tender scalp nodule that may resemble a BCC, particularly if ulcerated.
- Pallor of the optic disc, retinal haemorrhages and exudates, optic atrophy (late finding).

What should I do?
- Measure ESR and CRP: usually very high.
- Arrange a biopsy of the temporal artery, but disease is patchy, and the artery may look normal.
- ▶▶ Uncomplicated giant cell arteritis (no jaw or tongue claudication or visual symptoms): prednisolone 40–60mg/day, until resolution of symptoms and laboratory abnormalities. Visual loss or amaurosis fugax: IV methylprednisolone 500mg to 1g/day for 3 days.

Further reading

Morgan A and Schwartz R. *Int J Dermatol* 2010;49:750–6.

Thrombo-occlusive vasculopathies

These conditions are characterized by vascular occlusion without frank vasculitis (also see ➋ pp. 102–3).

⚠ Livedo reticularis (livedo racemosa)

Livedo reticularis is seen most often on the legs. The mottled, reddish purple, reticulated discoloration reflects the sluggish vascular flow in the superficial dermis. A continuous livedo network is likely to be physiological and will disappear when the skin is warmed.

A broken (discontinuous) persistent livedo reticularis is seen with:

- Hyperviscosity states: polycythaemia rubra vera, antiphospholipid syndrome (see Box 20.10) (see ➋ Type I cryoglobulinaemia, p. 444).
- Medium- or large-vessel vasculitis: connective tissue diseases, PAN, GPA (see ➋ p. 446).
- Cholesterol emboli and other emboli; calciphylaxis (see ➋ pp. 312–13).

What should I look for?

(See Fig. 20.4.)

- A mottled, reddish purple, reticulated discoloration, usually on the limbs.
- Retiform purpura (purpura in a reticulate or net-like distribution).
- Is the skin cold? Does the discoloration disappear when the skin is warmed, indicating a physiological change of no significance?
- Is the discoloration a continuous network or discontinuous?
- Signs of a vasculitis affecting medium or large cutaneous vessels, e.g. subcutaneous nodules or ulcers.

Differential diagnosis

- Erythema ab igne, a reticulated brown staining that can develop if the skin is exposed chronically to heat from a radiator, open fire, or hot water bottle (see Fig. 20.5).

What should I do?

- If the livedo is physiological, no investigation or treatment is required.
- If the livedo is discontinuous and persistent:
  - Screen for an underlying disease (see earlier in this section).
  - Take deep biopsies that extend into fat to demonstrate diagnostic pathology in arterioles or small arteries such as cholesterol emboli or hyaline thrombi.

Livedoid vasculopathy with ulceration

Synonyms: segmental hyalinizing vasculitis, livedo reticularis with summer/winter ulceration, livedoid vasculitis.

This thrombo-occlusive vasculopathy affects young to middle-aged women. Hyaline thrombi occlude small vessels in the upper and mid dermis, leading to painful ulceration that is chronic and recurrent (see ➋ pp. 314–15).

Further reading

Bachmeyer C and Elalamy I. *Clin Exp Dermatol* 2014;**39**:840–1.
Gonzalez-Santiago T and Davis M. *Dermatol Ther* 2012;**25**:183–94.
Keeling D et al. *Br J Haematol* 2012;**157**:47–58.

⚠ **Box 20.10 What is the antiphospholipid syndrome?**

This thrombo-occlusive vasculopathy presents most often in ♀. Anticardiolipin antibodies, lupus anticoagulant antibodies, and/or anti-β2 glycoprotein 1 antibodies cause microvascular occlusion. Many patients have SLE. Anticoagulants or antiplatelet agents are the mainstay of treatment. Efficacy and safety of novel anticoagulants are under investigation. Cutaneous features include:

- Livedo reticularis and retiform purpura; livedoid vasculopathy (see ➋ pp. 314–15).
- Purpuric lesions simulating vasculitis.
- Atrophie blanche-like scars.
- Raynaud phenomenon and digital gangrene.
- Nail fold ulcers, splinter haemorrhages.
- Superficial thrombophlebitis migrans, leg ulcers.
- Cutaneous necrosis which may be limited or, rarely, widespread.

Extracutaneous features include:
- Complications in pregnancy such as unexplained fetal deaths, premature births, or unexplained spontaneous abortions.
- Sneddon syndrome: cerebrovascular accidents with livedo reticularis and labile hypertension.
- Pulmonary embolus, DVT.

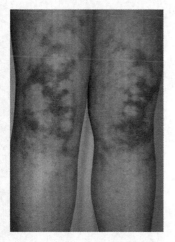

Fig. 20.4 Livedo reticularis in a discontinuous network.

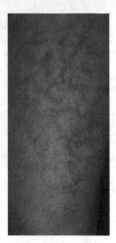

Fig. 20.5 Erythema ab igne: reticulate brownish pigmentation on the thigh of a patient who was snuggling up to a hot water bottle.

Panniculitis

Contents

Introduction

Inflammation of subcutaneous fat is known as panniculitis. Panniculitis is characterized by erythematous nodules. Depending on the cause of panniculitis, nodules may resolve without loss of fat and change in contour, or cause fat necrosis (that may discharge) and leave a depression.

The inflammation may commence in the fat or spread into the fat from the adjacent dermis. The panniculitides are classified histologically into predominantly septal or predominantly lobular patterns of inflammation, and some types are associated with vasculitis (see Box 21.1).

Some types of panniculitis, such as erythema nodosum, may indicate an underlying systemic disease.

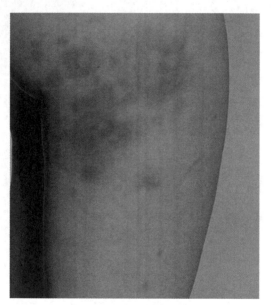

Fig. 21.1 Cold panniculitis in a young ♀ horse rider.

Further reading

Requena L et al. *J Am Acad Dermatol* 2001;**45**:163–83.
Requena L et al. *J Am Acad Dermatol* 2001;**45**:325–61

Box 21.1 Types of panniculitis

Septal panniculitis

With large-vessel vasculitis
- Superficial thrombophlebitis.
- Cutaneous PAN (see ➲ p. 450).

No vasculitis
- Erythema nodosum (see ➲ pp. 458–9).
- Rheumatoid nodule.
- Necrobiosis lipoidica (see ➲ p. 468).
- Scleroderma and eosinophilic fasciitis (see ➲ pp. 420–1).

Lobular panniculitis

With large-vessel vasculitis
- Nodular vasculitis (see ➲ pp. 460–1).

No vasculitis
- AAT deficiency (see ➲ p. 462).
- Cold panniculitis: seen most often in winter in plump, young ♀ horse riders wearing tight jodhpurs that provide insufficient insulation and restrict the blood supply to subcutaneous fat. Mottled, bluish red chilblain-like plaques appear on thighs ('Chiltern chaps') and buttocks ('Berkshire buttocks') (see Fig. 21.1). The plaques resolve without scarring. Riders should wear loose-fitting warm clothing.
- Sclerosing panniculitis (also known as lipodermatosclerosis)—seen on the lower leg in association with venous insufficiency (see ➲ p. 308).
- Calcific uraemic arteriolopathy (calciphylaxis) (see ➲ pp. 312–13).
- Lupus panniculitis (lupus profundus) (see ➲ Box 19.8, p. 405).
- Pancreatic panniculitis (see ➲ pp. 462–3).
- Infective panniculitis (infections of subcutaneous fat in immunosuppressed patients).
- Traumatic or factitious panniculitis.
- Polymer microemboli from the coating of intravascular devices.
- Cytophagic histiocytic panniculitis and subcutaneous T-cell lymphoma.

Weber–Christian disease

Weber–Christian disease is no longer considered to be a distinct entity. This term was used to describe a nodular, relapsing panniculitis with fever and lipoatrophy. Subsequently, most cases considered to be examples of Weber–Christian disease have been given more specific diagnoses.

White JW et al. *J Am Acad Dermatol* 1998;**39**:56–62 (discusses Weber–Christian panniculitis).

Erythema nodosum

What is erythema nodosum?
- EN is the commonest type of panniculitis. It is a septal panniculitis. Vasculitis is not a feature of typical EN.
- EN may be a delayed hypersensitivity response to infection or to an underlying inflammatory disease (see Box 21.2), but no cause is identified in about 1/3 of cases. Cases usually occur in the first half of the year, possibly because of an increase in streptococcal infections.
- Most cases appear between the second and fourth decades, with a peak incidence between the ages of 20 and 30. EN is commoner in women.
- Prognosis depends on the underlying disease. Idiopathic EN is self-limiting with an excellent prognosis. Relapses are uncommon.

What should I look for?
- Underlying triggers (see Box 21.2).
- A prodrome with fever, malaise, arthralgia, and headache.
- Tender, erythematous (no purpura), warm nodules, measuring 1–5cm or more in diameter (see Fig. 21.2).
- A symmetrical distribution on the shins, ankles, and knees (for differential diagnosis, see Box 21.3 and Table 21.1).
- Less often, nodules appear on the arms or trunk.
- EN does not ulcerate.
- Sometimes GI problems such as abdominal pain, vomiting, or diarrhoea.
- Nodules fade over 2–6 weeks (more quickly in children), leaving a purplish, bruise-like appearance that slowly resolves.
- Absence of scarring (nodules do not leave a depression—contour goes back to normal).
- A chronic migratory variant (subacute nodular migratory panniculitis, erythema nodosum migrans) is much less common and usually presents as a single tender, indurated, erythematous plaque that slowly enlarges peripherally, while clearing centrally.

What should I do?
- Check FBC, ESR, urinalysis, and chest radiography.
- Further investigations should be guided by the history, examination, and local prevalence of aetiological factors such as bacterial, viral, fungal, or protozoal infections.
- If required, take a deep elliptical biopsy that includes fat (a biopsy is usually unnecessary).
- Manage any underlying problem such as infection.
- Provide pain relief with NSAIDs.
- Elevation may relieve pain in acute disease.
- Support stockings control swelling and may speed resolution.
- Potassium iodide 300–900mg/day has been recommended in persistent disease.
- Rarely, oral corticosteroids are required, but exclude an infection before prescribing.

Box 21.2 Causes of erythema nodosum

No cause is identified in about 1/3 of cases. Consider:
- Infection: bacterial (often streptococcal in children), viral, protozoal, and fungal.
- Drugs, e.g. combined oral contraceptive pill, penicillins. BRAF inhibitors have been reported to induce EN-like nodules.
- Sarcoidosis (EN and bilateral hilar adenopathy) (see ➲ pp. 524–5).
- IBD (Crohn disease > ulcerative colitis).
- Pregnancy.
- Rheumatological disease, e.g. Behçet disease.
- Malignancy—rare, e.g. Hodgkin lymphoma, acute myeloid leukaemia.

Box 21.3 Differential diagnosis of erythema nodosum

If one or more erythematous nodules in an asymmetrical distribution, consider:
- Trauma.
- Cellulitis.
- Insect bite.
- Superficial thrombophlebitis—cord-like nodules usually on the side of one leg.

If symmetrical nodules, consider:
- Nodular vasculitis (erythema induratum of Bazin). The nodules, which tend to be on calves, rather than shins, ulcerate and heal with scarring (loss of fat) (see ➲ p. 460 and Table 21.1).

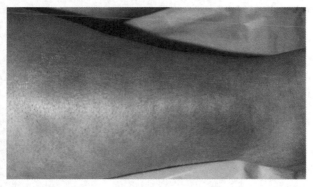

Fig. 21.2 Erythema nodosum with smooth, tender, erythematous nodules on both shins.

Further reading

Blake T et al. Dermatol Online J 2014;**20**:22376.
Gilchrist HI and Patterson JW. Dermatol Ther 2010;**23**:320–7.

Nodular vasculitis (erythema induratum of Bazin)

What is nodular vasculitis?

Nodular vasculitis is the commonest form of lobular panniculitis with vasculitis. It is considered to be a 'reactive disorder', but, in many patients, no underlying trigger is identified.

Bazin described this form of vasculitis in 1861, and a link with TB was recognized in the early 1900s. TB is still the commonest infectious trigger, and *Mycobacterium tuberculosis* DNA has been demonstrated in cutaneous biopsies.

Nodular vasculitis is commonest on the back of the legs of obese middle-aged women in whom chronic venous stasis, previous thrombophlebitis, and/or cooling may play some part in the localization to the leg. The condition tends to run a protracted course over many years.

What should I look for?

- History of recurrent nodules that form slowly and equally slowly resolve.
- Tender, erythematous, indurated nodules and plaques on the calves (rather than the shins) of fat legs where the skin is cyanotic and cold. Nodules develop most often in winter months.
- Ulceration of nodules (unlike EN; see Table 21.1).
- Atrophic scars (depressions) where ulcerated nodules have healed.
- Venous insufficiency of the lower legs (a frequent association).
- Any indications in history and examination of an underlying disease such as TB.

What should I do?

- Take a deep incisional biopsy to demonstrate the pathology.
- Exclude TB by chest radiography, Mantoux test, and/or a TB IFN-γ release assay (QuantiFERON® TB Gold test or T-SPOT® TB test).
- Treat the underlying disease, if identified.
- Control venous stasis by weight loss, compression bandages, elevation, and exercise.
- Relieve pain with NSAIDs.
- Corticosteroids are not usually indicated.

Table 21.1 Differential diagnosis

	Erythema nodosum	Nodular vasculitis
Presentation	Acute	Indolent
Distribution	Shins	Calves
Signs	Tender, warm, erythematous nodules	Tender, erythematous nodules and plaques that may ulcerate
Resolution	Resolves in a few weeks, leaving a bruise-like mark that slowly fades	Heals slowly over months, leaving an atrophic scar
Prognosis	Relapses uncommon	Relapse common. Course is protracted, lasting many years

Further reading

Gilchrist HI and Patterson JW. *Dermatol Ther* 2010;**23**:320–7.
Segura S et al. *J Am Acad Dermatol* 2008;**59**:839–51.

Uncommon causes of panniculitis

α-1-antitrypsin deficiency panniculitis

AAT is a circulating serine protease inhibitor (SERPINA1). AAT inhibits enzymes (e.g. trypsin, collagenase, elastase) involved in the proteolytic degradation of tissues, has effects on the immune system, and inhibits the activation of complement.

Mutations in the *AAT* gene may cause enzyme deficiency or abnormal enzyme function. Severe deficiency mainly affects Caucasians and has a prevalence of 1:2000–1:5000 in Europe. Patients may develop emphysema, pancreatitis, liver cirrhosis, glomerulonephritis, RA, vasculitis, and/or angio-oedema. Rarely, AAT deficiency is associated with relapsing lobular panniculitis accompanied by fat necrosis (seen in adults more often than children). Patients with partial deficiency of AAT may have panniculitis without systemic disease.

Enzyme function may be significantly impaired, despite normal serum levels of AAT, but most cases associated with panniculitis have the ZZ phenotype with AAT levels below normal.

What should I look for?
- Family history of AAT deficiency.
- Recurrent painful, erythematous plaques and nodules in a proximal distribution on the hips, thighs, and buttocks.
- Panniculitis that is induced or exacerbated by trauma.
- Characteristically, nodules suppurate with the release of oily material (uncommon in other forms of panniculitis).
- Associated diseases, including early-onset emphysema, hepatitis and/or cirrhosis, vasculitis (ANCA-positive), and angio-oedema.

What should I do?
- Take a deep biopsy from a fresh nodule to reveal suppurative lobular panniculitis.
- Only check the serum level of AAT and the AAT phenotype if the clinical and histological findings are compatible with panniculitis associated with AAT deficiency.
- Dapsone may be effective in mild cases (inhibits neutrophil migration and function).
- Oral tetracyclines (doxycycline 200mg bd) may have a direct effect on serine proteases released from neutrophils and can help some patients.
- NSAIDs and hydroxychloroquine have been recommended.
- Replacement therapy using IV infusions of AAT controls panniculitis effectively.

Pancreatic panniculitis

A characteristic form of panniculitis has been described (rarely) in association with a number of pancreatic diseases, including:
- Acute or chronic pancreatitis.
- Pancreatic islet cell tumours.
- Ductal adenocarcinoma.

- Acinar cell carcinoma.
- Post-traumatic pancreatitis.
- Pancreatic pseudocysts.

Circulating lipase and/or amylase may be responsible for destruction of fat. The cutaneous signs may present some months before the manifestations of pancreatic disease. Disseminated fat necrosis is associated with a high mortality.

What should I look for?
- Subcutaneous erythematous or reddish brown nodules, usually on the legs, but sometimes on the thighs, arms, buttock, and/or trunk (see Fig. 21.3).
- Nodules may soften in the centre.
- Nodules may be painful or painless.
- In mild cases, nodules heal with atrophic scarring.
- In severe cases, nodules may ulcerate and discharge sterile brown, oily material (necrotic fat).
- May be associated with arthritis (necrosis of periarticular fat) and pleural effusions.

What should I do?
- Search for evidence of pancreatic disease, including measurement of serum amylase.
- Biopsy a nodule. The histology of pancreatic panniculitis is characteristic with fat necrosis, basophilic granular material (fatty acids combine with calcium to form calcium soap), and 'ghost-like' cells (adipocytes with thick shadowy walls—the cell membrane resists lipase).
- Treat the underlying condition.

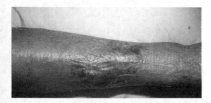

Fig. 21.3 Reddish brown nodules that discharged oily fluid in a patient with pancreatic cancer.

Further reading
de Serres F and Blanco I. *J Intern Med* 2014;**276**:311–35 (AAT deficiency).

Skin and diabetes and endocrinology

Contents

Relevant pages in other chapters
Flushing ➔ p. 521.
Erythrasma ➔ p. 132.
Bacterial folliculitis ➔ pp. 134–5.
Cellulitis ➔ pp. 138–9.
Candida ➔ p. 166.
Leg ulcers ➔ pp. 294–307.
Calcific uraemic arteriolopathy ➔ pp. 312–13.
Neuropathies ➔ pp. 548–50.
Melasma ➔ Box 30.1, p. 583.

Diabetes mellitus and the skin

Chronic diabetes affects microcirculation, as well as skin collagen, and cutaneous problems are common. These include specific manifestations of diabetes, complications such as neuropathy (see ➲ pp. 548–50), skin infections (see Box 22.1), and cutaneous adverse effects related to treatment. Type 1 diabetes (autoimmune) is less common than type 2 diabetes (defective insulin action or secretion).

Diabetes: what should I look for?

- Linear periungual telangiectasia without loss of capillary loops— compare with systemic sclerosis in which capillaries are lost.
- Periungual erythema, ragged cuticles, and tender fingertips.
- Diabetic hand syndrome: scleroderma-like thickening on the dorsum of the hands, with knuckle pads and papules on periungual skin and the sides of fingers; and sclerosing tenosynovitis of palmar flexor tendons, with stiffness of MCP and PIP joints. Mild flexion contractures may limit the ability to press the hand flat on a table or to oppose the palmar surfaces of fingers. May also have Dupuytren contractures and carpal tunnel syndrome.
- Diabetic dermopathy or shin spots (round or oval erythematous papules or pigmented scars on shins). Associated with microvascular complications.
- Feet: neuropathic ulcers (check shoes), onychomycosis, or tinea pedis.
- Necrobiosis lipoidica diabeticorum on shins. May ulcerate (see ➲ p. 468).
- Diabetic bullae: asymptomatic bullae on non-inflamed skin. Seen most often on legs and feet. Cause is unknown, but the differential includes bullous impetigo, PCT, and autoimmune blistering diseases. Bullae resolve without scarring in 2–3 weeks.
- Vitiligo: well-demarcated, smooth, depigmented macules/patches. Check for other autoimmune diseases (see ➲ pp. 486–7).
- Lipohypertrophy (like a lipoma) at sites of insulin injections. Lipoatrophy is uncommon, since recombinant human insulin introduced.
- Lipodystrophy (acquired or inherited)—very rare cause of insulin resistance with diabetes and hypertriglyceridaemia (see Box 22.4).
- Neuropathic itch (see ➲ pp. 548–9).
- Eruptive xanthoma (itchy, yellow papules on extensor surfaces and buttocks) associated with elevated triglycerides (see ➲ p. 470).
- Skin tags and (pseudo)acanthosis nigricans: velvety thickening in skinfolds—in obese patients with insulin resistance and high circulating insulin levels. Insulin has a growth hormone-like action on skin. Encourage patients to lose weight. Acanthosis nigricans may respond to a topical retinoid such as 0.05% tazarotene gel. (Also see ➲ HAIR-AN syndrome, p. 476.)
- Scleredema diabeticorum (see Box 22.2).
- Calcific uraemic arteriolopathy (see ➲ pp. 312–13).
- Acquired perforating dermatosis in diabetes with renal failure (see ➲ p. 494, and Fig. 23.2, p. 495).

Box 22.1 Cutaneous infections in diabetes mellitus

Candidal infections

- Look for scaly flexural erythema with satellite pustules. Chronic paronychia (inflammation of nail fold) may be caused by *Candida*.
- *Candida* causing angular cheilitis, vulvitis, or balanitis may be a presenting sign of diabetes. Pruritus vulvae or ani also common.

Dermatophyte infections

- Look for a well-demarcated scaly rash, often asymmetrical distribution, involving palms or soles. May also have onychomycosis.
- Ulceration caused by a thickened toenail digging into the adjacent toe or fissuring of dry scaly skin provide an entry portal for bacterial infection.

Bacterial infections

- Impetigo, folliculitis, and erysipelas may be severe and widespread in patients with diabetes.
- Erythrasma presents with a glazed erythema or hyperpigmentation in flexures. Look for coral pink fluorescence when examined with a Wood lamp (see ➔ p. 640).
- Life-threatening cutaneous infections may be caused by organisms such as *Pseudomonas aeruginosa* and *Clostridium* species, particularly when diabetes is not well controlled.

Box 22.2 What is scleredema diabeticorum?

This slowly progressive and persistent cutaneous mucinosis occurs in long-standing poorly controlled diabetes. Compare with scleredema of Buschke—dermal thickening on the face, arms, and hands develops suddenly after an infection and resolves in months or years. Look for:

- Thickening of the skin of the posterior neck and upper back, limiting mobility of the neck and shoulders. Occasionally, changes extend to the deltoid and lumbar regions.
- Non-pitting induration with a peau d'orange appearance.
- Sometimes reduced sensitivity to pain and touch.
- Normal FBC, unlike eosinophilic fasciitis (eosinophilia) (see ➔ p. 421).
- No paraprotein, unlike scleromyxoedema (paraproteinaemia) (see ➔ Box 26.10, p. 541).
- Histopathologically: swollen dermal collagen bundles separated by mucin. Skin biopsy not usually required to make the diagnosis.
- Phototherapy with UVA1 may reduce induration and improve mobility, but long-term controlled studies of therapy are needed.

Further reading

Murphy-Chutorian B et al. Endocrinol Metab Clin North Am 2013;42:869–98.
Van Hattem S et al. Cleveland Clin J Med 2008;75:774–86.

Necrobiosis lipoidica

Necrobiosis lipoidica occurs most often in women. It usually presents on shins but may affect other areas. Reddish yellow plaques enlarge slowly and are generally asymptomatic, unless they ulcerate. The pathogenesis of the granulomatous inflammation (see ➲ Box 33.5, p. 651) is uncertain, but many cases are associated with diabetes (necrobiosis lipoidica diabeticorum). It can precede the diagnosis of diabetes in up to 14% of patients. Necrobiosis lipoidica shares some features with granuloma annulare, another granulomatous condition, but one that is rarely associated with diabetes (see Box 22.3).

What should I look for?

- Oval, well-demarcated papules or plaques, usually on the shin (may be bilateral), that expand slowly and may coalesce (see Fig. 22.1).
- Reddish brown plaques that are smooth, shiny, and telangiectatic.
- The border is erythematous and may be scalloped in outline.
- In older plaques, the reddish centre is more yellow and may be atrophic, revealing deeper subcutaneous vessels (see Fig. 22.1).
- Plaques may ulcerate, but surrounding intact skin generally has some features of necrobiosis lipoidica.
- Some patients also have granuloma annulare (see Box 22.3 and Fig. 22.2).

What should I do?

- If necessary, take a deep elliptical biopsy to confirm the diagnosis, but the wound may not heal. The histological features, which overlap with those of granuloma annulare, include extensive dermal necrobiosis (alteration of collagen bundles) outlined by histiocytes and giant cells.
- Avoid trauma—use protective shin pads.
- Treatment options include topical and intralesional corticosteroids, and topical 0.1% tacrolimus, but response is variable.
- Topical corticosteroids, pentoxifylline, nicotinamide with minocycline, and ciclosporin have been advocated for ulcerated necrobiosis lipoidica.

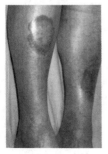

Fig. 22.1 Necrobiosis lipoidica.

Box 22.3 What is granuloma annulare?

- Granuloma annulare is a chronic non-infectious inflammatory condition. The cause is unknown, but rarely extensive disease is linked to diabetes. Sometimes patients also have necrobiosis lipoidica.
- Any age group can be affected, but granuloma annulare is commonest in children.
- One or more asymptomatic skin-coloured or erythematous ring-like marks appear on the skin, most often on limbs.
- Most people only have one or two annular lesions, but granuloma annulare may be widespread (disseminated) (see Fig. 22.2).
- In children, granuloma annulare tends to affect the back of the hands, ankles, or the dorsum of the feet.
- Stretch the skin, and you will see that the raised border is composed of coalescing papules that may be umbilicated.
- The surface is smooth (unlike tinea which is scaly).
- Rings slowly expand and develop a purplish red colour.
- The lesions may persist for several years but eventually fade to leave normal skin.
- Subcutaneous granuloma annulare presents as nodules, sometimes on the fingers when they may simulate rheumatoid nodules.
- The histological features (granulomatous inflammation with necrobiosis) overlap with those of necrobiosis lipoidica.
- Treatment is unsatisfactory but generally is not required. Topical corticosteroids, intralesional corticosteroids, oral retinoids, tetracyclines, and phototherapy have been used, with variable success.

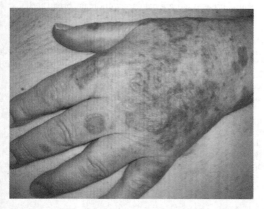

Fig. 22.2 Granuloma annulare with disseminated smooth, purplish papules and annular plaques.

Hyperlipoproteinaemias

The hyperlipoproteinaemias are classified according to which of the four classes of lipoproteins (chylomicrons; very low-density lipoprotein—VLDL; low-density lipoprotein—LDL; or β-VLDL) are elevated (see Table 22.1). Hyperlipoproteinaemia may be 1° or 2° to an underlying problem such as obesity, diabetes mellitus, renal disease, cholestatic liver disease, alcohol abuse, hypothyroidism, hyperuricaemia, or drugs. Lipodystrophy is a rare cause of diabetes with hypertriglyceridaemia (see Box 22.4).

Identification is important, because of the risk of coronary artery disease. Cutaneous xanthomas (lipid deposits in the skin) are a marker of hyperlipoproteinaemia. The type of xanthoma correlates with the underlying cause (see Table 22.1).

What should I look for?

- Eruptive xanthomas: clusters of yellowish papules with erythematous halos on the extensor surfaces of the arms and legs, shoulders, and buttocks. Itch is common, as they regress (1° and 2° hypertriglyceridaemia).
- Tendon xanthomas: firm subcutaneous nodules on the Achilles tendon and over other extensor tendons, including the dorsum of interphalangeal joints (knuckles), patellae, and elbows. May become inflamed. Skin is a normal colour and is not yellow (1° and 2° hypercholesterolaemia).
- Tuberous xanthomas: firm yellow papules and nodules found over large joints (knees, elbows), the heels, or the dorsum of interphalangeal joints (1° and 2° hyperlipidaemia).
- Plane xanthomas: yellow macules with a predilection for the face, upper trunk, and scars. Orange-yellow plane xanthomas may also be found in palmar creases (striate palmar xanthomas, 'bread and butter' palms)—type III and 2° hypercholesterolaemia. Generalized plane xanthoma may be found in myeloma (see ➔ p. 540).
- Xanthelasma: soft yellowish papules on eyelids or below the eyes. Common in the normal population and not a very specific sign, but may be associated with hypercholesterolaemia if present in young patients. Xanthelasmas are associated with cholestatic liver disease.
- Corneal arcus may be linked to familial hypercholesterolaemia but is more likely to be significant if present in adolescence or early adulthood.
- Lipaemia retinalis (pallor of the optic fundus with white retinal veins and arteries) seen in severe hypertriglyceridaemia.
- Signs of underlying disease such as diabetes, hypothyroidism, nephrotic syndrome, cholestatic liver disease, or, very rarely, lipodystrophy (see Box 22.4, p. 471).

Table 22.1 1° hyperlipidaemias and xanthomas

Fredrickson classification	Biochemistry	Signs
Type I familial hyperchylomicronaemia	Severe hypertriglyceridaemia (raised chylomicrons)	Eruptive xanthomas, lipaemia retinalis, hepatosplenomegaly
Type IIa Familial hypercholesterolaemia or familial defective apoB	Hypercholesterolaemia (raised LDL)	Tendon xanthomas, tuberous xanthomas
Type IIb familial combined hyperlipidaemia	Hypercholesterolaemia with hypertriglyceridaemia (raised LDL and VLDL)	Usually no xanthomas
Type III familial dysbetalipoproteinaemia (broad beta disease)	Hypercholesterolaemia with hypertriglyceridaemia (raised β-VLDL)	Plane xanthomas on palms, tuberous xanthomas
Type IV familial hypertriglyceridaemia (may be 2° to diabetes or excess alcohol)	Moderate hypertriglyceridaemia (raised VLDL)	Usually no xanthomas
Type V familial hypertriglyceridaemia	Severe hypertriglyceridaemia (raised chylomicrons and VLDL)	Eruptive xanthomas, lipaemia retinalis, hepatosplenomegaly

---

Box 22.4 Lipodystrophies

Acquired lipodystrophies
- Localized; 2° to pressure, injected drugs (corticosteroids), panniculitis, or unknown causes.
- HIV infection treated with protease inhibitors—subcutaneous fat lost from the face and limbs. Subcutaneous fat deposited on the trunk.
- Acquired partial lipodystrophy (Barraquer–Simons syndrome): loss of fat from the face, neck, arms, and trunk (cephalocaudal sequence). Excess fat on the lower limbs. Associated with low serum C3—impaired complement-mediated phagocytosis, resulting in increased risk of bacterial infections and membrano-proliferative glomerulonephritis (highest risk with low C3 and C3 nephritic factor)—onset up to 10 years after onset of lipodystrophy.
- Generalized panniculitis may be followed by fat loss with tender nodules.

⚠ *Inherited*: all rare and caused by different genetic mutations. Lipodystrophy may be complete or partial.

Complications of lipodystrophies may include insulin resistance, impaired glucose tolerance and diabetes, hypertriglyceridaemia, acute pancreatitis, and hepatic cirrhosis. Psychological distress is common.

Thyroid disorders and the skin

Hyperthyroidism: what cutaneous signs should I look for?

- Warm, moist skin.
- Palmar erythema.
- Onycholysis.
- Fine hair, sometimes with diffuse alopecia (may be predominantly parietal hair loss).
- Thyroid-associated ophthalmopathy—upper lid retraction, periorbital oedema, scleral injection, conjunctival oedema, and proptosis (50% of patients with Graves disease).
- Pretibial myxoedema (<5% of patients with Graves disease) (see Box 22.5, and Figs. 22.3 and 22.4).
- Autoimmune hyperthyroidism may be associated with vitiligo and/or alopecia areata (see ➍ pp. 486–7, pp. 488–9).
- Thyroid acropachy (<1% of patients with Graves disease) (see Box 22.6).
- Evidence of scratching (generalized pruritus is not common).
- Chronic urticaria.

Hypothyroidism: what cutaneous signs should I look for?

- Pale skin with a yellow tinge.
- Puffy face, especially the skin below the eyes.
- Puffy hands and feet (non-pitting).
- Cool peripheral extremities.
- Coarse, rough, dry skin, particularly on extensor surfaces of the limbs, e.g. shins. In severe cases, the changes may simulate ichthyosis.
- Reduced sweating.
- Coarse, dry, brittle hair.
- Diffuse alopecia (may be predominantly frontal hair loss).
- Thinning of outer third of eyebrows.
- Autoimmune hypothyroidism may also be associated with vitiligo and alopecia areata (see ➍ pp. 486–7, pp. 488–9).
- Eruptive and tuberous xanthomas (unusual; see ➍ p. 470).

Box 22.5 What is pretibial myxoedema?

Synonyms: localized myxoedema, thyroid dermopathy.

- Pretibial myxoedema is an autoimmune manifestation of Graves disease. Less often, it is seen in association with Hashimoto thyroiditis.
- All patients have high serum concentrations of antibodies to thyroid-stimulating hormone receptor. Humoral and cellular immune mechanisms may stimulate dermal fibroblasts with the production of large amounts of glycosaminoglycans.
- Pretibial myxoedema is preceded by ophthalmopathy and may be associated with thyroid acropachy (usually without bone changes).

Box 22.5 (*Contd.*)

- Look for:
  - Non-pitting erythematous or flesh-coloured indurated nodules or plaques on both shins. Nodules may also develop on the dorsum of feet, as well as other sites (see Fig. 22.3).
  - The surface has a waxy appearance.
  - The skin is not warm or tender (unlike cellulitis).
- Rarely, extensive infiltration by mucin causes gross non-pitting thickening of skin on the legs and foot. The thickened skin has a waxy, papular surface. Indurated folds may overhang the ankles, simulating the changes 2° to lymphoedema (see Fig. 22.4).
- Mild disease may be a cosmetic problem but does not require treatment.
- Potent topical or intralesional corticosteroids may be helpful in symptomatic disease.
- Lymphoedematous pretibial myxoedema may benefit from compression stockings.

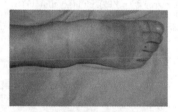

Fig. 22.3 Pretibial myxoedema: firm nodules and mild erythema.

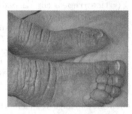

Fig. 22.4 Extensive pretibial myxoedema simulating lymphoedema (see ➔ p.316).

Box 22.6 What is thyroid acropachy?

- Thyroid acropachy is the triad of nail clubbing, swollen fingers, and a periosteal reaction.
- Typically, the periosteal reaction affects the metacarpal bones of the thumb, index, and little fingers, and their proximal and middle phalanges, as well as the first metatarsals.
- The periosteum of the long bones of the forearms and leg is involved less often.
- The periosteal reaction is usually asymptomatic but occasionally causes bone or joint pain.
- Acropachy is strongly associated with Graves disease, thyroid-associated ophthalmopathy, and pretibial myxoedema (thyroid dermopathy).

Hirsutism and hypertrichosis

Hirsutism is defined as excess terminal (coarse, pigmented) hair that appears in a ♂ pattern in a woman. It affects about 10% of Caucasian women (more in Mediterranean women) and usually results from subtle increases in androgens (see ➲ p. 380), but rarely may presage a serious underlying condition (see ➲ pp. 94–5 and Box 22.7).

In contrast, hypertrichosis is independent of androgens. The increased hair growth may be localized or generalized, and affects any part of the body. Hypertrichosis may be racial, hereditary, or be caused by drugs (see ➲ p. 380) and some disease (see ➲ pp. 94–5 and Box 22.7).

What should I ask?

- Enquire about onset, sites involved, and progression. Sudden onset and rapid progression may indicate a virilizing tumour (rare).
- What is the psychological impact? What treatments have been tried?
- Look for symptoms suggesting hyperandrogenism or polycystic ovary syndrome (PCOS), e.g. acne, androgenetic alopecia, menstrual irregularities, or infertility (see ➲ pp. 476–7), hyperprolactinaemia (galactorrhoea), adrenal pathology (see ➲ p. 482), pituitary tumour (visual disturbance, headache), late-onset congenital adrenal hyperplasia (hirsutism, prepuberty, premature pubarche, menstrual irregularity, 1° amenorrhea), or virilization (increased libido, deep voice).
- Drug history, including oral contraceptives (see ➲ p. 380 and Box 22.7).
- Family history of hirsutism, PCOS, androgenetic alopecia, or congenital adrenal hyperplasia.

What should I look for?

- Exclude hypertrichosis by ensuring excess hair is limited to androgen-dependent areas, and score using the Ferriman–Gallwey scale (see Box 22.8).
- Other cutaneous manifestations of excess androgens: ♀ pattern hair loss—the frontal hairline is preserved in women (unlike men), but hair on the vertex of the scalp thins diffusely (see ➲ p. 480); acne and seborrhoea (oily skin on the central face).
- Signs of PCOS (the commonest cause) or another underlying cause (see Box 22.7).
- ⚠ Signs of virilization: deep voice, cliteromegaly, breast atrophy, muscularity. If present, examine for an ovarian or adrenal mass.
- Signs of a visual field defect if you suspect a pituitary adenoma.

What should I do?

- Investigation is recommended in moderate or severe hirsutism; hirsutism of any severity if it is sudden in onset or progressing rapidly; and hirsutism associated with menstrual irregularity or infertility, central obesity, acanthosis nigricans, or cliteromegaly (see Box 22.9).
- For management of hirsutism, see ➲ pp. 478–9.
- Treat the underlying cause.

Further reading

Martin KA et al. J Clin Endocrinol Metab 2008;93:1105–20.

Box 22.7 Causes of hirsutism

- Idiopathic (normal menstrual cycle, normal androgens, but may have a subclinical abnormality in androgens or response to androgens).
- PCOS, the commonest hormonal cause, ovarian hyperandrogenism, or ovarian tumours (see ➜ pp. 476–7). SAHA syndrome—seborrhoea, acne, hirsutism, and androgenetic alopecia.
- HAIR-AN syndrome (see ➜ p. 476).
- Adrenal hyperandrogenism, including non-classical congenital adrenal hyperplasia (21-hydroxylase deficiency) and rarely virilizing tumours.
- Other endocrine disorders: Cushing syndrome or disease, acromegaly, or hyperprolactinaemia.
- Pregnancy-related hyperandrogenism.
- Drugs, including oral contraceptives with androgenic progestins (levonorgestrel, norgestrel, norethindrone), anabolic and androgenic steroids. (Non-androgenic drugs that cause hypertrichosis, rather than hirsutism, include ciclosporin, phenytoin, diazoxide, minocycline, and high-dose corticosteroids.)

Box 22.8 What is the Ferriman–Gallwey score?

- Hair growth is rated from 0 (no growth of terminal hair) to 4 (complete and heavy cover) in nine locations—upper lip, chin, chest, upper back, lower back, upper abdomen, lower abdomen, upper arms, and thighs.
- It is difficult to score accurately, as most women will have removed some of the excess hair.
- Score does not correlate closely with androgen level, probably because the response of the pilosebaceous unit to androgen is variable.
- Caucasian women: 8–15 = mild hirsutism.

Box 22.9 Investigation of hirsutism

Investigation should be guided by the clinical findings, but consider:
- Pregnancy test in patients with amenorrhoea.
- Total testosterone, ideally in early morning. Discuss with your laboratory—some have reliable assays that compute free testosterone by also measuring sex hormone-binding globulin (SHBG).
- Transvaginal ultrasound and luteinizing hormone/follicle-stimulating hormone levels and ratio for polycystic ovaries or ovarian neoplasm.
- Prolactin level to exclude hyperprolactinaemia.
- Early morning 17-hydroxyprogesterone (17-OHP) to exclude adrenal hyperandrogenism in high-risk populations (positive family history or ethnic groups at high risk—Ashkenazi Jews, Hispanics, and Slavs).
- Screen for Cushing syndrome/disease, thyroid disease, or acromegaly, if clinically indicated.
- Obese hirsute women: assess for type 2 diabetes and hyperlipidaemia (metabolic syndrome), as well as thyroid disease.

Polycystic ovary syndrome

Polycystic ovary (ovarian) syndrome (PCOS) is common (affects 5–10% of Caucasian women of reproductive age) and is the commonest hormonal cause of hirsutism, which may be the presenting complaint. Diagnostic criteria for PCOS are shown in Box 22.10.

PCOS is caused by a combination of genetic and non-hereditable factors, but the pathogenesis is incompletely understood (see Box 22.11).

Many patients also have the metabolic syndrome (central obesity, glucose or insulin abnormalities, dyslipidaemias, elevated blood pressure) and are at risk of cardiovascular disease (stroke, coronary artery disease, congestive heart failure). Lipodystrophy is a rare association (see Box 22.4).

What should I ask?

- Menstrual history/history of infertility?
- Family or personal history of diabetes, hyperlipidaemia, acne, or hirsutism?

What should I look for?

- Cutaneous manifestations of excess androgens:
  - Hirsutism: which may be mild (or altered by treatment).
  - ♀ pattern of hair loss: frontal hairline is preserved in women (unlike men), but hair on the vertex of the scalp thins diffusely.
  - Acne.
  - Seborrhoea: oily skin on central face (nose and forehead).
- Acanthosis nigricans usually 2° to obesity with insulin resistance.
- HAIR-AN syndrome: hyperandrogenism (acne), insulin resistance, and acanthosis nigricans. May also have hirsutism.
- Central obesity (record the waist–hip ratio or waist circumference).
- Evidence of the metabolic syndrome, including hypertension. Record the height and weight, and calculate the body mass index (BMI).
- Rarely lipodystrophy (see Box 22.4).

What should I do?

- Pregnancy test, in patients with amenorrhea.
- Measure plasma testosterone, ideally in early morning (normal or increased).
- Transvaginal ultrasound to detect polycystic ovaries.
- Luteinizing hormone (LH)/follicle-stimulating hormone (FSH) ratio >2 suggests PCOS, but, as the ratio is raised in <50% of cases, it is not a useful test for confirming PCOS.
- Fasting glucose and lipids (the metabolic syndrome is common).
- PCOS is the commonest cause of hirsutism, but consider excluding other causes of hirsutism, if clinically relevant (see Box 22.7).

Box 22.10 Diagnostic criteria for polycystic ovary syndrome

Diagnosis of PCOS requires two of the following three criteria:
- Polycystic ovaries (not pathognomonic).
- Oligo- or anovulation (menstrual irregularity, infertility).
- Biochemical and/or clinical signs of hyperandrogenism such as hirsutism, acne, or androgenetic alopecia.

Box 22.11 Factors involved in the pathogenesis of polycystic ovary syndrome

The pathogenesis is still incompletely understood but is multifactorial:
- Intrinsic dysfunction of ovaries and adrenal glands probably contributes to hyperandrogenaemia.
- Central obesity (40% of patients with PCOS):
  - Adipocytes containing excess triglycerides are insulin-resistant, and this triggers compensatory hyperinsulinaemia. Hyperinsulinaemia stimulates the production of ovarian androgens.
  - Increased conversion of androgen to oestrogen by adipocytes stimulates the release of LH and reduces FSH.
- LH also stimulates the production of ovarian androgens (testosterone, androstenedione, and dehydroepiandrosterone).
- Hyperinsulinaemia and elevated androgen inhibit the production of sex hormone-binding globulin (SHBG).
- Reduced SHBG leads to an increase in the proportion of plasma testosterone that is free (unbound) and therefore is available for conversion to dihydrotestosterone in the pilosebaceous unit (by the enzyme 5α-reductase).
- Dihydrotestosterone binds more strongly to the androgen receptor in follicles than testosterone and is the 1° mediator of androgenetic effects on the pilosebaceous unit (acne, hirsutism, androgenetic alopecia). Hyperinsulinaemia may increase the responsiveness of the pilosebaceous unit to androgen.

Further reading

Buzney E et al. J Am Acad Dermatol 2014;**71**:859.
Housman E and Reynolds RV. J Am Acad Dermatol 2014;**71**:847.

Management of hirsutism

Women with hirsutism may be too embarrassed to discuss the condition or what they have been doing to remove the excess hair. Hirsutism can have a major impact on quality of life, and many women will be anxious, have a low self-esteem, or have concerns about sexual self-worth.

Although there is no single easy answer, treatments can make a difference, and most women will value the opportunity to talk to a sensitive physician about what can be done. Any underlying cause of androgen excess should be controlled, and drugs contributing to hirsutism withdrawn. The choice of treatment for reducing or removing hair will depend on the patient's preference, the distribution and severity of hirsutism, and the cost of treatment (most are not provided through the NHS).

Topical treatments

- Bleaching with hydrogen peroxide preparations may make dark facial hair less obvious but can be irritant.
- Depilatory creams or foams containing thioglycolates that dissolve hair are widely available but smell unpleasant, are irritant, and are not very effective for coarse hair.
- Eflornithine cream (inhibitor of ornithine decarboxylase) applied bd reduces the rate of growth of hair after 6–8 weeks. May irritate or induce acne. Once treatment is discontinued, the hair growth returns to pretreatment levels. Eflornithine is helpful in combination with mechanical treatments.

Mechanical treatments

- Shaving: regrowing hairs have a blunt tip which may make them look thicker than before. Although women are prepared to shave their legs or axillae, most do not find it acceptable to shave the face. Shaving may cause a folliculitis, particularly on the thighs.
- Epilation: plucking, waxing, threading, or sugaring to extract hairs. Contrary to popular opinion, epilation does not make hairs grow back more thickly. Epilation is uncomfortable. Irritation and folliculitis are common. Post-inflammatory hyperpigmentation may be a problem in dark skin.
- Electrolysis is effective and can permanently destroy some hair follicles (about 60%), but the outcome depends on the skill of the operator. Complications include scarring and infection.
- Laser hair removal (photoepilation) is most effective for dark hairs on fair skin (laser energy is absorbed by melanin in the hair follicle, and not the surrounding epidermis). Treatment interrupts hair growth temporarily, but regrowing hairs may be finer and lighter. Some permanent hair loss may be achieved after repeated treatments. Laser treatment is considerably more expensive than electrolysis but is also more effective and faster.

Oral therapy

See Box 22.12.

Box 22.12 Oral therapy for hirsutism

- Combined oral contraceptive containing the progestin cyproterone acetate (2mg). Cyproterone acetate blocks the androgen receptor in the pilosebaceous unit and, to a lesser extent, the activity of 5α-reductase. First-line therapy for premenopausal women. Treat for at least 6 months. Adverse effects: liver toxicity, weight gain, fatigue, loss of libido, mastodynia, nausea, headaches, and depression. Monitor liver function.
- Spironolactone (androgen receptor antagonist) up to 100mg/day: monitor for hyperkalaemia. Treat for at least 6 months. Causes breast soreness and menstrual irregularities.
- Finasteride (inhibits 5α-reductase) 5mg/day. Treat for at least 6 months. Relatively contraindicated in premenopausal women due to teratogenic effects for $\male$ fetuses.
- Ensure that premenopausal women taking anti-androgens always use effective contraception to avoid the potential risk of feminization of a $\male$ fetus. Explain anti-androgens can be effective in the absence of abnormal androgen levels. Benefits lost within months of treatment withdrawal.
- Insulin-sensitizing drugs, e.g. metformin, lower insulin levels in hyperinsulinaemia by increasing sensitivity to insulin. Metformin also attenuates both hyperinsulinaemia and hyperandrogenaemia, and may reduce hirsutism in patients with PCOS but is less effective than spironolactone.

Further reading

Blume-Peytavi U and Hahn S. *Dermatol Ther* 2008;**21**:329–39.
Martin KA et al. *J Clin Endocrinol Metab* 2008;**93**:1105–20.
Somani N et al. *Dermatol Ther* 2008;**21**:376–91.
Wanitphakdeedecha R and Alster TS. *Dermatol Ther* 2008;**21**:392–401.

Male and female pattern hair loss

Synonyms: male pattern baldness, androgenetic alopecia, genetic hair loss.

Hair loss (alopecia) is common as people age, but the pattern of loss is different in males and females. Androgens play a pivotal role in male pattern hair loss, but their role in female pattern hair loss is less certain, and other mechanisms may be involved. Genetically determined susceptibility is important (prevalence varies in different populations).

Male pattern hair loss—what should I look for?
- About 25% of men begin to lose hair by age 30, and 50% by age 50.
- Androgens cause follicular miniaturization, with progressive decrease in the width of the hair shaft.
- Receding frontal hairline is common, particularly on the temples (may commence in the mid teens).
- Gradual thinning of the hair on the vertex is eventually followed by complete loss of hair over the vertex (loss may be preceded by curling and coarsening of hair—acquired progressive kinking).
- A rim of hair is retained around the back and sides of the scalp (occipital follicles are not dependent on androgens and are a source of follicles for hair transplants).

Female pattern hair loss—what should I look for?
- Female pattern loss occurs any time after the onset of puberty. Prevalence varies widely but increases to 29–42% in women aged >70.
- Some report increased shedding; others complain of gradual diffuse thinning over the crown, usually with sparing of the frontal hairline.
- Women may say 'I can see my scalp' or complain central parting gets sunburnt. There may be a family history of androgenetic alopecia.
- Density of hair on top of the scalp is reduced in a diffuse central pattern. Other patterns include accentuated loss frontally or loss localized to the vertex. Hair pull (see ➔ Box 3.3, p. 45) may be positive in early loss, but usually negative.
- Temporal thinning is common, but, unlike men, women do not progress to complete balding on the vertex. In advanced female pattern hair loss, when hair may be very sparse over the top of the scalp, a rim of hair is still retained along the frontal margin.
- Rapidly progressive hair loss in a male pattern suggests virilization—look for other signs/symptoms, e.g. oligomenorrhoea or amenorrhoea, hirsutism, severe acne, or cliteromegaly (see ➔ p. 474).
- Some hyperandrogenic women show female pattern of hair loss.
- Exclude other causes of diffuse non-scarring alopecia (see Boxes 22.13 and 22.14).
- Ask about menstrual history, dieting, recent illnesses, and drugs.

What should I do?
See Box 22.15.

Further reading
Olsen EA *et al. J Am Acad Dermatol* 2005;**52**:301–11.

Box 22.13 Differential diagnosis in diffuse non-scarring alopecia

- Female pattern hair loss.
- Telogen effluvium: seek a trigger in previous 2–5 months, including pregnancy. If acute, hair falls out in handfuls. Remits in 12 months. If chronic (lasts months to years), can be difficult to distinguish from female pattern hair loss.
- Diffuse alopecia areata: positive hair pull, may have lost hair at other sites (see ➡ p. 488). Dermoscopic features include cadaverized hairs, exclamation mark hairs, broken hairs (black dots), and yellow dots. Look for nail pitting and autoimmune thyroid disease.
- Traction alopecia: is the patient pulling hair back tightly?
- Systemic disease or drugs (see Box 22.14).

Box 22.14 Systemic causes of diffuse non-scarring alopecia

- Iron deficiency (often associated with heavy menses).
- Hypothyroidism (often frontal hair loss) or hyperthyroidism (often parietal hair loss), but may resemble female pattern hair loss.
- Hypoparathyroidism, hypopituitarism.
- SLE (frontal alopecia is commonest).
- Protein malnutrition, crash dieting, or anorexia nervosa.
- Severe chronic disease, including malignancy.
- Cytotoxic drugs, vitamin A, and oral retinoids.

Box 22.15 Management of male and female pattern hair loss

- If the woman has no symptoms or signs suggesting hyperandrogenaemia, investigation of the androgen status is not indicated.
- Investigate and treat coexisting problems, e.g iron deficiency.
- Explain to women that they are unlikely to go bald, shorter layered hair styles make hair look fuller, and boosting the volume of hair with rollers, mousses, or a gentle permanent wave will not increase hair loss—this reassurance may be all that is required.
- Explain that treatment will only have a modest impact (stabilizes loss, thickens residual hair shafts) but will not reverse hair loss.
- Topical 2% or 5% minoxidil solution or foam bd may produce some regrowth in men and women. Minoxidil should halt progression, while the treatment is being used, and can produce some regrowth and thickening. Treat for 12–24 months.
- Women—anti-androgens: the combined oral contraceptive containing the progestin cyproterone acetate, or spironolactone up to 100mg/day. Treat for at least 6 months (for management of hirsutism, see Box 22.12).
- Finasteride 1mg/day—for men and post-menopausal women.
- Monitor with photographs or hair counts (if shedding).
- Hair fibres for camouflage—these fibres stick to remaining hairs to create an appearance of fullness and mask the visible scalp.
- Wigs or hair transplantation are an option for some patients.

Other endocrinopathies

Panhypopituitarism

Cutaneous signs include:
- Smooth facial skin with fine wrinkles, loss of facial hair, reduced body hair.
- Decreased ability to tan and pale yellowish skin (deficiency of ACTH, which has a role in regulating melanin pigmentation).

Addison disease

1° adrenal failure is commonly caused by autoimmune adrenalitis or infection (TB, fungal, CMV, AIDS). High levels of circulating pituitary peptides, e.g. pro-opiomelanocortin, ACTH β-lipotropin, and melanocyte-stimulating hormone, induce melanocyte activity. Look for:
- Hyperpigmentation of sun-exposed skin.
- Hyperpigmentation in palmar creases, axillae, nipples, old scars, and sites of pressure or friction such as knuckles and waistline.
- Pigmented mucous membranes—lips (can occur up to 10 years before diagnosis, may be diffuse, speckled, or streaks), gums, buccal, vaginal, vulval, and anal.
- Darkening of melanocytic naevi and hair.
- If caused by autoimmune adrenalitis, you may find vitiligo.

Note: hyperpigmentation does not occur if adrenal failure is 2° to ACTH deficiency, e.g. after withdrawing oral glucocorticoids.

Cushing syndrome

Cushing syndrome is associated with inappropriately elevated free plasma glucocorticoid. For causes, see Box 22.16. Skin signs include:
- Central obesity with thin arms and legs. Dorsal neck and supraclavicular fat pads. Plethoric telangiectatic round 'moon' face.
- Hirsutism with fine hair on the cheeks.
- Atrophic skin with purple striae on the trunk, upper thighs, and arms.
- Easy bruising.
- Cutaneous fungal infections: pityriasis versicolor, widespread *Trichophyton rubrum* (nails, trunk, buttocks), nail candidiasis.
- Acne: pustules and perifollicular papules, but no comedones.
- Signs of virilism if adrenal tumour produces androgens (see ➔ p. 474).
- Hyperpigmentation if associated with high ACTH levels, e.g. in ectopic ACTH syndrome (see ➔ Addison disease, p. 482, and Nelson syndrome in Box 22.17).
- ⚠ Signs of Carney syndrome/McCune–Albright syndrome (see Box 22.16).

Acromegaly

Excess secretion of growth hormone by pituitary tumours. Look for:
- Thick greasy, coarse, furrowed skin on the face and neck.
- Frontal bossing, thick lips, and broad nose; doughy hands.
- Cutis verticis gyrata (thick ridges and furrows on the scalp).
- Hyperhidrosis (common). Hyperpigmentation: 40% of patients. Hirsutism: 50% of patients.

Multiple endocrine neoplasia

See Box 22.18.

Box 22.16 Causes of Cushing syndrome

- Cushing disease: pituitary-dependent bilateral adrenocortical hyperplasia, usually 2° to a pituitary adenoma. The commonest cause of Cushing syndrome (50–70% of patients).
- Adrenal adenomas or carcinomas (20–30% of patients).
- Iatrogenic.
- Ectopic ACTH: ACTH released by non-pituitary tumours, e.g. small-cell carcinoma of the bronchus (16% of patients).
- Carney syndrome: cutaneous and mucosal freckling, mesenchymal tumours (atrial myxoma), peripheral nerve and endocrine tumours.
- McCune–Albright syndrome: fibrous dysplasia and cutaneous pigmentation (large café au lait patches with an irregular outline), may be associated with pituitary, thyroid, adrenal, and gonadal hyperfunction.

⚠ Box 22.17 What is Nelson syndrome?

- This rare syndrome presents in patients with Cushing disease who have been treated by bilateral adrenalectomy.
- The pituitary adenoma, no longer inhibited by cortisol released from the adrenals, continues to enlarge and release ACTH.
- High levels of ACTH produce Addisonian hyperpigmentation.

⚠ Box 22.18 Multiple endocrine neoplasia

Multiple endocrine neoplasia type 1
- Inherited as AD.
- Predisposition to tumours of the parathyroid glands, anterior pituitary, pancreatic islets cells (gastrinoma, insulinoma).
- Cutaneous signs: multiple cutaneous angiofibromas (flesh-coloured papules), collagenoma (thickened yellow plaque), café au lait spots.

Multiple endocrine neoplasia type 2A
- Inherited as AD.
- Predisposition to medullary thyroid cancer, phaeochromocytoma, and 1° parathyroid hyperplasia.
- Cutaneous signs: cutaneous lichen amyloidosis (see ➲ Box 23.3, p. 497).

Multiple endocrine neoplasia type 2B
- Inherited as AD.
- Predisposition to medullary thyroid cancer and phaeochromocytoma.
- Intestine ganglioneuromas.
- Cutaneous signs: mucosal neuromas on the lips, tongue, buccal mucosa, gingiva, and palate. Café au lait spots. Marfanoid appearance (see ➲ p. 430).

Autoimmune polyendocrine syndromes

Interactions between genetic and environmental factors influence susceptibility. Vitiligo is common in all types (see Fig. 22.5).

⚠ Polyglandular autoimmune syndrome type 1

Synonym: autoimmune polyendocrinopathy–candidiasis–ectodermal dystrophy (APECED).

Very rare: mutation of autoimmune regulator gene on chromosome 21.

- At least two of: chronic mucocutaneous candidiasis (includes nails) often apparent in first few months of life, usually before age 5; chronic hypoparathyroidism (paraesthesiae, muscle twitching, or spasms, dry skin, brittle hair and nails)—onset usually before age 15; and/or Addison disease.
- Defect in T-lymphocytes demonstrated by skin anergy to *Candida* and tuberculin antigens.
- Associated conditions may include alopecia (totalis or areata) (see Fig. 22.6), vitiligo, hypergonadotropic hypogonadism, autoimmune thyroid disease, pernicious anaemia, chronic active hepatitis, and/or steatorrhoea (malabsorption), type 1 diabetes mellitus (rare—18%), IgA deficiency, ectodermal dysplasia.
- Malignant neoplasias, e.g. oral SCC, adenocarcinoma stomach.

⚠ Polyglandular autoimmune syndrome type 2

Rare, associated with HLA-DR3/DR4 = Schmidt syndrome.

- Addison disease (always present) and autoimmune thyroid disease and/or type 1 diabetes mellitus (>50%).
- Associations include alopecia (totalis or areata) (see Fig. 22.6), idiopathic heart block, vitiligo, 1° hypogonadism, autoimmune hepatitis, pernicious anaemia, Parkinson disease, IgA deficiency.

⚠ Polyglandular autoimmune syndrome type 3

(Has been subdivided into types A, B, C, and D.)

- Autoimmune thyroid disease (Hashimoto thyroiditis, idiopathic myxoedema, asymptomatic thyroiditis, Graves disease, endocrine ophthalmopathy, pretibial myxoedema) associated with another autoimmune disease (excluding Addison disease, and/or hypoparathyroidism).
- Examples of other diseases include vitiligo (common), type 1 diabetes mellitus, alopecia areata, pernicious anaemia, coeliac disease, myasthenia gravis, RA, or Sjögren syndrome.

⚠ Polyglandular autoimmune syndrome type 4

- Combination of organ-specific autoimmune diseases not included in other groups, e.g. vitiligo and alopecia, type 1 diabetes mellitus and vitiligo.

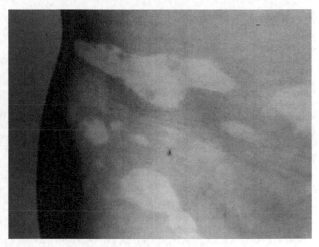

Fig. 22.5 Vitiligo: smooth depigmented patches.

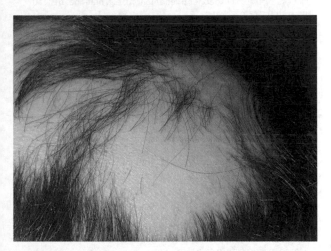

Fig. 22.6 Alopecia areata: well-circumscribed patches of non-scarring alopecia. The skin is not scaly or inflamed.

Further reading

Cutolo M. *Autoimmun Rev* 2014;**13**:85–9.

Vitiligo

Vitiligo is a common acquired skin condition in which epidermal melanocytes are lost, leading to complete loss of pigment, i.e. depigmentation, rather than hypopigmentation (partial pigment loss) (see Fig. 22.5). Average age of onset is 20 years, but vitiligo may commence in childhood. Up to a third report a family history of vitiligo. Psychological impact may be profound, particularly in individuals with darkly pigmented skin. Vitiligo is associated with various autoimmune diseases, including thyroid disease (see Box 22.19).

What should I look for?

- Smooth (no scale) white (depigmented) macules and/or patches.
- Are you sure that the pale skin is abnormal? Might it be possible that the rest of the skin is hyperpigmented? For example, melasma may be confused with facial vitiligo, when hyperpigmented facial lesions surround normal, but pale-looking, skin.
- Pigment loss may be non-segmental (localized, generalized, or acrofacial) or segmental (unilateral following a dermatomal distribution; one or more segments may be affected) (see Table 22.2).
- Non-segmental: common on fingers, wrists, axillae, groins, perioral and periorbital skin, and genitalia. Check sites sensitive to pressure, friction, or trauma (Koebner phenomenon), e.g. belt-line, beneath the watch strap.
- Rims of depigmented skin around melanocytic naevi—halo naevi— are ten times commoner in vitiligo. The melanocytic naevi regress, leaving depigmented macules (Fig. 17.5).
- Genital vitiligo—the patient may be too embarrassed to report the vitiligo. Lichen sclerosus may coexist with genital vitiligo (see ⮩ p. 288).
- White hairs on eyelashes and scalp, as well as white body hair within areas of vitiligo (leukotrichia).
- A 'trichrome' appearance with a white depigmented centre, a surrounding light brown zone of varying width, and dark brown normal skin. Seen rarely in developing patches in dark skin.
- Inflammation at the advancing edge of a macule—uncommon.
- Mucosae may be affected in patients with dark skin.

What should I do?

- Exclude other causes of pigment loss (see ⮩ pp. 89–90).
- Assess the psychological impact of vitiligo using DLQI (see ⮩ p. 32.
- Check thyroid function (high prevalence of thyroid antibodies).
- Examine the skin under Wood light to confirm diagnosis (the depigmented skin appears bright white), and determine the extent of disease, particularly in pale skin.
- Record the extent of vitiligo with photographs.
- Management is challenging—sun protection is essential (see Box 22.20).

Box 22.19 Autoimmune diseases associated with vitiligo

- Thyroid disease, type 1 diabetes mellitus, and adrenal insufficiency.
- Autoimmune polyendocrinopathy syndromes (see ➔ pp. 484–5).
- LE, RA, sarcoidosis, myasthenia gravis, pernicious anaemia, autoimmune hepatitis.
- Alopecia areata, psoriasis, LP, lichen sclerosus.

Table 22.2 Types of vitiligo

Non-segmental vitiligo	Segmental vitiligo
Late onset is commoner	Often begins in childhood when it may be difficult to distinguish from naevus depigmentosus (see ➔ p. 89)
Is progressive, with flare-ups	Has rapid onset but stabilizes. Halo naevi and leukotrichia are risk factors for progression to mixed vitiligo
Involves hair compartment late	Involves hair compartment early
Often associated with personal or family history of autoimmunity	Usually not accompanied by other autoimmune diseases

Box 22.20 Management of vitiligo

- Advise about sun protection (pale-skinned individuals should also use sunblocks to prevent normal skin from tanning, so that vitiligo is less obvious).
- Vitamin D supplements may be needed, as strict sun avoidance can reduce vitamin D levels (see ➔ Box 16.11, p. 339).
- Minimize trauma to the skin (vitiligo koebnerizes).
- Very potent (clobetasol propionate) topical corticosteroid cream or 0.1% tacrolimus ointment may induce repigmentation in vitiligo of recent onset.
- UVB phototherapy or PUVA may be indicated in adults with widespread disease that has not responded to conservative treatment, but prolonged courses are required, and the response is variable. Partial follicular repigmentation may be even more disfiguring, and normal skin darkens, making vitiligo more obvious.
- Skin grafts (highest repigmentation rates) or epidermal suspension transplants (cultured or non-cultured) have been advocated, particularly for segmental vitiligo.
- Offer cosmetic camouflage (patients can self-refer via ✆ https://www.changingfaces.org.uk/Home).
- Vitiligo support societies, e.g. ✆ http://www.vitiligosociety.org.uk.

Further reading

Gawkrodger DJ et al. Br J Dermatol 2008;**159**:1051–76.
Whitton ME et al. Cochrane Database Syst Rev 2010;**20**:CD003263.

Alopecia areata

Alopecia areata is a common (1–2% of the population) T-cell-mediated cause of non-scarring alopecia. Presents at any age but most often affects children and young adults when it may cause considerable psychological distress, particularly if widespread. Genetic and environmental factors are involved in the pathogenesis, and it is associated with autoimmune diseases, including vitiligo and autoimmune thyroiditis, as well as with atopy. T-cell clustering around the hair bulb of growing (anagen) hair follicles disturbs the normal cycle of hair growth. Hair follicles in the growing part of the cycle are pushed prematurely into the resting (telogen) phase. Affected follicles have potential for regrowth, as there is no scarring. Patients have circulating IgG antibodies to anagen hair follicles, but these may not be pathogenic.

Recent evidence implicates cytotoxic T-cells and the janus kinase (JAK) pathway in pathogenesis, and a potential role for JAK inhibitors in treatment. Disease is both dynamic and unpredictable. Stress may trigger onset. Severity ranges from transient loss in few patches to persistent loss of all scalp and body hair. It is chronic in 7–10% of patients.

Poor prognostic factors include:
- Young age of onset. Family history of alopecia areata (20% of patients).
- History of autoimmune diseases or atopy.
- Nail involvement. Extensive hair loss or ophiasic pattern of loss (see below). Recurrent episodes of hair loss or long-standing loss.

What should I look for?
- One or more well-circumscribed, smooth, round, or oval patches of non-scarring alopecia on the scalp (commonest pattern). Skin is not inflamed; patches are asymptomatic (for differential, see Box 22.21).
- Often sparing of grey or white hair. Regrowing hairs white at first.
- Exclamation-mark hairs (short and tapering to a point) seen at the edge of patches of hair loss. Easier to see using a dermatoscope: cadaverized hairs (black dots), yellow dots, and clustered short vellus hairs.
- In active disease, hair pull may be positive for telogen hairs (resting hairs) or dystrophic anagen hairs at the edge of the patch; >6 hairs are pulled out by the root, when a small clump is tugged gently but firmly (see ➔ Box 3.3, p. 45).
- Patches of hair loss in the beard area, loss of eyebrows or eyelashes.
- Nail pitting (about 10% of cases).
- Other patterns of loss include:
  - Band of loss around the periphery of the scalp (ophiasic pattern).
  - Diffuse thinning that resembles ♀ pattern hair loss (see ➔ p. 480).
  - Complete loss of scalp hair (alopecia totalis). Sudden onset of alopecia totalis can make a patient's hair appear to 'go white overnight', because white hairs are retained.
  - Complete loss of scalp hair and body hair (alopecia universalis).

What should I do?
See Boxes 22.21, 22.22, and 22.23.

Box 22.21 Alopecia areata: differential diagnosis

The characteristic dermoscopic findings of alopecia areata will help to exclude other diagnoses such as:
- Telogen effluvium: hair loss is generalized and not patchy.
- Tinea capitis: the scalp is erythematous and scaly, but signs may be subtle, particularly in infections caused by *T. tonsurans*.
- Trichotillomania (deliberate hair pulling): broken hairs or regrowing hairs are still firmly anchored to the scalp.
- Drug-induced anagen effluvium may mimic diffuse alopecia areata.
- ♀ pattern hair loss (see ⊃ p. 480) may mimic diffuse alopecia areata.
- SLE (usually frontal alopecia).
- 2° syphilis (patchy moth-eaten appearance).
- Early scarring alopecia (see ⊃ Box 3.2, p. 45).

Box 22.22 Investigations in alopecia areata

- Usually none required. Although autoimmune diseases are increased in frequency, current UK guidelines do not recommend routine screening. Serum 25-hydroxyvitamin D levels may be low and are inversely correlated with disease activity. If diagnosis is in doubt, consider:
  - Fungal culture of plucked hairs.
  - Skin biopsy: rarely needed, but can distinguish from ♀ pattern hair loss.
  - Serology for SLE and syphilis.

Box 22.23 Management of alopecia areata

- Difficult to treat. Some treatments induce hair growth, but none affects the course of disease or the long-term outcome.
- Remember that most patients (80%) have spontaneous regrowth of hair in any individual patch within 12 months of onset.
- Potent topical corticosteroids are safe and used widely, although there is limited evidence that they are effective. Intralesional corticosteroids temporarily stimulate tufts of hair growth, but repeated injections cause atrophy. Intralesional steroids near the eye may cause cataract or raised intraocular pressure, but lower concentrations can be used cautiously at these sites.
- Other treatments that have been tried include short courses of oral prednisolone, contact immunotherapy (50–60% can show a response, but patients with extensive hair loss are less likely to respond), dithranol and other irritants, and phototherapy (high relapse rates with PUVA). Patients with extensive loss or recurrent episodes may benefit from psychological support or contact Alopecia UK, available at ⟨http://www.alopeciaonline.org.uk⟩.
- For some, a wig or hairpiece may be the best option.

Further reading

Delamere FM et al. Cochrane Database Syst Rev 2008;2:CD004413.
Messenger AG et al. Br J Dermatol 2012;166:916–26.

Skin and renal disease

Contents

Relevant pages in other chapters
Calcific uraemic arteriolopathy (calciphylaxis) ➔ pp. 312–13
Porphyria ➔ p. 332 and pseudoporphyria ➔ p. 334
Vasculitis ➔ pp. 436–51
α-1-antitrypsin deficiency ➔ p. 462
Lipodystrophy ➔ Box 22.4, p. 471
Familial cancer syndromes ➔ pp. 542–4
Skin and rheumatology ➔ Ch. 19, p. 393

Skin changes in renal disease

General examination

- Dry skin; pale skin 2° to chronic anaemia.
- Yellow tinge to skin (accumulation of carotenoids, urochromes, and lipochromes) or diffuse hyperpigmentation (increased melanin).
- Macular purpura: increased vessel fragility, heparin during dialysis.
- Sparse body hair, diffuse alopecia, and/or dry hair.
- Nail changes (see below).
- Signs of scratching (see ➔ p. 494).
- Problems associated with AV fistula (see Box 23.1).

Nail changes

- Transverse white bands (Mees lines): acute kidney injury.
- Paired narrow transverse white lines on several nails (Muehrcke lines): hypoalbuminaemia in nephrotic syndrome. Bands fade if the nail plate is compressed, unlike Mees lines.
- 'Half-and-half' nails (proximal white, distal brownish-pink = Lindsay nails): uraemia.
- Less frequent changes seen in chronic kidney disease:
  - Absence of lunulae.
  - Splinter haemorrhages.
  - Brittle nails.
  - Koilonychia.

Other cutaneous problems

- Cutaneous vasculitis related to underlying problems such as SLE (see ➔ p. 436).
- Acquired perforating dermatosis (see ➔ p. 494).
- PCT and pseudoporphyria present with skin fragility, erosions, and blisters on exposed skin, usually the dorsum of the hands (see ➔ p. 332 and p. 334). Take a detailed drug history, as many drugs may be implicated in the pathogenesis of pseudoporphyria.
- Calcific uraemic arteriolopathy (calciphylaxis): a life-threatening condition, seen in patients on dialysis. Presents acutely with painful mottled erythema that becomes necrotic (see ➔ pp. 312–13).
- Nephrogenic systemic fibrosis (see ➔ p. 498); drug reactions (see ➔ pp. 366–7).
- Amyloidosis (see ➔ pp. 496 and Fig. 23.1).

Further reading

Chen ZJ et al. Clin Exp Dermatol 2009;34:679–83.

Box 23.1 Skin and iatrogenic arteriovenous fistulae

A number of skin conditions are associated with iatrogenic AV fistulae, and it is more difficult to achieve haemostasis during skin surgery on the same limb as the fistula.

- Viral warts may arise more commonly on the side of the AV fistula, probably as a result of the Koebner phenomenon.
- The presence of AV fistulae does not affect the distribution of cutaneous malignancies, e.g. SCC or BCC. However, those present on the same limb as the AV fistulae (in particular those distal to the fistulae) will require excision under general anaesthetic by surgeons with experience of managing haemostasis in these individuals.
- Acroangiodermatitis (pseudo-KS): confluent violaceous or brown-black papules cover large areas of the distal limb as a result of increased venous stasis, which results in AV channel formation. Oral erythromycin may help.
- Unilateral limited scleroderma-like features have been reported—skin thickening associated with Raynaud phenomenon, sclerodactyly, and painful cutaneous ulcers involving the arm with the AV fistula as a result of vascular steal phenomenon and occlusive arterial disease. Revascularization may lead to improvement.
- Stasis dermatitis of the affected hand.
- Diffuse dermal angiomatosis: a variant of reactive angioendotheliomatosis is uncommon and usually presents as irregular, painful ulcerations with a background of livedo reticularis-like changes. It is caused by ischaemia, and tying off the haemodialysis AV fistula may improve microcirculation, resulting in resolution of the lesions.

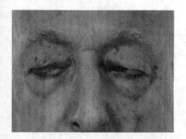

Fig. 23.1 Systemic amyloidosis: periorbital purpura. Reproduced with permission from Warrell D et al. (eds) Oxford Textbook of Medicine, 5th edn, 2010. Oxford: Oxford University Press.

Itch in chronic kidney disease

Uraemic pruritus

For management, see Box 23.2.

- Itching is a common and distressing problem both in chronic kidney disease and in those individuals receiving dialysis (60–90% of patients).
- Itch, whether intermittent or persistent, generalized or localized, may have a major impact on quality of life, e.g. insomnia, depression.
- Pathogenesis is unclear, but accumulation of metabolic toxins and immunological mechanisms may be involved. Dryness and impairment of integrity of the stratum corneum may also play some part.
- Signs include excoriations, skin thickening (lichen simplex) caused by chronic rubbing, and nodules (nodular prurigo; see ➲ p. 222).
- Always consider other causes of itching, including scabies; is anyone else in the family itchy? Check for burrows between fingers and on genitalia (see ➲ p. 172).

Acquired perforating dermatosis

Synonym: reactive perforating collagenosis.

- Most often seen in diabetic patients with chronic kidney disease.
- Scratching may play some part in the pathogenesis.
- Itchy dome-shaped nodules erupt on the trunk and extensor surfaces of limbs, each with a central depression filled with a crust (see Fig. 23.2).
- Skin biopsy shows collagen with other dermal components being eliminated through transepidermal channels ('perforations').
- Often resolves spontaneously.
- Topical steroids, occlusion, UVB, or retinoids may be helpful.

Box 23.2 Management of uraemic pruritus

Exclude other causes of itch, including drugs, scabies, iron deficiency, and thyroid disease (see ➲ pp. 60–1). Optimize dialysis, and control hyperparathyroidism and/or hyperphosphataemia. High-permeability haemodialysis can clear medium and large molecules acting as toxins.
Strategies worth trying include:

- Trim nails short to prevent damage to skin from scratching.
- Reduce the body temperature by using cool cotton clothing.
- Keep the room cool, particularly at night (avoid too many bedclothes).
- Avoid soap or excessive bathing (keep water temperature tepid).
- Copious emollients, as well as soap substitutes, to relieve dryness.
- Aqueous cream with 1% menthol.
- Occlusion with paste bandages such as Zipzoc®.

Box 23.2 *(Contd.)*

- Capsaicin 0.025% cream (initially causes a burning discomfort).
- Tacrolimus 0.03% or 0.1% ointment (potentially carcinogenic and not suitable for long-term treatment).
- Topical gamma-linolenic acid.
- Sedating antihistamines (non-sedating antihistamines are ineffective). Oral doxepin is a powerful antipruritic—start with low dose. Doxepin is metabolized via the liver cytochrome P450 pathway. Avoid if also prescribing macrolide antibiotics or imidazole antifungals.
- Phototherapy with UVB.
- Gabapentin or pregabalin.
- Other systemic treatments that have been used, with variable success, include colestyramine (inconsistent results, risk of acidosis), thalidomide, naltrexone, ondansetron, and sodium cromoglicate.

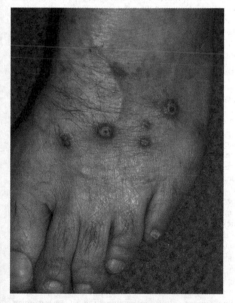

Fig. 23.2 Itchy dome-shaped nodules with a central hyperkeratotic plug in acquired perforating dermatosis.

Amyloidosis

What is amyloid?

The amyloidoses are disorders of protein folding. At least 20 different proteins can form the extracellular deposits of non-functional β-pleated sheets that typify amyloid fibrils. Fibrils stain with Congo red dye and produce apple-green birefringence under polarized light. Amyloid protein may be deposited in any tissue, including the kidney, GIT, heart, skin, muscle, brain, and/or blood vessels. Accumulation of protein eventually causes organ failure (often renal).

Reactive systemic amyloidosis (AA) develops in association with chronic inflammation, including chronic infections, e.g. leprosy, TB, or osteomyelitis, and chronic inflammatory diseases, e.g. RA and ankylosing spondylitis. Amyloidosis is also a frequent complication in patients with chronic kidney disease on maintenance haemodialysis. Rarely, systemic amyloidosis may be hereditary, e.g. as a result of autoinflammatory syndromes or in association with FMF (see ➜ p. 234).

Monoclonal Ig light-chain amyloidosis (AL), which has similar clinical features to AA, is seen in association with diseases involving B-lymphocytes such as multiple myeloma, B-cell lymphomas, and macroglobulinaemia.

The commonest forms of 1° localized cutaneous amyloidosis (macular and lichenoid) are caused by the deposition of keratin filaments in the skin and are not associated with systemic amyloidosis (see Box 23.3).

Systemic amyloidosis: what should I look for?

- Smooth yellowish or rather waxy, translucent-looking, but firm, papules, nodules, or plaques on the face (eyelids, nasolabial folds, perioral), neck, or trunk (chest, flexures, periumbilical). Some may be purpuric or become purpuric, if rubbed.
- Petechiae and/or purpura arising spontaneously.
- Pinch purpura: pinching or rubbing the skin causes purpura.
- Purpura of the face or neck induced by coughing or vomiting.
- Periorbital purpura, including 'post-proctoscopy palpebral purpura' (see Fig. 23.2) (purpura on the eyelids of patients who have been positioned head down for investigation by proctoscopy).
- Mucosal infiltration:
  - Smooth, pale, enlarged, indurated tongue (rare but virtually pathognomonic). The teeth may produce scalloped indentations on the sides of the tongue.
  - Thickened gingiva that bleed easily.
  - Pale red or yellow papules on buccal, conjunctival, nasal, vaginal, or anal mucosa.
- Hepatosplenomegaly.
- Evidence of systemic involvement such as nephrotic syndrome, renal disease, sensory or autonomic neuropathy, heart failure, arrhythmias, malabsorption, or GI haemorrhage.

Box 23.3 1° localized cutaneous amyloidosis

Lichen amyloidosis

Intensely itchy shiny or hyperkeratotic hyperpigmented papules, often on the shins. Commonest in South East Asia and South American countries.

Macular amyloidosis

- Itchy, oval, greyish brown, poorly defined patches with rather rippled or whorled patterns of hyperpigmentation. Often on the upper back.
- Macular and lichen amyloid are 2° to chronic rubbing or friction, sometimes with rough towels or brushes. Small globular deposits of amyloid, formed from keratin filaments, are found in the papillary dermis just beneath the BMZ.
- Macular and lichen amyloid may coexist. These forms of cutaneous amyloid are never associated with systemic amyloidosis.

⚠ *Familial 1° localized cutaneous amyloidosis* is a rare variant caused by missense mutations in the *OSMR* gene, encoding oncostatin M receptor β subunit, an II-b type cytokine receptor complex. The molecular studies have provided new insights into the pathogenesis of itch.

Nodular localized 1° cutaneous amyloidosis

- A very rare variant, usually presenting in the sixth or seventh decade, with one or more waxy translucent nodules or plaques that may become purpuric if traumatized. Bullous variant possible.
- Nodules are formed by deposits of Ig light chains (amyloid L protein, AL). AL infiltrates the dermis, subcutis, and blood vessel walls.
- Such patients must be screened for an underlying systemic disease and should be monitored if no systemic disease is identified, but few (<10%) will develop systemic amyloidosis.

Further reading

Tanaka A et al. Br J Dermatol 2009;161:127–4.
Woollons A and Black MM. Br J Dermatol 2001;145:105–9.

Nephrogenic systemic fibrosis

What is nephrogenic systemic fibrosis?

Nephrogenic systemic fibrosis (NSF) is a rare, but devastating, cutaneous fibrosing dermopathy seen in patients with end-stage kidney disease who have been exposed to the gadolinium-based contrast agents used in MRI. Onset usually within 2–10 weeks of exposure. NSF may affect the lungs, heart, liver, and muscles, as well as the skin and subcutaneous tissues. Complications, such as cardiomyopathy, pulmonary fibrosis, pulmonary hypertension, and/or diaphragmatic paralysis, may be fatal (mortality rate 30%).

Gadolinium is deposited in affected tissues. Circulating fibrocytes may be involved in the pathogenesis of fibrosis, and certain factors increase the risk of developing NSF (see Box 23.4).

What should I ask?

- Symptoms: progressive painful tightening of skin, leading to disabling joint contractures. Bone pain is common.
- Has the patient been investigated by a contrast-enhanced MRI in previous weeks or months?
- Explore other causes of skin thickening (see Box 23.5). For example, symptoms such as itch, Raynaud phenomenon, or difficulty swallowing suggest systemic sclerosis, rather than NSF.

What should I look for?

- Symmetrical erythematous, oedematous, hyperpigmented patches or plaques most often on the lower limbs, but may affect the trunk and upper limbs. The face and neck are spared.
- Papules, nodules, and/or well-demarcated indurated plaques with an irregular outline.
- Woody thickening of the skin and fascia gives a cobblestone or 'peau d'orange' appearance.
- Yellow scleral plaques, especially in patients under 45 years old.
- Normal nail folds (unlike systemic sclerosis).
- Flexion contractures of joints in association with skin thickening.

What should I do?

- Take a deep elliptical skin biopsy, looking for fibrosis, dermal fibroblast-like cells (CD34[positive]), thickening of collagen, and increased elastic and mucin.
- Consider a muscle biopsy.
- Exclude other causes of skin thickening (see Box 23.5):
  - FBC (no eosinophilia), and anti-Scl-70 and anti-centromere antibodies (absent). ANA may be positive in NSF and is not a helpful discriminator; paraproteins absent; thyroid antibodies absent.
- Echocardiogram, CXR, lung function to exclude systemic disease.
- For treatment, see Box 23.6. May improve if renal function improves.

Further reading

Daftari Besheli L et al. Clin Radiol 2014;69:661–8.
Idee JM et al. Crit Rev Toxicol 2014;44:895–913.

Box 23.4 Factors which predispose to developing nephrogenic systemic fibrosis

- Severe renal insufficiency (GFR <30mL/min/1.73m²).
- Acute kidney injury.
- Caution in patients with eGFR 30–59mL/min/1.73m².
- Erythropoiesis-stimulating agents.
- Acidosis.
- Recent surgery.
- Pro-inflammatory events such as infection.

Box 23.5 Differential diagnosis of nephrogenic systemic fibrosis

- Systemic sclerosis: localized cutaneous or diffuse cutaneous. Look for Raynaud phenomenon, hand signs, involvement of the face, and presence of specific antibodies (Scl-70, anti-centromere) (see ➲ Box 19.18, p. 414).
- Plaque morphoea (scleroderma): one lesion. Asymmetrical (see ➲ p. 420).
- Eosinophilic fasciitis (= subcutaneous morphoea): eosinophilia (see ➲ p. 421).
- Scleromyxoedema: associated with a monoclonal paraprotein. The face is involved (see ➲ Box 26.10, p. 541).
- Chronic GVHD (see ➲ pp. 534–6).
- Pretibial myxoedema: positive thyroid antibodies (see ➲ Box 22.5, p. 472.
- PCT (see ➲ p. 332).
- Other rare causes of skin thickening include Spanish toxic oil syndrome, vinyl chloride exposure, and eosinophilia–myalgia syndrome.
- Gadolinium-associated plaques: erythematous plaques, which may be pruritic, related to a type of gadolinium (gadodiamide) in the absence of NSF or chronic kidney disease.

Box 23.6 Treatment of nephrogenic systemic fibrosis

Generally, disease progresses relentlessly. Thickening and hardening of the skin has a major impact on quality of life.
These therapies have been tried:
- Topical corticosteroids, calcipotriol ointment.
- Oral corticosteroids, cyclophosphamide, ciclosporin.
- Phototherapy (UVA), extracorporeal photopheresis (see ➲ Box 26.7, p. 536).
- Other: high-dose IV Igs, plasmapheresis, tyrosine kinase inhibitors (imatinib mesylate), sirolimus.

Skin cancer in renal transplant recipients

⚠ Skin cancer, lymphoma/lymphoproliferative malignancies, and solid organ tumours are common in renal transplant recipients (RTRs) and are a leading cause of death. By 5 years after transplantation, the risk of developing an SCC is ~100 times greater than in an immunocompetent patient. Most patients have multiple cancers. Pathogenesis of skin cancer is multifactorial (see Box 23.7). Risk relates to the level, as well as chronicity, of immunosuppression, e.g. patients who receive ciclosporin, prednisolone, and azathioprine have a three times higher risk of SCC than those taking prednisolone and azathioprine alone. Switch of immunosuppressant drugs to mycophenolate mofetil and sirolimus may reduce the risk of future cancers but risk compromising graft function.

T-regulatory (Treg) cells (a subset of T-lymphocytes) suppress immune responses (facilitating cancer development) and inhibit graft rejection. There is now strong evidence for a potentially causal relationship between Treg cell numbers and cancer incidence in RTRs.

What should I look for?

- Photodamage: telangiectasia, solar elastosis, erythema, pigmentation. Common in fair-skinned individuals who are at greatest risk of skin cancer (see ➜ Box 3.1, p. 43).
- Persistent HPV-induced warts and pre-cancers, e.g. Bowen disease, solar keratoses on sun-exposed skin. Large numbers of seborrhoeic warts are linked to an increased risk of skin cancer.
- New warty papules or tender keratotic nodules on sun-exposed skin: SCCs are the commonest skin cancer (65- to 250-fold increase in risk) and may resemble viral warts. SCCs are significantly commoner in immunosuppressed patients than BCCs, a reversal of the usual ratio of three BCCs to one SCC. RTRs with SCC are at increased risk of developing internal malignancies.
- Other skin cancers include BCC (10- to 16-fold increase), malignant melanoma (3- to 8-fold increase), KS (84-fold increase, HHV-8-related), and Merkel cell cancer (polyomavirus-related).
- Non-melanoma skin cancers are commoner in fair-skinned individuals living in tropical or subtropical countries.
- Post-transplant lymphoproliferative disorders (mostly B-cell/EBV-related) rarely present in skin with erythematous patches or nodules.

Box 23.7 Pathogenesis of skin cancer in renal transplant recipients

- Chronic exposure to UVR (see ➜ p. 346).
- Impaired immunosurveillance—relates to the level of immunosuppression, as well as the length of time the patient has been immunosuppressed.
- Genetic factors, including skin type (see Table 2.1, p. 27).
- HPV may play a part in the pathogenesis of skin cancer. Transplant patients have high numbers of low- and medium-risk HPV types in skin.
- Other viruses, e.g. HHV-8 (KS), polyomavirus (Merkel cell cancer), EBV (post-transplant lymphoproliferative disorders, smooth muscle tumours).

What should I do?

- Clinical accuracy of diagnosis is poor: cancers may appear banal, but conversely warts or hypertrophic solar keratoses may simulate SCC. Have a high index of suspicion, and biopsy or excise changing lesions for histological examination, particularly new tender nodules on sun-exposed skin. Cancer on the lip and ear may be subtle.
- Ensure the patient understands the importance of rigorous sun protection, and reinforce the message regularly (see ➜ pp. 338–9).
- Ensure that patients with chronic kidney disease, who may eventually need a transplant, are educated about the importance of sun protection and regular self-examination.
- Examine all the skin of transplant recipients regularly; patients are best managed in dedicated transplant/immunosuppressed skin clinics.
- Oral acitretin 10–25mg/day may reduce the incidence of skin cancers.
- High-risk 1° skin cancers/locally invasive disease should be managed by reducing immunosuppression which must be undertaken with guidance from renal transplant physicians.

Further reading

Lakkis FG. *Nat Rev Nephrol* 2014;**10**:185–6.
Seckin D et al. *Am J Transplant* 2013;**13**:2146–53.

Fabry disease

Synonyms: Anderson–Fabry disease; angiokeratoma corporis diffusum.

⚠ Cutaneous signs may be an early manifestation of this rare X-linked lysosomal storage disease caused by a deficiency in α-galactosidase A. Globotriaosylceramide accumulates in endothelial cells, vascular smooth muscle, cutaneous fibroblasts and erector pilori muscles, myocardium, corneal epithelial cells, and organs such as the kidneys, heart, lungs, bowel, and eyes.

Complications include renal disease, angina, myocardial infarction, transient ischaemic attacks, and stroke. Severe neuropathic pain causes depression or even suicide. Before the introduction of enzyme replacement therapy, ♂ with Fabry disease died around age 40–50 years, and life expectancy was shortened in heterozygous ♀. Patients who have cutaneous angiokeratomas and telangiectasias are more likely to have major organ involvement. Prevalence may be higher than previously realized, e.g. 2–5% patients with cryptogenic stroke may have milder forms. Enzyme replacement therapy may improve quality of life by relieving symptoms, such as pain, and slowing the progression of disease, but it is not curative.

What should I ask?

- Patients complain of excruciating neuropathic pain (lancinating, burning) in extremities (onset in childhood, associated with small-fibre neuropathy). Exercise, heat, and alcohol make the pain worse.
- Asymptomatic telangiectasias and dark red papules (angiokeratomas) may appear in childhood and become more numerous with age.
- Reduced sweating (50% of ♂, 28% of ♀) or anhidrosis (25% of ♂, 4% of ♀) causes heat intolerance. Patients may collapse after exercise. Rarely, patients report hyperhidrosis.
- Other problems include hearing loss, visual loss, nausea, abdominal pain, and episodic diarrhoea/constipation, but presentation is variable.

What should I look for?

- Facial features: ♂ have prominent supraorbital ridges, frontal bossing, and thickening of the lips.
- Angiokeratomas (slightly keratotic vascular papules, like Campbell de Morgan spots) on the thighs, hips, buttocks, genitalia, and lower back and abdomen, i.e. between the knees and the umbilicus in a 'bathing trunk' distribution (66% of ♂, 36% of ♀).
- Telangiectases, vascular macules and/or papules distributed sparsely in other areas, e.g. palms and soles, fingers and toes, nail folds, vermillion border of the lips, and labial mucosa.
- Reversible oedema/lymphoedema of lower extremities (16–25% of ♂, 6–17% of ♀).

What should I do?

See Box 23.8.

Box 23.8 Confirming the diagnosis of Fabry disease

- Refer to ophthalmology for a slit-lamp examination to detect changes such as cornea verticillata (vortex opacities located in the superficial corneal layers), tortuous conjunctival and retinal vessels, or Fabry cataract (posterior lens opacities with a radiating appearance).
- Assess renal, cardiac, respiratory, and nervous systems.
- Males: measure α-galactosidase A levels in plasma or white cells.
- Genotype females.

Further reading

El-Abassi R et al. J Neurol Sci 2014;344(1–2):5–19.
Fabry Support & Information Group. Available at: ℞ http://www.fabry.org/ (patient support group).
Mehta A et al. QJM 2010;103:641–59.

Skin and gastroenterology

Contents

> **Relevant pages in other chapters**
> These conditions that may be associated with manifestations
> in the GIT are discussed in more detail elsewhere:

Cirrhosis

Mucocutaneous signs will depend on the cause of cirrhosis.

What should I look for?

- Colour change:
  - Dry yellow skin and yellow sclerae.
  - Hyperpigmentation of exposed skin.
  - Generalized hyperpigmentation, with sparing of the interscapular and scapular skin, has been described in primary biliary cirrhosis.
  - Generalized slate-grey pigmentation (melanin) or bronzed pigmentation of the legs (iron and melanin deposition)—'bronze diabetes'—in haemochromatosis.
  - Greyish skin and bluish lunulae in Wilson disease (also Kayser–Fleischer rings—copper in the limbus of the cornea).
- Excoriations. Itch may be very distressing, particularly in primary biliary cirrhosis. Precise cause unknown. Presumably relates to the impaired biliary excretion of an irritating substance or substances. Bile acids injected into the skin cause itch, but the intensity of pruritus is not related to the levels of bile acids. Lysophosphatidic acid (a potent neuronal activator) and autotaxin (the enzyme forming lysophosphatidic acid) may be involved in the pathogenesis of itch. Serum activity of autotaxin correlates with itch intensity. Biliary obstruction leads to increased intrahepatic synthesis of opioid peptides which are released into the circulation, but levels do not correlate with itch intensity. For the management of itch, see Box 24.1.
- Spider telangiectasia in the distribution of the superior vena cava.
- Bruising and purpura, gingival bleeding.
- ♂: loss of body hair (axillary, pubic) and gynaecomastia.
- White nails (Terry nails) or parallel white bands (Muehrcke lines).
- Nail clubbing.
- Palmar erythema, erythematous tips to fingers.
- Peripheral oedema and ascites.
- Dilated superficial veins on the abdomen and chest if portal hypertension.
- Xanthomas in primary biliary cirrhosis and hyperlipidaemia (see ➲ p. 470).
- Limited cutaneous systemic sclerosis may be associated with primary biliary cirrhosis (see ➲ p. 416).
- Signs of PCT (photosensitivity, skin fragility, blisters) associated with iron overload (haemochromatosis), alcoholic cirrhosis, and hepatitis C infection (see ➲ p. 332).
- Panniculitis in α-1 antitrypsin deficiency (see ➲ p. 462).

Box 24.1 Itch in 1° biliary cirrhosis

What should I do?

- Exclude other causes of itching, including drugs, scabies, iron deficiency, and thyroid disease (see ➋ pp. 60–1).
- Trim nails short to prevent damage to skin from scratching.
- Reduce body temperature by using cool cotton clothing and keeping the room cool, particularly at night (avoid too many bedclothes).
- Avoid soap or excessive bathing (water should not be too hot).
- Copious emollients, as well as soap substitutes, will relieve dryness.
- Aqueous cream with 1% menthol may be helpful.
- Ursodeoxycholic acid (UDCA), 13–15mg/kg/day, delays the progression of hepatic fibrosis in 1° biliary cirrhosis but may not relieve itch.
- Colestyramine 4–12g/day (binds bile acids and other biliary molecules). Take before and after breakfast (when the gall bladder empties). At least 4h should elapse between the administration of colestyramine and other medications.
- Rifampicin 150mg bd or tds (max dose 600mg/day) may help but may cause hepatitis.
- Other options include:
  - UVB phototherapy.
  - Sertraline (75–100mg/day), a serotonin reuptake inhibitor.
  - Naloxone (opioid antagonist). Start with low dose, and increase very gradually. May cause symptoms of narcotic withdrawal.
  - Plasmapheresis.
  - Nasobiliary drainage.

Further reading

Beuers U et al. *Hepatology* 2014;**60**:399–407 (review of itch in cholestasis).
Kremer AE et al. *Dig Dis* 2014;**32**:637–45 (pathogenesis and management of itch in cholestasis).

Inflammatory bowel disease

Cutaneous signs are common in both Crohn disease and ulcerative colitis, and may precede the diagnosis by several years. Abdominal stomas also cause skin problems (see Box 24.2).

What should I look for?

- Nail clubbing and palmar erythema.
- EN (see ➜ pp. 458–9).
- Aphthous ulcers and glossitis (see ➜ pp. 282–3).
- Thrombophlebitis.
- Perianal fissures, fistulae, and abscesses—more severe in Crohn disease than ulcerative colitis (see ➜ p. 510).
- Genital or orofacial Crohn disease (see ➜ p. 510). (Biopsy shows non-caseating sarcoidal granulomas with multinucleated giant cells in the dermis and subcutaneous tissue.)
- Peristomal dermatitis or folliculitis (see Box 24.2).
- Cutaneous adverse drug reactions, including reactions to sulfasalazine (patients may be photosensitive), azathioprine hypersensitivity (see ➜ p. 389), and reactions to anti-TNF agents (see ➜ p. 389).
- Manifestations of nutritional deficiency, including an acrodermatitis enteropathica-like syndrome (acquired zinc deficiency) (see ➜ p. 513).
- Psoriasis (increased prevalence in Crohn disease).
- Chronic palmoplantar pustulosis, sometimes linked to SAPHO syndrome (see ➜ p. 248).
- Neutrophilic dermatoses such as PG, including peristomal pyoderma (see ➜ p. 310 and Box 24.2), Sweet syndrome (see ➜ p. 518), and bowel-associated dermatosis–arthritis syndrome (see ➜ p. 519). ❶ Azathioprine hypersensitivity resembles Sweet syndrome.
- Pyostomatitis vegetans: a rare pustular disorder that is a marker of IBD and usually precedes the onset. Friable grey-yellow pustules may involve oral, vaginal, nasal, and rarely periocular mucosa. Ruptured pustules leave vegetating erosions or ulcers. Symptoms are mild. Differentiate from pemphigus by histology and IMF (see ➜ pp. 268–9). Skin involvement has been reported (pyodermatitis vegetans).
- Cutaneous granulomatous vasculitis (in Crohn disease).
- Vitiligo.
- Autoimmune bullous diseases: BP, linear IgA disease, and EBA (see ➜ pp. 270–2).
- Skin manifestations of systemic amyloidosis (see ➜ p. 496).

Extraintestinal non-cutaneous signs

- Inflammatory arthropathies with sacroiliitis, peripheral arthritis with or without enthesitis, tenosynovitis, and dactylitis. Some patients develop SAPHO syndrome (see ➜ p. 248).
- Episcleritis, scleritis, and uveitis.

Box 24.2 Skin and abdominal stomas

Skin disorders are reported in 2/3 of patients with an abdominal stoma. Hydrocolloids are used both for securing stoma devices and for protecting the skin. Stoma nurse specialists provide invaluable advice on care and suitable appliances. Problems include:

- Irritant dermatitis 2° to leakage or overfrequent bag changes: common and may be secondarily infected. Chronic irritation induces hyperkeratosis or erosions. Treat with topical corticosteroids. Sucralfate powder prevents further irritation and may promote healing. Rarely, chronic irritation induces intestinal metaplasia in the skin surrounding the stoma. Presents as mucosa-like change or friable granulomatous papules. Take a biopsy, as intestinal metaplasia may transform into adenocarcinoma.
- Skin infection: common, and all peristomal rashes should be swabbed for culture. Staphylococcal folliculitis usually occurs when shaving is used to help the bag adhere to hairy skin. Treat with antibiotics. Triclosan washes may be helpful (rinse off to prevent irritation under the bag).
- Allergic contact dermatitis: very uncommon, but consider patch testing to reassure the patient and stoma nurse.
- Peristomal psoriasis: treat with topical corticosteroids. A bag with a thicker hydrocolloid barrier may be helpful.
- Peristomal PG (rare): treat with a very potent topical corticosteroid or 0.1% tacrolimus (in carmellose sodium paste). May need systemic treatment, e.g. oral ciclosporin. Is the patient taking nicorandil—another cause of painful ulceration?
- Chronic papillomatous dermatitis (warty papules) around urostomies: caused by chronic urine leaks. Acetic acid soaks may be helpful.
- Peristomal lichen sclerosus (rare): most often around urostomies. Painful and may ulcerate (see ➜ pp. 288–9).

Topical corticosteroids

Creams, gels, or oils will impair adhesion of the bag. Apply betamethasone valerate (0.1%) lotion to the adhesive surface of the stoma appliance. Let alcohol evaporate before placing the appliance on the skin. Alternatively, spray on steroid powder from an aerosol inhaler.

Further reading

Al-Niaimi F and Lyon C. *Br J Dermatol* 2013;**168**:643–6 (urostomies).
Lyon CC et al. *Br J Dermatol* 2000;**143**:1248–60.
Lyon CC and Beck MH. Skin problems in ostomates. In: Goldsmith LA *et al.* (eds) *Fitzpatrick's Dermatology in General Medicine*, 8th edn, 2012. New York: McGraw-Hill.

Cutaneous Crohn disease

Signs may suggest lymphoedema, hereditary angio-oedema, cellulitis, chronic HSV infection, sarcoid, hidradenitis suppurativa (see ➲ p. 250) or a sexually transmitted infection such as syphilis.

What should I look for?

Three patterns of cutaneous Crohn disease are recognized.

Perianal

- Perianal: polypoid tags, moist plaques, erythema, swelling, induration, fissures, fistulae, scarring, abscesses, and sinus tracts.
- Aphthous ulcers in the anal canal, ulcers of the anal sphincter.

Orofacial

- Granulomatous infiltration of the oral mucosa with oedema, aphthous ulcers, and a 'cobblestone' papular hyperplasia (orofacial granulomatosis) (see Box 24.3).
- Angular cheilitis with fissuring.
- Gingival erythema and oedematous gingival nodules.
- Persistent swelling of the lips and/or cheeks.

Metastatic

- Metastatic disease is separated from the GIT by normal tissue.
- Swelling or induration of the genitalia sometimes with erythema (commoner in children).
- Genital papules, plaques, fissures, and ulcers.
- Erythematous papules, plaques, nodules, or ulcers exuding pus, mainly in the lower extremities and flexures.

What should I do?

- Faecal calprotectin may be a useful test in suspected IBD.
- Treatment options include:
  - Potent topical corticosteroids.
  - Tacrolimus 0.1% ointment.
  - Oral metronidazole 800–1500mg/day for at least 4 months.
  - Systemic corticosteroids.
  - Other immunosuppressants, e.g. methotrexate, azathioprine, ciclosporin.
  - TNF-α inhibitors, e.g. adalimumab, infliximab.

Box 24.3 What is orofacial granulomatosis?

- An uncommon condition in which facial lymphoedema is associated with non-caseating granulomas. Many patients have Crohn disease. Management is difficult.
- Presents with painless swelling of one or both lips.
- Swelling fluctuates initially but eventually persists.
- Other signs include intraoral swelling, painful mouth ulcers, mucosal tags, and tongue fissuring.
- Fissures in the lips or angular cheilitis are portals of entry for streptococcal infection which may damage lymphatics, exacerbating lymphoedema.
- Facial nerve paralysis occurs in Melkersson–Rosenthal syndrome.
- Investigations: exclude allergy (patch tests), Crohn disease, and sarcoid.
- Initial management: phenoxymethylpenicillin 250–500mg/day for at least 6 months to prevent infection, and topical steroids.
- Other treatments: intralesional steroids, oral steroids (short courses), immunomodulators such as methotrexate and thalidomide.
- Facial massage may reduce swelling.
- The role of oral allergens in pathogenesis and the efficacy of benzoate/cinnamon-free diets are controversial

Nutritional deficiencies

Starvation is the commonest cause of nutritional deficiency in the developing world. In Africa, one of every three children is underweight. Malnutrition contributes to more than 1/2 of the nearly 12 million deaths among the under-5s in developing countries each year.

In the developed world, patients who are seriously ill, are unable to care for themselves, or have problems, such as malabsorption, chronic alcoholism, chronic diarrhoea, or bowel fistulae, may also be malnourished. Some patients choose to restrict their diets, perhaps because of religious beliefs, concerns about food allergy, or eating disorders. Parents of children with atopic eczema may omit essential nutrients, such as milk, from the child's diet in the well-intentioned, but mistaken, belief that this may cure the eczema. Bariatric surgery, used to restrict the stomach's capacity in obesity, may cause nutritional deficiency. Rarely, genetic or metabolic defects cause nutritional deficiency (see ➲ cystic fibrosis in Box 24.6).

Cutaneous signs depend on the deficiency—protein, carbohydrate, vitamins, minerals, and/or essential trace elements. Some patients have a number of deficiencies.

Cutaneous signs in malabsorption

Increased faecal excretion of fat is associated with variable deficiency in proteins, minerals, trace elements, fat-soluble vitamins, and carbohydrates, as well as water. Look for combinations of:

- Itching, dry skin which may be very scaly (ichthyotic).
- Hyperpigmentation (chloasma-like facial, generalized Addisonian, or pellagra-like; see ➲ p. 513).
- Pallor (iron deficiency and anaemia).
- Brittle nails and hair loss.
- Scaly follicular papules (phrynoderma = toad skin). Mainly extensor surfaces of extremities (lack of vitamin A and other nutrients).
- Bruising, petechiae, oral bleeding (lack of vitamin K).
- Angular stomatitis, cheilitis, glossitis (smooth, sore, red tongue), mucosal erosions (lack of vitamin B complex or folic acid).
- Seborrhoeic dermatitis-like rash (lack of vitamin B complex).

Cutaneous signs in kwashiorkor

This common childhood disorder, seen in developing countries, is caused by protein malnutrition in the presence of reasonable calories. Kwashiorkor develops after the child is weaned (age 1–4), when diet is mainly starchy vegetables. Look for:

- Erythematous or purplish hyperkeratotic plaques with fissuring like 'flaky paint' or 'crazy paving'.
- Hypopigmented dry skin. Fine desquamation is common.
- Sparse dry, brittle hair.
- Normal dark brown hair becomes orangeish red. The flag sign— alternating bands of pale and dark hair—with intermittent protein intake.
- Cheilitis, angular stomatitis, oral erosions, vulvovaginitis.
- Swollen abdomen.
- Pitting oedema of lower extremities and muscle wasting.

Cutaneous signs in pellagra: niacin (vitamin B$_3$) deficiency

Characterized by dermatitis (only sign in 3% of patients), diarrhoea, and dementia. May complicate chronic alcoholism. Look for:
- Erythema and superficial scaling on sun-exposed skin that fades to leave reddish brown pigmentation.
  - 'Butterfly rash' (malar) on the face.
  - Well-demarcated erythema on anterior neck (Casal necklace).
- Erythema and scaling of skin exposed to heat, friction, or pressure.

Cutaneous signs in scurvy: vitamin C deficiency
- Follicular keratoses on the upper arms, back, buttocks, and lower extremities, containing 'corkscrew' coiled hairs.
- Petechiae, perifollicular haemorrhage, and bruising.
- Gingival hypertrophy and bleeding gums.
- Delayed wound healing.

Acrodermatitis enteropathica: zinc deficiency

Acrodermatitis enteropathica is an AR disorder in which intestinal absorption of zinc is inadequate. Usually presents 4–6 weeks after weaning but may develop earlier if the infant is not given breast milk, which enhances zinc absorption. Zinc deficiency has also been described following total parenteral nutrition without zinc and in association with alcoholism, Crohn disease, and chronic pancreatitis.

Zinc deficiency causes acral dermatitis, alopecia, and diarrhoea, as well as (in infants) failure to thrive with apathy and irritability. Look for:
- Vesiculobullous or pustular dermatitis on hands and feet.
- Pustular paronychia.
- Periorificial (perioral, periorbital, and perianal) crusted papules and plaques which may be pustular. Differentiate from impetigo (see p. 136) and necrolytic migratory erythema (see p. 516).
- Photophobia with blepharitis and conjunctivitis.
- Slow hair growth, generalized alopecia, and nail dystrophy with Beau lines in chronic zinc deficiency.
- Delayed healing of ulcers.
- 2° bacterial and fungal infections.

Cutaneous signs in essential fatty acid deficiency
- Dry leathery skin and follicular keratoses.
- Dry hair and brittle nails.
- Periorificial plaques resembling acrodermatitis enteropathica have been described, but patients may also be zinc-deficient.

Cutaneous signs in iron deficiency

In addition to the pallor of anaemia, iron deficiency may lead to:
- Hair loss and itching.

Cutaneous signs in vitamin D deficiency
- Calcinosis cutis (hard nodules) caused by 2° hyperparathyroidism.

Further reading

Ragunatha S et al. J Clin Diagn Res 2014;8:116–18 (treatment of phrynoderma).

Coeliac disease (coeliac sprue)

Coeliac disease is a gluten-sensitive enteropathy, primarily found in Caucasians, that is associated with IgA anti-gliadin, anti-endomysial, and anti-transglutaminase 2 antibodies. Genes for specific class II HLA-DQ2 and-DQ8 confer susceptibility to coeliac disease. Presentation varies but may include failure to thrive (children), delayed puberty, chronic diarrhoea, and abdominal distension or pain. Malabsorption leads to nutrient and mineral deficiencies with problems such as anaemia (folate and iron deficiency), osteomalacia, or osteoporosis. Symptoms are controlled by a gluten-free diet.

Coeliac disease is associated with an increased prevalence of other disorders, including splenic atrophy, autoimmune endocrine disorders (hypothyroidism, diabetes, and Addison disease), primary biliary cirrhosis, neurological disorders, and IgA deficiency (5% of patients). Patients have an increased risk of intestinal lymphoma and rarely other GI cancers. The risk is reduced by a strict gluten-free diet.

DH occurs in 10–20% of patients but is rare in children.

What is dermatitis herpetiformis?

DH is a rare IgA-mediated bullous disease that is associated with sensitivity to gluten. All patients have coeliac disease which is never severe and is usually subclinical. Serum IgA autoantibodies to epidermal transglutaminase 3 probably play some part in the pathogenesis (see ➔ p. 515). DH may be associated with other autoimmune diseases (see Box 24.4).

For more information, see ➔ pp. 274–5.

Box 24.4 Diseases associated with dermatitis herpetiformis

- Vitiligo and alopecia areata.
- Autoimmune thyroid disease (common), diabetes mellitus, Addison disease.
- SLE, Sjögren syndrome, RA.
- Acral petechiae, sometimes with a histology of leukocytoclastic vasculitis.
- ⚠ Intestinal lymphoma.

Pathogenesis of coeliac disease and dermatitis herpetiformis

- An inflammatory response to certain proteins in wheat (gliadin, the alcohol-soluble component of gluten) and related proteins in rye and barley damages the mucosa of the small intestine, leading to malabsorption. Oats do not cause problems, provided they have not been contaminated with wheat proteins when ground in the mill.
- Gluten peptides cross the intestinal epithelial barrier.
- Tissue transglutaminase (transglutaminase 2) in the small bowel binds to, and deaminates, gliadins, producing immunogenetic peptides that activate a T-cell response. Antigen-presenting cells expressing the HLA-DQ2 and HLA-DQ8 molecules have an increased affinity for these peptides.
- Activated gluten-specific T-cells stimulate B-cell production of IgA anti-gliadin and anti-transglutaminase 2 antibodies. (The antigen recognized by the anti-endomysial antibody is tissue transglutaminase.)
- Inflammation causes intestinal mucosal damage, crypt cell hyperproliferation, and villous atrophy.
- IgA antibodies to tissue transglutaminase cross-react with epidermal transglutaminase, but patients with DH also produce specific IgA antibodies to epidermal transglutaminase 3 (TG3).
- Anti-epidermal transglutaminase antibodies in immune complexes play a role in the pathogenesis of DH.

Further reading

Bolotin D and Petronic-Rosic V. *J Am Acad Dermatol* 2011;**64**:1017–24 and 1027–33.
Briani C et al. *Autoimmun Rev* 2008;**7**:644–50.
Kárpáti S. *J Dermatol Sci* 2004;**34**:83–90.
Rose C et al. *J Am Acad Dermatol* 2009;**61**:39–43.

Pancreatic disease

See Box 24.5 for cutaneous signs of pancreatic disease.

⚠ Necrolytic migratory erythema

This very rare, but striking, skin condition should prompt an urgent search for a glucagon-producing tumour in the pancreatic α cells. Unfortunately, many patients already have metastases at the time of diagnosis. The full syndrome includes necrolytic migratory erythema, diabetes mellitus (mild), stomatitis, cheilitis, weight loss, diarrhoea, venous thrombosis, and neuropsychiatric symptoms.

'Pseudoglucagonoma syndromes'—necrolytic migratory erythema has been described in association with other conditions, including pancreatic cancers, chronic pancreatitis, coeliac disease, jejunal adenocarcinoma, and hepatic cirrhosis.

What should I look for?
- Recurrent outbreaks of itchy, uncomfortable, erythematous papules or plaques most marked on the face, flexures, and sites of friction, but may be widespread.
- Superficial flaccid vesicles and bullae within erythematous patches. These rupture rapidly, leaving crusted erosions.
- The crusted edges of patches extend outward in serpiginous patterns.
- After 1–2 weeks, patches heal centrally, often leaving hyperpigmentation.
- Perioral erythematous crusted patches with peripheral scale.
- Genital or perianal skin may be involved, and some features may resemble acrodermatitis enteropathica (see ➲ p. 513).
- Patients may have glossitis.

What should I do?
- Check serum glucagon levels, which are markedly raised.
- Check serum zinc levels, which are normal.
- Take a skin biopsy from the edge of an early lesion. Histological features (which may be non-specific) include parakeratosis, subcorneal neutrophils, intracellular oedema in the upper layers of the epidermis, and degeneration (necrolysis) of superficial keratinocytes.
- Investigate for a pancreatic tumour initially by abdominal CT scan.

Cystic fibrosis

For cutaneous features, see Box 24.6.

Box 24.5 Pancreatic disease and the skin

- Acute pancreatitis may be associated with purpura in the left flank (Grey Turner sign) or periumbilical purpura (Cullen sign).
- Pancreatic panniculitis, probably caused by the escape of pancreatic enzymes from circulation, occurs in association with pancreatic disease such as acute or chronic pancreatitis, pancreatic islet cell tumour, ductal adenocarcinoma, and acinar cell carcinoma. The tender reddish brown subcutaneous nodules are found most often on the legs. Nodules often ulcerate, discharging oily brown liquefied fat (see ➡ pp. 462–3). Pancreatic enzymes may also cause fat necrosis at other sites, e.g. intramedullary, omental, peritoneal, and periarticular.
- Necrolytic migratory erythema—a glucagon-producing tumour in the pancreatic α cells (see ➡ p. 516).
- Manifestations of nutritional deficiency in cystic fibrosis (see Box 24.6).

Box 24.6 Cystic fibrosis

Cystic fibrosis is inherited in an AR pattern and is characterized by chronic bacterial infection of airways and sinuses, fat malabsorption, ♂ infertility, and elevated concentrations of chloride in sweat. Mutations in the cystic fibrosis transmembrane conductance regulator (CFTR) gene cause abnormalities in ion transport.

Cutaneous features include:
- Aquagenic skin wrinkling. Itchy or tingling oedematous white papules and plaques appear on the palms and soles within 2min of exposure to water. Remits within a few hours. Mechanism uncertain—elevated sweat chloride may increase keratin binding to water, or regulation of water membrane channels may be abnormal, or eccrine ducts may be dysfunctional.
- Nutrient deficiency dermatitis (age 2 weeks to 6 months). Features overlap with those of acrodermatitis enteropathica, essential fatty acid deficiency, and kwashiorkor (see ➡ p. 512). Erythematous papules (may be annular) present in the napkin area, and periorbital and perioral skin, but may spread to the extremities and progress to extensive desquamating plaques.
- Cutaneous adverse drug reactions (30% of patients), e.g. morbilliform, urticaria, angio-oedema, SJS, and leukocytoclastic vasculitis.
- Atopic eczema (increased prevalence).
- Cutaneous vasculitis.

Further reading

Bernstein ML et al. Paed Dermatol 2008;25:150–7.

Neutrophilic dermatoses

The neutrophilic dermatoses associated with bowel disease include PG (see ➲ p. 310), Sweet syndrome, neutrophilic dermatosis of the dorsal hands, and bowel-associated dermatosis–arthritis syndrome.

Sweet syndrome (acute febrile neutrophilic dermatosis)

This syndrome is characterized by intense neutrophilic infiltration of the skin. It is commoner in women.

Associations

- Infection: 70% of patients. Most often 1–3 weeks after infection of upper respiratory tract.
- Chronic inflammation: 15% of patients, e.g. IBD, connective tissue diseases such as polychondritis, sarcoidosis.
- ⚠ Malignancy: 10–20% of patients—particularly haematological malignancies, e.g. acute myelogenous leukaemia, myeloproliferative disease or myelodysplastic syndromes, lymphoma, and paraproteinaemias.
- Drugs, e.g. azathioprine, oral contraceptive, minocycline, diazepam, G-CSF, and bortezomib (a proteasome inhibitor).
- Immunodeficiency: 1° or 2°.
- Pregnancy.

What should I look for?

- Fever and neutrophilia with a raised ESR, often suggesting sepsis.
- Tender, well-demarcated, oedematous, erythematous papules and large plaques, most often on the face and upper trunk (differentiate from cellulitis or herpes infection, particularly if solitary lesion) (see Fig. 24.1).
- Surface may appear to be vesicular (pseudo-vesicles), reflecting the intense dermal oedema, but it is rare to find discrete vesicles or bullae that can be ruptured. Occasionally, plaques become pustular.
- Panniculitis: nodules rupture, releasing necrotic fat (uncommon).
- Iritis, episcleritis, and/or conjunctivitis.
- Arthralgia, polyarthritis, and myalgia.
- Oral mucosal ulcers (mimic aphthae) (uncommon).
- Patients may also have PG (see ➲ p. 310).

What should I do?

- Exclude infection by taking blood for culture and swabs from pustular skin lesions. Cultures are sterile in Sweet syndrome.
- Check FBC and ESR, and exclude an underlying disease.
- Take a skin biopsy from a well-developed plaque. In Sweet syndrome, you will find a dense dermal neutrophilic infiltrate with leukocytoclasis, but without vasculitis. Gram stain is negative.
- Treat with systemic corticosteroids (initially prednisolone 30mg/day) and very potent topical corticosteroids bd.
- Recurrences are common. Steroid-sparing agents that may be helpful include dapsone, colchicine, and ciclosporin.

Neutrophilic dermatosis of the dorsal hands

- Rare.
- Painful, erythematous papules, plaques, and haemorrhagic bullae limited to the dorsum of the hands.

- Like Sweet syndrome, may be associated with low-grade fever and arthralgia.
- Disease associations similar to Sweet syndrome.

Bowel-associated dermatosis–arthritis syndrome

The overgrowth of bacteria in a blind loop with the deposition of immune complexes is thought to trigger disease. The histopathological changes resemble those of Sweet syndrome.

Associations
- Bowel bypass surgery to treat morbid obesity.
- Extensive resection of the small bowel.
- Patients with an abnormal segment of bowel in diseases such as diverticulosis or IBD.

What should I look for?
- A history of GI disease or GI surgery.
- Crops of erythematous macules, purpuric papules, and small vesicopustules on the upper trunk and extremities.
- Migratory polyarthralgia or a non-erosive polyarthritis.
- Malaise and fever.

What should I do?
- Confirm diagnosis by skin biopsy which shows a neutrophilic dermatosis like Sweet syndrome.
- Correct the underlying cause.

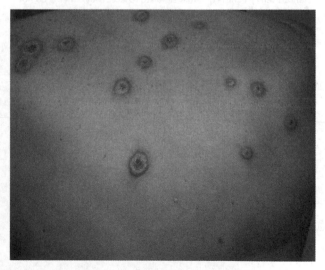

Fig. 24.1 Sweet syndrome: well-demarcated oedematous plaques.

Carcinoid syndrome

Carcinoid tumours are found most often in the GI tract (55%) and bronchopulmonary system (30%). Carcinoids arise from enterochromaffin cells of the GI tract, and the tumours release a variety of polypeptides, pyogenic amines, and prostaglandins, which are responsible for the carcinoid syndrome. Tumours are rare, and the syndrome even rarer, occurring in <10% of patients with a tumour.

What should I look for?

Features of carcinoid syndrome comprise:
- Episodic dry cutaneous flushing (85% of patients) lasting 20–30s.
- Flushes may last from hours to days in bronchial carcinoid.
- Flushes may be spontaneous or triggered by eating, alcohol, defecation, changes in temperature, emotional stress, or palpation of the liver.
- Flushing starts suddenly on the face, neck, and upper chest.
- A mild burning sensation is common, or the skin may be intensely itchy.
- Severe dry flushes may be accompanied by hypotension and tachycardia.
- Diarrhoea may be explosive and disabling.
- Wheezing and dyspnoea are common, particularly during episodes of flushing.
- Chronic disease leads to persistent brawny facial oedema and facial venous telangiectasia that may simulate rosacea, but patients do not have pustules or papules.
- Scleroderma-like fibrosis probably caused by impaired tryptophan metabolism.
- Pellagra (dietary tryptophan is diverted for synthesis of serotonin)— rough scaly skin, glossitis, angular stomatitis, and confusion.
- Signs of tricuspid regurgitation.

What should I do?

- Exclude common causes of a red face (see Box 24.7 and ➔ p. 72).
- If clinically indicated, measure 24-h urinary excretion of 5-hydroxyindoleacetic acid (HIAA) which is increased in carcinoid syndrome.
- Localize the tumour, e.g. abdominal CT.

Box 24.7 Flushing: what should I look for?

- Is flush wet (associated with sweating) or dry?
- Menopausal flushes (flashes) associated with sweating (wet).
- Fever—wet flushes, illness.
- Flushing of the face, chest, and neck is common in fair complexions, particularly Celts and northern Europeans. Triggered by emotion and exercise. Treatment options limited:
  - Reduce anxiety levels.
  - β-blockers (propranolol 10–40mg bd to tds).
  - Clonidine has been recommended.
- Easy flushing may precede the development of rosacea—look for papules, pustules, swelling, and telangiectasia (see → p. 254).
- Exclude seborrhoeic dermatitis, psoriasis, or contact dermatitis as a cause of facial redness.
- Exclude photosensitivity (drugs) or a photoaggravated dermatosis (cutaneous LE, atopic eczema) (see → pp. 322–4).
- Neurological causes, e.g. autonomic dysfunction in Parkinson disease, migraines, multiple sclerosis, and epilepsy.
- Rare causes of flushes:
  - Carcinoid syndrome: episodic dry flushes, abdominal pain, diarrhoea, dyspnoea, or hypotension (see → pp. 520–1).
  - Phaeochromocytoma: hypertension (sustained or episodic). Attacks of wet flushes, palpitations, nausea, vomiting; headache and sense of impending doom.
  - Medullary carcinoma of thyroid: telangiectasia of the face and arms.
  - Pancreatic cell tumour (VIPoma): watery diarrhoea, abdominal pain.
  - Renal cell carcinoma: haematuria.

Further reading

Izekison L et al. *J Am Acad Dermatol* 2005;55:209–11 (flushing—what to look for and how to manage).

Other rare gastrointestinal conditions

- *Hereditary haemorrhagic telangiectasia (Osler–Weber–Rendu disease)*: telangiectasias on skin and mucous membranes (stretch the lip to see the branching vessels); nail clubbing if the patient has pulmonary AV fistulae. Look for telangiectasias and a history of nasal bleeds in any patient with anaemia or melaena. Eighty percent of cases have a positive family history (autosomal inheritance). Patients may also have von Willebrand disease.
- *Blue rubber-bleb naevus syndrome*: cavernous haemangiomas in skin and GIT with GI bleeding.
- *Pseudoxanthoma elasticum*: GI bleeds are a major complication (see ➜ pp. 432–3).
- *Gardner syndrome—variant of familial adenomatous polyposis*: AD inheritance. Mutations in tumour suppressor gene *APC*. Premalignant colonic and rectal polyps, cancers—colorectal, duodenal, thyroid, adrenal, and hepatoblastoma. Epidermoid cysts, lipomas, desmoid tumour (see ➜ p. 543).
- *Peutz–Jeghers syndrome*: AD inheritance, mutation in *STK11* gene. Intestinal polyps and visceral cancers. Pigmented macules (lentigines) on the vermillion border of the lips, oral mucosa, perioral, perianal, and periorbital skin, over joints, and on palms and soles (see ➜ p. 543).
- *Cronkhite–Canada syndrome*: nail dystrophy, alopecia, and hyperpigmentation; intestinal polyps cause diarrhoea, malabsorption, and weight loss; rapidly fatal in 1/3 of patients.
- *Hereditary non-polyposis colorectal cancer (Lynch syndrome)*: AD inheritance. Germline mutations in mismatch repair genes *MLH1, MSH2, MSH6,* and *PMS2*. Colon cancers. Other malignancies: endometrial, urologic, small bowel, ovarian, hepatobiliary, and brain. Cutaneous signs in Muir–Torre variant: sebaceous tumours, multiple keratoacanthomas (see ➜ p. 544).
- *Degos disease*: crops of erythematous papules evolve into porcelain-white macules with an erythematous rim. An occlusive vasculopathy produces wedge-shaped infarcts in the skin. Similar pathology in the GIT or cerebral vessels may be fatal.
- *FMF*: abdominal pain, tender erythematous patches (like erysipelas), and arthritis (see ➜ p. 234).

Further reading

Shah KR et al. J Am Acad Dermatol 2013;68:189.e1–21.
Thrash B et al. J Am Acad Dermatol 2013;68:211.e1–33.

Chapter 25

Skin and chest diseases

Contents

> **Relevant pages in other chapters**

Sarcoidosis

Sarcoidosis is a granulomatous disease of unknown cause (see Box 25.1) that predominantly affects the lung (90%), but may involve virtually any organ. African/Caribbean patients tend to have more severe manifestations. Skin is affected in 25% of patients.

What should I look for?

Specific cutaneous lesions

Skin is easier to biopsy to confirm the diagnosis than internal organs, so look hard for skin signs. Cutaneous sarcoidosis is a great imitator. Specific cutaneous lesions have a granulomatous histology (see ➔ Box 33.5, p. 651) and may include:

- Asymptomatic translucent yellowish brown firm papules (often periorbital), nodules, or plaques (round, oval, or annular) (see Fig. 25.1) on an erythematous background. Smooth or scaly. May appear psoriasiform. Diascopy reveals yellow-brown colour (see Box 25.2). Usually resolve spontaneously.
- Changing scars: infiltration gives skin a purplish red colour (see Fig. 25.2). May be tender. Sarcoid may also involve tattoos.
- Firm subcutaneous nodules (Darier–Roussy sarcoid) most often on the forearms. Often associated with systemic disease.
- Lupus pernio: indolent reddish purple destructive plaques and nodules on the nose, cheeks, lips, and ears (sites where skin is cool). Commonest in women. Lesions may ulcerate and heal with telangiectatic scars (see Fig. 25.3). Poor prognosis. Associated with more severe pulmonary disease. May respond to oral lenalidomide.
- Alopecia: scarring or non-scarring.
- Ulcers, most often on legs: seen most often in African Americans.
- Ichthyosis-like scaling on legs (rarely generalized).
- Lichenoid (1–2%): violaceous or yellow/brown scaly papules on the face, trunk, and limbs. Histology: both granulomas and focal basal cell degeneration.
- Hypopigmented macules or patches, or hypopigmentation over papules.
- Nail involvement: nail plate dystrophy, including pitting, longitudinal ridging, opacity, and loss of nail plate. Periungual changes are unusual.
- Coarse trabecular bony changes in the distal phalanx are rare.

Non-specific cutaneous lesions

- Erythema nodosum is a 'reactive' panniculitis, which tends to be associated with an acute form of sarcoid. It resolves without treatment. Löfgren syndrome (EN with bilateral hilar adenopathy, fever, and acute ankle arthritis) is diagnostic of sarcoid (see ➔ p. 458).

Involvement of other organs

- Lungs: asymptomatic in 60%. May have cough, dyspnoea, or pleuritic chest pain. Ten to 30% develop chronic pulmonary disease. Pulmonary fibrosis causes respiratory failure.
- Eyes: blurring or loss of vision, painful red eye, or photophobia. Signs include macular oedema and papilloedema. Risk of permanent visual impairment.

- Lacrimal or salivary gland swelling (with dry eye/dry mouth).
- Peripheral lymphadenopathy.
- Heart (symptomatic in 5%): arrhythmias, conduction abnormalities, left ventricular dysfunction.
- CNS (symptomatic in up to 13%): palsy of cranial nerve VII, mono- or polyneuropathies.
- Liver: abnormal LFTs (raised alkaline phosphatase).
- Renal failure 2° to hypercalcuria or hypercalcaemia.

What should I do?

See 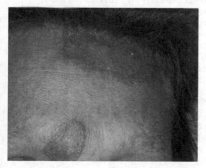 p. 526.

Box 25.1 Pathogenesis of sarcoidosis

- Genetic susceptibility: more severe in African Americans (black Americans) than white Americans.
- Chronic cell-mediated immune response to unknown antigen:
  - Activated macrophages and CD4⁺ T-lymphocytes release cytokines that trigger the formation of granulomas.
  - Elevated IFN-γ, IL-2, and IL-12.
  - Overproduction of TNF-α at the sites of disease.
- Relative anergy *in vivo*, possibly 2° to regulatory T-cells inhibiting IL-2 and T-cell proliferation.

Box 25.2 How to perform diascopy

- Gently press a glass slide onto a sarcoidal papule or plaque.
- The pressure enhances the yellow-brown 'apple jelly' colour by removing the background erythema.
- Cutaneous TB has a similar appearance.

Fig. 25.1 Reddish brown slightly scaly plaques with a raised border.

Management of cutaneous sarcoidosis

⚠ The diagnosis is one of exclusion. Always search hard for another explanation for the granulomatous histology, particularly mycobacterial or fungal diseases (see Box 25.3).

What should I do?

- Take a biopsy from a specific cutaneous lesion (much easier than taking a biopsy from an internal organ).
- If the histology is granulomatous, exclude mycobacterial and fungal infection by culture of the involved skin.
- Tuberculin skin test (may be anergic in sarcoid).
- FBC, renal function, and liver function.
- Serum and urinary calcium (risk of hypercalcaemia and hypercalciuria). 1-α hydroxylase is activated by macrophages in granulomas and converts 25-hydroxyvitamin D_3 to 1,25-dihydroxyvitamin D_3, the active form of the vitamin. Absorption of calcium from the gut increases, as does renal excretion.
- Although serum ACE may be elevated in active sarcoidosis, this test is insufficiently sensitive or specific to be of diagnostic help.
- Serum protein electrophoresis: 50% have a polyclonal hypergammaglobulinaemia. ⚠ If hypogammaglobulinaemia, check for variable common immunodeficiency or lymphoma.
- Chest radiograph and pulmonary function tests.
- Electrocardiogram (ECG).
- Refer for an ophthalmological assessment.

Treatment of cutaneous sarcoid

- No treatment required, if not symptomatic. Skin manifestations may resolve spontaneously.
- Very potent topical corticosteroids: may be used under a hydrocolloid occlusive dressing (see ⊃ p. 660). Fludroxycortide tape is an alternative.
- Intralesional triamcinolone (3–20mg/mL): repeated injections required.
- Topical 0.1% tacrolimus ointment.
- Systemic agents that have been recommended for cutaneous disease (few controlled trials) include:
  - Hydroxychloroquine 200–400mg/day (no more than 6.5mg/kg/day). Should see an optician annually.
  - Methotrexate 10–20mg/week.
  - Oral tetracyclines.
  - Oral prednisolone 20–40mg/day is indicated in recalcitrant extensive or destructive skin disease. May be combined with hydroxychloroquine or methotrexate.
  - Other drugs that have been advocated include isotretinoin, fumaric acid esters, leflunomide, mycophenolate mofetil, thalidomide, and infliximab.

Further reading

Judson MA. *Clin Rev Allergy Immunol* 2015;49:63–78.
Vorselaars AD et al. *Inflamm Allergy Drug Targets* 2013;12:369–77.

**Box 25.3 Cutaneous sarcoid: histological
differential diagnosis**

- Cutaneous TB and atypical mycobacterial infections.
- Deep fungal infection.
- Foreign body reaction: zirconium, beryllium, tattoo, paraffin, etc.
- Rheumatoid nodule.
- Leishmaniasis.
- Melkersson–Rosenthal syndrome: recurrent or persistent orofacial swellings (especially the lower lip and around the eyes), a fissured tongue, and intermittent paralysis of the peripheral facial nerve.

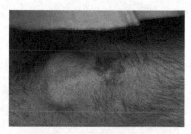

Fig. 25.2 Purplish red discoloration of an old scar 2° to sarcoidal infiltration.

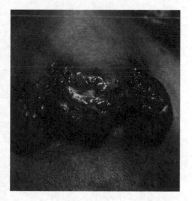

Fig. 25.3 Lupus pernio with destruction of the nose.

Skin and haematology/ oncology

Contents

Radiotherapy

Early reactions in radiation field

Acute side effects resolve within 4–6 weeks, usually without treatment, but moisturizers and soap substitutes may be helpful.

Reactions include:

- Erythematous, dry skin and mild oedema (like sunburn).
- Oedema, marked erythema, and moist desquamation.
- Blisters, ulcers, and haemorrhagic crusting (infrequent because doses of radiotherapy are more precisely controlled than in the past).
- Hyperpigmentation (commoner in darker skin).
- Hair loss.

Late reactions in radiation field

Late reactions in the radiation field may appear years after radiotherapy, and changes gradually progress. Reactions include:

- Telangiectasia, hypo- and hyperpigmentation.
- Epidermal atrophy and fragility.
- Necrosis leading to ulceration (may simulate malignancy).
- Dermal and subcutaneous fibrosis (within first 3 months).

Generalized skin diseases induced by radiation

- Herpes zoster.
- EM.
- Autoimmune blistering diseases (BP, pemphigus).

Skin diseases induced by radiation but localized to the radiation field

- Post-radiotherapy skin changes are more painful when affecting the breast, compared to other sites.
- Acneiform lesions with comedones.
- Lichenoid reactions, e.g. EM, GVHD, LP.
- BP.
- Fibrosing reactions:
  - Morphoea: abrupt onset with erythema and induration 1 month to 3 years after radiotherapy. Usually affects the breast. Treatment is not very effective, but topical, intralesional, and oral corticosteroids have been recommended.
  - Lichen sclerosus.
  - Post-irradiation pseudosclerodermatous panniculitis 1–8 months after megavoltage (deeply penetrating) radiotherapy. Usually affects the breast. May resemble metastatic disease. Can improve spontaneously.
- Vasculopathy with fibrosis, atherosclerosis, and rupture of vessels.
- Malignancy, e.g. BCCs, SCCs.
- Radiation recall dermatitis (see Box 26.1).
- Radiation-associated vascular lesions—morphological range from atypical vascular lesions to cutaneous angiosarcoma—usually following breast carcinoma.

Box 26.1 Radiation recall dermatitis

- Well-defined cutaneous reaction at a previously irradiated site.
- Resembles an acute radiation reaction. Mild reactions are characterized by erythema, scale, and pruritus. In more severe reactions, oedema and vesiculation may be followed by moist desquamation or haemorrhagic ulceration with necrosis.
- Drug therapy elicits a severe inflammatory response in the irradiated skin, often far exceeding the initial radiation dermatitis.
- Triggered most often by IV chemotherapy, especially taxanes and anthracyclines. Other triggers include antibiotics, anti-TB drugs, tamoxifen, and simvastatin.
- Recall may be triggered from a few days to 15 years after radiotherapy. Reactions tend to be more severe when the recall-triggering drug is given shortly after the end of radiotherapy.
- Interval between radiotherapy and the recall symptoms should exceed 7 days, if the radiation recall reaction is considered.
- Reaction settles, when the drug is withdrawn.
- Topical steroids help control inflammation.
- Response to re-challenge with the drug is unpredictable.
- Precise mechanism is unknown. Several hypotheses have been proposed: (1) Cytotoxic treatment induces a recall reaction in the remaining surviving cells; (2) mutation caused by radiotherapy yields more vulnerable cells that cannot tolerate cytotoxic treatment; (3) a vascular reaction occurs after radiotherapy; (4) an idiosyncratic drug hypersensitivity reaction—radiation can induce non-specific prolonged secretion of inflammatory mediators in irradiated tissues, e.g. IL-1, IL-6, platelet-derived growth factor β, TNF-α, or TGF-β, that could be upregulated when a precipitating factor (chemotherapy) is introduced.

Further reading

Brenn T and Fletcher CD. *Histopathology* 2006;**48**:106–14.
Reddy SM et al. *Semin Arthritis Rheum* 2005;**34**:728–34.
Requena L and Ferrándiz C. *Dermatol Clin* 2008;**26**:505–8, vii–viii.
Weaver J and Billings SD. *Semin Diagn Pathol* 2009;**26**:141–9.

Acute cutaneous graft-versus-host disease

What is graft-versus-host disease?

Haemopoietic stem cell transplants (HSCTs) are used to treat conditions such as leukaemia, myeloma, lymphoma, aplastic anaemia, and immunodeficiency. GVHD complicates >50% of allogeneic HSCTs and is caused by donor immunocompetent T-cells reacting against immunocompromised host tissues. New, less aggressive approaches (reduced-intensity conditioning and umbilical cord blood transplantation) have expanded the indications for HSCTs, and the prevalence of GVHD is rising. Donor lymphocyte infusions (DLIs) are used to induce remission in patients who relapse after allogeneic HSCT but also incur a risk of acute GVHD. Some GVHD may be desired for the graft-versus-malignancy effect, but chronic GVHD is a major cause of morbidity and mortality. For risk factors, see Box 26.2.

The boundary between acute and chronic GVHD is blurred, and diagnosis depends on clinical features, and not on timing post-transplant. Although the prevalence of acute GVHD is directly related to the degree of mismatch between HLA proteins in the donor and recipient, acute GVHD has been reported after autologous HSCT, because regulatory T-cells are depleted, allowing the autologous graft to recognize self-antigens.

What should I look for?

- Sudden onset of burning or pruritic morbilliform rash—often perifollicular initially.
- Macular blotchy erythema, initially affecting the palms and soles, and face.
- Commonly involves the pinnae, cheeks, lateral neck, and upper back. The scalp is usually spared. The patient may become erythrodermic.
- Mucosal involvement is frequent, especially conjunctival and oral.
- Generalized erythema, blistering, and erosions simulate TEN in severe acute GVHD (see ➔ p. 116).
- Other features:
  - Fever (culture-negative).
  - Abdominal pain, nausea, vomiting, and watery/bloody diarrhoea.
  - Abnormal liver function—raised bilirubin and alkaline phosphatase.

Box 26.2 Risk factors for graft-versus-host-disease

- Older age.
- History of acute GVHD increases the risk of chronic GVHD.
- HLA mismatch.
- Intense preparative regimen.
- Haemopoietic cells from peripheral blood, not bone marrow (more T-cells).
- Less aggressive immunosuppression after transplantation.
- Donor T-lymphocyte infusions (given to incite a graft-versus-malignancy effect).

What should I do?

- Consider alternative diagnoses, especially drug reactions (see Box 26.3).
- Exclude infection with cultures of blood, urine, sputum, and stool.
- If the diagnosis is uncertain, take a skin biopsy from a well-established perifollicular lesion, but the histology may not distinguish between a severe drug reaction and acute cutaneous GVHD.
- Potent topical corticosteroids may control mild acute cutaneous GVHD, but severe cases require high-dose systemic corticosteroids.
- Other treatment options include immunosuppressants, anti-TNFs, and extracorporeal photopheresis (ECP) (see Box 26.7).

Box 26.3 Morbilliform rash after haemopoietic stem cell transplant: differential diagnosis

- Drug eruption (including early TEN): chemotherapeutic agents, antibiotics, etc.
- Viral exanthema.
- EM 2° to herpes simplex infection.
- Acute GVHD.
- Eruption of lymphocyte recovery (ELR):
  - Occurs 1–4 weeks after chemotherapy, when immunocompetent lymphocytes return to peripheral circulation and skin.
  - Mild fever.
  - No mucosal involvement. No systemic involvement.
  - Rash fades spontaneously, with desquamation within 1–3 weeks.
- Engraftment syndrome (ES, capillary leak syndrome):
  - Occurs within 96h of engraftment. Neutrophil recovery is associated with cytokine release and neutrophil degranulation.
  - Described most often after autologous HSCT (may be confused with early acute GVHD in allogeneic HSCT).
  - Fever >38.3°C without infection.
  - Non-cardiogenic pulmonary oedema or haemorrhage with diffuse pulmonary infiltrates.
  - Generalized oedema with weight gain.
  - Multi-organ failure and increased mortality.
- Stem cell transplantation erythema (SCTE):
  - Occurs 3–15 days after HSCT.
  - Itchy, widespread, symmetrical, erythematous eruption. Discrete circular macules may become confluent. Marked at acral sites. May develop tender plaques, occasionally surrounded by microvesicles or pustules. No purpura or bullae. Lesions darken, then desquamate.

Further reading
Dignan FL et al. Br J Haematol 2012;158:30–45.

Chronic cutaneous graft-versus-host disease

Chronic GVHD has an insidious onset. It is multisystem, but the skin, mouth, and eyes are major targets. Donor-derived, alloreactive CD4-negative and CD8-positive T-cells are thought to play a part in the pathogenesis. Some aspects of chronic GVHD share features with other autoimmune diseases such as primary biliary cirrhosis, bronchiolitis obliterans, and Sjögren syndrome.

Patients should be cared for by a multidisciplinary team that includes ophthalmologists, dermatologists, and haematologists. Fifty percent have limited cutaneous disease and a good prognosis, but the outcome in widespread chronic cutaneous GVHD is poor (see Box 26.6).

What should I look for?

- Manifestations vary, and patients often have overlapping patterns of disease with a combination of lichenoid and sclerodermoid features.
- Check hair and nails, as well as skin (see Box 26.4).
- Examine mucosae, including genitalia (see Box 26.5).
- Assess joint mobility and impact of disease.
- ❶ These patients have been exposed to chemotherapy and prolonged immunosuppression and are at risk of cutaneous malignancies and/or unusual cutaneous infections (fungal, atypical mycobacterial).
- Other organ involvement includes:
  - GIT causing abdominal symptoms (diarrhoea) and weight loss.
  - Liver with abnormal LFTs.
  - Lungs causing shortness of breath (check lung function tests).

What should I do?

- Biopsy atypical cutaneous lesions to exclude malignancy/infection.
- Emollients and soap substitutes with antiseptics may reduce itch, improve the skin barrier, and reduce the risk of infection.
- Artificial saliva, topical local anaesthetic gels, and topical corticosteroids are indicated for painful oral disease (see ➋ Box 14.4, p. 283).
- Prescribe artificial tears for dry eyes.
- Lichenoid disease: potent corticosteroid ointments or 0.1% tacrolimus ointment bd may reduce inflammation.
- Sclerodermoid disease: UVB, PUVA, or UVA1 may be helpful in early disease. ECP may have a role in widespread disease (see Box 26.7). ECP may induce antigen-specific regulatory T-cells that suppress GVHD, but the mechanisms of action are not clear.
- The combination of systemic corticosteroids and immunosuppressive agents is generally used as first-line treatment. Complications, such as infection, increase mortality.
- Other treatments include mTOR inhibitors, rituximab, and imatinib. More trials are needed.

Box 26.4 Signs of chronic cutaneous graft-versus-host disease

- Lichenoid (like LP) (see Fig. 26.4):
  - Flat-topped violaceous papules that may be perifollicular and involve scars (sites of central lines, scars of herpes zoster).
  - Hands, forearm, trunk, nails, and mucosa are often involved.
  - May be photosensitive.
- Sclerodermoid GVHD (see Fig. 26.3):
  - Also tends to involve scars (koebnerization).
  - Lichen sclerosus-like. Hypopigmented with wrinkling and follicular plugging. Involves the neck, upper trunk, and vulva. Progresses to morphoeaform/sclerodermoid (generalized) pattern.
  - Morphoeaform. Single/multiple plaques may progress to generalized tight, thickened skin with contractures (see ➔ p. 420).
  - Disfiguring hypo- and hyperpigmentation is common.
  - Atrophy with fragility, blistering, and skin ulceration (significant morbidity).
  - Eosinophilic fasciitis-like disease with deep sclerosis and contractures (diagnostic). Acute onset of pain and oedema in extremities, sparing the hands and feet. Sometimes preceded by vigorous exercise. Peripheral eosinophilia in 60% (see ➔ p. 421).
- Appendageal involvement:
  - Brittle hair, premature greying, scarring alopecia.
  - Dystrophic nails, longitudinal ridging, thinning, fragility, scarring (pterygium), and loss of nails (like LP) (see Fig. 26.1).
  - Loss of body hair and sweat glands causes heat sensitivity.
- Other features that have been described:
  - Poikiloderma (diagnostic).
  - Asteatotic eczema or ichthyosis.
  - Intensely itchy, diffuse erythema with fine scaling and palmoplantar hyperkeratosis. Frequent impetiginization ('eczematoid' GVHD).
  - Keratosis pilaris-like rash.
  - Cutaneous focal mucinosis.
  - Eruptive angiomas, nodular fibromas.

Box 26.5 Mucosal involvement in chronic graft-versus-host disease

(See Fig. 26.2.)

- Mouth with LP-like lacy white buccal involvement (early diagnostic sign), ulceration, and fibrosis (late—patients report difficulty moving the tongue when chewing). Sicca syndrome causes pain, dryness, sensitivity, and dental caries. Viral or fungal infections, especially candidiasis, are common.
- Eyes with burning, irritation, dryness, and photophobia.
- Vaginal dryness, pain, erythema, LP-like changes (diagnostic), lichen sclerosus-like changes, and strictures.

Box 26.6 Poor prognostic factors for chronic graft-versus-host disease

- Increasing age.
- Prior acute GVHD (and progressive onset to chronic GVHD).
- Time from transplantation to chronic GVHD <5 months.
- Donor mismatch.
- Intermediate or advanced disease at transplantation.
- Type of GVHD prophylaxis.
- Gender mismatch.
- High serum bilirubin.
- Over 50% skin involvement.
- Platelet count $<100 \times 10^9$/L.

Box 26.7 What is extracorporeal photopheresis?

- The patient's blood is collected, and white blood cells (WBCs) are separated.
- RBC and plasma are returned to the patient.
- WBCs are photosensitized by mixing with a psoralen and then exposed to UVA, which induces apoptosis.
- Treated cells are then returned to the patient.
- Used as a second-line treatment for skin, mucous membrane, or liver GVHD.
- Initial treatment schedule is fortnightly paired treatments (two consecutive days) for a minimum of 3 months.
- Frequency of treatments is subsequently reduced, when a response is observed.

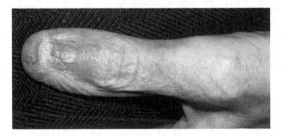

Fig. 26.1 Destruction of nails in lichenoid chronic graft-versus-host disease.

Further reading

Dignan FL et al. Br J Haematol 2012;**158**:46–61.
Ferrara J et al. Lancet 2009;**373**:1550–6.
Scarisbrick JJ et al. Br J Dermatol 2008;**158**:659–78.

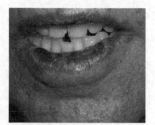

Fig. 26.2 Erosions and whitish discoloration of the lips simulate lichen planus in lichenoid graft-versus-host disease.

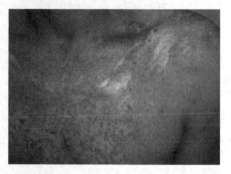

Fig. 26.3 The sclerodermoid variant of chronic graft-versus-host disease with tight indurated skin and both hypo- and hyperpigmentation.

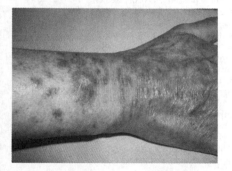

Fig. 26.4 The lichenoid variant of chronic graft-versus-host disease simulating lichen planus with purplish nodules and plaques.

Haematological diseases and skin

Polycythaemia rubra vera

- Itching or paraesthesiae, typically after a hot shower or bath.
- Erythromelalgia: attacks of burning pain in legs, often worse in bed, when the patient is unable to tolerate heat under bedclothes. Skin is erythematous but cool, and the legs may be swollen. Raised platelets. Aspirin is helpful. Resolves when polycythaemia controlled (see ➔ p. 551).

Essential thrombocythaemia

- Livedo reticularis and/or retiform purpura with painful leg ulcers 2° to vasculopathy (see ➔ pp. 314–15).
- Erythromelalgia (see above and ➔ p. 551).

Leukaemias and lymphomas

- Neutrophilic dermatoses: Sweet syndrome (see ➔ p. 518) and pyoderma gangrenosum (see ➔ p. 310).
- Interstitial granulomatous dermatitis (see ➔ p. 373).
- Cutaneous lymphoma, Sézary syndrome, and leukaemia cutis (see ➔ pp. 358–9).
- Adverse reactions in skin and nails 2° to chemotherapy (see ➔ pp. 382–3, pp. 384–7).
- ⚠ Paraneoplastic pemphigus (rare) (see ➔ pp. 268–9). Seen most often in chronic lymphocytic lymphoma (see Box 26.9), non-Hodgkin lymphoma, or Castleman disease (a rare lymphoproliferative disorder). Alemtuzumab may be helpful.

Rosai–Dorfman disease (sinus histiocytosis with massive lymphadenopathy)

- Presents with prominent painless cervical lymphadenopathy in ~90% of cases. Tends to affect children and young adults.
- Associated with fever, raised WCC and ESR, polyclonal hypergammaglobulinaemia, RBC autoantibodies, juvenile-onset diabetes, and asthma.
- Extranodal disease occurs in around 40% patients.
- Skin is the most commonly affected site—single or multiple, yellow, erythematous, or brown papules, nodules, or plaques commonly affecting the torso, followed by the head and neck.
- Usually runs a benign, self-limiting course.
- Rarely exists as purely the cutaneous Rosai–Dorfman disease (RDD) form (older women); no reported risk of developing systemic disease.
- Lesions can spontaneously resolve or persist, with variable response to therapy.
- Treatment options include surgical excision, topical or intralesional steroids, cryotherapy, or radiotherapy.

Hyperglobulinaemic purpura

Asymptomatic diffuse petechiae and purpuric macules at sites of pressure, minor trauma, or stasis. Purpura may be precipitated by exercise. Occasionally, paraesthesiae precede the rash. Occurs in association with chronic inflammatory diseases, including:

- LE, RA, and Sjögren syndrome.
- Sarcoidosis.
- Chronic hepatitis.
- Inflammatory bowel disease.
- Chronic infections.

Hypergammaglobulinaemias

Multiple myeloma

Skin lesions are uncommon and occur late in the course of disease.

- Plasma cell tumours: erythematous/purplish nodules—direct extension into the skin from an underlying bone disease or metastatic disease.
- Neutrophilic dermatoses, including subcorneal pustular dermatosis, erythema elevatum diutinum, urticarial vasculitis, Sweet syndrome, PG (IgA gammopathy). Also urticarial-like neutrophilic dermatosis reported—asymptomatic urticarial-like erythematous plaques, commonly affecting the trunk. Persists for days and may resolve with hyperpigmentation.
- Amyloidosis may have cutaneous manifestations (see ➲ p. 496).
- Type 1 cryoglobulinaemia: cold sensitivity, mottling, cyanosis, purpura, blisters, ulcers (occlusive vasculopathy) (see ➲ pp. 444–5).
- POEMS syndrome—rare (see Box 26.8).
- Follicular spicules, particularly on the nose. Also scalp and neck.
- Acquired cutis laxa—granuloma annulare-like plaques clinically.
- Papular mucinosis (see Box 26.10).

Waldenström macroglobulinaemia

- Epistaxis and oral mucosal bleeding.
- Cutaneous macroglobulinosis—flesh-coloured papules on extensors.
- Evidence of type 1 cryoglobulinaemia as in myeloma (IgG or IgM) (see ➲ p. 444).
- May be preceded by Schnitzler syndrome (IgM) (see ➲ Box 11.1, p. 229).

IgG4-related disease

- Characterized by raised levels of IgG4, tissue infiltration of IgG4-positive plasma cells, and presence of fibrosis.
- Affects multiple organs, including the pancreas, bile duct, lacrimal and salivary glands, thyroid.
- Skin lesions reported—mainly head and neck.
- Cutaneous disease responds to oral corticosteroids.
- IgG4 levels do not correlate with disease activity.

> ⚠ **Box 26.8 POEMS syndrome**
>
> A rare syndrome associated with plasma cell disorders, comprising:
> - *P*olyneuropathy: motor and sensory. Starts distally and spreads proximally.
> - *O*rganomegaly: liver, spleen, lymph nodes.
> - *E*ndocrinopathy: impotence, gynaecomastia, amenorrhoea (2° to raised oestrogen), diabetes, hypothyroidism, hyperprolactinaemia, hypoparathyroidism.
> - *M*onoclonal gammopathy, usually IgG.
> - *S*kin changes: hyperpigmentation, skin thickening, sclerodermoid changes, hypertrichosis, multiple cutaneous angiomas (glomeruloid histology, reflects the vascular endothelial growth factor expression), nail changes (clubbing, white nails), oedema, and hyperhidrosis.
> - Fifteen percent of patients have evidence of Castleman disease (giant—angiofollicular hyperplasia, multicentric plasma cell variant)—also associated with multiple cutaneous angiomas.

Box 26.9 Chronic lymphocytic leukaemia and the skin

Chronic lymphocytic leukaemia (CLL) infiltrating the skin occurs rarely but can manifest in a number of ways, including erythematous nodules and plaques. However, more commonly, CLL is associated with other skin conditions, and these patients have a high risk of subsequent skin cancers.

Increased risk of cutaneous malignancies
- Keratinocyte malignancies, e.g. BCC, SCC.
- Melanoma (worse prognosis).
- Merkel cell carcinoma (worse prognosis).
- Cutaneous T-cell lymphoma.
- Rare skin cancers, e.g. malignant fibrous histiocytoma, dermatofibrosarcoma protuberans.

Skin conditions associated with chronic lymphocytic leukaemia
- Generalized pruritus, petechiae/purpura.
- Sweet syndrome.
- Paraneoplastic pemphigus.
- Granuloma annulare.
- Cutaneous granulomatous vasculitis.
- Atypical presentations of herpesvirus infections.
- Exaggerated insect bite reactions.
- Linear IgA disease.
- Leukaemia cutis.

Box 26.10 Papular mucinosis

Uncommon mucinoses associated with a serum monoclonal IgG para-protein. A minority of patients develop myeloma. Mucin deposition in the dermis, fibroblast proliferation, and fibrosis.
- Lichen myxoedema: 2–3mm waxy, flat-topped, non-pruritic papules (may be linear) on the hands (palms spared), elbows, forearms, upper trunk, face, and neck.
- Scleromyxoedema: papules coalesce. Waxy indurated skin may resemble scleroderma. Involvement of the forehead produces furrowing and may mimic acromegaly (leonine facies). Thickening of skin limits movement of limbs and mouth opening; 'doughnut sign' (thickening over PIP joints with a central depression); 'Shar-Pei sign' (deep furrowing on the back). Systemic involvement can occur with mucin in the vocal cords, kidneys, pulmonary and coronary vessels, joints/muscles, and other organs.

Compare with scleredema (see ➲ Box 22.2, p. 467).

Familial cancer syndromes

Basal cell naevus syndrome (Gorlin syndrome)

- AD inheritance. Mutation in *PTCH1* tumour suppressor gene on 9q22.3–q31—upregulation in sonic-hedgehog pathway; targeted smoothened inhibitors (vismodegib) now available.
- Prevalence between 1 in 19 000 and 1 in 256 000.
- ❶ Consider diagnosis if BCC before age 20, or many BCCs out of proportion to skin type and history of sun exposure.
- Multiple BCCs resembling pigmented or non-pigmented 'moles', milia, dermal and epidermoid cysts, pits on palms and soles.
- Medulloblastoma (frequent and early onset; avoid radiotherapy which may induce BCCs within the field).
- Intracranial ectopic calcification.
- Skeletal abnormalities, including macrocephaly with frontal bossing, bifid ribs, short fourth metacarpal, and scoliosis.
- Odontogenic keratocysts of the jaws, cleft lip, and/or palate.
- May have ocular, genitourinary, auditory, cardiac, and/or respiratory abnormalities.

Melanoma/pancreatic cancer syndrome (familial atypical multiple mole melanoma–pancreatic cancer syndrome)

- Mutation of gene encoding cyclin-dependent kinase inhibitor-2A (*CDKN2A*) on chromosome 9p21. Rare. Prevalence uncertain.
- Malignant melanoma and pancreatic cancer.
- Large melanocytic naevi with irregular pigmentation and border.
- Possibly breast cancer.

Birt–Hogg–Dubé syndrome

- AD inheritance. Mutation in the 17p11.2 gene encoding folliculin.
- Prevalence estimated at about 1 in 200 000.
- Skin tags and benign hair follicle tumours (fibrofolliculomas and trichodiscomas) present as skin-coloured papules.
- Lung cysts and spontaneous pneumothorax.
- Renal carcinoma.

Cowden syndrome (multiple hamartoma syndrome)

- AD inheritance. Mutations in *PTEN/MMAC1* tumour suppressor gene on chromosome 10q22–23.
- Prevalence estimated at about 1 in 200 000.
- Prototype of PTEN–hamartoma tumour syndrome (see Box 26.11).
- Flesh-coloured papules on the head and neck (trichilemmomas).
- Smooth papules (cobblestone-like) on oral mucosal surfaces: labial, palatal, and gingival (benign fibromas). Furrowed tongue.
- Flat wart-like papules on the dorsum of hands and feet.
- Keratoses on palms, soles, and sides of feet.
- Lipomas and haemangiomas; café au lait spots.
- Fibrocystic breast disease and breast cancer, thyroid tumours, melanoma, endometrial cancer, lung cancer, GI polyps, and colon cancer.

Howel–Evans syndrome

- AD inheritance associated with mutation in *RHBDF2* (Rhomboid family member 2) gene (intramembranous serine protease) located at 17q25. Extremely rare—a few families.
- Keratoderma (thickened hyperkeratotic skin on palms and soles).
- Oral mucosal precancerous lesions, e.g. leukoplakia.
- Oesophageal cancer.

Hereditary leiomyomatosis/renal cell cancer syndrome

- AD inheritance. Mutation of gene encoding fumarate hydratase at locus 1q42.3–43 (>60% decrease in fumarate hydratase activity is diagnostic). Prevalence unknown.
- Leiomyomas of skin: firm reddish brown painful tumours of smooth muscle (benign) that may be in a band-like distribution or diffuse. Pilar subtype or angioleiomyomas. Also atypical smooth muscle tumours seen.
- Leiomyomas/leiomyosarcoma of the uterus. Increased risk of uterine fibroids at a young age.
- Papillary renal cell cancer—regular surveillance recommended.

Peutz–Jeghers syndrome

- AD inheritance. Mutations in the *STK11/LKB1* tumour suppressor gene on chromosome 19p13.3.
- Estimates of prevalence range from 1 in 25 000 to 1 in 300 000.
- Pigmented macules (lentigines) on perioral skin, lips, buccal mucosa, palms, and soles. Hamartomatous polyps throughout the GIT, particularly in the jejunum. Intussusception causes bleeding and pain.
- Increased risk of GI cancer, especially stomach and duodenum.
- Other cancers: pancreas, gall bladder, lung, breast, uterus, and ovary.

Gardner syndrome

- Variant of familial adenomatous polyposis coli.
- AD inheritance—mutation in adenomatosis polyposis coli gene (*APC*) at locus 5q21–22. APC protein is involved in the regulation of cell division.
- Estimates of prevalence range from 1 in 6850 to 1 in 31 250.
- Multiple epidermoid ('sebaceous') cysts on the face, scalp, and extremities—commonest skin finding.
- Also fibromas, desmoid tumours, lipomas, and leiomyomas.
- Adenomatous polyps throughout the colon, with high risk of colorectal cancer.
- Other cancers (thyroid, osteosarcoma, chondrosarcoma, liposarcoma, hepatoblastoma).
- Dental abnormalities (unerupted teeth, supernumerary teeth).
- Hypertrophy of retinal pigment epithelium.
- Osteomas of the mandible, skull, and, less often, long bones.

Muir–Torre syndrome

- AD inheritance. Variant of non-polyposis colon cancer syndrome (Lynch syndrome). Mutations in DNA mismatch repair genes. Prevalence uncertain.
- Many sebaceous gland tumours (hyperplasia, adenomas, carcinomas), keratoacanthomas with sebaceous differentiation.
- GI cancers. Also breast cancer, genitourinary cancer, and haematological malignancies.

Box 26.11 PTEN–hamartoma tumour syndrome

- Germline *PTEN* mutations (10q23.3) that lead to hamartoma formation occur in four rare allelic disorders. All are linked to an increased risk of malignancy in the breast, thyroid, and uterus:
  - Cowden syndrome.
  - Bannayan–Riley–Ruvulcaba syndrome—congenital disorder. Common findings include macrocephaly, lipomas, haemangiomas, pigmented macules of the penis, proximal myopathy, joint hyperextensibility ± developmental delay.
  - *PTEN*-related Proteus syndrome and Proteus-like syndrome. Some clinical overlap with Proteus syndrome (see ➲ Box 27.11, p. 561). Hamartomatous overgrowth of a variety of tissues.

Further reading

Hobert JA and Eng C. *Genet Med* 2009;11:687–94.
Jelsig AM et al. *Orphanet J Rare Dis* 2014;9:101.

Paraneoplastic skin changes

Most of these paraneoplastic phenomena are uncommon. Look for a commoner explanation for the skin changes.

- Nail clubbing with hypertrophic osteoarthropathy (phalanges)—lung cancer.
- Ichthyosis (dry scaly skin)—lymphoma/lymphoproliferative disease.
- Dermatomyositis (see ➔ pp. 408–9)—10–30% of adult patients have an associated malignancy.
- SCLE may be triggered by an underlying malignancy (rare) (see ➔ p. 402).
- Neutrophilic dermatoses (Sweet syndrome, PG) (see ➔ p. 310, pp. 518–19) (commonest association AML).
- Acanthosis nigricans: more often seen in insulin resistance and obesity (see ➔ pp. 466–7) than in malignancy (generally adenocarcinoma of the stomach). Flexural skin is hyperpigmented and thickened with a velvety texture. Skin tags are common. May be associated with a wrinkled ridged appearance on the palms (tripe palms).
- Diffuse pigmentation may be caused by an ACTH-secreting tumour (ectopic ACTH). Malignancies include SCC of the lung, carcinoid tumours, and pancreatic islet cell tumours.
- Carcinoid syndrome (rare)—episodic flushing eventually leads to persistent facial oedema and telangiectasia (see ➔ pp. 520–1).
- Necrolytic migratory erythema (rare)—seen in association with glucagonoma (α-cell tumours of the pancreas) (see ➔ p. 516).
- Eruptive seborrhoeic warts (sign of Leser–Trelat)—sudden appearance of large numbers of seborrhoeic warts is seen rarely in association with GI tract cancers, genitourinary cancers, and lymphoproliferative disease. Seborrhoeic warts are very common in the elderly and, in most patients, are of no significance. Eruptive seborrhoeic warts may also be triggered by widespread inflammatory skin diseases such as eczema.
- Bazex syndrome (acrokeratosis paraneoplastica). Psoriasiform rash on the ears, nose, cheeks, hands (palmar hyperkeratosis), feet, and knees, with nail dystrophy. Rare and associated with carcinomas of the larynx, pharynx, trachea, bronchus, or upper oesophagus.
- Acquired hypertrichosis lanuginosa. Long silky non-pigmented hair (lanugo hair) on the face and trunk. Most often associated with adenocarcinoma of the GI tract (rare). Consider other causes of hypertrichosis (increased hair growth on any part of the body, independent of androgens), including drugs and PCT (see ➔ p. 94).
- Paraneoplastic pemphigus (rare). Associated with B-cell lymphoma, thymoma, and Castleman disease (see ➔ Box 13.4, p. 269).
- Erythema gyratum repens. Urticated wavy erythematous bands like the grain of wood that advance outward by about 1cm a day. Most often associated with lung carcinoma (rare).

Further reading
Thiers BH et al. CA Cancer J Clin 2009;**59**:73–98.

Skin and neurology

Contents

Relevant pages in other chapters
Seborrhoeic dermatitis (common in Parkinson disease) ➔ p. 219
Neuropathic ulcers ➔ pp. 294–5
Porphyria ➔ pp. 330–1
Xeroderma pigmentosum ➔ pp. 336–7
Pompholyx induced by IV Ig ➔ p. 388
Rheumatology ➔ Chapter 19, pp. 393–433
Vasculitis ➔ Chapter 20, pp. 435–454
Amyloidosis ➔ pp. 496–7
Fabry disease ➔ p. 502–3
Sarcoidosis ➔ pp. p524–5
Congenital cutaneous lesions ➔ pp. 594–5
Vascular malformations ➔ pp. 600–1
Ectodermal dysplasias ➔ pp. 634–5
Sjogren-Larsson syndrome ➔ Box 32.2, p. 627
Ataxia telangiectasia ➔ p. 612
Immunodeficiency syndromes ➔ p. 612
Incontinentia pigmenti ➔ pp. 636–7
Pigmentary mosaicism ➔ Box 32.7, p. 637
Goltz syndrome ➔ Box 32.8, p. 637
Melkersson–Rosenthal syndrome ➔ Box 25.3, p. 527
Localized dysaesthesias ➔ pp. 568–9

Neuropathic pain and itch

Patients with localized itching or paraesthesiae usually attribute their puzzling symptoms to the skin. But sensory neuropathy may cause itch or contribute to itch in conditions such as chronic renal failure. (Also see ➲ parasitophobia, pp. 570–1; leprosy, p. 144; syphilis, pp. 146–7.)

What should I look for?

- Burning, tingling, stinging, hypoaesthesia, or hyperalgesia.
- Distribution: distal symmetrical (polyneuropathy), individual nerve territories (mononeuritis multiplex, e.g. vasculitis), dermatomal (radiculopathy), or one side of the body (central).
- Evidence of rubbing (lichen simplex) or scratching.
- Sensory loss—check light touch, vibration, proprioception, pain, and temperature (use a cold tuning fork). Asteatotic eczema may develop in hypoaesthetic skin.
- Motor/autonomic dysfunction in the distribution of sensory disturbance.

Causes of generalized neuropathic itch/pain

- Small-fibre neuropathy (Aδ and C-fibres), e.g. diabetes, amyloidosis, SLE, HIV. Fabry disease (Aδ fibres)—rare (see ➲ pp. 502–3).
- Centrally driven neuropathic itch has been described in association with brain tumours, strokes, spinal tumours, and multiple sclerosis.

Causes of localized neuropathic itch

- Peripheral nerve or root impingement may underlie puzzling conditions such as notalgia paraesthetica (see Box 27.2) and perhaps brachioradial pruritus (see Box 27.1)
- Herpes zoster may cause itch, as well as pain (see ➲ Box 7.7, p. 157).
- Trigeminal trophic syndrome (see Box 27.3).
- Keloids may be associated with neuropathic itch, but the cause is uncertain. Pain fibres may be trapped in proliferating collagen.

(Also see ➲ Localized dysaesthesias, pp. 568–9.)

Box 27.1 What is brachioradial pruritus?

- Brachioradial pruritus presents with tingling or burning, in addition to intractable itch, on the dorsolateral aspect of the arms.
- The condition is commonest in ♀.
- Symptoms are frequently bilateral.
- Although cervical spine abnormalities have been demonstrated in many patients, their relevance is unclear.
- Sun exposure often exacerbates symptoms.
- Application of ice packs may alleviate itch (ice pack sign).
- Capsaicin 0.075% cream, topical doxepin, lidocaine gel, oral gabapentin, or oral carbamazepine may be helpful.
- May be mimicked by drug-induced photosensitivity.

Box 27.2 What is notalgia paraesthetica?

- Notalgia paraesthetica is thought to be caused by impingement of the posterior rami of T2–T6 nerve roots, because it is associated with degenerative changes in the thoracic spine.
- Patients present with a localized area of itch and paraesthesiae over the lower border of the scapula. Other symptoms may include tingling, burning, formication, and hyperalgesia.
- The skin may be normal, lichenified, or pigmented. Notalgia paraesthetica has also been labelled a 'puzzling posterior pigmented pruritic patch'. Sensory examination may be normal, or the involved skin may be hypoaesthesic to pinprick or hyperaesthetic.
- Amyloid may be deposited within the affected skin (macular amyloid), probably 2° to chronic rubbing (see ➔ Box 23.3, p. 497).
- Capsaicin, which depletes neuropeptides from C-type sensory nerve fibres, may be helpful. Other options include topical local anaesthetic cream (e.g. lidocaine 2.5% with prilocaine 2.5%) or oral gabapentin.

Box 27.3 What is trigeminal trophic syndrome?

- Trigeminal trophic syndrome is an uncommon complication of damage to the trigeminal nerve. The syndrome most often follows trigeminal ablation by rhizotomy or alcohol injection into the Gasserian ganglion, but may be triggered by other causes of damage to the trigeminal nerve or its central connections such as cerebrovascular accidents, acoustic neuromas, syringobulbia, herpes zoster, or trauma.
- Irritating paraesthesiae or dysaesthesiae in the affected dermatome or a sensation of nasal congestion provoke compulsive self-mutilation. Picking and rubbing lead to ulceration.
- Patients may not be aware of their actions.
- Typically, ulcers involve the ala nasi, sometimes spreading to the adjacent lip and cheek. The scalp, forehead, ear, palate, or jaw may be affected.
- The tip of the nose (anterior ethmoidal nerve) and angle of the jaw (greater auricular nerve) are spared.
- Differential diagnosis includes infection (herpes simplex and zoster, deep fungal, syphilis, yaws, TB, leprosy), malignancy (BCC, SCC, lymphoma), vasculitis (granulomatosis with polyangiitis), and pyoderma gangrenosum.
- Biopsy shows non-specific inflammation.
- Management is difficult and requires a multidisciplinary approach.
- Educate the patient, and protect the skin with occlusive dressings. Carbamazepine, diazepam, and amitriptyline are of limited help. Surgical repair with a skin flap has been recommended.

Further reading

Hoeijmakers JG et al. Nat Rev Neurol 2012;8:369–79 (small-fibre neuropathies).
Mirzoyev SA and Davis MDP. Br J Dermatol 2013;169:1007–15.

Autonomic and motor dysfunction

Autonomic dysfunction and the skin

Autonomic dysfunction occurs in disease of peripheral small fibres (e.g. diabetes, vasculitis, HIV), disease affecting autonomic ganglia, and CNS disease (e.g. Parkinson disease, multiple system atrophy). Manifestations may be cardiac (e.g. postural hypotension, tachycardia, exercise intolerance), GI (e.g. dysphagia, abdominal pain, nausea, vomiting, malabsorption, diarrhoea, and constipation), genitourinary (e.g. erectile dysfunction), and metabolic (e.g. hypoglycaemia). Diabetes is one of the commonest causes of autonomic neuropathy, when it is usually accompanied by a sensory neuropathy.

Complex regional pain syndrome, a disabling condition that most often affects the hand, is associated with dysfunction of autonomic nerves. Skin abnormalities are common.

What should I look for?

- Alterations in microvascular skin circulation affect skin colour (erythema, cyanosis, oedema, delayed capillary refill, livedo reticularis) and may impair skin nutrition, contributing to dryness and cracking.
- Alterations in sweating.
- Dryness of the feet which predisposes to cracking and provides a portal of entry for infection. Diabetic patients with sudomotor dysfunction are more likely to develop foot ulcers (see ➜ Box 15.1, p. 295; and Fig. 15.4, p. 297).
- Gustatory sweating (hyperhidrosis associated with eating).
- Compensatory hyperhidrosis in normal skin if patients have a focal loss of sweating, e.g. in Ross syndrome (tonic pupil, areflexia, segmental hypohidrosis, or anhidrosis).
- Harlequin syndrome (see Box 27.4).

Box 27.4 Harlequin syndrome

- Caused by compromise of vasomotor and sudomotor sympathetic nerve supply to one side of the face. Half the face fails to flush during thermal or emotional stress. May also have tonic pupils, areflexia, and impaired sweating (Ross syndrome) on this side or Horner syndrome.
- Over-reaction of corresponding fibres on the intact side results in unilateral flushing and compensatory hyperhidrosis (sweating).
- Topical 0.5% glycopyrronium bromide or iontophoresis may reduce sweating.

Erythermalgia (erythromelalgia)

1° erythermalgia is a rare autosomal dominant channelopathy caused by gain-of-function mutations in *SCN9A*, the gene encoding the voltage-gated sodium channel NaV1.7. Hyperexcitable autonomic and nociceptive neurons cause incapacitating pain, refractory to analgesia. (Loss of function in *SCN9A* causes congenital insensitivity to pain.)

Acquired erythromelalgia is most often 2° to a myeloproliferative disorder associated with raised platelets (less often to autoimmune or rheumatological disease). Typically, aspirin relieves pain (see ➲ p. 538).

What should I look for?
- Intermittent attacks of severe burning pain, warmth, swelling, and redness of legs, feet, and occasionally hands.
- Bilateral and symmetrical symptoms and signs.
- Symptoms provoked by warmth, e.g. by bed clothes and exercise.
- Symptoms may last for minutes or hours.
- Skin may appear normal between attacks.
- Patients frequently give a history of soaking feet (and legs) in ice-cold water to relieve pain.
- Maceration with infections caused by prolonged immersion in water.

The motor system and the skin

Muscle weakness with abnormalities in gait or musculoskeletal deformity may lead to skin problems.

What should I look for?
- Callosities at pressure sites.
- Pressure sores caused by immobility.
- Use tone, power, coordination, and reflexes to determine whether pathology is central, peripheral, or both.
- ⚠ POEMS syndrome in patients with plasma cell disorders is a rare cause of motor and sensory neuropathy that starts distally and spreads proximally, mimicking chronic inflammatory demyelinating polyneuropathy (see ➲ Box 26.8, p. 540).

Further reading

Drenth JP *et al. Arch Dermatol* 2008;**144**:320–4. (p erythermalgia).
Kabani R and Brassard A. *JAMA Dermatol* 2014;**150**:640–2 (cutaneous findings in complex regional pain syndrome).
Lance J. *Pract Neurol* 2005;**5**:176–7 (Harlequin syndrome).

Neurofibromatosis type 1

Synonym: von Recklinghausen disease.

Neurofibromatosis type 1 (NF1), a RASopathy, is one of the commonest AD inherited conditions (1 in 3000 births). NF1 is caused by mutations in a large tumour suppressor gene encoding neurofibromin, a protein involved in the RAS/MAPK signalling pathways responsible for cell growth, proliferation, and differentiation.

NFI is associated with other conditions (see Box 27.5). The diagnosis is clinical. For some of the causes of café au lait spots, see Box 27.6. Lipomas or tissue overgrowth in Proteus syndrome (see ➲ Box 27.11, p. 561) may simulate the neurofibromas of NF1.

Diagnostic criteria: what should I look for?

Two or more of these clinical features establish the diagnosis:

- Six or more café au lait spots (macules or patches). Numbers increase in childhood. Spots in prepubertal children >5mm in diameter, but post-puberty >15mm. Usually have smooth outlines, but larger ones may be irregular. Intensity of colour varies, but most are pale brown. Fade in adulthood.
- Axillary or inguinal freckles, 1–3mm in diameter, develop later than café au lait spots. Freckling may also appear around the neck and in other skinfolds (for other causes of freckling, see ➲ p. 613).
- Two or more neurofibromas of any type, or one or more plexiform neurofibroma. Dermal neurofibromas also appear later than café au lait spots. Large numbers only develop in adulthood. They may occur at any skin site but usually spare exposed skin (e.g. face), except in severe cases (see Fig. 27.1). Apply gentle pressure to small neurofibromas, and they sink down into the skin, 'buttonholing'—a virtually pathognomonic sign. Neurofibromas are soft and may become pedunculated. Patients may develop thousands of disfiguring neurofibromas. subcutaneous neurofibromas may involve major peripheral nerves or nerve roots. Plexiform neurofibromas (usually congenital) track along nerves or infiltrate subcutaneous tissues, and are associated with local hypertrophy of bone and soft tissues. Overlying skin may be hyperpigmented, with increased hair growth (hypertrichosis).
- An optic pathway glioma.
- Two or more Lisch nodules (melanocytic hamartomas of the iris). The yellowish-brown nodules within the iris appear before neurofibromas and will confirm the diagnosis. They are easier to see with a slit-lamp than with the naked eye, so refer to an ophthalmologist.
- Sphenoid wing dysplasia or thinning of the cortex of long bones, with or without pseudarthrosis.
- First-degree relative with NF1 diagnosed by the presence of two or more of the above criteria.

Further reading

Boyd KP et al. J Am Acad Dermatol 2009;**61**:1–14 (review).
Ferrari F et al. JAMA Dermatol 2014;**150**:42–6 (early cutaneous signs in children).
Hirbe AC and Gutmann DH. Lancet Neurol 2014;**13**:834–43 (review).

Box 27.5 Other features associated with neurofibromatosis type 1

- Epilepsy and learning difficulties (often mild).
- Neurofibromas in bone or GIT (may bleed), spinal neurofibromas, glioblastomas. Malignant peripheral nerve sheath tumours often in plexiform neurofibromas (heralded by pain or rapid growth). (Dermal neurofibromas do not undergo sarcomatous change.)
- Phaeochromocytoma, duodenal carcinoids.
- Cardiovascular anomalies, e.g. pulmonary, renal, or cerebral artery stenosis, coarctation of the aorta. Rarely cutaneous vasculopathy.
- Skeletal deformity, e.g. scoliosis, leg bowing, short stature.
- Other tumours, e.g. GI stromal tumours, breast cancer, rhabdomyosarcomas, childhood leukaemia.
- Cutaneous features in young children that suggest NF1:
  - Multiple juvenile xanthogranulomas—yellow-brown papules or nodules. Resolve spontaneously.
  - Naevus anaemicus—multiple, usually on the neck and upper chest (see ➔ p. 562).

Box 27.6 Café au lait spots

Use UV (Wood) light to accentuate epidermal pigmentation in individuals with pale skin, so that café au lait spots are easier to see (see ➔ p. 640). Light brown, evenly pigmented, well-defined, flat café au lait spots occur in a variety of situations and rare syndromes:
- Ten percent of normal people have one or two café au lait spots.
- NF1: six or more café au lait spots.
- NF2: rarely >5 café au lait spots (see ➔ p. 554).
- Segmental NF1: café au lait spots localized to one segment of the body (mosaicism for mutation) (see ➔ pp. 554–5).
- Tuberous sclerosis: <6 café au lait spots (see ➔ pp. 556–7).
- McCune–Albright syndrome: <6 café au lait spots. Darker brown with a more irregular outline (like a map) and larger than in NF1. Usually unilateral (do not cross the midline) and most often trunk or proximal limbs. No axillary freckling. Also precocious puberty, endocrine abnormalities. Caused by mosaicism for activating mutations in the guanine nucleotide-binding protein, α-stimulating activity polypeptide (GNAS) gene. Mutations stimulate adenylate cyclase activity and cyclic adenosine monophosphate (cAMP) levels in multiple tissues. Always somatic—lethal if involves the germline.
- Cowden syndrome (see ➔ p. 542); Carney complex (see ➔ p. 613); multiple lentigines syndrome: multiple lentigines, sometimes café au lait spots (see ➔ p. 613).
- MEN type 1 and type 2B (see ➔ Box 22.18, p. 483).
- Autosomal mismatch repair gene mutations, ring chromosome syndromes, and DNA repair syndromes such as ataxia telangiectasia (see ➔ p. 612).
- Proteus syndrome (see Box 27.11, p. 561).

Other neurofibromatoses

Neurofibromatosis type 2

Neurofibromatosis type 2 (NF2) is a rare condition inherited as an AD disorder (incidence about 1 in 40 000). The NF2 tumour suppressor gene encodes the FERM domain protein (Merlin), which promotes the formation of intercellular contacts and regulates cell proliferation. The diagnosis is confirmed, if the individual has bilateral vestibular schwannomas or a family history of NF2 in a first-degree relative plus a unilateral vestibular schwannoma diagnosed by age 30 or any two of: meningioma, glioma, schwannoma, juvenile posterior subcapsular lenticular opacities/juvenile cataracts.

What should I look for?
- Café au lait spots: rarely >5, so do not meet criteria for NF1.
- Peripheral nerve tumours: less frequent than in NF1. Most often small (<2cm) discrete plaques with a rough surface (may be pigmented or hypertrichotic) or subcutaneous schwannomas. Dermal neurofibroma-like tumours are uncommon and few in number.

Segmental neurofibromatosis 1

Patients mosaic for a somatic mutation in the *NF1* gene have features of NF1 limited to one or a few body segments. Children may present with unilateral lentigines in the axilla or groin or a group of café au lait spots anywhere on the body.

The clinical features are determined by the timing of the mutation during the development of the embryo, but it is unusual to see both neurofibromas and café au lait spots. The segmental bands of neurofibromas probably follow the dermatomes (see Fig. 27.1), but pigmentary changes are more likely to follow the lines of Blaschko (see ⮕ p. 63).

Such patients rarely experience the complications found in generalized NF1 but should be advised about the low risk of having a child with generalized NF1.

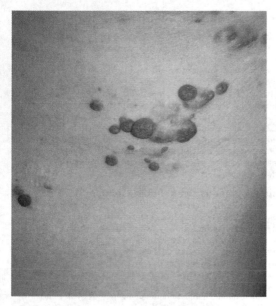

Fig. 27.1 Soft neurofibromas in a linear band in a patient with segmental neurofibromatosis.

Further reading
Cooper J and Giancotti FG. *FEBS Lett* 2014;**588**:2743–52 (molecular insights).

Tuberous sclerosis complex and skin

Synonyms: Bourneville disease, Pringle disease, epiloia.

A dominantly inherited condition (prevalence around 1 in 10 000) associated with learning difficulties (50% of cases) and epilepsy (35% of cases), as well as involvement of almost any organ (see ➔ p. 558). Ten to 20% of children with infantile spasms have tuberous sclerosis.

Two-thirds of cases are sporadic mutations. One of two tumour suppressor genes is involved in the pathogenesis of the hamartomas that are the hallmark of the disease. Mutations in *TSC1* (protein product hamartin) or *TSC2* (protein product tuberin) lead to upregulation of the mTOR pathway with uncontrolled cell growth. mTOR inhibitors, e.g. sirolimus or everolimus, may be helpful. Cutaneous signs, especially hypopigmented macules, may be of considerable help in making the diagnosis, particularly in children.

What mucocutaneous signs should I look for?

- Hypopigmented macules on the trunk and limbs. May be present at birth. Few or scattered widely in a confetti-like pattern. Hair within macules is hypopigmented (look for white streak in scalp hair). Ash leaf patch is a misnomer, as macules may be any shape. Cutaneous hypopigmentation is accentuated by examination of the skin under Wood light. But remember other causes of hypopigmentation, particularly post-inflammatory hypopigmentation (see Box 27.7).
- Forehead plaques (may be present at birth) on the scalp, face, or neck. Initially resemble capillary haemangiomas but evolve into firm, red, or yellowish brown plaques, with a histology of angiofibromas.
- Facial angiofibromas ('adenoma sebaceum') on nasolabial folds and cheeks. The erythematous papules and/or nodules appear in 85% of individuals after age 5 and slowly increase in number. Associated with telangiectasia. Often misdiagnosed as acne or rosacea—but no pustules (see ➔ p. 254). May respond to topical mTOR inhibitors.
- Shagreen patch (connective tissue naevus with increased collagen). Rare in infancy, but usually appear in adolescence. The orange-red patches develop most often on the lower back or thigh, varying in size from a few mm to 15cm. Dermal thickening may give the skin the feel of soft rubber. Surface may be dimpled like orange peel or slightly rough (resembles untanned leather or pig skin). Small 'gooseflesh' bumps may surround a larger central patch.
- Periungual fibromas (garlic clove tumours). Check toes, as well as fingers. The small, smooth, fleshy tumours arise from beneath the nail fold and may press down on the nail plate to produce a longitudinal groove. A single fibroma may occur in a normal individual (see Fig. 27.2).
- Skin tags around the neck: molluscum fibrosum pendulum.
- Subcutaneous occipital angiofibromas.

Box 27.7 Pale macules and patches

Hypopigmented macules or patches

Loss of pigment is partial. Skin is creamy, rather than bright white. A few hypopigmented macules may occur in normal individuals. Large numbers are more likely to be associated with an underlying condition (see ➲ pp. 89–90). You should decide:

- Was pigment loss preceded by inflammation? Post-inflammatory hypopigmentation is common in dark-coloured skin.
- Is the skin scaly? Consider pityriasis versicolor in young adults (see ➲ pp. 168–9).
- Is the texture normal? Localized scleroderma causes hypopigmentation, but skin is thickened (see ➲ pp. 420–1).
- One to 5% of normal individuals have a congenital naevus depigmentosus (despite the name, pigment loss is partial).

Depigmented macules or patches

The skin has a bright white tone and is a brighter white than hypopigmented skin, when examined under Wood light.

- Vitiligo is the commonest cause of acquired smooth depigmented macules or patches (see ➲ p. 486).

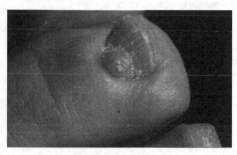

Fig. 27.2 Periungual fibroma in a child with tuberous sclerosis complex. Reproduced with permission from Lewis-Jones, Sue (ed). Paediatric Dermatology, Oxford University Press 2010.

- Oral angiofibromas on lips, gingiva, dorsum of the tongue, palate.
- Café au lait spots (<6) occasionally.
- Folliculocystic and collagen hamartoma. Papule or plaque studded with comedo-like openings. May occur on the scalp, trunk, or limb.

Further reading

Balestri R et al. J Eur Acad Dermatol Venereol 2015;**29**:14–20 (topical rapamycin).
Dill PE et al. Pediatric Neurol 2014;**51**:109–13 (topical everolimus).
Inoki K and Guan K-L. Hum Mol Genet 2009;**18**:R94–100.
Meetin RR et al. Brain Dev 2014;**36**:306–14 (manifestations in children)

Tuberous sclerosis complex and other organs

Tuberous sclerosis complex can involve numerous organs (see Box 27.8).

Box 27.8 Organ involvement in tuberous sclerosis complex

- Skin (see ➲ pp. 556–7).
- CNS: cortical 'tubers' (giant cell astrocytoma) associated with epilepsy (infantile spasms, partial seizures, absence seizures, and tonic–clonic seizures); behavioural problems, e.g. autism, hyperactivity, and/or learning disorders; and focal neurological deficits, e.g. mild hemiparesis. Giant cell astrocytoma may cause life-threatening raised intracranial pressure.
- Retinal astrocytomas (25% of patients): often asymptomatic.
- Cardiac rhabdomyomas (60% of patients at birth). Detect by echocardiography. May be multiple. Often asymptomatic and may regress. May cause heart failure (e.g. by outflow obstruction), arrhythmia, including Wolff–Parkinson–White syndrome, thromboembolism, or sudden cardiac death.
- Renal angiomyolipomas may cause haematuria.
- Renal cancer is rare. Renal cysts may cause hypertension and renal failure. *TSC2* is localized very close to the gene for AD polycystic kidney disease, and some patients have both conditions, but renal cysts also occur in tuberous sclerosis.
- Pulmonary lymphangioleiomyomatosis causes pneumothorax, haemoptysis, and respiratory insufficiency.
- Bone cysts and periosteal new bone formation—asymptomatic.

Epidermal naevus syndromes

These neurocutaneous syndromes are defined as the presence of epidermal and adnexal hamartomas associated with extracutaneous disease, most often involving the CNS, eyes, or skeletal system. Phenotypes vary, and understanding is evolving, but each syndrome probably reflects a different cutaneous mosaicism (see pp. 620–621, and Boxes 27.9 and 27.10). Extensive epidermal naevi, centrofacial epidermal naevi, or scalp epidermal naevi may be more likely to be associated with neurological or ophthalmological manifestations.

What should I look for?
- Linear epidermal or sebaceous naevus in Blaschko lines (see ➜ p. 620):
  - Verrucous (keratinocyte) epidermal naevus: pink, yellow, or brown linear array of papules usually present at birth. Becomes darker, more raised, and wart-like with age. Less common on the head and neck than the trunk or limbs. If on the scalp, may be associated with alopecia or abnormal hair (e.g. woolly hair naevus). Also see Proteus syndrome in Box 27.11.
  - Sebaceous naevus: yellowish smooth waxy plaque present at birth. Most often on the face or scalp (overlying hair is absent). Become more prominent in adolescence, when sebaceous glands enlarge. (Round or oval sebaceous naevi are commoner than linear lesions and much less likely to be associated with neurological problems, probably because linear lesions arise earlier in development.) (see ➜ Fig. 31.2, p. 595.)
- Other skin signs:
  - Hypo- or hyperpigmentation or café au lait macules.
  - Scalp aplasia cutis (see ➜ pp. 594–5, and Fig. 31.1, p. 595).
- CNS abnormalities, including:
  - Seizures, infantile spasms, or hemiparesis.
  - Intellectual disability or developmental delay.
- Eye problems, including:
  - Strabismus, lipodermoids, choristomas (congenital overgrowth of ectopic tissue), and colobomas (congenital defect when part of the eye does not form—may affect the choroid, iris, lens, optic nerve, or retina).
- Skeletal abnormalities, including:
  - Bony hypoplasia, bone cysts, abnormal skull shape, limb hypertrophy, kyphoscoliosis.
  - Spontaneous fractures, hypophosphataemic vitamin D-resistant rickets (described in association with both keratinocyte and sebaceous epidermal naevi).

Further reading
Happle R. *J Am Acad Dermatol* 1991;25:550–6.
Sugarman JL. *Semin Cutan Med Surg* 2007;26:221–30.

Box 27.9 Sebaceous naevus syndrome (uncommon)

Linear or extensive sebaceous naevus of the head (often centrofacial), with neurological and/or ocular abnormalities that may include:
- Intellectual disability.
- Seizures, especially infantile spasms, hemiparesis.
- Choristomas, colobomas.
- Skull asymmetry on the same side as the naevus.

All children with large sebaceous naevi should be assessed for neurological or ophthalmological problems.

2° tumours derived from adnexal structures may develop within sebaceous naevi. These are usually benign.

Box 27.10 Phacomatosis pigmentokeratotica (rare)

A combination of a linear sebaceous naevus in the lines of Blaschko and a speckled lentiginous melanocytic naevus in a checkerboard pattern (the pigmented patches do not cross the midline).
Associated problems may include:
- Mild intellectual disability and seizures.
- Segmental sensory abnormalities and segmental hyperhidrosis on the same side as the speckled lentiginous melanocytic naevus.
- Deafness.
- Ptosis and strabismus.
- Hemiatrophy with muscle weakness.

⚠ Box 27.11 Proteus syndrome (very rare)

Named after the Greek demigod Proteus, who could change his appearance. The condition is characterized by asymmetrical overgrowth (macrosomia) in a variety of tissues. Individual digits, limbs, or half of the body may be grossly enlarged. Before the features were delineated, patients were often considered to have NF1. The elephant man Joseph Merrick probably had severe Proteus syndrome, rather than neurofibromatosis. Intelligence is usually normal. Clinical features vary but may include:
- Hemifacial macrosomia or macroglossia.
- Skeletal anomalies, including hemihypertrophy, limb gigantism, and asymmetrical macrodactyly.
- Linear verrucous epidermal naevi following the lines of Blaschko.
- Vascular malformations, especially port wine stains.
- Connective tissue naevi, causing localized 'cerebriform' thickening of palmar or plantar soft tissues—may be misdiagnosed as plexiform neurofibroma, lipomas, or lipoatrophy.
- Visceral hamartomas.
- Choristoma of the eye.
- Café au lait macules have been reported.

Capillary malformations

Slow-flow capillary malformations (CMs) in the skin present at birth as port wine stains (PWS) (see Fig 31.4, p. 601). PWS are caused by a somatic activating mutation in the gene *GNAQ*. Rarely, PWS develop later in life. These vascular malformations never regress and may be associated with overgrowth of underlying tissues or ocular or neurological problems. In adults, PWS darken to deep purple and, on the face, may become hypertrophic. Laser surgery may be an effective cosmetic treatment, if carried out in infancy.

What should I look for?

- A red patch, present at birth, that enlarges with the growth of the child. Facial PWS are now thought to follow the embryonic vasculature of the face, rather than innervation by the trigeminal nerve.
- ❶ Neurological and ocular abnormalities in patients with facial PWS, involving the forehead and upper eyelid (Sturge–Weber syndrome) (see Fig. 31.4, p. 601 and Box 27.12).
- Naevus anaemicus with a well-defined serpiginous outline. A naevus anaemicus does not go red, if the skin is rubbed, but stands out more clearly from surrounding erythematous skin. Diascopy can also be used to confirm the diagnosis (see ➔ p. 641). Found in phakomatosis pigmentovascularis (see Box 27.13). May be sporadic.
- Naevus spilus or dermal melanocytosis (Mongolian spot) (see ➔ Fig. 31.10, p. 615), suggesting phakomatosis pigmentovascularis (see Box 27.13).
- Overgrowth of an affected limb: Klippel–Trenaunay (CM plus venous ± lymphatic malformations) or Parkes–Weber (CM plus AV malformation) syndrome.
- ⚠ Evidence of occult spinal dysraphism in patients with a midline lumbosacral PWS. Look for other signs such as a midline pit or dimple above the gluteal cleft, sinus, fibroma, or tuft of hair (faun's tail). Confirm with MRI. (Also see ➔ p. 594.)

Further reading

Dasgupta D and Fishman SJ. *Semin Pediatr Surg* 2014;23:158–61 (International Society for the Study of Vascular Anomalies classification).

Shirley MD et al. *N Engl J Med* 2013;368:1971–9 (mutation in PWS).

Waelchli R et al. *Br J Dermatol* 2014;171:861–7 (classification of PWS and prediction of Sturge–Weber syndrome).

Box 27.12 Sturge–Weber syndrome

(see ➲ Fig. 31.4, p. 601.) Neurological and ocular abnormalities occur in 10–15% of patients with a facial PWS involving the forehead (defined as any part of the forehead from the midline to an imaginary line between the outer canthus of the eye and the top of the ear, including the upper eyelids). The PWS is often extensive and may be bilateral.

- ⚠ Ocular problems 2° to choroidal vascular malformations include:
  - ❶ Glaucoma—may be congenital (buphthalmos). May develop slowly or present acutely with a cloudy cornea. This is a medical emergency. Need annual checks of pressures.
  - Retinal detachment.
  - Choroidal haemorrhage.
- Neurological problems associated with leptomeningeal vascular malformations, atrophy, and calcification of the affected cerebral hemisphere, absence of superficial cortical veins, and/or dilated deep-draining veins may include:
  - Seizures on the opposite side of the body or generalized.
  - Stroke-like episodes.
  - Neurodevelopmental delay.
  - Emotional or behavioural problems, attention deficit.
  - Headache.

❶ Refer for an urgent ophthalmology review (ideally on the first day of life) and a neurological assessment, including a brain MRI with gadolinium contrast (within the first 3 months of life). Prophylactic treatment with aspirin may be indicated, if MRI is abnormal.

Box 27.13 What is phakomatosis pigmentovascularis?

Definition: association of a widespread vascular naevus with an extensive pigmentary naevus. Associated with extracutaneous defects. A number of types have been described, including:

- Mongolian spots, dermal melanocytosis, and one or more PWS. Patients may also have naevus anaemicus and hypoplastic nails. Associations include CNS defects, ocular anomalies, asymmetrical length of the limbs, and dysplastic veins or lymph vessels.
- Naevus spilus (speckled lentiginous naevus) and a pale pink telangiectatic naevus. May be associated with unilateral lymphoedema, hemiparesis, seizures, or asymmetrical length of the legs.
- Naevus cesius (blue spot, aberrant Mongolian spot) and cutis marmorata telangiectatica congenita (reticulated vascular skin markings present since birth). Reported in association with asymmetry of hemispheres and ventricles, limb hyperplasia.

Other neurocutaneous disorders

Biotinidase deficiency

Rare AR inherited metabolic disorder. Prevented by treatment with biotin. May not present until adolescence. Partial deficiency may not present, unless the child is stressed.

Neurological problems include hypotonia, seizures, ataxia, developmental delay, hearing loss, and visual problems such as optic atrophy. Also hyperventilation, laryngeal stridor, and apnoea.

What should I look for?

- Eczematous periorificial skin rash—around the mouth, nose, and eyes. Differentiate from candidiasis and acrodermatitis enteropathica (see ➋ p. 513).
- Alopecia—total or partial.
- Recurrent viral or fungal skin infections.

Further reading

Wolf B. *Genet Med* 2012;**14**:565–75.

Skin and psychiatry

Contents

Relevant pages in other chapters
Porphyria ➔ pp. 330–1
Neuropathic pain and itch ➔ p. 648

Self-induced dermatoses

Self-mutilation

Lip licking, hair pulling (trichotillomania), and nail-biting are common childhood habits, with a good prognosis, that are not usually linked to an emotional disorder, but self-mutilation is used by some adults, usually young women, to relieve emotional stress. Tensions involving family or work may precede the onset. Self-mutilation may also be associated with learning difficulties and psychiatric conditions such as personality, eating, or mood disorders. Although patients may know what they are doing, they cannot easily stop the damaging behaviour. Serious self-harm associated with suicidal intent is a different problem.

- Cutting is probably the commonest form of episodic self-mutilation. Cuts are made in privacy to relieve tension and usually kept hidden.
- Obsessive–compulsive disorder—repeated hand-washing may lead to irritant contact hand dermatitis (see ⮕ p. 214).
- Endless picking, scratching, or gouging previously normal skin (psychogenic pruritus). Management is challenging (see Box 28.1, and ⮕ Box 10.5, p. 223).
- Acne excoriée (compulsive picking of mild acne lesions (see ⮕ pp. 242–3). A form of psychogenic pruritus. May be associated with obsessive–compulsive disorder or other body image disorders, e.g. anorexia nervosa. Self-inflicted scarring reinforces negative self-image.

Factitious disorders in dermatology

Deliberate and highly visible self-induced damage (dermatitis artefacta) may be used by patients who want to adopt the sick role and attract attention from other people, particularly doctors. Presents most often in young women (adolescence, early adulthood) and is usually an indirect 'cry for help' associated with stress, psychological illness, or psychiatric problems such as eating disorders. May complicate pre-existing skin disease.

- Lesions appear abruptly (often overnight) on normal-looking, exposed, and highly visible skin that is accessible to the patient, e.g. face, left side in a right-handed patient. Pattern is asymmetrical.
- History is vague, 'hollow', and unconvincing.
- Morphology depends on how lesions are induced, but well-defined, irregular, jagged, rather geometric outlines are common and unlike the smooth outlines of an endogenous skin disease. Signs may include crusted erosions, erythematous patches, blisters, sometimes with a linear streak suggesting contact with a caustic liquid that has dripped, purpura (produced by suction), ulcers, and oedema.
- Alternative diagnoses should always be considered (see Box 28.2).
- Patients deny damaging their skin, appear to lack insight into the problem, and are often reluctant to accept psychiatric help.
- Ideally, all patients should be managed by a multidisciplinary psychodermatology team.
- Confrontation, with the offer of support, may precipitate a different pattern of destructive behaviour or, very rarely, suicide.

Box 28.1 Management of psychogenic pruritus

- Assess thoughts and emotions before, during, and after the excoriation episode; enquire about sleep patterns, history of depression, suicidal ideations, and self-mutilating behaviours; and record previous use of psychiatric medications, as well as their effect on itch.
- What drugs is the patient taking? Any history of substance abuse?
- Do not accept a diagnosis of psychogenic pruritus, without excluding other contributory factors, especially scabies (see ➲ p. 172), no matter how long the history of itch.
- Exclude systemic causes of itch—iron deficiency, thyroid disease, renal failure, chronic liver disease, malignancies, HIV (see ➲ pp. 60–1).
- Look for excoriations, nodules, or ulcers on the skin that can be reached by the patient—typically the centre of the back is spared.
- Refer to a psychologist or psychiatrist for management of underlying psychological or psychiatric problem.
- Patients with an organic basis for itch may also have a psychogenic component and might benefit from psychological support.
- Trim nails.
- Prescribe soap substitutes and emollients, if the skin is dry (see ➲ p. 655).
- Occlusion, e.g. with Zipzoc®, will protect the skin from further damage (see ➲ pp. 660–1).
- Systemic options include antidepressants such as SSRIs or low-dose tricyclic antidepressants (amitriptyline, doxepin) which act as 'neuromodulators'. These drugs are often poorly tolerated, so start with a very low dose, e.g. amitriptyline 10mg at night.
- Topical corticosteroids are not helpful, unless the skin is inflamed.

Box 28.2 Dermatitis artefacta: differential diagnosis

- Physical or sexual abuse.
- Contact dermatitis: allergic or irritant.
- Phytophotodermatitis.
- Infection: bacterial, viral, fungal.
- Fixed drug eruption.
- Pyoderma gangrenosum.

Further reading

Gieler U et al. Acta Derm Venereol 2013;93:4–12 (terminology and classification).
Mohandas P et al. Br J Dermatol 2013;169:600–6 (artefactual skin disease and psychodermatology team).
Yosipovitch G and Samuel LS. Dermatol Ther 2008;21:32–41.

Localized dysaesthesias

Some patients complain of localized itching, tingling, or burning, without objective physical findings. These sensations may be linked to small-fibre neuropathies (see ➲ p. 548 and Box 28.3).

Frequently, these dysaesthesias are associated with underlying psychological factors, and they are exacerbated by stress. Women are affected more often than men. Some patients have fears of cancer or may have an associated body dysmorphic disorder (see ➲ p. 570).

Patients seek relief by trying a wide range of topical medicaments, and the conditions may be complicated by iatrogenic problems such as corticosteroid-induced skin atrophy or contact dermatitis (irritant or allergic).

The most frequent presentations are:

- Tingling, itching, or burning in the scalp.
- Burning scrotum.
- Burning vulva (vulvodynia).
- Burning mouth syndrome (often associated with an unpleasant taste) or glossodynia (usually affecting the anterior portion of the tongue).

What should I do?

- Set aside enough time to listen to the patient's concerns (this consultation is likely to be lengthy).
- Exclude an easily treatable cause for the symptoms such as irritant contact dermatitis. Refer for patch testing to exclude allergy.
- Check FBC, iron studies, and thyroid function.
- Discuss the diagnosis with a neurologist, if you suspect an underlying small-fibre neuropathy. Is there any loss of sweating? New diagnostic techniques include measurement of nerve fibre density in a skin biopsy.
- Reassure the patient that you understand the problem and that the condition is well described—sometimes patients have been dismissed by other professionals and despair of getting help.
- Explain that the skin/mucosa looks entirely normal and that the sensations may be a result of very sensitive nerve endings (whether this is true or not, it can be a helpful way of looking at things).
- If appropriate, reassure the patient that symptoms are not a sign of cancer or another serious disease.
- Prescribe soothing topical treatments such as emollients and soap substitutes (see ➲ p. 655).
- Avoid potent topical corticosteroids.
- A low dose of amitriptyline can be very helpful but may be poorly tolerated, so start with a very low dose (amitriptyline 10mg at night). Doxepin is an alternative. Explain that these drugs are prescribed for their action as 'neuromodulators', rather than antidepressants.
- Psychological support: a support group or cognitive behavioural therapy may be helpful.

Box 28.3 Causes of small fibre-neuropathies

Many small-fibre neuropathies are idiopathic, but consider:
- Diabetes, hypothyroidism.
- Chronic renal failure.
- LE and other connective tissue disease.
- Amyloidosis.
- Sarcoidosis.
- Leprosy, EBV, HIV, HCV.
- Malignancy.
- Drugs and toxins: alcohol, antiretroviral drugs, bortezomib, metronidazole, nitrofurantoin.
- Fabry disease.

Further reading

Flores S et al. Br J Dermatol 2015;**172**:412–18 (small-fibre neuropathies).
Hoeijmakers JG et al. Nat Rev Neurol 2012;**8**:369–79 (small-fibre neuropathies).
Yosipovitch G and Samuel LS. Dermatol Ther 2008;**21**:32–41.

Delusions

What is a delusion?
See Box 28.4.

Body dysmorphic disorder
Synonyms: dysmorphophobia; dermatologic non-disease.

Patients with a normal appearance become preoccupied by imaginary problems such as too much or too little hair, scars, vascular marks, acne, facial redness, or facial asymmetry. Patients attribute their personal failings at work or social difficulties to the 'defect' and may be tempted to spend large sums of money in an attempt to alleviate the 'problem'. Some young women devastated by what they perceive to be 'severe' acne may demand repeated courses of isotretinoin.

What should I do?
- Avoid doing anything that might produce changes such as redness, scars, or pigment that will cause even more dissatisfaction. Cosmetic surgery is unlikely to satisfy the patient.
- Encourage the patient to see a psychologist or psychiatrist for mental health assessment, especially if considering cosmetic surgery.
- Sadly, these patients are rarely satisfied with any treatment, have little psychological insight, and are most unlikely to accept that nothing is wrong.

Delusional infestation
Synonym: delusional parasitosis

Patients hold a fixed, but false, belief that they are infected with living pathogens, e.g. parasites, bacteria, mites, worms, or insects, as well as inanimate materials, e.g. fibres, crystals, needles, or 'Morgellons' (an Internet-induced disease). Delusions may be shared by one or more family members or close friends. The delusion may follow a real infestation or be linked to recreational drug abuse, dementia, or an underlying organic disease, but commonly no cause is found.

The patient will demonstrate skin signs (caused by scratching or picking) and describe how pathogens, e.g. 'insects' or 'threads', have been extracted from the skin. You are likely to be presented with a 'specimen sign'—a small container containing carefully collected 'proof' of infestation, e.g. particles of skin, hair, cloth, or plant.

What should I do?
- Search for true infestation, and study all specimens thoroughly to reassure the patient and establish trust.
- Acknowledge and discuss the 'skin sensations'.
- Exclude other causes of thought disorders or formication (crawling sensations), including abuse of alcohol or recreational drugs such as cocaine or amphetamine. Treat any underlying disease.
- Encourage the patient to accept help from a psychodermatologist or psychiatrist (this may be difficult).
- Prescribe antipsychotic drugs (see Box 28.5).

Box 28.4 Terminology

Definitions

- *Hypochondriasis*: an excessive and persistent fear of having a serious physical illness. Fears usually develop in response to minor physical abnormalities. The person is amenable to reassurance, but the impact of reassurance is only temporary.
- *Delusion*: a false personal belief that is not subject to reason or contradictory evidence and is not explained by a person's usual cultural and religious concepts. A delusion may be firmly maintained in the face of incontrovertible evidence that it is false.
- *Delusions of hypochondriasis*: a fixed belief that a problem is due to a serious physical disease, despite evidence to the contrary.

Box 28.5 Management of delusional infestation

- Prescribe soothing topical treatments, e.g. emollients.
- Counsel the patient, and explain why an antipsychotic may be helpful to control 'skin sensations'.
- Discuss the side effects of antipsychotic drugs—smaller doses are needed for delusional infestation than for schizophrenia.
- Atypical antipsychotic drugs, such as risperidone (a small dose, e.g. 0.5–1mg/day may be effective) or olanzapine (5–10mg/day), are better tolerated and safer than other antipsychotics. Aripiprazole (5–15mg/day) has also been recommended.
- Pimozide <6mg/day was the traditional treatment but has more extrapyramidal adverse effects, and, in higher doses, is associated with cardiotoxicity, including prolongation of the QT interval and sudden death.

Further reading

Ahmed A and Bewley A. *Br J Dermatol* 2013;**169**:607–10 (delusional infestation).
Freudenmann RW et al. *Br J Dermatol* 2012;**167**:247–51 (delusional infestation).

Eating disorders and skin

Cutaneous symptoms or signs may be the first presentation of anorexia nervosa (restrictive type) or bulimia nervosa (restrictive with inappropriate compensatory behaviour such as self-induced vomiting or laxative and diuretic abuse), conditions in which patients, usually young women, fear fatness and pursue thinness.

Cutaneous features may be caused by starvation (skin changes are most frequent in patients with a BMI of ≤16kg/m^2), adverse effects of drugs taken to induce weight loss, or complications related to self-induced vomiting. Hypothyroidism and vitamin deficiency contribute to changes, and cutaneous manifestations may resemble those seen in HIV infection.

Patients may also have other skin conditions related to an underlying psychiatric disease such as a self-induced dermatosis (see ➔ pp. 566–7).

What should I look for?

Cutaneous signs of starvation
- Loss of subcutaneous fat, pitting oedema (pretibial or pedal).
- Dry skin with fine scaling or asteatotic eczema (see ➔ p. 220).
- Generalized pruritus, sometimes with prurigo (see ➔ p. 222).
- Cheilitis, acne.
- Generalized hyperpigmentation or melasma (pigment localized to the face) (see ➔ Box 30.1, p. 583).
- Cold intolerance with acrocyanosis and perniosis.
- Paronychia, brittle nails, and/or interdigital intertrigo.
- Dry brittle scalp hair, diffuse hair loss (telogen effluvium), and/or hypertrichosis with fine lanugo-like body hair.
- Acquired striae distensae.
- Orange palms (carotenoderma).
- Pellagra (niacin deficiency), scurvy (vitamin C deficiency), acrodermatitis enteropathica (zinc deficiency) (see ➔ p. 513).
- Petechiae and purpura in association with hypoplastic bone marrow and thrombocytopenia.
- Poor wound healing.

Drug-related adverse effects
- Fixed drug eruption (e.g. phenolphthalein-containing laxatives).
- Photosensitivity with thiazide diuretics.
- Finger clubbing associated with laxative abuse.

Complications of self-induced vomiting
- Single or multiple calluses on knuckles (Russell sign).
- Dental enamel erosion and gingivitis.
- Benign, usually bilateral, painless parotid gland enlargement.
- Transient facial purpura from increased intrathoracic pressure.
- Subcutaneous emphysema and/or spontaneous pneumomediastinum.

Further reading
Strumia R. *Clin Dermatol* 2013;31:80–5.

Skin in older people

Contents

Ageing skin

The changes observed in old skin are caused by a combination of intrinsic and extrinsic ageing. Skin undergoes genetically programmed senescence (intrinsic ageing), but exposed skin is also modified by environmental factors (extrinsic ageing), the most important of which is UV light (photoageing) (see ➔ p. 43). Mechanical trauma and chemicals, such as nicotine, also alter skin. Changes are cumulative. Compare the appearance of sun-protected intrinsically aged skin on a covered site, such as the buttock, with exposed extrinsically aged, photodamaged skin (face, forearm, back of the hand).

Intrinsic ageing

- Abnormal epidermal barrier function and abnormal lipids lead to increased permeability and water loss with dryness and fissuring.
- Variable epidermal thickness with loss of rete ridges reduces epidermal adhesion and predisposes to blistering.
- Loss and fragmentation of dermal collagen fibrils and degenerate elastin result in thin weak skin, inelasticity, and fine wrinkles (see Box 29.1).
- Fewer active melanocytes impair photoprotection.
- Fifty percent decrease in Langerhans cells impairs cell-mediated immunity.
- Age-related alterations in dermal extracellular matrix (ECM) may provide a microenvironment that supports the development of skin cancers.
- Reduced dermal microvasculature and changes in ECM contribute to delayed wound healing.
- Benign neoplasia, e.g. cherry angiomas, seborrhoeic warts.

Photoageing

UVR accelerates the intrinsic ageing process, including the accumulation of fragmented connective tissue fibres (collagen and elastin), and is responsible for many of the signs we associate with old age, including deep wrinkles, leathery appearance, purpura, and dyspigmentation (see ➔ Box 3.1, p. 43; and Box 29.1).

Further reading

Fisher GJ et al. Br J Dermatol 2014;**171**:446–9.
Quan T and Fisher GJ. Gerontology 2015;**61**:427–34.

Box 29.1 Collagen synthesis in ageing skin

- Collagen-rich ECM is synthesized by dermal fibroblasts. Collagen production is upregulated in stretched fibroblasts attached to specific binding sites on collagen fibrils.
- Fibroblasts also produce matrix metalloproteinases (MMPs) that degrade collagen.
- TGF-β upregulates collagen synthesis by fibroblasts and downregulates the activity of MMPs.
- Young sun-protected skin has low levels of MMP activity.
- Ageing skin: downregulation of TGF-β signalling and elevation of MMPs result in the loss of ECM and skin thinning.
- Elevated cysteine-rich protein 61 (CCN1) may contribute to skin ageing by reducing the synthesis of dermal ECM and promoting the activity of MMPs.
- MMPs do not degrade cross-linked collagen fibrils, and these slowly accumulate in the dermis with ageing. Fragmented collagen lacks binding sites for fibroblasts. Fibroblasts that cannot attach adequately to collagen downregulate the production of collagen but upregulate MMPs, leading to further fragmentation.
- Photoageing: UV exposure also reduces collagen synthesis and accelerates collagen fibril breakdown by increasing the level of MMPs, adding to the impact of intrinsic ageing.

Common conditions in older patients

Old skin, much like the skin of neonates, is easily irritated or traumatized, and should be handled gently. Although no one dies of old skin, skin disease lowers quality of life.

Examine all the skin in older patients (see Box 29.3).

What should I look for?

Common skin conditions in older people include:
- Dry itchy skin.
- Eczema: asteatotic, varicose, seborrhoeic, contact (irritant > allergic). Chronic eczematous eruptions may be associated with drugs such as calcium channel blockers or thiazides.
- Skin infections, particularly fungal in skin creases.
- Toenail dystrophy: poor vision or reduced mobility may mean that patients cannot cut their toenails (filing is safer than cutting or clipping). Fungal infection may complicate problems such as onychogryphosis (thick distorted nails).
- Scabies.
- Adverse drug reactions.
- Leg ulcers, pressure sores or traumatic erosions, and blisters.
- Premalignant changes, skin cancers, and benign skin tumours.

What should I do?

- Management may be challenging in older people (see Box 29.2).
- Poor hearing, vision, or memory may interfere with adherence to treatment plans, so keep the treatment simple.
- In some circumstances, it may be much more practical for the older patient to take a systemic treatment, despite the risk of adverse effects, than to apply topical treatments.
- Provide information sheets (in large print, if necessary) and a written treatment plan.

Box 29.2 Practicalities of treatment in older patients

- Impaired mobility may make it difficult to reach parts of the skin or to apply topical treatments.
- Difficulties bathing or showering or washing the scalp.
- Risk of falls if the bath is slippery, e.g. 2° to bath oils.
- Reactions to topical treatments: irritancy > allergy.
- Incontinence contributing to an irritant contact dermatitis.
- Immobility and obesity may contribute to intertrigo (sweating and irritation of skin in flexures).
- Poor vision may make it difficult to apply treatments correctly.
- Poor memory and difficulty following guidance.
- Interactions between systemic medicaments.
- Sedating antihistamines may cause confusion or falls.
- Information may have to be passed on to a carer, who is not present at the consultation.

**Box 29.3 Assessing older patients:
a dermatological checklist**

- Sun damage and skin cancer are common in older people: inspect all the skin, but pay particular attention to sun-exposed skin on the face, scalp, and ears.
- Inspect the skin under wigs or hairpieces.
- Do spectacles or hearing aids fit comfortably, without traumatizing the skin? Look behind the ears.
- When were false teeth last checked by a dentist? Angular cheilitis is common in individuals with ill-fitting dentures.
- Inspect the nails: can the patient cut (or file—much safer!) their fingernails and toenails? Should the patient see a podiatrist or chiropodist? It is easier to cut thick nails if they have been softened by soaking in warm water, e.g. after a bath.
- Painful subungual corns, particularly if containing a focus of haemorrhage, may simulate malignancy.
- Inspect the skinfolds and perineum: intertrigo is common in older patients. Causes include irritant contact dermatitis 2° to incontinence, as well as infection (*Candida* or tinea).
- Look at areas subjected to pressure, particularly the sacrum, and check cushions or wheelchairs, as well as shoes.
- Remove bandages: do not accept the diagnosis of 'leg ulcer', without examining the ulcer. BCCs on the leg are frequently misdiagnosed as 'ulcers'.
- Are compression bandages or stockings applied correctly, so that they run smoothly from the base of the toes to just below the knee (and stay in place)? Is there ridging or blistering of the skin beneath the bandage, suggesting poor bandaging technique? (see ➜ Box 15.10, p. 307; Box 34.4, p. 661; Fig. 34.1, p. 661.)
- Are the legs oedematous and eczematous, because the patient is immobile and spending much of the day in a sitting position ('armchair legs')? Would periods of elevation or compression stockings be helpful?
- Ensure that the skin is not being traumatized by appliances, such as indwelling urinary catheters, or by adhesive tape.

Dry itchy skin and asteatotic eczema

Most older people have dry itchy skin (xerosis) that is easily irritated. Symptoms often deteriorate after admission to hospital, because the skin is dried out by enthusiastic washing with soap, a low humidity, and central heating. Some patients with very dry skin develop asteatotic eczema. Itch may be distressing, interfering with sleep and significantly impacting on quality of life (see ➔ Fig. 10.2, p. 220).

What should I ask?

- Find out precisely what the patient or carer is using to wash the skin or is putting in the bath.
- Is the patient putting anything on the skin? Check precisely how any treatments have been used (see ➔ pp. 30–1).
- Take a full history, including a drug history (see ➔ pp. 18–21).
- Is anyone else itchy? Remember the old lady with 'a rash' who is in the same nursing home, the spouse with 'hand dermatitis', or the grandchild with 'eczema' may well have scabies.

What should I look for?

- Dry, slightly scaly skin.
- Asteatotic eczema: the skin is very dry and has a network of shallow erythematous fissures in the epidermis that produce an appearance that resembles 'crazy paving' (eczema craquelé). Asteatotic eczema usually starts on the shins but may spread in a patchy fashion to the thighs and trunk. Intensity of itch varies (see ➔ Fig. 10.2, p. 220).
- Some very itchy patients may have 2° changes such as excoriations or nodules (prurigo nodularis) where the skin is being scratched (the centre of the back is usually spared) (see ➔ p. 222, and Fig. 10.6, p. 223).
- Look for evidence of an infestation such as scabies (burrows or crusting between the fingers). Older patients with scabies may have a widespread crusted scaly rash—Norwegian scabies (see ➔ p. 172 and Box 8.1, p. 173).
- Signs of another skin disease, e.g. bullous pemphigoid, an autoimmune blistering disease that commonly presents in older people. Itchy, erythematous, 'urticated' papules may appear months before the tense blisters (pre-pemphigoid) (see ➔ p. 270).

What should I do?

- Investigate to exclude a systemic cause for the itch (see Box 29.4).
- Soap substitutes and emollients should be sufficient to settle the irritation in most patients with dry skin (see ➔ p. 655 and Box 29.5).
- Prescribe a mild or moderately potent topical corticosteroid ointment to use bd on inflamed skin (see ➔ p. 656).
- If the itch persists, despite these measures, check the treatment is being used correctly (is the skin still dry?); look for scabies again, and re-evaluate for a systemic disease, before considering the possibility of a psychogenic component to the itch (see ➔ Box 28.1, p. 567).

Box 29.4 Causes of itch in older patients

- Dry skin with asteatotic eczema, particularly on the shins.
- Another 1° skin disease—remember pre-pemphigoid (see ➋ p. 270) or infestation (scabies) (see ➋ p. 172).
- Systemic disease:
  - Iron deficiency.
  - Thyroid disease.
  - Cholestatic jaundice.
  - Chronic renal failure.
  - Polycythaemia.
  - Lymphoma, myeloma.
- Drugs:
  - Statins (also cause dryness).
  - ACE inhibitors.
  - Opiates.
  - Barbiturates.
  - Antidepressants.
  - Calcium channel blockers and, less often, thiazides cause chronic eczematous eruptions in older people.

Box 29.5 Managing dry itchy skin

- Trim nails to prevent damage to skin from scratching.
- Avoid soap or excessive bathing (water should not be too hot).
- Prescribe a creamy emollient for daytime use and a greasier emollient for the evening. Show the patient or carer how to use the treatment (see ➋ p. 655).
- Recommend a soap substitute but beware of making the bath or shower slippery, and avoid other bath additives (see ➋ p. 655).
- Aqueous cream with 1% menthol or crotamiton lotion may relieve itch if emollients are not effective.
- Occlude very itchy skin with a paste bandage or Zipzoc® stocking. This is soothing and protects the skin from fingernails (see ➋ pp. 660–1).
- Consider prescribing a sedating antihistamine, but risk of confusion or falls in older patients.
- Consider wet wraps (see ➋ p. 662).

Skin and pregnancy

Contents

Relevant pages in other chapters
Subacute cutaneous lupus erythematosus ➔ Box 19.7, p. 403
Antiphospholipid syndrome ➔ Box 20.10, p. 453

Skin in pregnancy

The changes in skin and hair that occur during pregnancy are linked to the physiological hormonal changes during gestation, including:
- Synthesis of human chorionic gonadotrophin (peaks at week 12).
- Production of progesterone and oestrogen from the corpus luteum.
- Alterations in thyroid function and increased output of gonadotrophins and ACTH.

What skin signs should I look for?

- Hyperpigmentation: more marked in women with dark hair. Some pigment tends to persist post-partum in dark-skinned women.
  - Nipples, areolae, axillae, vulva, perianal, and scars.
  - Abdomen: a central line of pigmentation (linea nigra) that is usually most marked below the umbilicus but may extend higher.
  - Face: the 'mask of pregnancy' (melasma) (see Box 30.1).
  - Increased numbers of melanocytic naevi (moles) and darkening or enlargement of pre-existing melanocytic naevi and freckles (see Box 30.4).
  - Generalized hyperpigmentation (less common than focal).
- Vascular: increased vascular permeability and proliferation:
  - Palmar erythema.
  - Cutis marmorata, purpura, and petechiae affecting the legs.
  - Spider naevi predominantly in areas drained by the superior vena cava (face, neck, arms, and hands). Capillary haemangiomas usually on the head and neck. Also pyogenic granulomas of the oral mucosa.
  - Varicose veins: lower legs, vulva (also haemorrhoids).
- Connective tissue:
  - Striae gravidarum/distensae ('stretch marks') predominantly on the abdomen and breasts. Appear in the third trimester. Initially pink or purple and fade, leaving white depressed bands. Never disappear entirely.
  - Skin tags (molluscum fibrosum gravidarum) on the neck and axillae; involute partially after delivery.
- Hair:
  - Thickening of hair during pregnancy.
  - Diffuse loss (telogen effluvium) 2–4 months post-partum, causing thinning of hair (not baldness). Shedding continues for 6–24 weeks, and then hair regrows (see p. 24 and p. 44).
- Nail:
  - Ridging, splitting, distal onycholysis, longitudinal melanonychia.
- Excoriations:
  - One in five pregnant women develop itching (commonly first/second trimester)—may be localized or generalized (see pp. 584–5).
  - A shift to Th2 cytokines in pregnancy may trigger atopic eczema, even in patients with no previous history of atopy.

Box 30.1 Melasma

Synonym: chloasma.

- Melasma is increased pigmentation that is most often centrofacial (forehead, cheeks, upper lip, chin) or malar (cheeks), but may involve the mandibular ramus or forearms. Pigment is brown and distributed in blotchy, smooth, flat patches.
- Exposure to sunlight increases pigmentation.
- Melasma occurs most often in pregnancy or in women taking oral contraceptives, but may be seen in men (particularly Asian men) and women who are not taking any hormones.
- The melanin pigment may be mainly epidermal (contrast is accentuated by examination of the skin using Wood light), dermal (no accentuation under Wood light), or mixed (see ➲ p. 640).
- The differential diagnosis includes post-inflammatory hyperpigmentation, including pigmentation 2° to contact dermatitis. Ask if a rash or itching preceded the colour change.
- Tends to fade post-partum, particularly in fair-skinned women.
- Rigorous photoprotection (hats, sunblock creams) is crucial in management (see ➲ pp. 338–9).
- Avoid irritating the skin, particularly dark-coloured skin, as this may increase hyperpigmentation (post-inflammatory hyperpigmentation).
- Persistent epidermal melasma may be treated for 6–12 months with 20% azelaic acid cream or 0.05% tretinoin cream (may irritate) or creams containing 2–4% hydroquinone in combination with tretinoin and a mild corticosteroid to prevent irritation, but response may be disappointing.
- Oral tranexamic acid 250mg bd demonstrated utility as an adjunct.
- Sun protection must be continued during treatment and even after pigment has faded.
- Avoid prolonged treatment with creams containing >4% hydroquinone, as these can cause exogenous ochronosis with permanent hyperpigmentation, particularly in dark-skinned patients.
- Cosmetic camouflage may be helpful (✆ www.changingfaces.org.uk/Skin-Camouflage).
- Dermal melasma is unresponsive to treatment.

Further reading

Arrese M et al. Expert Rev Mol Med 2008;10:e9.
Geenes V and Williamson C. World J Gastroenterol 2009;15:2049–66.
Vaughan Jones S et al. BMJ 2014;348:g3489.

Pregnancy-specific dermatoses

What should I ask?
- When did symptoms start—before or after the onset of the third trimester?
- Is there a rash—where did it start, e.g. in striae? Any blisters?
- Any past or family history of skin problems or atopy?
    - Exacerbation of pre-existing inflammatory skin disease common.
    - Any rash in previous pregnancies or when taking the contraceptive pill?

What should I look for?
Evidence of scratching without a 1° rash
Excoriations or firm erythematous nodules (prurigo), but background skin is not inflamed or scaly. The centre of the back is usually spared.
- Search for other causes of itching such as scabies (see Box 30.2).
- Is the patient jaundiced? Intrahepatic cholestasis of pregnancy is associated with risk to the fetus (see Box 30.3).

With a 1° rash (30–50%)
Erythematous scaly skin, wheals, or blisters. Consider:
- *Atopic eruption of pregnancy* (common). Starts earlier than other specific dermatoses (before third trimester). The scaly, erythematous, eczematous rash is often flexural. Some patients also have prurigo or follicular papules. Commonly recurs in subsequent pregnancies.
- *Polymorphic eruption of pregnancy.* Starts late in pregnancy or immediately post-partum. Smooth, erythematous, 'urticated' papules and plaques (like wheals, but do not come and go) appear in abdominal striae. *Spares the periumbilical skin*. May exhibit Koebner phenomenon (rash in scars). Occasional vesicles, usually associated with scratching. Rash spreads to buttocks/proximal thighs and distal sites. Commonest in primigravidas (linked to excessive maternal weight gain) and multiple gestation pregnancies. Resolves within 4–6 weeks spontaneously. No effect on the mother or fetus.
- △ *Pemphigoid (herpes) gestationis* (rare). Autoimmune blistering disease that usually starts in the second or third trimester. IgG antibodies bind to BP180 in hemidesmosomes of the BMZ of skin. Crops of urticated, erythematous papules, vesicles, or tense bullae on the abdomen. *Involves the periumbilical skin*. Spreads to the trunk and limbs. Usually settles 4 weeks post-partum but may persist for longer. May recur and be more severe in subsequent pregnancies. Recurrence may occur with hormonal treatment or menstruation. Associated with small-for-date babies; 10% of infants have a transient rash (see ➔ pp. 270–271).

What should I do?
- Check LFTs and serum bile acid levels to exclude intrahepatic cholestasis (see Box 30.3).
- Take a skin biopsy for histology and direct IMF to distinguish polymorphic eruption of pregnancy from pemphigoid gestationis. In

pemphigoid gestationis, direct IMF shows linear deposition of C3, with or without IgG, at the dermo-epidermal junction. Direct IMF is negative in polymorphic eruption of pregnancy.

- Treat with emollients (1% menthol in aqueous cream), potent topical corticosteroids (see ➡ p. 655 and p. 656), and, if needed, chlorphenamine. Prednisolone (0.5–1mg/kg/day) may be required in pemphigoid gestationis.

Box 30.2 Causes of itch in pregnancy

- Consider causes unrelated to pregnancy (see ➡ p. 660) such as:
  - Infestations (scabies) or infections (viral, bacterial, or fungal).
  - Systemic disease (renal, hepatic, haematological, HIV).
  - Drugs.
  - Contact dermatitis.
  - Exacerbation of a pre-existing dermatosis.
- Intrahepatic cholestasis of pregnancy (see Box 30.3). Onset usually in third trimester.
- Specific dermatosis of pregnancy (see ➡ p. 584):
  - Atopic eruption of pregnancy (includes eczema in pregnancy, prurigo of pregnancy, and pruritic folliculitis of pregnancy). The commonest dermatosis of pregnancy. Onset early in pregnancy.
  - Polymorphic eruption of pregnancy—common. Also known as pruritic urticarial papules and plaques of pregnancy (PUPP). Onset late in pregnancy or immediately post-partum.
  - Pemphigoid gestationis (rare). Onset in second or third trimester.

Box 30.3 Intrahepatic cholestasis of pregnancy

- Intrahepatic cholestasis (raised serum bile acids) causes itching—often nocturnal and affects palms and soles.
- Itch may recur in subsequent pregnancies. Abnormal biliary transport is probably caused by a combination of genetic factors, the cholestatic effect of sex hormones (mainly oestrogens), and environmental factors (seasonal, dietary, geographic). May also be caused by the contraceptive pill.
- Itch usually commences around 25–32 weeks of gestation but clears promptly post-partum. Worse in twin pregnancies.
- Serum bile acids, alkaline phosphatase, and aminotransferases are raised. Jaundice occurs in 10–25% of patients.
- ⚠ Associated with placental insufficiency, premature labour, and sudden fetal death. Placental anoxia may be caused by decreased fetal elimination of toxic bile acids. Fetal monitoring essential.
- Ursodeoxycholic acid alleviates itch, improves liver enzymes, and prolongs the duration of pregnancy.
- Other options include emollients, 1% menthol in aqueous cream, and sedating systemic antihistamines (chlorphenamine).

Other skin conditions in pregnancy

For other skin conditions and pregnancy, see Box 30.4.

> ### Box 30.4 Other skin diseases in pregnancy
>
> *Melanoma in pregnancy*
> - Moles may naturally darken during pregnancy. Apply the ABCDE rule—any suspicious changing or new melanocytic naevus should be excised (see ➔ p. 354). Melanoma incidence is not increased during pregnancy. There is no effect on survival in women diagnosed with localized malignant melanoma (MM) during pregnancy (prognosis related to AJCC staging prognostic factors; see ➔ Table 17.1, p. 355). Pregnancies prior or subsequent to a diagnosis of MM do not impact prognosis. Risk of metastasis to the placenta and/or fetus is extremely low and occurs exclusively in women with widespread metastatic disease (AJCC stage IV; see ➔ Table 17.1, p. 355). There is no enhanced risk of developing MM associated with oral contraceptive pill use or hormone replacement therapy.
>
> *Systemic lupus erythematosus*
> - Increased risk of flares during pregnancy. Corticosteroids are the treatment of choice but do not prevent flares. Associated with increased risk of miscarriage, fetal loss, pre-eclampsia, preterm delivery, and fetal growth restriction. Anti-Ro antibodies can cross the placenta, with 5% risk of cutaneous neonatal LE—scaly, annular eruption on the face/scalp within first 2 weeks of life. Rash disappears spontaneously within 6 months; scarring unusual. Congenital heart block, detected *in utero* at around 16–18 weeks gestation, incurs a risk of perinatal mortality. (See ➔ Box 19.7, p. 403.)
>
> *Psoriasis*
> - Typically improves but, in 10–20%, can worsen. Increased risk of low-birthweight infants in women with severe psoriasis. Treatment includes emollients, topical corticosteroids, localized calcipotriol, and UVB. Ciclosporin and anti-TNF therapies can be used under specialist supervision for very severe disease. (See ➔ pp. 202–3)
>
> *Acne vulgaris*
> - Often improves in early pregnancy but worsens in third trimester. Avoid topical and systemic retinoids (teratogenic). Oral erythromycin is the first choice for treatment after 1st trimester (cardiac risk to the neonate, if used in early pregnancy). Azithromycin or clarithromycin preferred in first trimester. Acne neonatorum may occur as a result of transfer of maternal androgens across the placenta during the final trimester. (See ➔ p. 246.)

Box 30.4 (*Contd.*)

Rosacea
- Often worsens during pregnancy. Topical azelaic acid and metronidazole can be used. Oral erythromycin in second/third trimesters. (See ➲ p. 254.)

Pityriasis rosea
- Associated with HHV-6 infection. Conservative management. (See ➲ p. 151.)

Erythema nodosum
- Can be triggered during pregnancy with tender, erythematous nodules/plaques over legs. Supportive treatment. Resistant or severe cases may justify a short course of oral prednisolone. (See ➲ p. 458.)

Safety of treatments in pregnancy

Most drugs are not studied in pregnancy, and there are little data about safety of common medications in pregnancy. Congenital malformations may occur during the first trimester—the greatest risk is from weeks 3 to 11 of pregnancy. Drugs should only be prescribed, if benefits outweigh the risks, but remember suboptimal treatment of the mother might also be harmful to the unborn child.

Topical medicaments

- Antifungals: safe when used topically.
- Corticosteroids: mild to potent topical corticosteroids are safe to use in pregnancy. Large amounts (>300g during entire pregnancy) of very potent topical corticosteroids may be linked to low birthweight.
- Calcipotriene (topical vitamin D): no data, probably safe topically.
- Coal tar: limited data. Avoid in first trimester.
- Retinoids: contraindicated.
- Tacrolimus: no data, probably safe when used topically.

Oral medicaments

- Antibiotics: penicillins, erythromycin, clindamycin—appear safe.
- Antivirals: aciclovir, valaciclovir, famciclovir—appear safe.
- Antihistamines: chlorphenamine—probably safe. Cetirizine appears safe in third trimester.
- Antifungals: avoid itraconazole (risk of abortion). Terbinafine: no data.
- Azathioprine: risks not established but may be associated with low birthweight or spontaneous abortion. Avoid, if possible.
- Ciclosporin: may be associated with prematurity, growth retardation, or impaired immune function. Avoid, if possible.
- Dapsone: folic acid should be given throughout pregnancy. Risk of neonatal haemolysis and methaemoglobinaemia. May cause kernicterus—avoid in late pregnancy.
- Prednisolone: 88% of prednisolone is inactivated, as it crosses the placenta. Short-term treatment is safe. Prolonged or repeated treatment may be associated with intrauterine growth restriction.
- Methotrexate: teratogenic. Avoid in pregnancy. ♂ and ♀ should use effective contraception during treatment and for at least 3 months after stopping the drug. May also reduce fertility.
- Retinoids: teratogenic. ♀ must use effective contraception during treatment. Acitretin: continue contraception for at least 2 years after withdrawing treatment. Isotretinoin: continue contraception for at least 1 month after withdrawing treatment.
- Adalimumab: appears safe, but limited data.

Further reading

Chi CC et al. *JAMA Dermatol* 2013;**149**:1274–80.
Murase JE et al. *J Am Acad Dermatol* 2014;**70**:401–14 (part I) and 417–26 (part II).

Skin in infancy and childhood

Contents

Relevant pages in other chapters

Skin of the neonate: the first 28 days

The skin of a full-term infant

- Fine desquamation at 24–48h of age. Increased desquamation in post-mature babies. Persists up to 1 week. WSP is a safe emollient.
- Increased heat loss with reduced vasoconstriction.
- Permeable, particularly if occluded or in high temperatures or humidity. Topical agents are easily absorbed and may be toxic.
- Wash with unperfumed, neutral-pH cleanser. Rinse and dry completely. Aqueous chlorhexidine is a safe antimicrobial.
- Minimal eccrine sweating, more on the forehead than trunk and limbs. Emotional sweating (palms, soles) in response to pain or hunger.

The skin of a premature infant

- Thin, very fragile skin prone to mechanical injury (e.g. from tapes or electrodes) may leave scars, apparent after a few months. Protect injuries with occlusive dressings. Avoid adhesive tapes.
- Very permeable. Large transepidermal water loss (20–50% of body weight in 24h). Loss is increased by phototherapy and heat.
- Immature thermal homeostasis—loss of body heat. No sweating.

Some transient neonatal skin changes

- Vascular changes:
  - Cutis marmorata. A physiological net-like (reticulate) pattern of purplish red mottling that disappears on warming.
  - Capillary ectasia (salmon patch) on the nape (stork bite), eyelids (angels' kisses), and/or glabella. Most resolve in months or years. May persist on the nape of the neck.
  - Petechiae on upper body caused by pressure during delivery.
  - Harlequin colour change (rare). Reddening of dependent side of body, with sharp midline demarcation and blanching of the upper side. Episodes last seconds to minutes. Seen most often in premature infants lying on one side. Episodes cease after 3 weeks.
- Sebaceous hyperplasia: creamy papules on nose. Last a few weeks.
- Milia: 1–2mm firm, yellowish papules on face. Last a few months.
- Pigmented macules:
  - Mongolian spots (dermal melanosis). Blue-grey macules on the sacrum or low back. Most often in black or Asian neonates. May be multiple and can be confused with bruises. Disappear by age 4 (see Fig. 31.10).
- Blisters and pustules (see ➔ p. 592).
- Perianal dermatitis:
  - Erythematous macules, 2–3mm, that may be eroded or bleed. Occurs between days 4 and 7. Commoner in premature infants. Associated with feeds of formula milk (see ➔ p. 604).

⚠ More worrying signs

- Perinatal injury (see Box 31.1).
- Subcutaneous nodules or plaques (see Box 31.2).
- Purpuric macules or nodules (see Box 31.3).

Box 31.1 Cutaneous signs of perinatal injury

- Caput succedaneum: swelling over presenting part of scalp caused by pressure on the head during labour. Vacuum extraction—haematoma and oedema. Forceps—facial erythema or abrasions.
- Needle marks: hypopigmented speckles. Heel pricks may leave calcified nodules. Scalp electrodes may leave cuts, superficial ulcers, or, uncommonly, abscesses.
- Ring of alopecia 'halo scalp ring' caused by pressure during labour. Usually over the vertex and associated with caput succedaneum. Sometimes necrosis. If severe, may leave permanent scarring alopecia.
- Amniocentesis scars: more apparent after a few weeks; 1–5mm cutaneous dimple-like scars. Most often on extremities.

Box 31.2 Subcutaneous nodules or plaques in neonates

Neonate appears well

Subcutaneous fat necrosis. One or more circumscribed, firm, mobile subcutaneous nodules in first few months of life. Most often on the back or buttocks. Sign of preceding fetal stress, hypothermia, or difficult labour with ischaemic fat injury. May calcify or ulcerate. Usually resolves within 6 months. Prognosis good, but monitor for hypercalcaemia.

Sick neonate

⚠ Sclerema neonatorum. Generalized yellowish hardening of the skin that occurs in very sick preterm neonates. Treat the underlying condition, and, if the infant survives, hardening resolves.

⚠ Box 31.3 Blueberry muffin baby

Bluish purple, non-blanching (purpuric) macules, papules, and/or nodules are produced by extramedullary erythropoiesis in the dermis. Usually involves the head, neck, and trunk. Causes include:
- Congenital infections, e.g. toxoplasmosis, other, rubella, cytomegalovirus (commonest), herpes simplex ('TORCH').
- Haematological disease, e.g. haemolytic disease of the newborn, hereditary spherocytosis, twin–twin transfusion syndrome.
- Malignancy/proliferative diseases, e.g. leukaemia, neuroblastoma, congenital rhabdomyosarcoma, Langerhans cell histiocytosis.

Investigate to determine the cause (including skin biopsy) (see ➲Box 33.4, p. 649), and manage the underlying condition.

Pustules and blisters

Blisters are discussed in detail in ➲ Chapter 13, pp. 259–75, but here we consider some problems specific to infants and children. Blisters may evolve into pustules. Consider infection, infestation, dermatitis, or trauma, before much less common or very rare blistering diseases.

What should I ask?

- Is the child sick—any fever, lethargy, loss of appetite?
  - Could blisters/pustules be caused by a systemic disease or drug?
- When did the problem start—neonatal or childhood?
- Is the problem localized or generalized?
- What triggers blisters or pustules?
  - Are sun-exposed sites affected more than covered sites?
  - Is the skin fragile? Do blisters occur at sites of friction, e.g. feet? Or in heat? (Sweating may exacerbate EB; see ➲ pp. 624–5).
  - Are mucosal surfaces affected?
- Any post-inflammatory pigment, scarring, or milia?
- Is there a family history of skin problems, e.g. maternal autoimmune blistering disease (IgG autoantibodies cross the placenta and may cause transient blisters in the neonate)?

Neonatal vesicles, pustules, or papulopustules

See Box 31.4.

Vesicles, pustules, or papulopustules in childhood

- Infections and infestations:
  - Scabies: vesicopustules on palms and soles in infants usually at least 4 weeks of age. Is the mother itchy? (see ➲ p. 172).
  - Virus: HSV, including eczema herpeticum (see ➲ p. 152), VZV, CMV, EBV, Coxsackie virus (hand–foot–mouth disease).
  - Bacterial: *Staphylococcus aureus* (bullous impetigo, SSSS; see ➲ pp. 136–7), *Streptococcus, E. coli, Haemophilus influenzae, Klebsiella pneumoniae*.
- Contact dermatitis, including phytophotodermatitis (see ➲ Box 16.4, p. 327).
- Trauma, including burns (see ➲ p. 110).
- Erythema multiforme (see ➲ p. 111).
- Drug-related: phototoxic or photoallergic (see ➲ p. 326), SJS or TEN (see ➲ pp. 116–20).
- Mastocytosis (see Box 31.5).
- Rare: EB (see ➲ pp. 624–5, and p. 593), photosensitivity (see ➲ Box 16.5, p. 329), acrodermatitis enteropathica (zinc deficiency—unusual before age 4 weeks; see ➲ p. 513), autoimmune (see ➲ pp. 260–75).

What should I do?

- Identify the 1° lesions: vesicle or pustule. Remember these may evolve into erosions or ulcers.
- Exclude infection: culture fluid or pus for bacteria, *Candida*, and herpesvirus.
- A Tzank smear may help you to make the diagnosis (see ➲ p. 647).

Box 31.4 Vesicular and pustular eruptions in neonates

Swabs sterile

- Erythema toxicum neonatorum: onset age 1–3 days. Mainly trunk. One to 2mm yellowish papules or pustules with an erythematous halo (like flea bites). Fluctuates. Resolves in 2–3 days. Eosinophils in smear (very common).
- Transient pustular melanosis: usually in black neonates. Present at birth. Flaccid, 1–2mm pustules on the chin, neck, and trunk evolve to pigmented macules. Persists a few months. Neutrophils in smear.
- Miliaria: clear, fragile vesicles, papules, or pustules caused by occlusion of sweat ducts. Induced by heat and high humidity.
- Sucking blisters or trauma, including burns.
- Aplasia cutis may look bullous (see Box 31.6).
- Acropustulosis of infancy: crops of very itchy vesicles and pustules on hands and feet. Usually black neonates (neutrophils in Tzank smear). Lasts 1–2 years (uncommon). Exclude scabies (see ➡ p. 172).
- Benign cephalic pustulosis (neonatal 'acne'): pustules on the face and scalp. No comedones. Onset age 2 weeks. Persists about 2 months. May be reaction to *Pityrosporum* yeasts (see ➡ p. 602).
- Rare: maternal immunobullous disease (IgG autoantibodies cross the placenta), EB, incontinentia pigmenti (eosinophils in Tzank smear; look for linear pattern; examine the mother) (see ➡ pp. 636–7).

⚠ *Infection: neonate may not appear unwell*

- Bacterial infection, e.g. staphylococcal/streptococcal impetigo (common), SSSS (see ➡ pp. 136–7), listeriosis (rare cause of pustules and petechiae).
- Cutaneous candidiasis (may be congenital).
- HSV or VZV: look for scars (multinucleated giant keratinocytes in Tzank smear) (see ➡ p. 647).

Box 31.5 What is mastocytosis?

Uncommon conditions in which mast cells accumulate in skin and other organs. Linked to mutations in *KIT* gene. Systemic mast cell disease (raised serum tryptase) is extremely rare in children.

Presentations in childhood:
- Mastocytoma: localized reddish yellow macule, plaque, or nodule. Develops in infancy. Swells and may blister when rubbed (Darier sign). Blistering less frequent with age. Nodules resolve slowly.
- Urticaria pigmentosa: freckle-like macules. Urticate (become erythematous and raised), if rubbed. Improves by adolescence.
- Diffuse cutaneous mastocytosis: very rare. Mast cells disseminated widely in skin. Skin may be erythematous, leathery, or normal. Generalized blistering in infants aged <3, may mimic SSSS. Systemic symptoms include itch, flushing, hypotension, syncope, diarrhoea, and dyspnoea. Tends to improve with age.

Congenital cutaneous lesions

⚠ Midline congenital skin lesions on the spine may be a marker for occult spinal dysraphism (incomplete fusion of midline mesenchymal, bony, or neural structures). Cord tethering is a common complication. Ask about a family history of neural tube defects. Midline lesions on the face or scalp may have intracranial connections. Consider imaging, if clinically suspicious.

Back or perianal skin: what should I look for?

Occult spinal dysraphism is more likely in the presence of two or more cutaneous signs. Look for neurological symptoms or signs (may be subtle or none in neonate) and urogenital or anorectal abnormalities. Suggestive signs include:

- Lumbosacral markers, e.g. deep or large midline dimples >2.5cm from the anus or dermal sinus tract (may leak cerebrospinal fluid), localized tuft or patch of hypertrichosis (faun's tail), aplasia cutis, skin tags (check the gluteal cleft), lipoma, telangiectatic patch (PWS) or haemangioma near the midline.
- Asymmetrical curved gluteal cleft.
- Palpable vertebral defects.

Face or scalp: what should I look for?

- Midline dermoid cyst (firm subcutaneous nodule): those on the nose or occipital scalp are most likely to have intracranial extension. Punctum with hairs increases the chance of intracranial connection.
- Midline nasal mass or pit ± overlying skin discoloration may have an intracranial connection. Hair may protrude from the pit.
- Nasal glioma: firm, non-compressible blue or skin-coloured nodule on the side of the nose. May widen the nasal bone with hypertelorism. May have intracranial connection.
- Cephalocoeles: midline, 1–4cm, bluish, compressible, subcutaneous nodule on the nose (encephalocoele) or scalp (most often occipital) or circular area of alopecia, with a translucent membrane (may look bullous). Indications of possible intracranial involvement:
  - Enlarges with crying. May be pulsatile.
  - Transilluminates.
  - Scalp—overlying PWS (see Fig. 31.1).
  - Scalp—hair collar sign: a rim of dark coarse hair around the bald patch. This marker for ectopic neural tissue is also seen in membranous aplasia cutis congenita (see Fig. 31.1). If hair collar present, image to look for skull defect and to exclude cephalocoele. If no connection, may either be heterotopic brain tissue (meningothelial and/or glial tissue in subcutaneous tissue or dermis) or membranous aplasia cutis congenita (see Box 31.6).
- Sebaceous naevus: yellowish plaque with loss of hair. Most often oval. If linear (following Blaschko lines), may be associated with neurological problems (see ➜ p. 560 and Fig. 31.2).

Box 31.6 What is aplasia cutis congenita?

In this rare condition, localized areas of skin are absent at birth. Can occur anywhere. Aetiology is uncertain but may relate to incomplete closure of embryonic fusion lines.

- Aplasia cutis congenita has been classified into nine groups. All, but group 1 (commonest type), have associated abnormalities.
- Most cases are sporadic, rarely inherited in an AD or AR pattern.
- Usually presents as a 1–2cm circular or oval bald patch near the vertex of the scalp. Rarely affects the face (focal facial dermal hypoplasia) and other areas.
- Appearance varies—most often a bald patch appears to be covered by a shiny translucent membrane (membranous aplasia cutis), but the skin may be eroded, deeply ulcerated, or scarred.
- Membranous aplasia cutis is usually surrounded by a hair collar (see ➜ pp. 594–5 and Fig. 31.1).
- On scalp, may be associated with an underlying skull defect.
- May be >1 lesion.
- Extensive aplasia cutis of the trunk is associated with fetus papyraceus (defects may be caused by placental infarcts after death of a twin fetus). Also malformations in other organs.
- Differential diagnosis: obstetric trauma (e.g. forceps injury), HSV or VZV infection, EB (rare).

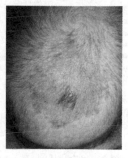

Fig. 31.1 Membranous aplasia cutis congenita with dark hair collar and surrounding capillary malformation.

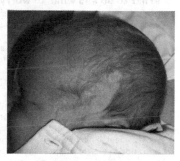

Fig. 31.2 Linear sebaceous naevus— yellowish smooth plaque and absence of overlying hair.

Further reading

Baselga E et al. Pediatr Dermatol 2005;22:13–17.
Bellet JS. Semin Perinatol 2013;37:20–5.
Frieden IJ. J Am Acad Dermatol 1986;14:646–60.
Guggisberg D et al. Arch Dermatol 2004;140:1109–15.

Infantile haemangioma

Synonyms: strawberry haemangioma, capillary haemangioma.

Infantile haemangiomas are common benign proliferative tumours, both disfiguring and alarming. To differentiate from other vascular tumours and malformations (see ➔ p. 598, pp. 600–1), endothelial cells in infantile haemangiomas are glucose transporter 1 (GLUT1)-positive (biopsy rarely required).

What should I look for?

- Seen most often in girls and preterm babies (may be multiple).
- Fifty percent occur on the head and neck.
- Infantile haemangiomas are not apparent at birth, but parents may notice a pale, telangiectatic or erythematous macule (may resemble a PWS).
- Bright red, dome-shaped nodules or plaques evolve in the first month of life. Some have a deeper bluish component (see Fig. 31.3).
- Growth phase: rapid for 3–4 months; slow for 6–18 months. Deep components grow for longer.
- Involution. Colour slowly fades; nodules soften and shrink; 50–60% involute completely by age 5 years, 70–75% by age 7 years, and 90% by age 9 years. Residual changes may include pallor and lax skin.
- Deeper components may persist.

⚠ What to do and when to worry

- Most do not require treatment, regressing spontaneously, without significant sequelae. Discuss the likely outcome with the parents. Photographs may be useful to document evolution and resolution.
- A minority of enlarging infantile haemangiomas need early treatment to prevent disfigurement or organ compromise (see Box 31.7).
  - Periocular: may obstruct vision and lead to permanent amblyopia. Refer for urgent visual assessment. MRI if displacement of the globe or thickening of the lid.
  - Mandibular or neck area: internal infantile haemangiomas may cause airway obstruction. If noisy breathing, stridor, or difficulty breathing when feeding, refer for urgent ENT assessment.
  - Lips: infantile haemangiomas may interfere with the ability to suck.
- Ulceration in the growth phase (see Box 31.8).
- Plaque-like facial haemangioma may be associated with PHACE (Posterior fossa malformations, Haemangioma, Arterial abnormalities, Coarctation of the aorta, and Eye abnormalities). Called PHACES if also Sternal clefting and/or Supraumbilical raphe.
- Plaque-like lumbosacral haemangioma: look for tags or dimples in the genital and sacral areas. May be associated with spinal dysraphism and/or multiple congenital anomalies (see ➔ p. 594).
- Large plaque-like haemangiomas are more likely to be associated with a systemic problem. Investigate with imaging, e.g. magnetic resonance angiography (MRA), MRI.
- Five or more cutaneous haemangiomas: rarely associated with disseminated haemangiomatosis (liver, heart, and other internal organs). Most not life-threatening. Age >6 months: unlikely to be problems.
- Bleeding disorder: review the diagnosis. (See Box 31.9.)

Box 31.7 Management of infantile haemangiomas

An enlarging infantile haemangioma may lead to irreversible disfigurement (central face, nasal tip, lips) or compromise organ function. β-blockers are the treatment of choice, ideally from age 4–6 weeks.

- Propranolol: gradually increase from 1mg/kg/day to 2mg/kg/day in three equal doses. Continue for 12–18 months. Well tolerated. Side effects include hypoglycaemia (feed regularly) and sleep disturbance. Risk of rebound growth of infantile haemangioma on stopping treatment.
- Use with caution in PHACE: risk of stroke if arterial anomalies.
- Topical timolol maleate 0.5% solution may have a role.
- Other options:
  - Topical potent corticosteroid or imiquimod for superficial periorbital infantile haemangiomas.
  - Intralesional corticosteroids in localized infantile haemangiomas—nasal tip, lip.

Box 31.8 Ulcerated infantile haemangiomas

- Large infantile haemangiomas growing rapidly may ulcerate, particularly infantile haemangiomas affecting anogenital skin, the neck, or the lower lip. Appearance of a grey-white colour on the surface of infantile haemangioma may herald ulceration.
- Ulceration is painful, particularly in the anogenital region.
- Ulcers usually heal in 2–3 weeks, but deep ulcers cause scarring.
- Bleeding is usually minimal.
- Monitor for infection (uncommon)—spreading erythema, warmth, and pain—and swab for bacterial culture.
- Treatment options:
  - Wound care: soak off crusts; apply white soft paraffin to protect skin.
  - Antibiotic ointments. Occlusive dressings.
  - Topical lidocaine has been advocated for pain relief (pea-sized amount, no more than qds).
  - Paracetamol for pain control.
  - Oral propranolol is now the treatment of choice (see Box 31.7).
  - Topical potent or very potent corticosteroid ointment may relieve pain and speed involution, as well as re-epithelialization.
  - Pulsed dye laser may relieve pain and speed healing.

Further reading

Luu M and Frieden IJ. *Br J Dermatol* 2013;**169**:20–30 (reviews infantile haemangioma and propranolol).
Solman L et al. *Arch Dis Child* 2014;**99**:1132–6 (propranolol protocol).

Other vascular tumours

Infantile haemangioma, the commonest infantile vascular tumour, should be differentiated from other vascular tumours, mostly much less common, including:

- Pyogenic granuloma: very common in childhood, but rare in infants <3 months of age. Friable vascular papule, often on the head or neck. Bleeds readily (see ➲ p. 343).
- Eruptive pseudoangiomatosis: sudden eruption of vascular papules. Usually facial. Age infancy to 6 years. Possibly viral aetiology. Resolves in 1–2 weeks.
- Glomangiomas: many bluish nodules (some may be congenital). Numbers increase slowly. Familial, AD inheritance.
- Congenital haemangiomas (CHs): rare. Resemble infantile haemangiomas, but fully developed at birth. May regress (RICH) by 12–14 months or no involution (NICH). Endothelial cells GLUT1-negative, unlike infantile haemangioma.
- Verrucous haemangioma: congenital linear vascular plaque with overlying hyperkeratosis. Mainly limbs. Wilms tumour antigen (WT1) and GLUT1-positive. Has some features of a vascular malformation (see ➲ pp. 600–1).
- Tufted angioma and kaposiform haemangioendothelioma: rare. Enlarging purplish red patches, indurated plaques, and/or nodules. Partial lymphatic endothelial immunophenotype. Associated with Kasabach–Merritt syndrome (see Box 31.9).

Box 31.9 What is Kasabach–Merritt syndrome?

The rare association of a vascular tumour with thrombocytopenia (platelet trapping in tumour) and sometimes microangiopathic haemolytic anaemia and a 2° consumptive coagulopathy.

- Occurs with some rare enlarging vascular tumours of infancy/childhood, e.g. tufted angioma and kaposiform haemangioendothelioma (not seen in infantile haemangioma).
- Podoplanin-positive endothelium in tumours binds CLEC-2 receptor on platelets, activates platelets and initiates clotting in tumour.
- ⚠ Look for a purplish, tender, rapidly enlarging deep dermal nodule or plaque surrounded by petechiae or bruising and prolonged bleeding at other sites.
- May be life-threatening. Check FBC with film (low platelets, fragmented RBC) and fibrinogen level.

Further reading

Colmenero I and Hoeger PH. *Br J Dermatol* 2014;**171**:474–84.
Hoeger PH and Colmenero I. *Br J Dermatol* 2014;**171**:466–73.

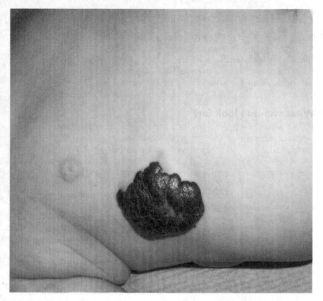

Fig. 31.3 A large infantile haemangioma with both superficial and deep components. The superficial component will resolve, but some of the deeper component may persist.

Vascular malformations

Malformations may be predominantly capillary, venous, lymphatic, arterial, or AV, or any combination of these. Distribution may be localized or diffuse. Malformations may be present at birth or only become apparent in childhood. Unlike infantile haemangiomas, most malformations do not involute but persist and may slowly worsen with age. Many capillary malformations occur in CM–AV malformation syndrome (see Box 31.10).

What should I look for?

- Port wine stain (PWS): malformation with dilated capillaries. Somatic mosaic activating mutation in GNAQ in affected tissue. May be associated with complex vascular syndromes:
    - Limb PWS may be associated with Klippel–Trenaunay (varicose veins, capillary, or mixed capillary–lymphatic malformation) or Parkes–Weber (multiple AV shunts) syndromes. Look for varicosities, haemangiomas, lymphangiomas, and hypertrophy, with gradual asymmetrical lengthening of the affected limb.
    - ❶ Facial PWS involving the forehead and upper eyelid may be linked to Sturge–Weber syndrome (see ➋ p. 562 and Fig. 31.4). Seizures are a frequent complication. Early and regular ophthalmological review required to detect glaucoma.
- Cutis marmorata telangiectatica congenita: very rare malformation with dilated capillaries and veins in the dermis and subcutis.
    - A network of purplish red bands with some telangiectasia. Persists when skin is warm.
    - Involved skin may be atrophic and may ulcerate.
    - Girth of the involved limb may be reduced—less fat, muscles, and/or bone.
    - Rarely associated with other congenital problems.
    - Fades partially over years.
- Venous—slow flow: elevated D-dimer levels.
    - Subtle bluish compressible vessels—no thrill or bruit.
    - May swell when dependent.
    - Can be associated with chronic localized or diffuse intravascular coagulopathy. ❶ In patients with large venous malformations, minor surgery may trigger DIC.
- AV—fast flow: normal D-dimer levels.
    - Most often head and neck.
    - May be subtle initially, like a PWS.
    - Look for local warmth, subtle thickening. Rarely a thrill or bruit.
    - Potentially life-threatening haemorrhage.
- Lymphatic: normal D-dimer levels.
    - Cystic hygroma: mass, usually in the neck or axilla that presents in the neonate. Collections of dilated lymphatics in the dermis, with superficial vesicles that intermittently leak clear fluid.
    - Localized group of vesicles: lymphangioma circumscriptum. These appear during childhood. Commonest on the proximal limbs and limb girdle.

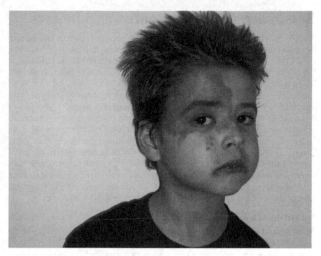

Fig. 31.4 The distribution of facial port wine stain probably follows the embryonic vasculature of the face, rather than the innervation of the trigeminal nerve. Facial port wine stain involving the forehead may be associated with cerebral and ocular vascular malformations (Sturge–Weber syndrome). Complications include seizures, stroke, and glaucoma (see ➲ p. 562).

Box 31.10 Capillary malformation–arteriovenous malformation syndrome

AD disorder, usually with loss-of-function *RASA1* mutations, but clinically and genetically variable. Features include:
- Numerous CMs—congenital and acquired (more with age). Multifocal and randomly distributed; 1–3cm in diameter, and oval or circular. Often surrounded by a pale halo.
- Less often large or irregular CMs.
- Partial or total absence of vellus hair over CMs.
- Punctate red spots surrounded by pale halos on upper extremities.
- Grouped telangiectasias on the neck/upper trunk.
- Naevus anaemicus has been noted in some cases.
- AV malformations and/or AV fistulae in one-third. Involve the skin, muscle, bone, spine, and brain. Risk of cerebral haemorrhage and sensorimotor deficits. MRI may be indicated to exclude intracranial and spinal AV malformations, if the diagnosis is suspected.

Further reading

Martin-Santiago A et al. Br J Dermatol 2015;**172**:450–4.
Orme CM et al. Paediatr Dermatol 2013;**30**:409–15.

Red scaly skin in neonates and infants

Atopic eczema (dermatitis), the commonest cause of redness and itching in children, does not usually present until around the age of 3 months (see ⊃ p. 606). Neonates with red scaly skin are much more likely to have infantile seborrhoeic dermatitis, which presents in the first month and usually clears after 3 or 4 months.

⚠ Severe generalized erythema and scale (neonatal erythroderma) associated with failure to thrive is rare but suggests an underlying problem (see Boxes 31.11 and 31.12). In some forms of ichthyosis, the neonate is born encased in a tight, smooth, shiny collodion membrane (collodion baby). The tight skin causes dysmorphic features, including ectropion (lower eyelid turned outwards), eclabium (lip turned outwards), malformed ears, and flexion contractures. In both erythroderma and collodion babies, the barrier function of the skin is abnormal, leading to fluid loss, infection, poor thermoregulation, and absorption of topical agents. Use bland emollients, and control humidity (see ⊃ pp. 626–7).

Infantile seborrhoeic dermatitis

What should I look for?
- A well infant, not particularly itchy (atopic eczema is very itchy).
- A greasy, erythematous, scaly, orange-red papular rash involving the face, scalp ('cradle cap'), and flexures. Look in skinfolds, particularly around the neck and in the napkin area (usually spared in atopic eczema) (see Fig. 31.6). Irritant napkin dermatitis involves convex surfaces and spares the skinfolds (see Box 31.12 and Fig. 31.5). Rash may be secondarily infected by *Candida*. Some infants develop tiny sterile pustules (see neonatal acne in Box 31.4).

What should I do?
- Explain that the condition should clear by about 4 months of age.
- Bath with emollients to reduce scale and crust. Avoid soaps which may irritate the skin.
- A mild topical corticosteroid combined with an antifungal bd will reduce redness. Avoid more potent corticosteroids.
- Remove scalp scale with olive oil or an emollient such as Hydromol® ointment.

Langerhans cell histiocytosis

This rare disease may be misdiagnosed as infantile seborrhoeic dermatitis. ⚠ Purpura and ulceration should alert you to 'something different'. A skin biopsy will confirm the diagnosis. Look for:
- Erythematous pink or brown, scaly, crusted papules on the trunk, in the napkin area, and in flexures that may become confluent.
- Purpuric papules that may ulcerate and weep.
- Scaling and crusting on the scalp. The scalp bleeds, when scale is removed (a useful sign).
- Fever (sometimes).
- Isolated skin involvement may regress spontaneously, but refer for assessment and treatment.

Box 31.11 Scaly skin—differential diagnosis

Common

- Atopic eczema (see ➔ pp. 606–7).
- Seborrhoeic dermatitis (see ➔ p. 602).
- Scabies (see ➔ p. 172).
- Keratosis pilaris: scaly follicular papules on lateral aspects of arms and thighs, and sometimes cheeks. Not itchy. Skin feels rough.
- Psoriasis (much less common than eczema in childhood) (see ➔ pp. 189–208). Usually a family history of psoriasis.
- Ichthyosis vulgaris: fine pale scale, increased skin markings on palms. Presents after age 3 months. Mutation in filaggrin gene.

Rare

- Langerhans cell histiocytosis (see ➔ p. 602). Refer to a specialist for assessment and treatment.
- Netherton syndrome: erythroderma (diffusely red and scaly), failure to thrive, hypernatraemic dehydration, and sparse hair. Mutations in *SPINK5* gene that encodes the lymphoepithelial Kazal-type 5 serine protease inhibitor (LEKTI) lead to uncontrolled proteolytic degradation of the corneodesmosomes and a thin, highly permeable stratum corneum. May find characteristic hair shaft abnormality—trichorrhexis invaginata (bamboo hair) on the scalp or eyebrow, and later a characteristic rash—ichthyosis linearis circumflexa. Also raised IgE, atopy, and food allergies. Skin very permeable—risk of infection and absorption of topical agents.
  - ⚠ Avoid topical corticosteroids or topical calcineurin inhibitors.
- Nutritional deficiency, including:
  - Zinc deficiency (see ➔ p. 513): well-demarcated periorificial and perineal glazed erythema, paronychia, dermatitis on the fingers and toes.
  - Cystic fibrosis: periorificial and perineal rash like in zinc deficiency (see ➔ Box 24.6, p. 517)
  - Biotin deficiency: eczematous or psoriasiform rash around the eyes, face, and perineum. Also vomiting, seizures, developmental delay, hypotonia, ataxia.
- Immunodeficiency (see ➔ p. 612).

⚠ Box 31.12 Features that should make you re-evaluate the diagnosis of atopic eczema or seborrhoeic dermatitis

- Congenital onset.
- Erythroderma, large scaling plaques, or indurated skin.
- Purpura or ulceration.
- Failure to thrive, diarrhoea.
- Repeated infections.
- Poor response to emollients and mild/moderately potent topical corticosteroids.

Napkin rashes

Atopic eczema, the commonest form of dermatitis in infancy, tends to spare the moist skin in the napkin area. Instead, most napkin rashes are caused by urine and/or faeces irritating macerated skin (irritant contact dermatitis). Prevalence has fallen, because highly absorbent nappies wick moisture away from the skin.

What should I look for?

- Irritant dermatitis occurs between the ages of 3 weeks and 2 years. The rash involves the convex surfaces (e.g. buttocks) in contact with the napkin and spares skinfolds. The erythematous skin may have a rather glazed shiny appearance (see Fig. 31.5). Severe chronic irritant dermatitis may be associated with well-demarcated erosions (Jacquet dermatitis) or extensive papules.
- *Candida* napkin dermatitis, in infants aged 6–24 months, starts in skinfolds but may extend to involve the entire perineum. Look for satellite papules (less often pustules) and oral candidiasis.
- Infantile seborrhoeic dermatitis is an asymptomatic rash that usually presents around age 4–6 weeks. Look for well-demarcated erythematous patches, without much scale, in skinfolds. Inspect the scalp, face, and axillae (see ➲ p. 602 and Fig. 31.6). May be difficult to differentiate from napkin psoriasis (see Box 31.13).
- Allergy to preservatives in wet wipes may present as dermatitis.
- Erosive perianal eruption is caused by diarrhoea, often in breastfed infants aged 6 weeks to 3 months. The rash is characterized by erythema, with well-demarcated superficial erosions.
- Staphylococcal impetigo may present with flaccid bullae in the napkin area, often in the first few weeks of life.
- Group A streptococcal dermatitis (infants, >6 months) causes painful perianal erythema (may involve inguinal folds) (see ➲ p. 132).

What should I do?

- Culture skin swabs for *Candida* and bacteria.
- Minimize irritation of the skin:
  - Wash skin with plain water and a soap substitute.
  - Ensure that baby wipes are alcohol- and fragrance-free.
  - Change the napkin, as soon as it is soiled by faeces.
  - Avoid talcum powders which may irritate the skin.
- Paraffin-based ointments, such as Hydromol® or 50% WSP in liquid paraffin, hydrate the skin and act as a barrier to external irritants.
- Treat inflamed skin with twice-daily applications of an ointment containing 1% hydrocortisone, in combination with an antifungal agent such as miconazole or clotrimazole.
- Treat bacterial infection with oral antibiotics.
- Rashes unresponsive to treatment: think again (see Box 31.13).

Further reading

Stamatas GN and Tierney NK. *Pediatr Dermatol* 2014;31:1–7.

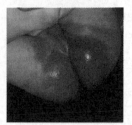

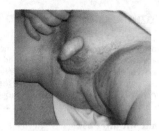

Fig. 31.5 Painful irritant dermatitis with a shiny glazed erythema that spares the skinfolds.

Fig. 31.6 Seborrhoeic dermatitis favours the skinfolds.

Box 31.13 Napkin rash unresponsive to standard treatment

- Find out how the skin in the napkin area is being washed, how often the napkin is being changed, what wipes are being used (could this be allergic contact dermatitis?), and what ointments are being applied.
- Take skin swabs, and culture for *Candida* and bacteria … again.
- Psoriasis responds poorly to treatments used for napkin dermatitis. The well-demarcated, but asymptomatic, erythema has minimal scale. Napkin psoriasis tends to start on the convex surfaces of the buttocks but may spread to the flexures, trunk, face, and scalp. Most infants do not have evidence of psoriasis in nails. Any family history of psoriasis? The rash is difficult to differentiate from infantile seborrhoeic dermatitis, but seborrhoeic dermatitis is usually controlled after 2–4 weeks of treatment. Aim to keep the skin comfortable using emollients and mild topical corticosteroids, rather than clear psoriasis.
- Dermatophyte infection ('ringworm') presents with well-demarcated scaly, erythematous papules and plaques, usually in toddlers, rather than infants. Sometimes there are pustules. Often involves the thighs and lower abdomen, as well as the napkin area. Has anyone in the family got tinea pedis? Take a skin scrape for mycology (see ➡ p. 164).
- Blisters or erosions? SSSS, caused by a circulating exfoliative exotoxin, presents with a tender peeling erythema, sometimes limited to the napkin area (see ➡ p. 112). Allergic contact dermatitis is uncommon in infants but may present as a vesicular eruption in infants aged >6 months. Rarely, autoimmune blistering diseases may present in the napkin area in infancy.
- Purpura or ulceration? Langerhans cell histiocytosis involves the flexures and the napkin area, but may also affect the scalp, the skin behind the ears, and the trunk (see ➡ p. 602).
- Zinc deficiency presents with psoriasiform dermatitis around the mouth, as well as in the napkin area. Look for paronychia, sparse hair, and failure to thrive, as well as recurrent *Candida* infections (see ➡ p. 513).

Atopic eczema (atopic dermatitis)

Atopic eczema is a chronic itchy skin condition that affects 20–25% of children in Western Europe. Prevalence is increasing. Atopic eczema usually starts in infancy. Most have mild disease. Disease clears in about 50% of children by puberty. Others have a chronic and recurrent lifelong illness. Pathogenesis is multifactorial (see Box 31.14). The prevalences of bronchial asthma and allergic rhinitis are increased in atopic patients, and skin-prick tests are positive to many common environmental allergens.

What should I ask?

Explore:

- Age of onset (usually age 2–3 months) and distribution of eczema.
- Response to previous and current treatments.
- Impact on the child and family/carers (especially on sleep).
- Growth, development, and progress at nursery/school.
- Dietary history, including any dietary manipulation.
- Immediate reactions (urticaria, wheeze, angio-oedema) to foods.
- Exposure to trigger factors, including heat and irritants such as wool clothing, soaps, shampoos, bubble baths, and shower gels. Allergic dermatitis is unusual in children, but irritant reactions to creams are common.
- Contact with airborne allergens such as house dust mite and pet dander (more important in older infants/children).
- Personal and family history of atopy (e.g. asthma, allergic rhinitis).

What should I do?

- Confirm the diagnosis: usually clear-cut, but remember scabies in any itchy child. For diagnostic criteria, see Box 31.15, and Figs. 31.7, 31.8, and 31.9).
- Make a global assessment: mild, moderate, or severe—based on symptoms (such as itching and sleep disturbance); the quantities or strengths of treatment, clinical signs, and the area affected.
- Record impact on quality of life of the child/family (see ➍ pp. 32–4).
- Using 'POEM' (patient-orientated eczema measure), get the patient's view (see ✍ www.nottingham.ac.uk/dermatology/POEM.htm).
- Scores, such as EASI (Eczema Area and Severity Index) or SCORAD (SCORing Atopic Dermatitis), will help to monitor response to treatment objectively.
- Crusted weeping eczema or pustules: swab for bacterial culture.
- Pain, grouped vesicles or small well-defined crusted erosions: exclude herpes simplex infection (eczema herpeticum), a medical emergency (see ➍ Box 7.2, p. 154).
- Immediate reactions to foods: refer for further investigation, if clinically indicated (see Box 31.18).
- Refer for patch testing, if you suspect allergic contact dermatitis, but irritancy is much commoner than allergy.
- Approaches to management, including top tips, are discussed on ➍ pp. 608–9 and pp. 610–11.

Box 31.14 Pathogenesis of atopic eczema

- Genetic and environmental factors interact.
- Atopic diseases are common in the family of affected individuals. Risk is more closely related to inheritance of maternal than paternal genes.
- No single atopic gene has been identified, but potential loci have been mapped to chromosomes 1q, 3q, 3p, 17q, and 20p, among others.
- Defective barrier function and innate immunity seem likely to play a role in the pathogenesis. Loss-of-function mutations in the gene for filaggrin, an epidermal barrier protein, predispose to atopic eczema, and the lipid/protein ratio is reduced in the stratum corneum. Defective stratum corneum may allow pathogens/allergens to penetrate the skin and trigger a hyperactive immune response, with activation of T-lymphocytes, dendritic cells, macrophages, keratinocytes, mast cells, and eosinophils. Pro-inflammatory cytokines and chemokines may perpetuate disease.
- Skin shows increased susceptibility to colonization by *Staphylococcus aureus*, which may also damage the skin barrier.
- *S. aureus* enterotoxins with superantigenic activity may play some part by activating T-cells and macrophages.

Box 31.15 UK criteria for diagnosis of atopic eczema

A child with an itchy skin condition in last 12 months, plus three or more of the following:
- Visible flexural dermatitis involving the skin creases such as the bends of the elbows or behind the knees (or visible dermatitis on the cheeks and/or extensor areas in children aged 18 months or younger).
- Personal history of flexural dermatitis (or dermatitis on the cheeks and/or extensor areas in children aged 18 months or younger).
- Personal history of dry skin in last 12 months.
- Personal history of asthma or allergic rhinitis (or history of atopic disease in a first-degree relative if child aged <4 years).
- Onset before age of 2 years (not used in children <4 years of age).

Further reading

Cork MJ et al. *J Invest Dermatol* 2009;**129**:1892–908.

Margolis JS et al. *JAMA Dermatol* 2014;**150**:593–600.

National Institute for Health and Care Excellence (2007). *Atopic eczema in under 12s. diagnosis and management.* Available at: ℘ https://www.nice.org.uk/guidance/cg57.

Nottingham Support Group for Carers of Children with Eczema. *Information.* Available at: ℘ http://www.nottinghameczema.org.uk/nsgcce/information/index.aspx.

Werfel T. *J Invest Dermatol* 2009;**129**:1878–91.

Managing atopic eczema: top tips

Living with and managing atopic eczema is challenging for child and family. The psychosocial burden can be profound. Aim to address concerns and to educate (see Box 31.16), so that the child /family have the tools to manage this distressing chronic disease.

- Intractable itch/scratch. Relieve dryness, and control eczema. Protect skin from damage—suggest stroking or pinching skin to relieve itch; use occlusion. Therapeutic stories, in which the child is champion, may facilitate behavioural change, improve self-esteem, and help the child engage with treatment (overcoming 'Evil Eric Eczema').
- Complaints that the skin 'reacts to'/'is allergic to' emollients. Irritation of inflamed skin is much commoner than allergy. Ointments may be tolerated less well than creams. Suggest trying a creamy emollient on normal skin for a few days, before applying to eczematous skin. Explain that, if normal skin does not react, allergy is unlikely. Control acute eczema with topical corticosteroids or calcineurin inhibitors, and then apply emollients.
- Steroid phobia. Some parents refuse to use 'bad' topical steroids (a misconception that may have been reinforced by other health-care professionals). Explain the different strengths of steroids and the proper use of topical steroids (see ➜ p. 610). State the specific quantity of topical corticosteroid you expect to be used over 1 or 2 weeks.
- Once eczema is controlled, empower the child and family by introducing proactive therapy, i.e. low-dose, intermittent applications of anti-inflammatory therapy to previously affected skin ('hot spots') (see Box 31.17).
- 'He has a food allergy'. Find out exactly what the parent means and what has been observed (see Box 31.18). Inappropriate withdrawal of foods may cause nutritional deficiencies. Most children with mild eczema do not need investigation for food allergies.
- Recurrent 2° bacterial infection (oozing golden-crusted patches), usually with *S. aureus*. Use antibacterial emollients, e.g. products containing benzalkonium chloride and/or chlorhexidine, to cleanse the skin and remove crusts. Bleach baths (1/4 cup of household bleach in a half bathtub of water) for 5–10min, 2–3×/week may reduce bacterial colonization. Treat nasal carriage of *S. aureus* (child and family) with topical mupiricin. Short courses of oral antibiotics may be required.
- Molluscum contagiosum. May be spread by scratching. Reassure the child/parent that molluscum will go, but this may take some time, particularly if topical steroids are being used. Flares of eczema around molluscum may herald regression. (Also see ➜ p. 158.)
- Attention-deficit/hyperactivity disorder (ADHD). Caring for children with eczema is exhausting. Some are just itchy and active, but others, in particular those with more severe eczema, may have ADHD. Consider referral to a child psychologist.

Box 31.16 Child/parent education

Adherence to treatment is difficult. Education is crucial, and the help of a dermatology nurse invaluable.

- Explore beliefs, fears, preferences, and hopes.
- Identify barriers to adherence, e.g. steroid phobia, time for treatment, complexity of regimen, cost, and discomfort.
- Agree educational objectives, e.g. proper use of topical steroids.
- Implement a written action plan.

Box 31.17 Proactive therapy for atopic eczema

Normal-looking non-lesional skin in patients is not normal—there is subclinical inflammation, as well as a barrier defect. Proactive therapy targets invisible inflammation in problem areas and reduces overall use of topical anti-inflammatory therapy.

- After clearance of visible eczema, continue to apply anti-inflammatory therapy, e.g. a potent topical corticosteroid ointment or 0.1% tacrolimus ointment, to previously affected skin (hot spots or problem areas) ×2/week.
- Continue daily application of emollients to all skin.

Box 31.18 Food allergy

- Consider food allergy in children with atopic eczema who have reacted previously to a food with immediate symptoms (e.g. urticaria, wheeze, angio-oedema), or in infants and young children with moderate or severe atopic eczema that has not been controlled by optimum management, particularly if associated with gut dysmotility (colic, vomiting, altered bowel habit) or failure to thrive. Refer to a paediatric allergist.
- Most children will grow out of food allergies, except allergy to nuts. Food allergy is very unlikely to play any part in the pathogenesis of atopic eczema in adults.

Further reading

Gillette C and Wallenberg A (2014). Br J Dermatol 170(Suppl S1):19–24 (proactive therapy).
Naidoo RJ and Williams HC (2013). Paed Dermatol 30:765–7 (therapeutic use of stories).
University of Nottingham, Centre of Evidence-Based Dermatology. Psychology and eczema. Available at: ℛ www.nottingham.ac.uk/research/groups/cebd/resources/psychology-and-eczema.aspx (story templates).

Atopic eczema: gaining control

Step 1: Listen and explain

- Explore beliefs, fears, and hopes, and answer questions
  (see ➡ pp. 606–7 and pp. 30–31).
- Discuss the multifactorial cause, particularly the abnormal skin
  barrier, and trigger factors, including soaps and bubble baths.
- Provide written information about eczema and support groups.
- Explain that treatment can control, but not cure, eczema.
- Reassure that most children improve, as they grow older.
- Explain that eczema will fluctuate and can be frustrating to treat.
- Discuss how to recognize flares of eczema and infections, including
  eczema herpeticum (rare).

Step 2: Emollients, antiseptics and soap substitutes

- Emollients are the cornerstone of management and should be used
  all over the body, even when eczema has cleared. Supply a range of
  unperfumed emollients. The best emollient is the one the patient
  likes. Creamy emollients, rather than ointments, may be preferred
  for daytime use. Prescribe in large quantities (>500g/week) to be
  used liberally and frequently (see ➡ p. 655).
- Use an emollient as a soap substitute.
- Reduce bacterial colonization with antibacterial emollients,
  e.g. products containing benzalkonium chloride and/or chlorhexidine
  or bleach baths (see ➡ p. 608).

Step 3: Topical anti-inflammatories and other treatments

- Discuss and demonstrate the use of topical corticosteroids. Explain
  that topical corticosteroids, unlike emollients, should only be applied
  to eczematous skin. (Apply 20–30min after emollient.) Explain how
  to step up and step down the strength of treatment. Show how to
  measure the application in fingertip units (FTUs) (see ➡ Box 34.3,
  p. 658).
- Most mild infantile atopic eczema can be controlled with mild to
  moderate corticosteroid ointments used once daily. Ointments are
  preferable to creams, as they are less likely to irritate the skin. Mild
  corticosteroid ointments can be used safely on the face.
- Potent topical corticosteroids or topical calcineurin inhibitors may be
  needed ×1/day for 7–14 days for more active disease.
- Very potent corticosteroid ointments should not be prescribed,
  without the guidance of a specialist.
- Once eczema is controlled, switch to proactive therapy
  (see Box 31.17).
- Wraps or paste bandages can help children with very itchy skin
  (see ➡ p. 660, and Box 34.4, p. 661).
- Treat 2° bacterial infection with antibiotics.
- Treatments, such as UVB, methotrexate, azathioprine, or ciclosporin,
  may be indicated in severe chronic atopic eczema.
- Prednisolone should be avoided, except for acute severe flares.

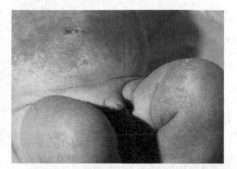

Fig. 31.7 Atopic eczema typically spares the napkin area.

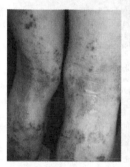

Fig. 31.8 Atopic eczema with secondary bacterial infection causing crusting and weeping.

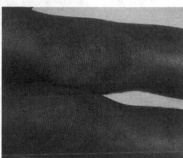

Fig. 31.9 Lichenification with increased skin markings secondary to chronic rubbing.

Step 4: General measures

- Involve a dermatology nurse to provide education and support.
- Discuss strategies to deal with problems such as sleep disturbance, irritability, or clingy behaviour.
- Eliminate irritants and other trigger factors—no pets in the bedroom!
- Use loose-fitting cotton clothing.
- Keep the bedroom cool, and avoid too much bedding.
- A sedating antihistamine may be helpful at night—but the impact may be disappointing.

Further reading

National Institute for Health and Care Excellence (2007). *Atopic eczema in under 12s: diagnosis and management.* Available at: ℘ http://www.nice.org.uk/CG57.

Cutaneous signs in rare syndromes

Immunodeficiency syndromes

⚠ Cutaneous signs may provide a valuable early clue to the diagnosis of these rare syndromes which may present insidiously. Problems suggesting immunodeficiency include recurrent, prolonged, or severe infections at more than one site, infections with unusual organisms, and infections poorly responsive to antibiotics (often requiring IV antibiotics).

Look for failure to thrive, chronic diarrhoea, and hepatosplenomegaly. Infants with severe T-cell immunodeficiency develop GVHD 2° to maternal engraftment at or around the time of delivery and may become erythrodermic. These patients also have an increased risk of malignancy.

- Omenn syndrome: AR. Severe combined immunodeficiency. Generalized eczema, failure to thrive, alopecia, eosinophilia, diarrhoea, repeated infections. Also hepatosplenomegaly and lymphadenopathy.
- Wiskott–Aldrich syndrome: X-linked disorder. Severe atopic eczema in first few months of life is associated with recurrent pyogenic infections and bleeding (petechiae, bruising), due to thrombocytopenia. May present with epistaxis and bloody diarrhoea.
- Ataxia telangiectasia: AR. Ataxia noticed in infancy. Oculocutaneous signs develop from age 3, conjunctival bulbar telangiectasias (by age 6), and cutaneous telangiectasias (ears, eyelids, malar, anterior chest, flexures). Also premature ageing of the skin (loss of fat), café au lait macules, hypertrichosis, chronic seborrhoeic dermatitis, and painful cutaneous granulomas (non-infectious). May have sinopulmonary infections, growth retardation, intellectual disability, and endocrine abnormalities.
- Hyper IgE syndrome (Job syndrome, Buckley syndrome): AD. *STAT3* mutations. Recurrent severe cutaneous and sinopulmonary infections in association with papulopustular dermatitis in first few months of life. 'Cold' abscesses with limited erythema. Also repeated fractures and retained 1° teeth. Elevated IgE levels (>2 000IU/L) and eosinophilia.
- Chronic mucocutaneous candidiasis. Most do not have positive family history. Progressive *Candida* infections of the skin, nails, and mucous membranes. May be associated with polyglandular autoimmune syndrome type 1 (autoimmune polyendocrinopathy–candidiasis–ectodermal dystrophy = APECED) (see ➔ p. 484).
- Chronic granulomatous disease: X-linked or AR. Chronic staphylococcal infections of skin, suppurative lymphadenitis, bronchopneumonia, hepatosplenomegaly, chronic diarrhoea, and malabsorption.
- Chediak–Higashi syndrome: AR. Silvery sheen to hair, partial albinism (strabismus and nystagmus), photophobia, hyperpigmented exposed skin, severe recurrent infections, and progressive neurological deterioration.

Multiple lentigines

What is a lentigo? (plural: lentigines or lentigos)

Lentigines are small (1–3mm in diameter), well-circumscribed, flat, brown to black 'freckles' that may appear on any body site. Lentigines do not fade when the skin is no longer exposed to sun, and are not necessarily triggered by sun exposure.

Some normal individuals have numerous lentigines, but, in a child with 'freckles', you should consider:

- Neurofibromatosis 1—a RASopathy: freckling in skinfolds (see ➡ p. 552). Incidence around 1 in 3000.
- Segmental neurofibromatosis 1: unilateral lentigines in the axilla or groin (see ➡ pp. 554–5). Incidence about 1 in 40 000.
- XP: premature sun damage with many lentigines mainly on sun-exposed skin. High risk of early-onset skin cancers, including malignant melanoma (see ➡ pp. 336–7). Rare—incidence around 1 in 250 000 to 1 in 500 000.
- Peutz–Jeghers syndrome: freckling on vermillion borders of the lips, oral mucosa, perioral, perianal, and periorbital skin, over joints, and on palms and soles (see ➡ p. 543). Incidence uncertain—estimates range from 1 in 25 000 to 1 in 300 000.
- Carney complex (includes NAME and LAMB syndromes): mucocutaneous pigmentation (lentigines on the lips, conjunctiva, inner or outer canthi, vaginal and penile mucosa, blue naevi; may have small café au lait spots that tend to fade with age), myxomas (cardiac, cutaneous—eyelid, external ear, nipple), breast myxomatosis or ductal adenoma, endocrine tumours (1° pigmented nodular adrenocortical disease, pituitary adenoma, testicular neoplasms, thyroid adenoma or carcinoma, ovarian cysts), psammomatous melanotic schwannoma, osteochondromyxoma. Inactivating mutation in regulatory subunit 1Λ of protein kinase A gene (PRKAR1A) located at 17q22-24 in 2/3 of cases (very rare indeed).
- Multiple lentigines syndrome—a RASopathy (previously known as LEOPARD syndrome). Lentigines (hundreds of freckle-like spots all over the skin), Electrocardiographic cardiac conduction defects, Ocular telorism, Pulmonary stenosis, Abnormalities of genitalia, Retardation of growth, Deafness. Mutations in protein tyrosine phosphatase, non-receptor type 11 gene (*PTPN11*) in 90% cases (very rare indeed).

This list is not exhaustive, and other rare syndromes are associated with multiple lentigines, either in a generalized or localized distribution.

Physical and sexual abuse

Sadly some children are abused, and it is important to recognize cutaneous signs that may indicate abuse—but it is equally important to realize that some dermatoses can be confused with abuse. Record all signs, and refer urgently to a paediatrician with expertise in this area, if you suspect abuse. The welfare of the child should be your 1° concern.

What should I look for?

- Carer has delayed seeking medical help.
- Inconsistent history, incompatible with the injury or signs.
- Parental hostility or lack of interest.
- Sad, withdrawn, or frightened child.
- A child displaying frequent sexualized behaviour.
- Physical abuse—the upper head and body are frequently targeted in cases of deliberate physical injury. Look for:
  - Many bruises of different ages, often in clusters.
  - Pinch marks on the ear or petechiae on the pinna.
  - Linear slap marks, belt marks, finger impressions, or buckle marks.
  - Cigarette burns to the face or hands, or burns to the lower limbs (child held forcibly in scalding water).
- Sexual abuse:
  - Pregnancy.
  - HIV infection or another sexually transmitted disease in the absence of perinatal acquisition. Anogenital warts in children may be acquired by autoinnoculation, but the possibility of sexual abuse should be considered, particularly in children <2 years (see ➋ p. 160).
  - Signs of acute penetrating anogenital trauma, including acute hymenal injury, laceration, bruising, or perianal lacerations.
  - Genital abrasions, lacerations, bites, suction marks, or burns.

Dermatological conditions that may simulate abuse

- Mongolian blue spots (present at birth or soon after) may simulate bruises (see ➋ p. 344 and Fig. 31.10), as may the blue/black pigmentation in naevus of Ota (face) or naevus of Ito (upper trunk).
- Bullous impetigo may simulate cigarette burns (see ➋ Fig. 6.1, p. 130).
- SSSS, as the name suggests, can simulate scalds (see ➋ Fig. 6.2, p. 131).
- Phytophotodermatitis with blistering in linear streaks may simulate burns, or the residual pigmented streaks may simulate linear bruising (see ➋ Fig. 31.11, and Box 16.4, p. 327).
- Angio-oedema with swelling of the face or lips may simulate an early bruise (see ➋ p. 104).
- Cutaneous vasculitis with purpura may simulate bruises (see ➋ p. 442).
- Group A streptococcal perineal infection with itch, pain, erythema, discharge, and localized bleeding may suggest sexual abuse (see ➋ p. 132).
- Lichen sclerosus with haemorrhage may suggest sexual abuse (see ➋ p. 288).
- EB (rare) with skin fragility and blistering may suggest physical injury (see ➋ pp. 624–5).

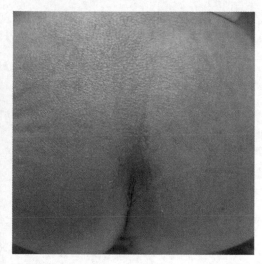

Fig. 31.10 Mongolian blue spot.

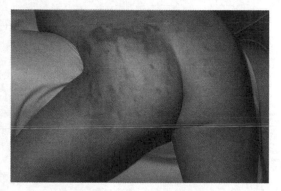

Fig. 31.11 Phytophotodermatitis. Linear pigmentation was preceded by streaky erythema and blisters where the sun-exposed skin had been in contact with the juice of a plant that contained psoralen.

Further reading

Department for Education, Home Office, Department for Communities and Local Government, Department of Health, Foreign & Commonwealth Office, Official Solicitor and Public Trustee, and Ofsted. *Safeguarding children*. Available at: ℘ https://www.gov.uk/childrens-services/safeguarding-children.

Skin and genetics

Contents

Genetic basis of skin diseases

Dermatogenetics is a rapidly expanding field. This chapter provides an introduction to a few of the many single gene disorders affecting the skin, hair, and/or nails—the genodermatoses.

Monogenic disorders

An understanding of the molecular basis of single-gene 'Mendelian' skin diseases has provided insights into the structure and function of normal skin, as well as the pathogenesis of some acquired diseases (e.g. autoimmune blistering diseases; see ➲ Table 13.2, p. 264). For the molecular basis of some monogenic skin disorders, see Table 32.1.

A clinical disorder (phenotype) is dominant when the condition is manifest in heterozygotes (two different alleles), and recessive when the trait is only manifest in homozygotes (two identical alleles). AD traits usually involve structural proteins, whereas AR traits commonly involve enzymes. Generally, it is possible to predict the likelihood of disease in monogenic disorders, based on analysis of the genotype, but some dominantly inherited disorders show age-dependent penetrance (features are not present at birth but evolve with time), whereas others show incomplete penetrance (not all those having the mutation develop the disease).

Genotype–phenotype correlation

Correlation can be difficult. Different mutations in a single gene may cause different clinical disorders; mutations in different genes may lead to similar phenotypes (genetic heterogeneity), and the same mutation (genotype) within a family may lead to disorders of different severity (different expressivity). In a few autosomal dominantly inherited diseases, severity increases in successive generations (anticipation). Some genes are expressed differently, if inherited from the mother than from the father (imprinting). Most X-linked traits are expressed more severely in men (who are hemizygous) than in women.

Contiguous gene syndromes

If large deletions affect several neighbouring genes, several disorders may be transmitted together, simulating a monogenic disorder.

Polygenic disorders

Genome-wide association studies in large populations have identified many hundreds of genetic variants (markers) associated with a susceptibility to many common genetically complex diseases such as diabetes, autism, psoriasis, and atopic eczema, as well as to physical traits such as height and pigmentation (colour of skin, hair, and eyes).

In contrast to single-gene disorders, environmental factors and gene–gene interactions (epistasis) play much greater roles in determining the risk of disease, so it is not possible to predict the likelihood of a complex disease based solely on the genotype.

Table 32.1 Molecular basis of some genodermatoses

Genodermatosis	Molecular basis	Signs
Darier disease	Calcium pump defect—SERCA2	Warty papules
Hailey–Hailey disease	Calcium pump defect—SPCA1	Blisters, fragility
Lamellar ichthyosis group	Transglutaminase defects	Scale, redness
Epidermolysis bullosa (EB) group	Defects in keratinocyte adhesion or collagen	Blisters, fragility
Keratoderma, ichthyosis with deafness (KID)	Connexin 26 defect	Keratoderma, deafness
Erythrokeratoderma variabilis (EKV)	Connexin 31 defect	Erythema, hyperkeratotic plaques
Some ichthyoses	Lipid metabolism defect	Scaly skin
X-linked recessive ichthyosis	Steroid sulfatase defect	Scaly skin
Netherton syndrome	Protease defect	Scaly skin, atopy
Papillon–Lefevre syndrome	Protease defect	Keratoderma, infections
Ehlers–Danlos group	Collagen defects	Hypermobile joints, stretchy or translucent skin
Cutis laxa group	Elastin or fibulin defects	Lax skin
Marfan syndrome	Fibrillin-1 defect	Musculoskeletal, cardiovascular, and ocular disorders
Goltz syndrome	Porcupine homologue defect (mosaicism—lethal if homozygous)	Atrophic skin, congenital defects
P63-associated disorders, e.g. ankyloblepharon–ectodermal defects–cleft lip/palate syndrome (AEC)	Mutations in *p63*, a transcription regulator of genes involved in various cell–matrix and cell–cell adhesion complexes in epidermis	Overlapping features include ectodermal dysplasia, cleft lip/palate, and limb abnormalities. AEC: also congenital erythroderma, skin fragility, and erosions
Schopf–Schulz–Passarge syndrome	*WNT10A* mutations disrupt Wnt/β catenin signalling involved in development of skin, hair, nails, and teeth	Eyelid cysts, palmoplantar keratoderma with hyperhidrosis. Nail, hair, and teeth abnormalities

Mosaicism

What is mosaicism?

Somatic mosaicism is caused by a mutation arising early in embryogenesis that is propagated in only a limited number of cells. The outcome is a partial phenotype, i.e. only some of the cells express the disease. In ♀, random X-inactivation (lyonization) results in functional X-chromosome mosaicism.

Skin disorders reflecting mosaicism in keratinocytes follow predictable patterns (Blaschko lines) (see Fig. 32.1). Individuals who are mosaic for a condition can only transmit the disorder to the next generation (who will inherit the non-mosaic form), if the mosaicism also affects cells in the germline (ovary, testis). Involvement of germline cells is hypothesized to be more likely in individuals with extensive skin involvement. Mutations arising early in development may be associated with widespread abnormalities in skin and other organs.

For examples of cutaneous mosaicism, see ➔ pp. 636–7.

What are Blaschko lines?

(see ➔ inside back cover for diagram.)

Alfred Blaschko was a dermatologist from Berlin who observed that epidermal naevi and some acquired skin diseases followed similar patterns: linear on the limbs, arcs on the chest, S-shapes on the abdomen, or V-shapes near the midline of the back. The patterns were not related to dermatomes (segments of skin defined by sensory innervations) or any known cause of linear skin markings such as Langer lines of cleavage, axial lines separating cranial and caudal dermatomes, lymphatic drainage, vascular flow, embryonic clefts, or pigmentary demarcation lines (see ➔ pp. 62–3). The lines probably reflect keratinocyte mosaicism and correspond to the pathways followed by keratinocytes migrating from the neural crest during embryogenesis.

How do I recognize cutaneous mosaicism?

Five patterns have been described (see Fig. 32.1). The pattern is influenced by the pathway of migration of the affected cell, as well as other factors such as the timing of the mutation:

- Keratinocyte: Blaschko-linear pattern. Each clone of keratinocytes forms a continuous line, as the cells migrate outwards by directional proliferation following surface forces.
- Melanoblast: block or phylloid but may be Blaschko-linear patterns. Melanoblasts migrate as single cells and proliferate locally in skin.
- Nerve cells: dermatomal. Nerve cells migrate along future dermatomes.
- Mesodermal tissues (blood vessels, fibroblasts): segmental or dermatomal. Cells migrate within segments or dermatomes.

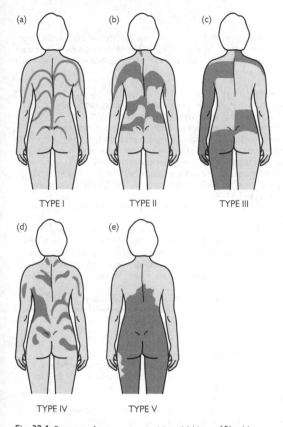

TYPE I TYPE II TYPE III

TYPE IV TYPE V

Fig. 32.1 Patterns of cutaneous mosaicism. (a) Lines of Blaschko, narrow bands. (b) Lines of Blaschko, broad bands. (c) Checkerboard pattern. (d) Phylloid pattern. (e) Patchy pattern without midline separation.

Further reading

Bolognia JL et al. *J Am Acad Dermatol* 1994;**31**:157–90.
Happle R. *Acta Pædiatrica* 2006;**Suppl 451**:16–23.
Paller AS. *J Clin Invest* 2004;**114**:1407–9.
Torrelo A et al. *Eur J Dermatol* 2005;**15**:439–50.

The genetic consultation

If you suspect an inherited disease, discussion should be handled sensitively because of the implications for other family members, but also because of the guilt that transmission of an inherited condition can engender in a parent.

What should I do?

- The medical history should include details of pregnancy, labour, signs at birth (was the skin abnormal?), and development.
- Take a thorough family history, ideally across at least three generations, including details of the youngest generations.
- Document consanguinity—relationships between second cousins or closer greatly increase the risk of recessive disease.
- Establish diagnoses as precisely as possible in other family members, avoiding vague terms such as 'cancer'. Also see ➔ Familial cancer syndromes, pp. 542–4.
- Draw a family tree showing affected and unaffected individuals (see Figs. 32.2 and 32.3).
- Document the physical findings in the patient—is all the skin affected, or are some areas spared, e.g. the flexures? Is there a pattern to the involvement, e.g. Blaschko lines, dermatomal? Are palms and soles affected? Examine the hair, nails, and teeth, as well as the skin.
- Examine so-called 'unaffected' family members carefully, looking for subtle clinical signs.
- Consider referring the patient and/or family to a clinical geneticist, so that the diagnosis can be confirmed by further investigation. Genetic testing will be guided by the clinical diagnosis.

Genetic counselling

- The help of a clinical geneticist is invaluable.
- The diagnosis may have serious implications for family members. In general, it is appropriate to encourage an affected individual to share their personal information with members of the family (with the support of a geneticist).
- Potential disclosure of genetic information to other members of a family raises issues of both consent and confidentiality.

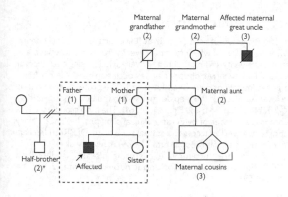

Maternal grandfather (2)   Maternal grandmother (2)   Affected maternal great uncle (3)

Father (1)   Mother (1)   Maternal aunt (2)

Half-brother (2)*   Affected   Sister   Maternal cousins (3)

(1) = First degree relative
(2) = Second degree relative
(3) = Third degree relative
*   Half siblings may be regarded as a first degree relative for the purposes of risk assessment (e.g. family history of colorectal cancer, breast cancer, inherited cardiovascular conditions) if the family history is from the shared parent.

Fig 32.2 Family tree to show immediate and extended family and degree of relatedness. Reproduced with permission from Bradley-Smith et al., *Oxford Handbook of Genetics*, 2009, Oxford: Oxford University Press.

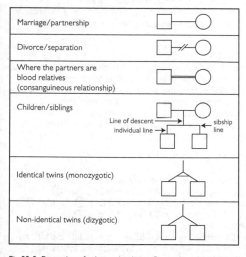

Marriage/partnership	
Divorce/separation	
Where the partners are blood relatives (consanguineous relationship)	
Children/siblings	Line of descent → individual line → ← sibship line
Identical twins (monozygotic)	
Non-identical twins (dizygotic)	

Fig 32.3 Examples of relationship lines. Reproduced with permission from Bradley-Smith et al., *Oxford Handbook of Genetics*, 2009, Oxford: Oxford University Press.

Inherited epidermolysis bullosa

A heterogeneous group of rare (1 in 17 000 live births) genetically determined blistering disorders, which range in severity from mild to severe and life-threatening. Severity and natural history vary within a single subtype or family. Sepsis, failure to thrive, or upper airway occlusion may be lethal. Many causative genes/mutations have been identified. The protein defect determines the level of blistering: intra-epidermal, within the BMZ, or subepidermal (see ➜ Table 13.1, p. 264; and Fig. 13.1, p. 261). The main groups (see Box 32.1) encompass a number of even rarer clinical subtypes. Multidisciplinary care is important, as well as access to a specialist EB team. DEBRA (UK charity) supports patients and families (⌗ http://www.debra.org.uk/).

Acquired EB, a rare autoimmune blistering disease, is described on ➜ p. 272. For more information about neonates with blisters, see ➜ Box 31.4, p. 593.

What should I ask or look for?
- Sites and precipitating factors, e.g. mechanical (pressure points, footwear), hot weather.
- Pain and/or itch (may be as distressing as pain).
- Change with age—lessening of blistering?
- Family history—is transmission likely to be AD or AR?
- Blisters—localization and severity. Erosions—excess granulation tissue.
- Milia, scarring, pigmentation, or eruptive naevi at sites of old blisters.
- Keratoderma, dystrophic or absent nails; alopecia.
- Teeth—enamel hypoplasia, caries.
- Extracutaneous involvement, e.g. oral mucosal involvement, oesophageal strictures, pseudosyndactyly, anaemia, growth retardation.
- Photosensitivity, poikiloderma, atrophic skin on dorsum of hands.
- SCCs (see ➜ p. 350).

How is the diagnosis confirmed?
- Diagnosis depends on clinical, immunohistochemical, and ultrastructural findings, but accurate diagnosis may be difficult in newborns.
- The major EB group and probable protein affected are determined by a combination of the phenotype, mode of transmission, and ultrastructural level of cleavage (IMF antigen mapping and/or transmission electron microscopy of a newly induced blister).
- Mutational analysis for subclassification and genetic counselling.

Neonates with suspected epidermolysis bullosa: what should I do?
- For causes of blisters in neonates, see ➜ Box 31.4, p. 593. Most other blisters are not present at birth. Exclude SSSS (see ➜ p. 112). Consider incontinentia pigmenti (rare) (see ➜ pp. 636–7) and epidermolytic ichthyosis (see ➜ Box 32.2, p. 627).
- Arrange for clinical photographs.
- ▶▶ Contact an EB centre urgently, if EB is suspected. In the UK, an EB clinical nurse specialist will visit to provide immediate training to parents/nursing staff on how to manage blistering and limit skin damage. If indicated, the nurse will perform skin biopsies and take blood samples (from child and family) for mutational analysis.

Box 32.1 Main groups of epidermolysis bullosa

Epidermolysis bullosa simplex—commonest form of epidermolysis bullosa
- Blisters within the epidermis. Usually keratin 5 or keratin 14 defects in basal keratinocytes. Rarely plectin defect. Usually AD transmission (can be AR).
- Mechanical fragility.
- Localized subtype: onset in early childhood, blisters on palms and soles, worse in hot weather.
- Generalized subtypes (mild or severe): onset at birth, keratoderma on palms/soles (may be relatively free of blisters), rarely scarring.
- Rarely with plectin defects—pyloric atresia, muscular dystrophy.

Junctional epidermolysis bullosa
- Blisters in mid portion of BMZ (lamina lucida). Laminin-332 (most often) or collagen XVII or integrin defects. AR transmission.
- Onset at birth, generalized or localized.
- Severe forms—death within first 2 years.
- Blisters (excess granulation tissue if severe), dystrophic/absent nails (occasionally atrophic scarring, milia).
- Other in severe—anaemia, growth retardation, enamel hypoplasia, caries, ocular problems, respiratory tract problems.

Dystrophic epidermolysis bullosa
- Blisters in upper dermis. Collagen VII defects. AD or AR transmission.
- Onset at birth, generalized.
- Blisters, atrophic scarring, milia, dystrophic/absent nails, alopecia.
- Contractures, pseudosyndactyly (usually in recessive forms).
- Other—anaemia, growth retardation, malnutrition, soft tissue abnormalities, caries, ocular problems.
- Eruptive melanocytic naevi at sites of old blisters (EB naevi) in recessive forms.
- Recessive forms: increased risk of SCCs—metastatic SCC lethal.

Kindler syndrome
- Mixed levels of blistering. Kindlin-1 (focal adhesion protein) defects. AD or AR transmission.
- Onset at birth, generalized.
- Blisters improve with age, dystrophic/absent nails, keratoderma.
- Photosensitivity, progressive poikiloderma, skin atrophy. especially on dorsum of hands (present in childhood).
- Other—soft tissue abnormalities, oral mucosal inflammation, oesophageal/urethral strictures, ectropion.
- Digital webbing, pseudoainhum, digital tapering.
- Increased risk of SCCs after age 30.

Further reading

Fine J-D et al. J Am Acad Dermatol 2014;70:1103–26 (diagnosis and classification).

The ichthyoses

A large group of disorders (inherited and acquired) characterized by a thick stratum corneum (usually) and scaly skin. Skin barrier defects underlie the pathogenesis, with mutations affecting cornification, the cell envelope, intercellular lipid layers, gap junctions, and intracellular signalling. Skin loses water, and the defensive barrier to outside agents is reduced. Ichthyosis may improve in humid summer months, deteriorating in winter. The commoner patterns are described below (for rarer ichthyoses, see Box 32.2). Emollients are the first-line therapy. Acquired ichthyosis has a variety of causes, including malignancy, hypothyroidism, drugs, nutritional deficiency, and neurological disease.

Ichthyosis vulgaris

- Commonest and mildest form of ichthyosis.
- AD transmission, mutations in gene encoding fillagrin.
- Onset: age 6 months (not present at birth).
- Fine, small whitish scales on extensor surfaces.
- Spares flexures: axillae, popliteal and antecubital fossae.
- More marked on the limbs than the trunk. Usually spares the face.
- Marked palmar creases (hyperlinear palms).
- Linked to atopic eczema.

Recessive X-linked ichthyosis

- Affects 1 in 5000 ♂.
- Deficiency in steroid sulfatase. Low maternal oestriol (produced by the placenta) in the mother of the affected fetus is linked to failure to initiate labour or to progress labour (forceps delivery, Caesarian).
- Onset birth to age 3 weeks as excessive neonatal desquamation.
- Large, dark brown adherent scales over the limbs, trunk, and scalp. Most obvious on extensor surfaces and sides/posterior neck ('dirty neck').
- Spares the antecubital and popliteal fossae, but affects the axillae.
- Spares the face, apart from pre-auricular skin.
- Palms and soles unaffected—not hyperlinear.
- Other—corneal opacities, testicular maldescent.
- Contiguous gene syndromes include Kallmann syndrome (hypogonadotrophic hypogonadism and anosmia).

Lamellar ichthyosis/congenital ichthyosiform erythroderma

- AR congenital ichthyoses. A spectrum of disease caused by mutations in at least seven genes. *TGM1* (encoding transglutaminase 1) causes most lamellar ichthyosis.
- Presents as collodion baby—outcome unpredictable (see Box 32.3).
- Mild disease—generalized fine white scale and variable redness (erythroderma) with ectropion. Severe disease—generalized thick brown scaling. Palmoplantar hyperkeratosis is common.
- Alopecia—advise on sun protection.
- Hypohidrosis affects temperature regulation.
- May be very disabling—psychological help is important.
- Oral retinoids are helpful.

Box 32.2 Rare inherited ichthyoses

- Epidermolytic ichthyosis (bullous congenital ichthyosiform erythroderma/epidermolytic hyperkeratosis). AD transmission. Mutations affect keratin 1 or keratin 10. Presents at birth with blisters or erosions. Differentiate from staphylococcal scalded skin (see ➔ p. 112) or EB. Later, dark thick scales.
- Superficial epidermolytic ichthyosis (ichthyosis bullosa of Siemens). AD transmission. Mutations affect keratin 2. Mild ichthyosis over joints, flexures, dorsum of the hands and feet. Superficial blistering and peeling of the stratum corneum in patches.
- Netherton syndrome. AR transmission. Mutations in SPINK5 gene. Severe neonatal erythroderma and failure to thrive. Evolves to an itchy ichthyosis—ichthyosis linearis circumflexa—with double-edged scale. Hair shaft abnormalities (trichorrhexis invaginata = bamboo hair)—check eyebrows. Link to atopy (see ➔ Box 31.11,p. 603).
- Harlequin ichthyosis. Extremely rare, very severe. AR transmission, congenital. Mutations in ABCA12 gene. Born prematurely as a collodion baby, with an armour-like casing often enveloping the hands/feet. Ectropion, eclabium, and underdeveloped nose and ears. Severe ichthyosis if survives.
- Sjögren–Larsson syndrome. AR transmission. Mutations in ALDH3A2. Deficient microsomal fatty aldehyde dehydrogenase leads to accumulation of fatty aldehydes and fatty alcohols. Clinical signs include congenital ichthyosis, bilateral spastic paresis (legs > arms), and intellectual disability.

Box 32.3 Collodion babies

- Baby (often premature) is encased in a tight, shiny membrane: the ectropion prevents the eyes from closing (protects the cornea); the eclabium (everted lips) interferes with sucking; may impair breathing.
- Impaired barrier function—heat loss, dehydration, and infection.
- Membrane dries slowly and peels off over weeks. Then the underlying disease (which may be mild ichthyosis) develops.
- Contact a specialist for an urgent opinion. Nurse in a humidified incubator. Monitor the temperature. Apply emollients several times per day, e.g. WSP, Emollin® spray. May need tube feeding if sucking impaired. Involve parents in the care of the baby.
- AR congenital ichthyoses are the commonest cause.
- Also consider trichothiodystrophy, neutral lipid storage disease, and Sjögren–Larsson syndrome (all very much less likely).

Further reading

Craiglow BG. *Semin Perinatol* 2013;37:26–31.
Oji V et al. *J Am Acad Dermatol* 2010;63:607–41.
Prado R et al. *J Am Acad Dermatol* 2012;67:1362–74 (collodion babies: management).

Darier disease and Hailey–Hailey disease

What is Darier disease?

Synonym: Darier–White disease.

This autosomal dominantly inherited disease usually presents in childhood or adolescence and pursues a chronic, relapsing course. Prevalence is around 1 in 36 000. Mutations in *ATP2A2*, a gene encoding the endoplasmic reticulum calcium pump SERCA2, cause impaired keratinocyte adhesion (acantholysis) with dyskeratosis. Severe disfiguring and disabling disease may be linked to major depression.

What should I look for?

- Warty brownish papules, coalescing into crusted plaques, in a seborrhoeic distribution (central trunk, forehead, scalp, flexures)) (see Fig. 32.4).
- Papules may follow Blaschko lines in individuals who are mosaic for the mutation (see ➔ p. 620 and Fig. 32.1).
- Itch, discomfort, and, if severe, malodour.
- Nails: fragility, red or white linear bands, V-shaped notches.
- Pits or keratotic papules on palms and/or soles.
- Flat, wart-like papules on the back of the hands and/or feet (acrokeratosis verruciformis).
- Painful fissures, blisters, and erosions in some patients (simulating Hailey–Hailey disease (see Box 32.4 and Fig. 32.5).
- Oral mucosal papules in some patients.

What should I do?

- Take a skin biopsy to look for acantholysis and dyskeratosis. (Differentiation from Hailey–Hailey disease may depend on the clinical presentation; see Box 32.4.)
- Patients are at risk of widespread herpes simplex infection—advise on how to recognize (unusual pain, blisters, erosions, poor response to usual treatment).
- Advise on avoiding disease triggers—heat, UVB.
- Prescribe:
  - Emollients containing urea to reduce hyperkeratosis.
  - Topical antiseptics to reduce bacterial colonization.
  - In limited disease: topical retinoid with a topical corticosteroid.
  - In extensive disease: oral alitretinoin, acitretin, or isotretinoin reduce itch, hyperkeratosis, and malodour—contraception essential (see ➔ p. 669).

Box 32.4 What is Hailey-Hailey disease?

Synonym: benign familial pemphigus.

- Autosomal dominantly inherited skin disease caused by mutations in *ATP2C1*, a gene encoding a calcium pump in the Golgi apparatus.
- Presents in late teens to early 20s with painful eroded, fragile skin/blisters at sites of friction (neck, flexures). Often misdiagnosed as 'eczema'; 2° bacterial infection is common (see Fig. 32.5).
- Pursues a chronic, relapsing course.
- Biopsy reveals acantholysis resembling autoimmune pemphigus, but IMF is negative. Also consider Darier disease (see ➲ p. 628).
- Management:
  - Reduce friction—loose-fitting cool clothing.
  - Control infection—antibiotics, antiseptics.
  - Potent/ultrapotent topical corticosteroids may be helpful.
  - Pain relief.
  - Consider patch testing for medicament allergy in chronic cases.
  - Herpes simplex infection may cause severe pain in eroded skin—advise on how to recognize (unusual pain, poor response to topical corticosteroid).

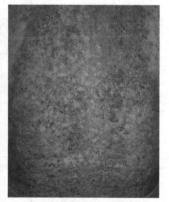

Fig 32.4 Darier disease—warty papules coalescing into greasy, hyperkeratotic, malodorous plaques on the trunk.

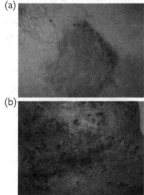

Fig 32.5 Hailey–Hailey disease. (a) Painful crusted erosions heal, leaving post-inflammatory pigmentation. (b) Extensive Hailey–Haily disease with widespread erosions, simulating an autoimmune blistering disease such as pemphigus.

Palmoplantar keratodermas

Disorders characterized by thickening of the epidermis on palms and soles (see Fig. 32.6). Mutations may affect keratins, the production of a cornified envelope (loricrin, transglutaminase), desmosomes, connexins, or transmembrane signal transduction (cathepsin C). Patterns of palmoplantar keratoderma (PPK) overlap.

What should I do?

- Ask when PPK developed and if there is a family history.
- If PPK is acquired, rather than inherited, is it caused by a dermatosis such as psoriasis, eczema, or LP? Rarely, acquired keratoderma is drug-induced, e.g. vemurafenib (see ⭘ p. 384), or paraneoplastic (cancer of the lung, breast, colon, or kidney).
- Ask about hyperhidrosis of the palms/soles—a troublesome association.
- Document the pattern of PPK—diffuse, focal (localized thickening), or punctate (numerous keratotic papules).
- Does the thickening extend from the palm/sole across the line of transgradience onto the dorsum of the hand/foot (transgradient PPK)?
- Are the nails affected?
- Check for 2° dermatophyte infection with skin scrapes—treat with systemic antifungals (may need repeated courses).
- Keratolytics, mechanical removal, or oral retinoids may be helpful.

For features in some types of PPK (all are rare), see Tables 32.2, 32.3, 32.4, and 32.5,.

Table 32.2 Diffuse palmoplantar keratoderma

Type	Gene product	Inheritance	Clinical information
Epidermolytic (Vorner)	Keratin 9	AD	Thick, yellow skin. Commonest PPK.
Non-epidermolytic (Unna–Thost)	Keratin 1	AD	Clinically identical. No transgradience
Mal de Meleda (see Fig. 32.6)	SLURP-1	AR	Rare. Transgradient PPK. Malodor. Plaques over elbows and knees. Nail dystrophy, perioral erythema. 2° infection common

Table 32.3 Diffuse palmoplantar keratoderma with other features

Type	Gene product	Inheritance	Clinical information
Papillon–Lefèvre syndrome	Cathepsin C	AR	Transgradient PPK, periodontitis, premature loss of teeth, psoriasiform plaques, systemic pyogenic infections
Mutilating (Vohwinkel syndrome)	Connexin 26	AD	Diffuse with honeycomb appearance. Pseudoainhum (constricting bands on fingers). Sensorineural deafness
Naxos disease	Plakoglobin	AR	Woolly hair, arrhythmias, and cardiomyopathy (right ventricle) in adolescence

Table 32.4 Focal palmoplantar keratoderma

Type	Gene product	Inheritance	Clinical information
Striate/areata	Desmoglein 1 Desmoplakin Keratin 1	AD	Signs vary. Painful localized thickening at pressure points on soles (like callosities) or linear (striate) hyperkeratosis on palms/fingers
Pachyonychia congenita	Keratins 6a, 6b, 6c, 16, or 17	AD	PPK (plantar pain) and thick nails. Often with follicular hyperkeratosis, oral leukokeratosis or cysts, e.g. steatocystoma, eruptive vellus hair cysts
Carvajal syndrome	Desmoplakin	AR (usually)	Striate PPK, cardiomyopathy, woolly hair

Table 32.5 Punctate type

Type	Gene product	Inheritance	Clinical information
Punctate	?	AD	Numerous 1–10mm keratotic papules, often resembling viral warts
Acrokeratoelastoidosis	?	AD	Skin-coloured papules on borders of palms and fingers

Erythrokeratoderma

A group of rare genodermatoses, traditionally divided into two main types—erythrokeratoderma variabilis (EKV) and progressive symmetric erythrokeratoderma (PSEK)—but phenotypes overlap, and both have been linked to the same mutation in a connexin gene. The term erythrokeratodermia variabilis et progressiva (EKVP) was proposed to encompass the range of phenotypes. Connexin defects have been linked to deafness, as well as other neurological problems, so it is not surprising that erythrokeratoderma-like changes have been described in association with neurological deficits, including deafness.

Erythrokeratodermia variabilis et progressiva

- Transmission AD (rarely AR). Mutations in gap junction genes, including those encoding connexin proteins 30.3, 31, and 43 in some cases, but genetically heterogeneous.
- Onset at birth or early childhood. Rarely later.
- Signs vary but may include:
  - Erythematous patches changing in size and shape. May have annular or serpiginous configurations. Patches may itch or burn. Most often on the face, buttocks, and extensor surfaces of the limbs. Last hours or days. May be followed by fine white scale (unlike urticaria). Triggered by heat, emotion, mechanical irritation. Erythema becomes less obvious in adulthood.
  - Fixed, well-demarcated reddish hyperkeratotic plaques on the trunk, buttocks, and extensor limbs. Fairly or very symmetrical. Plaques tend to extend until puberty, then stabilize and persist into adulthood (see Fig. 32.7).
  - PPK in some patients.
- The histological features in skin biopsies are non-specific.
- Emollients, keratolytics, or oral retinoids may be helpful.

Further reading

Boyden LM et al. J Invest Dermatol 2015;**135**:1540–7.
Rogers M. Australas J Dermatol 2005;**46**:127–43.
van Steensel MAM et al. Am J Med Genet A 2009;**149A**:657–61.

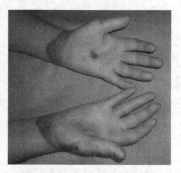

Fig 32.6 Diffuse palmar keratoderma in Mal de Meleda syndrome.

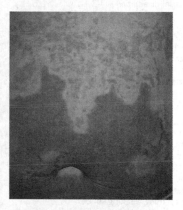

Fig 32.7 Erythrokeratoderma variabilis with well-demarcated hyperkeratotic plaques on the trunk.

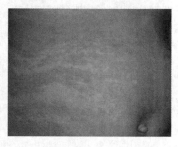

Fig 32.8 Pigmentary mosaicism with hyperpigmentation following Blaschko lines.

Ectodermal dysplasias

What are ectodermal dysplasias?

- A very diverse group of rare (7 in 10 000 births) inherited disorders affecting ectodermal tissues, including neuroectoderm. Over 200 ectodermal dysplasias (EDs) have been described. Transmission AD or AR.
- For molecular pathways in EDs, see Box 32.5.
- Developmental abnormalities in two or more ectodermal structures, most often hair, teeth, nails, or sweat glands.
- Other ectodermal structures may be affected: mammary/thyroid gland, thymus, anterior pituitary, adrenal medulla, CNS, external ear, melanocytes, cornea, conjunctiva, lacrimal gland/duct.
- Abnormal interactions between the ectoderm and mesoderm may cause mesodermal abnormalities.
- Occasionally linked to intellectual disability.
- Also see incontinentia pigmenti (see ➔ pp. 636–7).

X-linked hypohidrotic ectodermal dysplasia

Commonest form of ED—1 per 100 000 births. Defective ectodysplasin-A (mutations in *EDA1* gene). Activation of nuclear factor kappa B (NF-κB) signalling by ectodysplasin is required for the formation of ectodermal structures. Subtypes: transmission AD or AR; hypohidrotic ED (HED) linked to immunodeficiency.

What should I look for?

- Hair—sparse, fine blond hair in childhood. Grows slowly. Scanty eyebrows. Eyelashes may be normal or reduced. Usually no hair on the body or limbs. 2° sexual hair normal or reduced.
- Teeth—missing or malformed (often peg-shaped). Delayed dentition.
- Nails—normal or fragile.
- Sweating—reduced or absent. Hyperthermia on exercise. Febrile seizures in infants. Heat intolerance—patients describe drinking cold fluids, cooling skin by wetting clothing, seeking shade.
- Skin—peeling at birth (may resemble collodion baby). Periorbital wrinkling and pigmentation. Dry skin. Atopic eczema is common. No keratoderma.
- Craniofacial—frontal bossing, sunken nasal bridge, thick everted lips, large ears.
- Mucosal glands—reduced or absent in respiratory tract and GIT, leading to nasal obstruction, recurrent respiratory infections, wheezing, feeding problems in infancy, dysphagia, GI reflux, constipation.
- Lacrimal glands—reduced tears. Dry eyes, photophobia, corneal damage.
- Female carriers—tooth abnormalities, mild hypohidrosis, variable hypotrichosis (look for alopecia and dry skin in Blaschko lines).

Box 32.5 **Molecular pathways disrupted in ectodermal dysplasias**

- Group 1: defective signalling between the ectoderm and mesenchyme leads to hypoplasia or aplasia of ectodermal structures, e.g. mutations in *EDA1* affect activation of the transcription factor NF-κB, or mutations in *WNT10A* affect Wnt/β catenin signalling (see Box 32.6).
- Group 2: abnormal function of a structural protein in the cell membrane leads to abnormal growth of ectodermal structures, e.g. connexins in hidrotic ED (hair loss, nail dystrophy, and PPK) and keratitis–ichthyosis–deafness syndrome (nail dystrophy, alopecia, delayed teeth, ichthyosis, sensorineural deafness).

Box 32.6 **WNT10A syndromes (all rare)**

Wnt/β catenin signalling plays a crucial role in cell development. *WNT10A* mutations have been linked to:
- Schopf–Schulz–Passarge syndrome (AR): eyelid cysts (apocrine hidrocystomas) and PPK with hyperhidrosis. Variable nail, hair and teeth abnormalities.
- Odonto-onycho-dermal dysplasia (AR): oligodontia, nail dystrophy, hypotrichosis, erythematous lesions of the face, smooth tongue with reduced fungiform and filiform papillae, PPK with hyperhidrosis.
- HED (less often than *EDAI* gene).
- Tooth agenesis of varying types.

What should I do?
- ❶ Advise how to prevent hyperthermia—wet clothing, cool drinks, air conditioning (school/home). Advise on sun protection—hats.
- Refer the family to UK support network (🖰 www. ectodermaldysplasia.org).
- Involve a multidisciplinary team in care.

Further reading

García-Martín P et al. Actas Dermosifiliogr 2013;104:451–70.

Incontinentia pigmenti

Incontinentia pigmenti (IP) is a rare ectodermal dysplasia, usually lethal in ♂, caused by mutations in NF-κB essential modulator gene (*IKBKG/ NEMO*) on the X chromosome. ♀ are mosaics (random X chromosome inactivation). NEMO protein has a key role in the NF-κB signalling pathway involved in many functions, including cell survival. Loss of NEMO—cells are more sensitive to apoptosis.

What should I look for?

The skin lesions following Blaschko lines are diagnostic. Typically, the presentation evolves through four stages, but these may overlap, or the first/second stage (s) may not manifest at all:

- *Stage 1. Linear erythematous or vesiculobullous eruption* on the limbs or trunk, within 6 weeks of birth. May be present at birth. Blisters usually clear in 6 months. Recurring crops of blisters may be associated with a circulating eosinophilia. Smear from blisters will show eosinophils. Differential includes: erythema toxicum, infection (herpes simplex/zoster, or varicella), but the child is well. EB (rare).
- *Stage 2. Verrucous stage* with a linear hyperkeratotic or pustular rash, mostly acral (fingers, ankles), which commences around age 2 months and may persist for up to 3 years.
- *Stage 3. Linear streaks or swirls of macular hyperpigmentation* usually by age 6 months, fade during adolescence, and disappear by around 16 years. Differentiate from pigmentary mosaicism (see Box 32.7) or Goltz syndrome (see Box 32.8).
- *Stage 4. Persistent atrophic stage* in adult ♀ with pale, hairless patches or streaks, most often on arms and legs (rare in children). More obvious on suntanned skin.

Other ectodermal/neuroectodermal tissues affected in about 80%:
- Nails: ridging, pitting, and/or onychomycosis-like thickening.
- Hair: scarring alopecia or sparse eyelashes/eyebrows.
- Sweat glands: linear absence.
- Teeth: delayed dentition, missing or conical/peg-shaped teeth.
- Breast: asymmetrical development or supernumerary nipples.
- Ocular (20–37%): strabismus, retinopathy, congenital cataract, or microphthalmia.
- CNS (30%): seizures, spastic paresis, motor delay, intellectual disability, or microcephaly.

What should I do?

- Take a full medical history from the mother, and specifically enquire about miscarriages (♂ infants) or dental problems.
- Examine the mother for subtle pigment change on the limbs.
- Take a skin biopsy from the involved skin in the infant. Inflammatory stage shows eosinophilic spongiosis and dyskeratotic keratinocytes.
- Refer for genetic counselling and neurological, ophthalmological, and dental assessment.

Box 32.7 Pigmentary mosaicism

Synonyms: chromosomal mosaicism, hypomelanosis of Ito, IP achromi-ans, linear and whorled naevoid hypermelanosis.

A heterogeneous condition affecting both sexes. Signs reflect genetic mosaicism. Skin may be hypo- or hyperpigmented.

What should I look for?

- Linear or whorled hypo- or hyperpigmentation present from birth and following Blaschko lines (see ➔ p. 621 and Fig. 32.8). Pigment change is easier to see under UV (Wood) light (no inflammation or blisters, unlike incontinentia pigmenti).
- Areas of hypopigmentation may be hypohidrotic or anhidrotic (demonstrated using a starch iodine test).
- Hair abnormalities in some patients, e.g. colour or textural variation or alopecia.
- Nervous system involvement in some patients, e.g. epilepsy, autistic behaviour, or learning disability.
- Skeletal abnormalities in some patients, e.g. joint contractures, kyphoscoliosis, or digital abnormalities.
- Ocular abnormalities in some patients, e.g. micropthalmia, iris coloboma, or heterochromia of the iris.
- Dental abnormalities in some patients, e.g. hypodontia, absent teeth.

Box 32.8 Focal dermal hypoplasia (Goltz syndrome)

Rare X-linked dominantly inherited ED, usually lethal in ♂. Mutations in *PORCN* gene involved in signalling during embryonic tissue develop-ment. Random inactivation of X chromosome causes mosaicism, with distribution of skin lesions in Blaschko lines. Post-zygotic mosaicism may lead to an affected male.

What should I look for?

- Congenital linear hypo- or hyperpigmented lesions following Blaschko lines (no inflammation or blisters, unlike IP).
- Streaky atrophy of affected skin, with telangiectasia and herniation of fat 2° to loss of dermis.
- Hyperkeratosis, aplasia cutis (see ➔ Box 31.6, p. 595), and scarring within lesions.
- Skeletal abnormalities, including limb reduction, cleft hand or foot deformities, syndactyly, short stature, asymmetrical growth.
- Ocular abnormalities, including strabismus and microphthalmia.
- Malformed teeth.
- Less often, renal anomalies or congenital heart defects.

Further reading

Conte MI et al. *Hum Mutat* 2014;35:165–77 (reviews IP).

Special tools and investigations

Contents

Relevant pages in other chapters

Tools in the clinic

Dermoscopy

Synonyms: dermatoscopy, epiluminescence microscopy, skin surface microscopy.

- The dermatoscope is a hand-held instrument with a bright halogen beam that illuminates and magnifies (10×) intra- and some subepidermal structures, including the superficial vascular plexus. A smear of alcohol, water, or mineral oil on the surface of the lesion eliminates surface reflection and makes the horny layer translucent.
- Dermoscopy was developed as a non-invasive aid for assessing melanocytic skin tumours *in vivo*. Certain features in the pigment network correlate with malignancy (see ➔ p. 342 and p. 344).
- Dermoscopy can also help in the diagnosis of non-pigmented skin tumours such as haemangiomas or BCCs (see ➔ p. 350).
- Dermoscopy is increasingly being used in medical dermatology. For example, the extra magnification has been advocated to visualize nail fold capillaries in patients with possible vasculitis or a connective tissue disorder (see ➔ Box 19.19, p. 415), find the mites in suspected scabies (see ➔ Box 8.2, p. 175), and assess the cause of alopecia (see ➔ p. 488).
- Dermoscopy can be used to screen hair shafts for abnormalities in conditions such as Netherton syndrome (see ➔ Box 31.11, p. 603).

For more information, see ℘ http://www.dermoscopy.co.uk and ℘ http://www.dermoscopy-ids.org/.

Wood light (black light)

- The light emits UVR in the long-wave UVA region.
- Hypopigmentation is more obvious under Wood light, and examination may be particularly helpful in assessing a child with possible tuberous sclerosis for the presence of hypopigmented macules (see ➔ Box 27.7, p. 557).
- Depigmented skin, e.g. vitiligo, fluoresces a bright ivory-white, unlike hypopigmented skin which just looks pale.
- Epidermal hyperpigmentation is accentuated by Wood light, but pigment that is mainly in the dermis is not accentuated (see ➔ Box 30.1, p. 583).
- Some cutaneous infections fluoresce:
  - Tinea capitis caused by *Microsporum audouini* or *Microsporum canis*: light bright green fluorescence.
  - Pityriasis versicolor: yellow fluorescence.
  - Erythrasma: coral pink fluorescence.
  - *Pseudomonas*: green fluorescence.
- Urine containing porphyrins fluoresces pink (see ➔ p. 332).

Diascopy

A diascope is a flat glass plate (most often a microscope slide) through which one examines superficial skin lesions after applying gentle pressure to reduce or remove erythema.

- Diascopy distinguishes between inflammatory and haemorrhagic lesions. A glass slide pressed down on the skin will blanch the erythema of an inflammatory lesion or the redness of a vascular tumour. Bleeding into the skin (petechiae or purpura) does not blanch.
- Diascopy is recommended for assessing the reddish brown granulomatous lesions in sarcoid (see ➔ p. 524) or cutaneous TB (see ➔ p. 144). Gentle pressure enhances the yellow-brown 'apple jelly' colour of the dermal nodules by removing the background erythema.
- Diascopy will also differentiate a naevus anaemicus (where vasoconstriction gives the skin a pale colour; see ➔ p. 562) from a patch of hypopigmented or depigmented skin, e.g. vitiligo. A naevus anaemicus is no longer detectable, when a glass slide is pressed down gently onto the skin. The naevus anaemicus merges into the normal surrounding skin, which is blanched by gentle pressure. Hypopigmented or depigmented skin is still detectable.

Testing for allergy

What is patch testing?

- Dermatitis may be caused by delayed (type IV) hypersensitivity, and this type of allergy is detected by patch testing.
- Hypersensitivity is confirmed by allergic contact dermatitis developing under a patch containing the allergen to which the individual is sensitized. The reaction develops gradually over several days.
- The screening battery of patch tests contains standardized dilutions of allergens such as rubber allergens, neomycin and other medicaments, fragrance allergens, lanolin, and nickel.
- Patch tests are generally put onto the skin of the back (day 0) and are usually read on day 2 and again on day 4.
- Photopatch testing may be required for suspected photoallergic dermatitis. Two identical batteries of allergens are applied to the skin, but one side is irradiated with UVA after 24–48h.
- It takes expertise to correctly select the allergens for testing, to read the tests, but especially to determine the significance of the results.

Who should I refer for patch testing?

- Patients with persistent eczematous eruptions, particularly long-standing facial dermatitis, hand dermatitis, or perianal pruritus.
- Patients with chronic leg ulcers who may become sensitized to the constituents of dressings, bandages, or topical medicaments (see ➲ p. 302).

What is skin-prick testing?

- Skin-prick testing detects immediate (type I) hypersensitivity.
- Patients should stop taking antihistamines at least 48h before the test.
- Drops of allergens in standardized dilutions are placed on marked areas on the forearm, and gentle intradermal punctures are made through each drop with separate sterile fine needles. Positive and negative controls are performed with histamine and saline, respectively.
- Type I hypersensitivity is manifested by an urticarial wheal of 4mm or more that is usually apparent after 10–15min.
- The risk of anaphylaxis is small, but tests should only be carried out by an experienced individual with facilities for resuscitation.
- Specific IgE quantification is an alternative investigation (see Box 33.1).

Who should I refer for skin-prick testing?

- Prick testing is used in the investigation of some patients with acute urticarial reactions, but the relevance of positive results may be difficult to interpret (see ➲ Box 11.3, p. 233).
- Prick testing is not indicated in most patients with dermatitis, apart from those with hand dermatitis who may have a type I hypersensitivity to natural rubber latex, in addition to delayed (type IV) hypersensitivity to natural rubber latex or rubber additives.

Box 33.1 What is specific IgE quantification?

- The test is used to measure total and specific IgE levels to inhaled and ingested antigens.
- The test is performed on a blood specimen so, unlike skin-prick tests, does not present a risk of anaphylaxis.
- Specific IgE quantification may be indicated in patients with suspected food allergies, e.g. immediate reactions such as urticaria, lip swelling, or wheeze.
- Like skin-prick tests, the significance of positive results may be difficult to interpret, particularly in atopic individuals who tend to have multiple type I reactions.

Specimens for bacterial or viral culture

Surface swabs will identify harmless resident surface microbial species, e.g. coagulase-negative staphylococci such as *Staphylococcus epidermidis*, micrococcus species, and some subsurface organisms, as well as pathogenic organisms, e.g. *Staphylococcus aureus* or group A β-haemolytic streptococci. Inevitably, you only sample a small area of skin.

How to take a skin swab for bacterial culture

- Whenever possible, take a sample from pus, exudates, or eroded skin or tissue (see Box 33.2), rather than from the surface of intact skin.
- In individuals with recurrent skin infections, you may also wish to sample uninvolved skin, nose, axillae, and groins.
- To maximize detection from dry areas, first moisten the head of the swab with sterile saline or sterile water.
- Apply reasonably firm pressure to the skin with the swab.
- Put the swab into transport medium designed for bacterial culture.
- Label your sample, and complete the labelled request form. Provide clinical details, and, if necessary, ask for the culture of specific organisms, e.g. anaerobes.

Surface swabs in chronic leg ulcers

Any chronic cutaneous ulcer will be colonized by large numbers of organisms. In most cases, 'routine swabs for culture' are unhelpful. The role of bacteria in delaying healing or causing pain is controversial, but surface culture may be indicated in specific situations:

- Heavy malodorous exudate.
- Painful ulcer.
- Non-healing ulcer.
- Cellulitis (even in this situation, surface swabs may not be very informative).

How to take a skin swab for viral culture

In general, you will be trying to prove if the patient has cutaneous infection with HSV or VZV.

- Please check that you have the right culture medium, before you start (e.g. a small bottle of pink fluid that should be kept in a fridge in the ward or outpatient department). The commonest mistake is to put the swab into transport medium designed for bacteria.
- Put on sterile gloves.
- Look for a fresh vesicle, and gently de-roof with a scalpel. Try to retain some of the roof on the blade, and wipe onto your swab.
- Collect a sample of the fluid on the swab, and rub the swab firmly across the base of the vesicle.
- Place the swab in the viral culture medium.
- Alternatively, you can aspirate some fluid using a needle and syringe. Put the fluid directly into the viral culture medium.
- Label your sample; complete the request form, and provide clinical details. PCR can usually provide a rapid result.

Box 33.2 Culture of a skin biopsy

Culture of tissue is more informative than surface swabs, when dealing with deep cutaneous infections. Consider the need to exclude infection, and obtain suitable culture media (or sterile saline) before you start the biopsy, particularly with immunosuppressed patients. It may be helpful to obtain advice about suitable media from a microbiologist.

Send a sample for histological examination, as well as sending tissue for culture, in these situations:

- ⚠ Any persistent undiagnosed skin lesion (nodule, plaque, blister, ulcer) in an immunosuppressed patient.
- Pyoderma gangrenosum.
- Granulomatous inflammation to exclude deep fungal infection or mycobacterial infection (TB, atypical mycobacteria).
- Chronic non-healing ulcers, particularly in immunosuppressed patients. Virology (herpes simplex) is as important as bacteriology in this situation.

Skin scrapes and smears

Superficial fungal infections

Skin scrapes or brushings in scaly rashes

- Use a glass slide or a No. 15 scalpel blade, and gently scrape the active scaly edge, rather than the centre of the lesion. You are just trying to scrape off scale, not to draw blood.
- Scrape onto dark paper, so you can see the sample, and also scrape some scale onto a glass slide, so you can inspect this for hyphae yourself (see ➲ Microscopy in clinic below).
- Fold up and seal the paper containing your sample—no transport medium is required. Label the specimen, and complete the request form, providing clinical details.
- In suspected tinea capitis, pluck hair, and brush scale off the scalp with a disposable (unpasted!) toothbrush. The toothbrush in its container can be sent directly to the laboratory.
- Microscopy (see later in this section) will provide a rapid result, but it will probably take 4–6 weeks for results of culture.

Sampling dystrophic toenails

- Nails infected by fungus are discoloured, thickened, and fragile.
- Clip off samples of the crumbling nail using nail clippers, and also scoop out some of the soft debris beneath the nail.
- Transport the samples in paper, just as you do for skin scrapes.
- In superficial white onychomycosis, scrape a sample from the discoloured surface of the nail.

Microscopy in clinic

Scrapes or nail clippings may be examined for hyphae using light micros-copy, after dissolving scales, hairs, or nails in potassium hydroxide (KOH).

- Place the scrapings, hair, or nail clippings onto a glass slide, and cover with a coverslip.
- Drop a few drops of a solution of 20% KOH with 40% dimethyl sulfoxide (DMSO) in distilled water onto the slide, and allow it to spread under the coverslip. (No heat is needed, if DMSO is included.)
- Leave the sample in suspension for a few minutes (nails are thicker than skin or hair and should be left for a couple of hours).
- Examine for branching fungal hyphae running across sheets of keratinocytes, using a low-power (×25) objective lens with the iris diaphragm closed and the condenser lowered to increase contrast.

Deep fungal infection

- You will need to take a skin biopsy, and culture the tissue (see Box 33.2).

Tzanck preparation (smear for cytology)

Cytology may be helpful in blistering rashes, particularly if you suspect infection with HSV or VZV. If you are experienced, you can get a preliminary result in the outpatient room. Tzanck preparations (cytological smears) are used infrequently in the UK.

How to make a Tzanck preparation
- You will need a glass slide and a No. 10 or 15 scalpel blade.
- Put on sterile gloves.
- De-roof a fresh blister, and gently scrape the base (you only need tissue fluid and keratinocytes—try not to contaminate the smear with blood). Smear the contents of your blade onto a glass slide.
- Air-dry; fix with methanol, and stain with Giemsa, toluidine blue, or Wright's stain.
- Examine under a light microscope (×40 magnification).
- HSV or VZV infection: multinucleated giant keratinocytes confirm the diagnosis, but laboratory tests, such as PCR, are a more accurate diagnostic tool and have superseded Tzanck preparations.
- Tzanck preparations may help to differentiate subepidermal from intra-epidermal blistering in autoimmune blistering diseases such as BP (subepidermal, no keratinocytes in Tzanck preparation) or pemphigus vulgaris (intra-epidermal, acantholytic rounded-up keratinocytes in Tzanck preparation). The gold standard is histology with IMF studies (see ➔ Box 13.1, p. 267).
- Tzanck preparations have been advocated to differentiate SSSS from TEN. The presence of keratinocytes in the smear suggests SSSS (the blister is in the granular layer, and some intact epidermis is retained in the floor of the blister). In TEN, the blister is subepidermal, so there are no keratinocytes on the floor of the blister, and a Tzanck preparation from the base of the blister will not have any keratinocytes. The preparation must be made from freshly denuded dermis, because, once the epidermis starts to regenerate, keratinocytes will be found in the smear. In practice, it is not usually difficult to differentiate the diseases, particularly if the patient has mucosal involvement (a feature of TEN, not SSSS) (see ➔ p. 112, p. 116).

Skin biopsy in inflammatory conditions

Taking a skin biopsy is not technically difficult, but it may be more challenging to provide the pathologist with a differential diagnosis, to know what sort of biopsy to take, and to choose the right site.

What sort of biopsy

- Pathologists prefer elliptical biopsies (see Box 33.3), because they provide more tissue than a punch biopsy (see Box 33.4), but a deep (uncrushed) 4mm punch biopsy is adequate in some situations.
- Take a deep elliptical biopsy in panniculitis, when you need to examine fat lobules. The fat often shears off in punch biopsies.
- Punch biopsies are particularly suitable for investigating alopecia, as the specimen is examined using both horizontal and vertical sectioning. Ensure you insert the punch deeply along the length of the hair follicle (see ➔ Box 3.2, p. 45).
- For the investigation of blistering diseases, an intact blister is preferred (see ➔ Box 13.1, p. 267).

Where to take the biopsy

- Generally, choose a well-developed 1° lesion, avoiding 2° changes such as excoriations. If the rash has a variety of morphologies, you may wish to take several biopsies.
- Try to avoid taking biopsies from the leg (poor healing) or the cape area, i.e. shoulders, upper back, and central chest (risk of keloid).
- When taking a facial biopsy, use the direction of natural wrinkles to disguise the scar. Ask the patient to screw up his/her face to determine the direction of the incisional biopsy or the position of the punch biopsy.
- In blistering diseases, take the biopsy from a small early intact blister. If you select a large blister, the roof of the specimen may be lost during processing. In old blisters, re-epithelialization at the base of subepidermal blisters can mimic intra-epidermal blisters.
- If you suspect a condition, such as CTCL, it is worth taking multiple incisional biopsies. Be prepared to repeat the biopsies on several occasions over a number of years, before your clinical suspicions are confirmed.

Working with the pathologist

- You are not setting a mind-reading exercise for your pathology colleague! You had the advantage of seeing the patient, so describe the rash on the request form, and tell the pathologist what diagnoses you are considering, what sort of lesion you have biopsied (fresh, well-developed, blister, papule, etc.), and the site of the biopsy.
- Become familiar with the terms commonly used to describe pathological changes in the skin (see ➔ p. 650).
- Histopathology, like all of medicine, is an art, as well as a science. If the diagnosis provided by the pathologist does not fit the clinical findings, you both need to think again. Ideally, you should sit down with the pathologist to review the skin biopsies alongside the clinical photographs. You will learn a lot by discussing the case.

Box 33.3 Elliptical biopsy: how to do it

- The biopsy should either remove an entire lesion or extend from normal skin into the centre of the lesion. The longitudinal axis of the incision should run parallel to the wrinkle lines (face) or Langers lines (trunk, limbs; see ➲ p. 8) and measure 1cm in length.
- Mark out an elongated diamond shape with a sterile skin marker, prior to infiltration of local anaesthetic.
- Clean the skin, and infiltrate local anaesthetic (see Box 33.4).
- Incise vertically down into subcutaneous tissue, using a No. 15 scalpel blade. Lift up the specimen at a corner, and peel back, cutting the base with the scalpel. Do not crush the specimen.
- Close with interrupted or intradermal sutures.

Box 33.4 Punch biopsy: how to do it

- Mark the biopsy site.
- In children, 2.5% lidocaine plus 2.5% prilocaine cream (EMLA®), applied under occlusion for 40–60min, reduces the pain of infiltration:
  - Infants <3 months: maximum dose = 1g.
  - Infants >3 months: maximum dose = 2g.
- Consider restraining infants by wrapping firmly in a sheet.
- Lidocaine 1% with adrenaline 1 in 200 000 is suitable for most sites (avoid in digits). Warm the local anaesthetic to body temperature, prior to infiltration, and infiltrate slowly to minimize discomfort.
- Local anaesthetic in infants:
  - Lidocaine 1% without adrenaline: up to 3mg/kg (maximum for a 5kg infant = 1.5mL).
  - Lidocaine 1% with adrenaline 1 in 200 000: up to 5mg/kg (maximum for a 5kg infant = 2.5mL).
- Allow 20–30min for the anaesthetic and adrenaline to act, before taking the biopsy. Go away, and do something else.
- Do not attempt to check if the skin is numb by jabbing with a needle. Instead, ask an adult patient to tell you if the procedure is uncomfortable.
- Stabilize the skin. Insert the punch slowly down into fat, watching the patient's face. (The expression will tell you if it is painful.)
- Minimal pressure is needed, particularly in children or elderly people with thin skin. Disposable punches are very sharp.
- Depress the skin firmly on each side of the wound, so the specimen pops up, and lift it out on the tip of your scissors—you may need to cut the base with a sharp pair of scissors. Do not damage the specimen by crushing it with forceps or spearing it with a needle!
- If needed, only handle the specimen with a skin hook.
- Usually, sutures are not required if you have used adrenaline. Haemostasis can be obtained using topical 20% aluminium chloride or a piece of calcium alginate dressing in the wound and pressure.

What does the pathologist mean?

Epidermis

- *Acanthosis*: thickening of the epidermis.
- *Papillomatosis*: projections of the dermal papillae and the overlying epidermis above the surface of the surrounding skin.
- *Hyperkeratosis*: increased thickness of the stratum corneum.
- *Dyskeratosis*: abnormal keratinization of keratinocytes.
- *Parakeratosis*: flattened nuclei retained within the stratum corneum. Linked to hyperproliferation and altered differentiation, e.g. psoriasis.
- *Scale crust*: a mix of serum, variable numbers of inflammatory cells, and parakeratotic cells in the stratum corneum.
- *Spongiosis*: intercellular oedema causes widening of spaces between keratinocytes. The adhesion junctions between keratinocytes rupture, and vesicles form in the epidermis. Common in eczema.
- *Acantholysis*: loss of cohesion between keratinocytes. The individual keratinocytes round up and separate from each other, e.g. in the autoimmune blistering disease pemphigus.
- *Ballooning degeneration*: swelling and vacuolization of keratinocytes is followed by acantholysis (see earlier). Common in cutaneous HSV and VZV infections.
- *Necrosis*: cell death resulting from acute cellular injury, e.g. ischaemia.
- *Apoptosis*: programmed cell death. Excess apoptosis causes atrophy; insufficient apoptosis is linked to uncontrolled cell proliferation.
- *Colloid or Civatte body*: an eosinophilic round body in the basal layer of the epidermis or in the upper papillary dermis. The end result of apoptosis of a keratinocyte. Seen in lichenoid reactions (see ➔ p. 224).
- *Epidermotropism*: lymphocytes in the lower layers of the epidermis.
- *Vesicle*: fluid-filled cavity, either within or just below the epidermis.

Dermis

- *Lichenoid reaction or interface dermatitis*: a band-like infiltrate of inflammatory cells in the papillary dermis, which is often associated with basal keratinocyte apoptosis (see ➔ p. 224) and pigment incontinence.
- *Pigment incontinence*: melanin released from basal keratinocytes is deposited in the upper dermis. The pigment may be found within macrophages (melanophages) or free in the dermis. Pigment incontinence is a sign of damage to the basal layer of the epidermis.
- *Fibrinoid necrosis*: extravasation of fibrin into the wall of a blood vessel or its immediate surroundings. A feature of cutaneous vasculitis.
- *Leukocytoclasis*: disintegration of white blood cells, usually neutrophils, with small dark staining nuclear fragments in the dermis (nuclear dust). Associated with activation of neutrophils in conditions such as small-vessel cutaneous vasculitis (leukocytoclastic vasculitis), neutrophilic dermatoses, or dermatitis herpetiformis.
- *Granulomatous inflammation*: see Box 33.5.
- *Necrobiosis*: indistinct appearance of collagen fibres associated with accumulation of mucopolysaccharides. (The term necrobiosis is also used to mean death of cells.)

Box 33.5 Granulomatous inflammation

This is chronic dermal inflammation in which collections of histiocytes are organized into relatively discrete granulomas, sometimes in the presence of multinucleated giant cells. The pattern of inflammation and the presence of features, such as necrobiosis or suppuration, will provide clues to the underlying diagnosis. The pathologist will use polarized light to detect birefringent foreign material and will perform special stains for organisms. You should consider sending material for culture.

Types of granuloma include:

- *Sarcoidal granuloma* (few lymphocytes, 'naked' granuloma): consider sarcoidosis and some types of foreign body reaction (silica, tattoo pigments, zirconium, and beryllium).
- *Tuberculoid granuloma* (granulomas surrounded by a cuff of lymphocytes): think of TB, leprosy, leishmaniasis, or cutaneous Crohn disease.
- *Necrobiotic granuloma* (altered collagen surrounded by histiocytes and sometimes multinucleated giant cells): consider rheumatoid nodule, granuloma annulare, or necrobiosis lipoidica.
- *Suppurative granuloma* (neutrophils in the centre of the granuloma): think of *Mycobacterium marinum* and deep fungal infections.
- *Foreign body granuloma* (a granuloma forms around the foreign body material): localized granulomatous inflammation may be triggered by exogenous foreign bodies or endogenous material such as a ruptured hair follicle or cyst.

Medical management

Contents

Relevant pages in other chapters
Management of leg ulcers ➜ p. 306
Photoprotection ➜ pp. 338–9
Management of atopic eczema in children ➜ pp. 608–10
Skin failure and emergency dermatology ➜ pp. 100–26
Psoriasis ➜ pp. 202–04

General principles of topical treatment

Undertreatment is more common than overuse of topical medicaments. Patients (and ward nurses) are most likely to adhere to simple treatment plans that have been negotiated and explained. Provide a written treatment plan, if you can, in addition to the prescription.

What to tell the patient and/or carer

- Explore anxieties, and reassure (steroid phobia is common).
- Explain how often to apply the treatment and when to apply the treatment—particularly if using >1 medicament. Should both be applied at once, or should applications be separated?
- Ensure that the patient understands what to use and where to apply (provide a written treatment plan).
- Explain how much to use, and demonstrate how to use the treatment.
- Explain the adverse effects and how these may be minimized.
- Discuss the expected outcome of treatment—when might something happen and how much improvement is likely?
- Explain how long to continue treatment.
- Ensure the patient knows how and when to step up or step down the strength of treatment (if this is an option).

The prescription

- Specify the base (ointment, cream, gel, lotion, foam) and quantity (see Box 34.1).
- Prescribe tubs (500g), not tubes (25–30g), of emollient.
- Specify the site and frequency of application. You may need to provide >1 strength or type of treatment for different body sites.
- Potency of a topical corticosteroid preparation is dependent on the formulation, as well as the corticosteroid, so it is acceptable to prescribe using proprietary names, rather than generic names. This ensures that you know exactly what else is in the preparation, including vehicle and preservatives—important in patients with allergies.
- Inpatients: if the patient needs regular applications of an emollient or a topical corticosteroid, please do not add the prescription on the 'when necessary' (PRN) part of the drug chart. Ensure that nurses understand the importance of the topical treatment and that someone helps the patient to apply the treatment as prescribed (most often bd, but emollients may be required tds or qds).

Box 34.1 Quantities required in adults for a single daily application for 2 weeks

- Face and neck: 15–30g
- Both hands: 15–30g
- Scalp: 15–30g
- Both arms: 30–60g
- Both legs: 100g
- Trunk: 100g
- Groins and genitalia: 15–30g

Moisturizers and soap substitutes

Indications: dry, flaky, itchy skin, e.g. eczema, psoriasis. Note: there are many equivalent products to the ones listed below. Determine what is available locally, before you choose moisturizers and soap substitutes.

Emollients (moisturizers)

- Emollients soothe dry, itchy skin, but effects are short-lived, so apply frequently and liberally to all the skin.
- Best applied after a shower or bath, when the skin is moist.
- The best emollient is the one the patient likes! Offer a selection.
- Preparations:
  - Light creams (e.g. Dermol® cream, Cetraben® cream, Diprobase® cream, Doublebase®) or lotions (Dermol 500®).
  - Dermol® products contain benzalkonium chloride and are useful if 2° infection is a problem, e.g. in atopic eczema.
  - Greasy preparations (e.g. Hydromol® ointment, Epaderm® ointment, emulsifying ointment, 50% WSP in liquid paraffin, Emollin® or Dermamist® spray).
- Adverse effects:
  - Ointments are less likely to irritate or sensitize skin than creams.
  - Ointments are messy to use, and some patients find that greasy preparations make them hot and itchy.
  - Irritants in creams may cause transient burning or erythema.
  - Allergy to emollients is uncommon, but patients occasionally become allergic to excipients in creams, such as cetostearyl alcohol, parabens, and sodium metabisulfite, or to fragrances.
  - Folliculitis: smear the emollient in the direction of hair growth, and allow to soak into the skin. Advise not to rub the emollient into the skin, to minimize irritation or blockage of hair follicles.
  - Fire hazard: emulsifying ointment or 50% liquid paraffin in WSP can be ignited by a naked flame. The risk is greater, when applied to large areas of the body and if clothing/dressings are soaked with ointment.

Soap substitutes

- Useful in dry, itchy skin conditions.
- Aqueous cream is a better soap substitute than an emollient.
- Hydromol® ointment or Epaderm® ointment are greasy and effective soap substitutes.

Bath additives

- Patients (and carers) like to add oils to the bath. Most contain emollients that help to soothe dry, itchy skin, e.g. Balneum® range, Dermol® range, Oilatum® range.
- It is easy to moisturize all the skin with a bath oil.
- Emollient ointments and creams applied directly to the skin are probably more effective than bath additives in patients with very dry skin.
- Bath oils may make the bath very slippery—a problem in the elderly and the very young. Aveeno® Bath Oil turns milky in water and can be used for these patients, as the risk of slipping is much lower.

Topical corticosteroids

Indications: inflammatory conditions such as insect bites, acute or chronic eczema, localized psoriasis, including flexural and scalp psoriasis. Topical corticosteroids are of no value in treating urticaria.

Potency

Prescribe a corticosteroid strong enough to control the problem, and aim to gradually reduce the strength and frequency of application. Absorption is greatest where the skin is thin and in intertriginous areas, e.g. vulva, groins, and axilla. Use a milder corticosteroid in these areas. Avoid potent or very potent corticosteroids on the face, except in special circumstances, e.g. acute contact dermatitis, chronic cutaneous LE.

Commonly used topical corticosteroids include:

- Mild:
  - Hydrocortisone 0.5%, 1%, or 2.5%.
  - Hydrocortisone with antibiotic.
  - Hydrocortisone with antifungal (used for inflamed flexural rashes when candidiasis may complicate treatment with corticosteroid).
- Moderate:
  - Betamethasone valerate cream 0.025%, clobetasone butyrate 0.05%.
  - Moderate with antibacterials and antifungals (clobetasone butyrate 0.05%, oxytetracycline 3% (as calcium salt), nystatin 100 000 units).
- Potent:
  - Betamethasone valerate 0.1%, mometasone furoate 0.1%, hydrocortisone butyrate 0.1%.
  - Potent with antimicrobials.
  - Potent with salicylic acid, e.g. betamethasone 0.05% with salicylic acid 3%.
- Very potent:
  - Clobetasol propionate 0.05%, diflucortolone valerate 0.3%.

How to apply

- No more frequently than twice daily; once daily is often sufficient (see Box 34.2).
- Spread thinly on the affected skin. One FTU (~500mg) is sufficient to cover an area that is twice that of the flat adult palm (see Box 34.3).
- Apply about 20–30min after (or before) any emollient.
- Undertreatment because of steroid phobia is a common cause of treatment failure. Show the patient how to use the treatment.

For more information about treatment of children, see ➔ p. 610.

Adverse effects of topical corticosteroids

- *Mild* and *moderately potent* topical corticosteroids are associated with few side effects and are safe to use in children and on the thin skin of the face and flexures.
- *Potent* and *very potent* topical steroids—local side effects include:
  - Spread and worsening of untreated skin infection, including dermatophyte infections (tinea incognito) (see ➋ p. 164).
  - Thinning of the skin which may be restored over a period after stopping treatment, but the original structure may never return. Commoner on flexural skin where the skin is already thin. In general, avoid potent and very potent corticosteroids in flexures.
  - Irreversible striae atrophica and telangiectasia—also commoner in flexures.
  - Acne, worsening of acne or rosacea, or perioral dermatitis (see ➋ pp. 256–7). In general, avoid potent/very potent corticosteroids on the face.
  - Hypopigmentation which may be reversible. More often, the loss of colour is 2° to the skin condition (post-inflammatory hypopigmentation) than the treatment.
  - Rarely, prolonged topical treatment with large quantities of a very potent corticosteroid has been reported to cause adrenal suppression or Cushing syndrome.
  - Absorption with the risk of adverse effects is increased by occlusion.

Box 34.2 Get control and keep control—maintenance therapy for eczema

(see ➋ pp. 218–223 and pp. 608–610).

Eczema is chronic, but its severity can fluctuate. Many patients report a rapid flare shortly after using topical steroids, which leaves the skin looking apparently unaffected. Evidence suggests that, in atopic individuals, subclinical eczema persists and results in early relapse. To manage this, you should recommend the following:

- Get control: treat visible eczema with emollients and topical steroids every day for 2 weeks.
- Keep control: eczema appears to have cleared; use topical steroids for 2 consecutive days (e.g. weekend therapy), but continue with emollients daily.
- If the skin flares, return to 'Get control' step. Over time, the frequency of flares will reduce.

Box 34.3 Rough guide to the amount of topical corticosteroid

One FTU is the amount of cream or ointment squeezed from a standard tube (5mm nozzle) along the palmar surface of the distal phalanx of an adult index finger from the very tip to the crease of the DIP joint.

1 FTU weighs ~0.5g and will cover a surface area equivalent to the palmar surface of two adult hands (including the fingers).

In children, the FTU of cream or ointment is measured on an adult index finger, before being rubbed onto a child. 1 FTU treats an area of skin on a child equivalent to twice the size of the palmar surface of an adult's hand with the fingers together. Estimate the amount of topical steroid to use by using your (adult) hand to determine the area of skin affected on the child.

Tubes usually contain 30g (60 FTUs) or 100g (200 FTUs). All measurements assume the tube has a standard 5mm nozzle.

3- to 6-month-old child
- Entire face and neck: 1 FTU.
- An entire arm and hand: 1 FTU.
- An entire leg and foot: 1.5 FTUs.
- The entire front of the chest and abdomen: 1 FTU.
- The entire back, including buttocks: 1.5 FTUs.

1- to 2-year-old child
- Entire face and neck: 1.5 FTUs.
- An entire arm and hand: 1.5 FTUs.
- An entire leg and foot: 2 FTUs.
- The entire front of the chest and abdomen: 2 FTUs.
- The entire back, including buttocks: 3 FTUs.

3- to 5-year-old child
- Entire face and neck: 1.5 FTUs.
- An entire arm and hand: 2 FTUs.
- An entire leg and foot: 3 FTUs.
- The entire front of the chest and abdomen: 3 FTUs.
- The entire back, including buttocks: 3.5 FTUs.

Adult
- A hand and fingers (front and back): 1 FTU.
- A foot (all over): 2 FTUs.
- Front of the chest and abdomen: 7 FTUs.
- Back and buttocks: 7 FTUs.
- Face and neck: 2.5 FTUs.
- An entire arm and hand: 4 FTUs.
- An entire leg and foot: 8 FTUs.
- Entire body: about 40 FTUs.

Occlusion

Occlusion cools and soothes itchy skin, also protects the skin by preventing the damage wrought by fingernails, particularly at night. Consider occlusion in chronically itchy conditions, when endless rubbing has thickened the skin (lichenification; see ➔ Fig. 31.9, p. 611) or resulted in nodules (prurigo; see ➔ p. 222). Occlusion softens scaly skin and enhances the penetration of topical corticosteroids applied under the dressing or bandage. Do not occlude infected skin.

Occlusive dressings

- For a localized area of chronic irritation, prescribe a self-adhesive hydrocolloid dressing in combination with a potent or very potent topical corticosteroid ointment.
- Apply the ointment thinly to the active area.
- Cut a piece of the sticky hydrocolloid to cover the affected area and 1cm of surrounding skin. Trim the corners, so it is an oval shape.
- Apply the dressing, and hold it in place firmly for several minutes, until it warms up, becomes tacky, and sticks firmly to the skin.
- Advise the patient to leave the dressing in place for about 6 days (the patient can bathe or shower as normal), and then remove it to give the skin a 24-h 'breathing' period. Then the patient should apply more ointment and another dressing.
- Continue treatment, until the itch and inflammation settles. This may take a few weeks or several months.

Medicated stockings

- Zipzoc® are tubular rayon stockings impregnated with ointment containing 20% zinc oxide. Zipzoc® were developed for patients with chronic leg ulcers, but the stockings have proved extremely useful in patients, including children, with chronic eczema.
- The stockings are easy to use. Simply cut to length, and pull on.
- Corticosteroid ointment may be applied beneath the stocking.
- An overlying cotton tubular bandage will prevent staining of clothing or bedding.
- It may be possible to remove and reuse a Zipzoc® on several consecutive nights.

Medicated paste bandages

- The bandage may be impregnated with coal tar, icthammol, calamine, or zinc paste. Paste bandages are particularly useful for managing gravitational eczema associated with chronic venous leg ulcers, when they can be used under compression bandages (see Fig. 34.1).
- An emollient or topical corticosteroid ointment may be applied to areas of eczema beneath the bandage.
- Paste bandages, unlike Zipzoc®, are tricky to apply properly (see Box 34.4).

Box 34.4 Applying a paste bandage

- Paste bandages are an old-fashioned, but effective, method of occluding a whole limb.
- Clean the skin, and apply an emollient and/or a topical corticosteroid ointment, if required.
- If the paste bandage is simply wrapped around the limb in a continuous spiral, as it dries, it may tighten and restrict blood supply.
- Either cut up the bandage and wrap around the leg in single overlapping strips or use the pleating method of bandaging (see Fig. 34.1). Wrap the bandage around the limb once in one direction, until the ends meet, and then fold the bandage back upon itself, and apply in the opposite direction, slightly overlapping the previous turn of the bandage. Continue up the limb, reversing the direction of each turn of the bandage to avoid a circumferential band.
- A cohesive elastic bandage, such as Coban®, applied over the paste bandage will hold everything in place.
- Leave for up to 1 week.
- The patient should use a clean polythene bin liner to protect the bandage in the shower or bath.

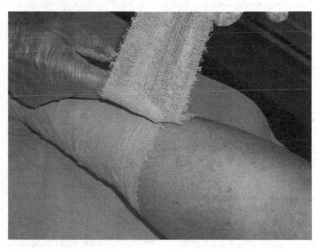

Fig. 34.1 Bandaging technique.

Further reading

The British Dermatological Nursing Group. *How to apply paste bandages*. Available at: ℗ http://www.bdng.org.uk/documents/How_to_Apply_Paste_BandagesBDNG.pdf.

Soaks, wet dressings, and 'wet wraps'

Astringent lotions are used to clean, dry, and soothe weeping eczema or blistering eruptions. Solutions are antiseptic and are also used to reduce bacterial contamination in chronic ulcers. The limb is soaked for 10–20min once or twice a day. You do not need anything more complicated than a plastic bucket and a bin liner, but you will have to explain to the patient and/or carer exactly what to do.

Wet dressings are a cooling and antiseptic alternative to soaks that may be used on an area that is difficult to soak in a bucket. Dip clean gauze in the solution, and apply as a compress to the affected skin several times a day. 'Wet wraps' may be used for short periods to relieve itching in conditions such as acute atopic eczema, particularly in infants. The wraps reduce itch by cooling the skin but also enhance the effect of topical treatments, including moisturizers, and protect itchy skin from fingernails. Do not use wet wraps if there are any signs of cutaneous infection.

Preparations for weeping eczematous skin or blistering

- Potassium permanganate (available in the UK as Permitabs®). Line a bucket with a clean bin liner, and half-fill with tap water. Put on gloves; add 1 Permitab® to the water, and agitate to ensure the potassium permanganate dissolves completely. Undissolved crystals at the bottom of the container could burn the skin. Dilute with more water, continuing to stir, until you have a uniform pale pink solution, the colour of rosé wine (1 Permitab® dissolved in 4L of water = 0.01% solution). The solution will stain fabric, skin, and nails brown. Coat nails with petroleum jelly, prior to soaking, to avoid staining. Remove brown stains on the skin with lemon juice. Potassium permanganate solution may be added to a bath—but the bath will be stained permanently!
- Silver nitrate 0.5% solution.
- Aluminium acetate solution 0.13–0.5% (Burow solution). This is available in the USA as tablets or powder for dissolving in water.

Preparations for chronic leg ulcers

(Also see ➔ p. 306.)

- Prontosan® wound irrigation solution is an antibacterial wash which contains betaine (surfactant) and polyhexanide (antimicrobial).
- Potassium permanganate solution—discussed earlier in this section.
- Acetic acid—2 tablespoonfuls of vinegar to 1 pint of tap water—is useful for chronic leg ulcers colonized with *Pseudomonas* (indicated by malodorous bright green dressings).
- Wet gauze dressings soaked in the antiseptic solution may be applied to the ulcer and kept wet for 20min.

Further reading

British Association of Dermatologists. Patient information leaflets. Available at: ℬ http://www.bad.org.uk.

Systemic drugs in dermatology

We provide no more than pointers to using these drugs—please read detailed prescribing guidelines and local protocols. Involve the patient in any decision about his/her treatment (see ➜ p. 31, Box 2.11). Discuss how long the drug will take to act and what the outcome might be, but offer written, as well as verbal, information. Explain the importance of monitoring, and encourage patients to keep their own record, either hand-held or electronic. The patient should bring this to clinic visits. Generally, you will share monitoring with the GP, according to a local protocol—read this, so you know what is expected of you. In many departments, specialist nurses monitor patients on systemic treatment, but the prescriber has overall responsibility.

Antihistamines

- Non-sedating: chronic urticaria, e.g. fexofenadine, cetirizine, loratadine, rupatadine.
- Sedating: for itching, e.g. hydroxyzine, chlorphenamine, but treat any underlying skin problem or systemic disease causing the itch. Caution in elderly.

Azathioprine

Azathioprine is an anti-inflammatory and immunosuppressant drug that is converted to 6-mercaptopurine (6-MP). Some 6-MP is catabolized to inactive metabolites by enzymes such as thiopurine methyltransferase (TPMT). Other pathways produce 6-MP metabolites that interfere with cell division and function of T- and B-cells. Dose: 2–2.5mg/kg/day.

What should I do?

- Measure TPMT activity or check the genotype, before starting treatment. A mutation in the *TPMT* gene lowers enzyme activity and increases the risk of myelosuppression. Approximately one in ten of the population is heterozygous (intermediate activity), and one in 100 homozygous (low activity) for the mutation. Prescribe a low dose, if the TPMT activity is reduced.
- Warn about nausea and diarrhoea. Limit alcohol intake.
- Warn about the increased risk of malignancy, including skin cancer, with long-term treatment. Advise the patient to use sun protection (see ➜ pp. 338–9).
- Monitor for hepatotoxicity and myelosuppression, initially with weekly FBC and LFT. Increased risk of pancytopenia with allopurinol.
- Avoid live vaccines, e.g. oral polio, BCG, rubella. Influenza and pneumococcal vaccines are safe and are recommended.

Ciclosporin

Ciclosporin is an immunosuppressant drug that blocks calcineurin, thus preventing the activation of T-cells. It is metabolized by the cytochrome P450 pathway and is susceptible to interaction with other drugs inhibiting or inducing these enzymes. Duration of treatment should be <2 years, whenever possible. Dose: 2.5–5mg/kg/day.

What should I do?
- Exclude contraindications: hypertension, renal impairment, active infection, or malignancy, except cured non-melanoma skin cancer.
- Urinalysis, FBC, renal function, LFTs, and fasting lipids.
- Measure blood pressure and creatinine twice, before starting treatment.
- Warn about hypertension and nephrotoxicity, as well as nausea, diarrhoea, gum hypertrophy, hirsutism, tremor, and burning sensation in hands and feet.
- Warn about increased risk of malignancy, including skin cancer, with long-term treatment (particularly if previous PUVA). Advise the patient to use sun protection (see ➲ pp. 338–9). Advise cervical smear, if appropriate.
- Warn about drugs or foods which may increase (e.g. cimetidine, erythromycin, grapefruit juice) or decrease (e.g. carbamazepine, phenytoin, St John's wort) ciclosporin levels. Avoid nephrotoxic drugs, e.g. NSAIDs and ACE inhibitors or potassium-sparing diuretics (increase risk of hyperkalaemia). Ciclosporin increases the risk of statin-induced myositis.
- Avoid live vaccines, e.g. oral polio, BCG, rubella. Influenza and pneumococcal vaccines are safe and are recommended.
- Prescribe one brand, as different preparations differ in bioavailability.
- Monitor blood pressure and renal function 2-weekly initially. Once stable, monitor monthly. Reduce the dose, if creatinine rises 30% above the baseline. Treat hypertension with a calcium antagonist, e.g. nifedipine or amlodipine.

Colchicine

Colchicine is extracted from the autumn crocus *Colchicum autumnale*. Colchicine has anti-inflammatory effects and decreases neutrophil degranulation. Dose: 0.5–2mg/day.

What should I do?
Warn patients about diarrhoea, the commonest adverse effect. GI adverse effects are related to higher doses. Other adverse effects include bone marrow suppression, peripheral neuropathy, myopathy, and hair loss.

Corticosteroids

Corticosteroids are potent anti-inflammatory drugs that exert their effects by binding to intracellular glucocorticoid receptors and regulating anything from ten to 100 genes involved in inflammation. Short-term courses of prednisolone 20–30mg/day, tapered over 2–3 weeks, may control acute inflammation. Some conditions require long-term treatment, high doses (up to 60mg/day), or pulses of IV methylprednisolone. Do not stop topical treatments, including emollients and topical corticosteroids, if you prescribe oral corticosteroids for a skin problem.

What should I do?
- Patients will be worried about adverse effects—discuss these, and help the patient to weigh up risks and benefits. Adverse effects are related to the dose and duration of treatment. The commonest are weight gain, osteoporosis, dyspepsia, easy bruising, thinning of skin, myopathy, mood changes, cataracts, menstrual irregularity, diabetes, hypertension, susceptibility to infections, and, in children, growth suppression.
- Advise patients on long-term treatment not to stop medication suddenly and to carry a steroid treatment card.
- Monitor weight, blood pressure, and blood glucose while on treatment.
- Live vaccinations are not recommended if taking high doses of oral corticosteroids (40mg prednisolone daily for >1 week), but encourage influenza and pneumococcal vaccination.
- Consider bone protection with a bisphosphonate and calcium/vitamin D. Check Royal College of Physicians guidelines for patients who are starting a course of at least 3 months of corticosteroids (℗ https://www.rcplondon.ac.uk). Bone protection (oral bisphosphonate with calcium and vitamin D supplements) should be given to high-risk patients (e.g. aged ≥65 or a previous fragility fracture), without requiring bone densitometry, although this may be useful for long-term follow-up. In other patients, measure bone density, and start a bisphosphonate if the T-score is −1.5 or lower. Consider calcium and vitamin D supplementation in all patients, but particularly if photosensitive and using sun blocks, e.g. patients with SLE.

Dapsone

Dapsone is a sulfone drug with anti-neutrophilic properties (inhibits neutrophil myeloperoxidase). Dose: 50–150mg/day.

What should I do?
- Ask about allergy to sulfonamides (dapsone contraindicated).
- Check for glucose-6-phosphate dehydrogenase (G6PD) deficiency in people of Mediterranean, African, and Asian ancestry.
- Warn about nausea, headache, or blue discoloration of fingertips and lips (methaemoglobinaemia). More serious, but rare, problems include agranulocytosis, peripheral motor neuropathy (weak hands and feet), and hypersensitivity ('DRESS'—fever, rash, lymphadenopathy 1–2 months after starting treatment; see ➔ pp. 122–3).
- Contraindications include liver disease, anaemia, allergy to sulfonamides, porphyria, and G6PD deficiency.
- Start with a low dose (50mg/day), and increase slowly, if tolerated.
- Monitor FBC, and liver and renal function. Initially the haemoglobin will fall. Dapsone always causes some haemolysis.
- Monitor for motor neuropathy by asking the patient to walk on tiptoes and then on heels.

Fumaric acid esters

Fumaderm (a mixture of fumaric acid esters, FAEs) is an unlicensed drug in the UK but is available on a doctor-named patient basis for treatment of moderate to severe psoriasis in adults. FAEs are licensed for treatment of psoriasis in some countries. FAEs have an anti-inflammatory action but also promote keratinocyte differentiation and inhibit keratinocyte proliferation. Dose is increased gradually over 9 weeks to a maximum of two tablets tds. It takes 4–6 weeks before any benefit is noted.

What should I do?
- Contraindications include severe GI disease, severe kidney or liver disease, haematological disorder, pregnancy, and breastfeeding.
- GI adverse effects may limit the dose, but usually well tolerated, provided dose increased slowly.
- Adverse effects include diarrhoea, abdominal cramps, nausea, flushing (worse at onset of treatment), and headaches.
- Monitor FBC (may cause mild leucopenia/lymphopenia, eosinophilia), liver function (transient rise in liver enzymes), and renal function, including urinalysis (rarely causes proteinuria, haematuria, and rise in creatinine). Repeat weekly for 1 month, and then monthly, if no abnormalities.
- Generally avoid concomitant use of ciclosporin, methotrexate, retinoids, psoralen, or phototherapy. Avoid other renal toxic drugs. Reduce dose if leucocytes $<3.0 \times 10^9$/L, or lymphocytes $<0.5 \times 10^9$/L, or persistent eosinophilia $\geq 25\%$, or creatinine 30% above baseline, or proteinuria. Stop if abnormality persists or further deterioration.

Hydroxychloroquine

Hydroxychloroquine is an antimalarial with anti-inflammatory properties. Dose: 200–400mg/day. Maximum dose = 6.5mg/kg/day.

What should I do?
- Advise to take with food to reduce nausea.
- Retinal toxicity is a rare adverse effect that is avoided by using a dose of no more than 6.5mg/kg daily. Patients should see an optician annually. Refer to an ophthalmologist, if the patient develops visual problems.
- Check FBC, and renal and liver function before starting. Reduce the dose in renal and hepatic impairment.

Mepacrine

Mepacrine is another antimalarial used on its own or sometimes in conjunction with hydroxychloroquine. Dose: 50–100mg/day.

What should I do?
- Warn about transient orange discoloration of the skin and urine (disappears on stopping the drug), dizziness, nausea, diarrhoea, and headache.
- Liver and bone marrow toxicity are rare. No retinal toxicity.
- Contraindications include porphyria and liver disease.
- Check FBC and LFTs twice a year.

Methotrexate

Methotrexate is a folic acid analogue with anti-inflammatory properties. It inhibits the enzyme dihydrofolate reductase, which reduces dihydrofolate to tetrahydrofolate. Tetrahydrofolate is required for the synthesis of DNA precursors. Methotrexate is thought to inhibit the proliferation of lymphocytes involved in inflammation. Dose: 5–25mg once a week.

What should I do?

- Contraindications include excessive alcohol intake, significant renal or hepatic impairment, active acute infection, immunodeficiency, blood dyscrasias, breastfeeding, pregnancy, and lactation.
- Prior to starting therapy, check FBC, liver function, and renal function. Enquire about alcohol use—recommend limiting or, ideally, avoiding entirely.
- Check CXR if any risk of prior lung disease.
- Screening for liver fibrosis can be done by measuring serum type III procollagen peptide (PIIINP). However, many patients with arthritis have a raised PIIINP, despite a normal liver biopsy, so PIIINP is not helpful in this population. There is increasing literature supporting the use of fibroscans as an alternative screening tool.
- Methotrexate is teratogenic—men and women should use contraception and stop the drug for at least 3 months before conception.
- Warn about common adverse effects, e.g. nausea, diarrhoea, hair loss, and less common serious adverse effects: mouth ulcers, bone marrow or liver or lung toxicity (lung toxicity is very uncommon in psoriasis).
- Ensure the patient has 2.5mg tablets, not 10mg tablets, which look the same. Prescribe a test dose (2.5–5mg), and check FBC after 1 week. If normal, prescribe the full weekly dose (usually 12.5–15mg/ week). Reduce the dose in renal impairment or the elderly.
- Prescribe folic acid (≥5mg/week) to reduce mucosal/GI toxicity.
- Monitor FBC and LFTs, ideally weekly, while the dose is adjusted. Once the dose is stable, check FBC and liver function 1- to 3-monthly.
- Check renal function and PIIINP 6-monthly.
- Consider liver biopsy if LFTs are persistently elevated.
- Nausea may limit the dose. Take with food; try splitting the dose over 12h; take at night, or try ondansetron (antiemetic) prior to methotrexate. Subcutaneous methotrexate may be better tolerated than oral.
- Patients with mouth ulcers, sore throat, fever, epistaxis, unexpected bleeding, or bruising should have urgent FBC and LFTs. Investigate breathlessness with CXR to exclude pneumonitis.
- Avoid co-trimoxazole and trimethoprim (antifolate effects).
- Avoid live vaccines, e.g. oral polio, BCG, rubella. Influenza and pneumococcal vaccines are safe and are recommended.

Mycophenolate mofetil

Mycophenolate mofetil is an immunosuppressant that is converted to the active agent mycophenolic acid, which inhibits lymphocyte proliferation and antibody production. Dose: 1–3g/day.

What should I do?
- Check FBC, and renal and liver function before starting, and monitor during treatment (weekly initially and then every 1–3 months).
- Warn patients about adverse effects of nausea, diarrhoea, and anaemia.
- Advise patients to use sun protection (increased risk of skin cancers if taken in conjunction with other immunosuppressants).
- Avoid pregnancy during treatment and for 6 weeks after stopping.

Retinoids

The retinoids are analogues of vitamin A that regulate gene transcription via intracellular nuclear receptors. They have diverse effects on cell differentiation and proliferation, immune function, and embryonic development. Acitretin (a metabolite of etretinate) is used in disorders of keratinization, e.g. severe psoriasis. Oral isotretinoin (0.25–1 mg/kg/ day) is used in severe acne. Acitretin is also used to reduce the risk of skin cancers developing in organ transplant recipients. Alitretinoin is used to treat severe chronic hand eczema.

What should I do?
- Oral retinoids are teratogenic and must be avoided in pregnancy. You will be expected to follow a protocol for prescribing, dispensing, and monitoring these drugs. Women of childbearing age must sign a consent form, agree to use secure contraception (two types are recommended), and agree to have monthly pregnancy tests. Contraception should be continued for at least 1 month after stopping isotretinoin, and 2 years after stopping acitretin. In practice, acitretin is rarely used in women of childbearing age.
- Common adverse effects include dryness of mucous membranes and skin, muscle aches and pains, photosensitivity, raised serum triglycerides or cholesterol, and raised liver enzymes. Headache and flushing are additional side effects observed with alitretinoin.
- Check plasma lipids (fasting) and liver function prior to starting treatment, and then monitor 1- to 3-monthly, depending on the retinoid prescribed.

Thalidomide

Thalidomide was used in the 1950s as a sedative and antiemetic, but phocomelia was a tragic adverse effect, and, by 1961, the drug had been withdrawn worldwide. Thalidomide has anti-inflammatory and immunomodulatory actions that may be mediated by inhibition of TNF-α.

What should I do?
- The risk of birth defects is 100% if the drug is taken in the first 21–36 days of gestation. Thalidomide must be prescribed and dispensed in accordance with the Thalidomide Celgene® Pregnancy Prevention Programme. Prescribers must read the Programme information and complete the appropriate forms. Pharmacists must register with Celgene®. For more information, see ℰ http://www.celgene. co.uk/content/uploads/sites/3/Thalidomide_Celgene_Healthcare_ Professional_Booklet.pdf.

- Follow the protocol for prescribing, dispensing, and monitoring thalidomide.
- Patients must give written consent. Women of childbearing age must use two forms of contraception and have monthly pregnancy tests.
- Another serious adverse effect is a peripheral sensory neuropathy that is irreversible. Patients have painful paraesthesiae of the hands and feet. Refer for pretreatment nerve conduction studies, and monitor 6-monthly during treatment.

We cannot provide more than a brief introduction to the principles of treatment. Patient information leaflets about most of the topical and systemic treatments mentioned here can be downloaded from the website of the British Association of Dermatologists (⅋ http://www.bad. org.uk). This information may also help carers, including ward nurses, unfamiliar with managing skin problems.

Further reading

British Association of Dermatologists. Patient information leaflets and clinical guidelines. Available at: ⅋ http://www.bad.org.uk.

British Association of Dermatologists. *Clinical guidelines*. Available at: ⅋ http://www.bad.org. uk/healthcare-professionals/clinical-standards/clinical-guidelines.

Chandler D and Bewley A. *Pharmaceuticals* 2013;6:557–78.

Medicines Complete. *British National Formulary*. Available at: ⅋ https://www.medicinescomplete.com/about/.

Wakelin SH, Maibach HI, Archer CB. *Handbook of Systemic Drug Treatment in Dermatology*, 2nd edn, 2015. Oxford: Wiley-Blackwell.

Biologics in dermatology

See Box 34.5.

Box 34.5 Biologics in dermatology

Biologic drugs include monoclonal antibodies and a variety of protein drugs, which alter the activity of cytokines, enzymes, and growth factors. They can be a useful alternative when standard treatments have failed, but are expensive, and their immunosuppressive properties can increase the risk of infections, in particular *Mycobacterium tuberculosis*. There is also a potential increase in the risk of malignancies.

Tumour necrosis factor inhibitors

Infliximab, adalimumab, golimumab, and certolizumab are anti-TNF monoclonal antibodies. Etanercept is a TNF receptor fusion protein.

Indications: Inflammatory skin conditions, e.g. psoriasis, hidradenitis suppurativa.

Adverse cutaneous effects include plaque, guttate, erythrodermic, and pustular psoriasis, and sarcoid-like granulomatosis (also occurs in lungs).

Interleukin antagonists

Ustekinumab is a monoclonal antibody, which binds to the p40 subunit of IL-12 and IL-23. Indications: plaque psoriasis. Can trigger pustular psoriasis.

Secukinumab is an anti-IL-17A monoclonal antibody. Also used for psoriasis.

Anakinra (IL-1 receptor antagonist) and canakinumab (IL-1β monoclonal antibody) are used for auto-inflammatory syndromes.

Newer agents include dupilimumab (IL-4 and IL-13 blocker) that may have benefits for atopic eczema.

Phosphodiesterase 4 inhibitors

Apremilast is a PDE 4 inhibitor under investigation for treatment of psoriasis.

B-cell therapies

Rituximab is a chimeric human/murine monoclonal antibody against CD20, a surface molecule expressed on B-lymphocytes. Rituximab prevents the development of antibody-producing cells.

Indications include connective tissue diseases, e.g. SLE, or bullous disease.

Immunoglobulin inhibitors

Omalizumab is a monoclonal antibody to IgE Fc region developed for treatment of asthma and chronic spontaneous urticaria.

Resources

Contents

Resources

The British Association of Dermatologists
🔗 http://www.bad.org.uk

The British Association of Dermatologists (BAD) is the professional organization for dermatologists in the UK and Irish Republic. The website has excellent resources for doctors, as well as for patients—check it out. The site includes these pages, amongst others.

For the public
The pages include patient information leaflets that not only explain many skin conditions, but also include information about drugs and topical treatments. The leaflets are easy to download. Nurses may also find some of this information helpful. The pages devoted to skin cancer and sun safety address topics such as sunbeds, sunscreens, and vitamin D, as well as skin cancers. The site also provides an extensive list of local, national, and international patient support groups.

Health-care professionals
You can access clinical guidelines as PDF documents. Also lists unlicensed dermatological preparations—'Specials'.

Psoriasis
Resources for assessment and management of patients with psoriasis, including assessment forms such as PASI, DLQI and PEST.

Education
A section for medical students, medical trainees, and dermatology trainees, as well as teachers of dermatology. The resources include intranet lectures for medical students, a dermatology handbook for medical students and junior doctors, and a smartphone app.

Specialist groups
Provides links to specialist societies, e.g. medical dermatology, paediatric dermatology, cutaneous allergy, and dermatological surgery.

DermNet NZ
🔗 http://www.dermnetnz.org/sitemap.html

Comprehensive resource for information about skin conditions and their treatment, including excellent pictures.

American Academy of Dermatology
🔗 http://www.aad.org/

Explore the Academy's website for educational resources, including clinical guidelines, fact sheets, and videos (for the public) about managing skin conditions.

Additional resources
- For online atlases, see Box 35.1.
- For evidence-based dermatology, see Box 35.2.
- For more information about skin cancer, dermoscopy, and British Skin Foundation, see Box 35.3.

Box 35.1 Online atlases

- DermQuest: teaching and learning resources. ℘ https://www.dermquest.com/
- Primary Care Dermatology Society. ℘ http://www.pcds.org.uk
- DermNet NZ. ℘ http://www.dermnetnz.org/
- DermIS. ℘ http://www.dermis.net/dermisroot/en/home/index.htm
- Dermatoweb.net: Spanish text. ℘ http://dermatoweb2.udl.es/
- Loyola University Dermatology Medical Education Website. ℘ http://www.meddean.luc.edu/lumen/MedEd/medicine/dermatology/melton/atlas.htm
- eMedicine: for review articles in Medscape CME. Registration is free. ℘ http://emedicine.medscape.com/dermatology

Box 35.2 Evidence-based dermatology

- Clinical guidelines published by NICE. ℘ http://www.nice.org.uk/
- The Cochrane Collaboration—an international independent organization dedicated to providing accurate information about effective health care. The Cochrane Library includes reviews of the management of some common skin problems. ℘ http://cochrane.co.uk/en/collaboration.html
- Centre of Evidence Based Dermatology: includes links to Cochrane Skin group, UK Dermatology Clinical Trials Network (℘ http://www.ukdctn.org/), *UK Diagnostic Criteria for Atopic Dermatitis* manual, and NHS Evidence—skin disorders. Also provides access to *Dermatology Health Care Needs Assessment Report* (2009). ℘ http://www.nottingham.ac.uk/research/groups/cebd/resources/index.aspx

Box 35.3 Miscellaneous information

Skin cancer

- Skin cancer resource. ℘ http://www.cancerresearchuk.org/about-cancer/type/skin-cancer/

Dermoscopy

- Dermoscopy: images and training. ℘ www.dermoscopy.co.uk or ℘ http://www.dermoscopy-ids.org/

Electronic textbook

- *The Electronic Textbook of Dermatology*. ℘ http://www.telemedicine.org/stamford.htm

British Skin Foundation

Charity committed to raising funds for research into skin disease. ℘ http://www.britishskinfoundation.org.uk/

Dermatology textbooks

Reference textbooks

Ashton R, Leppard B, Cooper H. *Differential diagnosis in Dermatology*, 4th edn, 2014. London: Radcliffe Publishing Ltd.

Bolognia J, Jorizzo J, Shaffer J (eds) *Dermatology*, 3rd edn, 2012. London: Mosby Elsevier Ltd.

Bolognia JL, Schaffer JV, Duncan KO, Ko C. *Dermatology Essentials*, 2014. London: Saunders Publishing Group.

Braverman I. *Skin Signs of Systemic Disease*, 3rd edn, 1998. Philadelphia: WB Saunders (*well worth dipping into if you can find it*).

du Vivier A and McKee PH. *Atlas of Clinical Dermatology*, 4th edn, 2013. London: Saunders.

Griffiths C, Barker J, Bleiker T, Chalmers R, Creamer D (eds) *Rook's Textbook of Dermatology*, 9th edn, 2016. Oxford: Wiley Blackwell.

Ogg G. Diseases of the skin (Chapter 23). In: Warrell D, Cox T, Firth J. (eds) *Oxford Textbook of Medicine*, 5th edn, 2010. Oxford: Oxford University Press.

Specialist dermatology

Archer CB. *Ethnic Dermatology*, 2nd edn, 2008. London: Inform Healthcare.

Baran R, Dawber RPR, de Berker DAR. *Baran and Dawber's Diseases of the Nails and their Management*, 4th edn, 2012. Oxford: Wiley-Blackwell.

Bowling J. *Diagnostic Dermoscopy: The Illustrated Guide*, 2011. Oxford: Wiley-Blackwell.

Ferguson J and Dover J. *Photodermatology*, 2006. Oxford: Wiley-Blackwell.

Fowler J and Zirwas M. *Fisher's Contact Dermatitis*, 7th edn, 2016. New York: McGraw-Hill Medical.

Irvine A, Höger P, Yan A. *Harper's Textbook of Pediatric Dermatology*, 3rd edn, 2011. Oxford: Wiley-Blackwell.

Lewis-Jones S (ed). *Paediatric Dermatology (Oxford Specialist Handbooks)*, 2010. Oxford: Oxford University Press.

Neill S and Lewis F. *Ridley's The Vulva*, 3rd edn, 2009. Oxford: Wiley-Blackwell.

Olsen EA (ed). *Disorders of Hair Growth: Diagnosis and Treatment*, 2nd edn, 2003. New York: McGraw-Hill.

Management

Lebwohl MG, Heymann WR, Berth-Jones J, Coulson I. *Treatment of Skin Disease: Comprehensive Therapeutic Strategies*, 4th edn, 2013. London: Saunders Elsevier Ltd.

Wakelin SH, Maibach HI, Archer CB. *Handbook of Systemic Drug Treatment in Dermatology*, 2nd edn, 2015. Oxford: Wiley-Blackwell.

Williams H, Bigby M Herxheimer A *et al*. *Evidence-based Dermatology*, 3rd edn, 2014. Oxford: Wiley-Blackwell.

Introductory textbooks

Morris-Jones R (ed). *ABC of Dermatology (ABC Series)*, 6th edn, 2014. Oxford: Wiley-Blackwell.

Weller R, Hunter H, Mann M. *Clinical Dermatology*, 5th edn, 2015. Oxford: Wiley-Blackwell.

Index